Advances in Intelligent Systems and Computing

Volume 654

Series editor

Janusz Kacprzyk, Polish Academy of Sciences, Warsaw, Poland
e-mail: kacprzyk@ibspan.waw.pl

About this Series

The series "Advances in Intelligent Systems and Computing" contains publications on theory, applications, and design methods of Intelligent Systems and Intelligent Computing. Virtually all disciplines such as engineering, natural sciences, computer and information science, ICT, economics, business, e-commerce, environment, healthcare, life science are covered. The list of topics spans all the areas of modern intelligent systems and computing.

The publications within "Advances in Intelligent Systems and Computing" are primarily textbooks and proceedings of important conferences, symposia and congresses. They cover significant recent developments in the field, both of a foundational and applicable character. An important characteristic feature of the series is the short publication time and world-wide distribution. This permits a rapid and broad dissemination of research results.

More information about this series at http://www.springer.com/series/11156

V.B. Aggarwal · Vasudha Bhatnagar
Durgesh Kumar Mishra
Editors

Big Data Analytics

Proceedings of CSI 2015

Springer

Editors
V.B. Aggarwal
Jagan Institute of Management Studies
New Delhi, Delhi
India

Vasudha Bhatnagar
Department of Computer Science
University of Delhi
New Delhi, Delhi
India

Durgesh Kumar Mishra
Microsoft Innovation Centre
Sri Aurobindo Institute of Technology
Indore, Madhya Pradesh
India

ISSN 2194-5357 ISSN 2194-5365 (electronic)
Advances in Intelligent Systems and Computing
ISBN 978-981-10-6619-1 ISBN 978-981-10-6620-7 (eBook)
https://doi.org/10.1007/978-981-10-6620-7

Library of Congress Control Number: 2017952513

Printed on acid-free paper

This Springer imprint is published by Springer Nature
The registered company is Springer Nature Singapore Pte Ltd.
The registered company address is: 152 Beach Road, #21-01/04 Gateway East, Singapore 189721, Singapore

Preface

The last decade has witnessed remarkable changes in IT industry, virtually in all domains. The 50th Annual Convention, CSI-2015, on the theme "Digital Life" was organized as a part of CSI-2015, by CSI at Delhi, the national capital of the country, during December 02–05, 2015. Its concept was formed with an objective to keep ICT community abreast of emerging paradigms in the areas of computing technologies and more importantly looking at its impact on the society.

Information and Communication Technology (ICT) comprises of three main components: infrastructure, services, and product. These components include the Internet, infrastructure-based/infrastructure-less wireless networks, mobile terminals, and other communication mediums. ICT is gaining popularity due to rapid growth in communication capabilities for real-time-based applications. New user requirements and services entail mechanisms for enabling systems to intelligently process speech- and language-based input from human users. CSI-2015 attracted over 1500 papers from researchers and practitioners from academia, industry and government agencies, from all over of the world, thereby making the job of the Programme Committee extremely difficult. After a series of tough review exercises by a team of over 700 experts, 565 papers were accepted for presentation in CSI-2015 during the 3 days of the convention under ten parallel tracks. The Programme Committee, in consultation with Springer, the world's largest publisher of scientific documents, decided to publish the proceedings of the presented papers, after the convention, in ten topical volumes, under ASIC series of the Springer, as detailed hereunder:

1. Volume # 1: ICT Based Innovations
2. Volume # 2: Next Generation Networks
3. Volume # 3: Nature Inspired Computing
4. Volume # 4: Speech and Language Processing for Human-Machine Communications
5. Volume # 5: Sensors and Image Processing
6. Volume # 6: Big Data Analytics

7. Volume # 7: Systems and Architecture
8. Volume # 8: Cyber Security
9. Volume # 9: Software Engineering
10. Volume # 10: Silicon Photonics and High Performance Computing

We are pleased to present before you the proceedings of the Volume # 6 on "Big Data Analytics". The title "Big Data Analytics" discusses the new models applied for Big Data Analytics. It traces the different business interests in the field of Big Data Analytics from the perspective of decision-makers. The title also evaluates the uses of data analytics in understanding the need of customer base in various organizations.

Big data is a new buzzword due to the generation of data from a diversity of sources. The volume, variety and velocity of data coming into an organization from both structured and unstructured data sources continue to reach unprecedented levels. This phenomenal growth implies that one must not only understand the big data in order to decipher the information that truly counts, but one must also understand the possibilities and opportunities of data analytics.

Big data analytics is the process of examining big data to uncover hidden patterns, unknown correlations and other useful information that can be used to make better decisions. With big data analytics, data scientists and others can analyse huge volumes of data that conventional analytics and business intelligence solutions cannot touch. The title "Big Data Analytics" analyses the different aspects of big data research and how the same is being applied across organizations to handle their data for decision-making and different types of analytics for different business strategies.

This volume is designed to bring together researchers and practitioners from academia and industry to focus on extending the understanding and establishing new collaborations in these areas. It is the outcome of the hard work of the editorial team, who have relentlessly worked with the authors and steered up the same to compile this volume. It will be a useful source of reference for the future researchers in this domain. Under the CSI-2015 umbrella, we received over 500 papers for this volume, out of which 74 papers are being published, after a rigorous review processes, carried out in multiple cycles.

On behalf of organizing team, it is a matter of great pleasure that CSI-2015 has received an overwhelming response from various professionals from across the country. The organizers of CSI-2015 are thankful to the members of *Advisory Committee, Programme Committee and Organizing Committee* for their all-round guidance, encouragement and continuous support. We express our sincere gratitude to the learned *Keynote Speakers* for support and help extended to make this event a grand success. Our sincere thanks are also due to our *Review Committee Members* and the *Editorial Board* for their untiring efforts in reviewing the manuscripts, giving suggestions and valuable inputs for shaping this volume. We hope that all the participants/delegates will be benefitted academically and wish them all the best for their future endeavours.

We also take the opportunity to thank the entire team from Springer, who have worked tirelessly and made the publication of the volume a reality. Last but not least, we thank the team from Bharati Vidyapeeth's Institute of Computer Applications and Management (BVICAM), New Delhi, for their untiring support, without which the compilation of this huge volume would not have been possible.

New Delhi, India V.B. Aggarwal
New Delhi, India Vasudha Bhatnagar
Indore, India Durgesh Kumar Mishra
March 2017

The Organization of CSI-2015

Chief Patron

Padmashree Dr. R. Chidambaram, *Principal Scientific Advisor, Government of India*

Patrons

Prof. S.V. Raghavan, Department of Computer Science, IIT Madras, Chennai
Prof. Ashutosh Sharma, Secretary, Department of Science and Technology, Ministry of Science and Technology, Government of India

Chair, Programme Committee
Prof. K.K. Aggarwal, Founder Vice Chancellor, GGSIP University, New Delhi

Secretary, Programme Committee
Prof. M.N. Hoda, Director, Bharati Vidyapeeth's Institute of Computer Applications and Management (BVICAM), New Delhi

Advisory Committee

- Padma Bhushan Dr. F.C. Kohli, Co-Founder, TCS
- Mr. Ravindra Nath, CMD, National Small Industries Corporation, New Delhi
- Dr. Omkar Rai, Director General, Software Technological Parks of India (STPI), New Delhi
- Adv. Pavan Duggal, Noted Cyber Law Advocate, Supreme Courts of India
- Prof. Bipin Mehta, President, CSI
- Prof. Anirban Basu, Vice President—cum- President Elect, CSI
- Shri Sanjay Mohapatra, Secretary, CSI
- Prof. Yogesh Singh, Vice Chancellor, Delhi Technological University, Delhi
- Prof. S.K. Gupta, Department of Computer Science and Engineering, IIT, Delhi

- Prof. P.B. Sharma, Founder Vice Chancellor, Delhi Technological University, Delhi
- Mr. Prakash Kumar, IAS, Chief Executive Officer, Goods and Services Tax Network (GSTN)
- Mr. R.S. Mani, Group Head, National Knowledge Networks (NKN), NIC, Government of India, New Delhi

Editorial Board

Contents

About the Editors

Dr. V.B. Aggarwal from 1981 to 88 was the Founder Head, Department of Computer Science, University of Delhi, India, where he introduced the 3-year postgraduate (PG) programme, Master of Computer Applications (MCA), from 1982 to 1985. In 1973, he was awarded his Ph.D. by the University of Illinois, Urbana, USA. He continued his research work in the areas of supercomputers and array processors. In the USA, he taught for seven years as a faculty member at three universities. As a life member of the Computer Society of India (CSI), he has held various offices at the Delhi Chapter, including chapter vice-chairman and chairman, since 1979. In February 2014, he received the prestigious "Chapter Patron Award 2013" for Delhi Chapter by the CSI Awards Committee. Dr. Aggarwal has authored more than 18 Computer Publications, which are very popular among school students.

Prof. Vasudha Bhatnagar is a Professor at the Department of Computer Science, University of Delhi, India. She is actively involved in research in the field of knowledge discovery and data mining (KDD). Her broad area of interest is intelligent data analysis. She is particularly interested in developing process models for knowledge discovery in databases and data mining algorithms. Her further interests include problems pertaining to modelling of changes in discovered knowledge in evolving (streaming) data sets, handling user subjectivity in KDD, projected clustering, outlier detection, classification and cluster ensembles. She is currently studying graphs as tool for modelling biology problems and texts.

Dr. Durgesh Kumar Mishra is a Professor (CSE) and Director of the Microsoft Innovation Centre at Shri Aurobindo Institute of Technology, Indore, India. He has 24 years of teaching and research experience and has published over 100 research papers. He is a Senior Member of IEEE and Chairman, Computer Society of India

(CSI) Division IV. He has held positions including Chairman, IEEE MP-Subsection and Chairman, IEEE Computer Society, Bombay Chapter. He has delivered invited talks at IEEE International conferences and serves on the Editorial Board of many national and international refereed journals. He is also a Member of the Bureau of Indian Standards (BIS), Government of India.

Need for Developing Intelligent Interfaces for Big Data Analytics in the Microfinance Industry

Purav Parikh and Pragya Singh

Abstract The main objective of the paper is to provide a multidimensional perspective of the microfinance industry where one finds that several different components such as "Sustainable Rural employment", "Data Analysis for the Micro Finance Industry", and Theory of Maslow's Need Hierarchy interrelate and work hand in hand. There is a strong correlation between Maslow's need hierarchy theory of motivation and assessing the changes in demand for financial services in the microfinance industry. How ICT and data analytics could help in efficiently tracking the change in demand and thus help the microfinance institutions in better demand forecasting as well as acquisition and management of resources, which are shared commonly, between various stakeholders, is the focus of this research paper. The paper is structured in sections starting with an introduction of the microfinance industry. It is then followed by the literature review, which explains a few of the concepts in theory to form the base. Other sections include discussion and policy implications followed by conclusion and future research which focuses more on the IT interventions and the need for advance level and integrated systems design for efficient delivery of financial services, better policy planning, and optimized use of real-time information for analytical decision-making, at the MFI level for the microfinance industry to achieve its goal of financial inclusion.

Keywords Microfinance industry · Big data · Data analytics · Real time · Motivation · MIPC · Human–computer interactions · ICT

P. Parikh (✉) · P. Singh
Department of Management Studies, Indian Institute of Information Technology, Allahabad, India
e-mail: puravparikh@gmail.com

P. Singh
e-mail: pragyabhardwaj23@gmail.com

V.B. Aggarwal et al. (eds.), *Big Data Analytics*, Advances in Intelligent Systems and Computing 654, https://doi.org/10.1007/978-981-10-6620-7_1

1 Introduction

Microfinance industry as we know it today is changing the lives of people who depend on it for various financial services not only in India but globally as well. Whether it is a small size or a marginal loan amount, or a savings account, crop loan, or for fulfilling social events of life such as birth or death ceremonies, marriages and likewise. Schumpeterian has defined microfinance service provider as an entrepreneur, in a sense that the form of business he is involved is social but innovative in nature. The fact is that by venturing into such a business he is not only running the business, but also solving a social problem, and creating new relationships using innovative business models which involve ground level actions for empowering people in different ways [1].

This research paper focuses on the aspect the use of data analytics in the MFIs (MFIs hereafter) for analyzing and tracking the user needs and necessities. The paper is structured in forms of sections, such as literature review, which relates more towards the need hierarchy theory of motivation as defined by Maslow (1943). The contextual correlation of this theory is significant in serving the microfinance sector customers as their needs and aspirations keep on changing from time to time. The section covers in detail about the connections of this theory and its applicability in the microfinance industry, in particular at the MFIs level. Followed by it is the method of study, which is analytical and based on the information obtained from the secondary data sources such as scholarly articles, periodical, working papers, report publications, as well as recent studies conducted by the researchers in India and abroad. The rest of the sections such as discussion and policy implications, followed by conclusion and future research, talks more about the ICT interventions for efficient delivery of financial services for the microfinance industry and in particular, the MFIs.

2 Literature Review

Maslow (1943) said that, "*A musician must make music, an artist must paint, a poet must write, if he is to be ultimately happy. What a man can be, he must be. This need we may call self actualization*". This definition as proposed by Maslow indicates that there is a strong relationship with the entrepreneur and the business he operates. At the same time, this also indicates the fact that the self-actualizing entrepreneur is also looked upon in this world for producing most innovative ideas, products and services, for the benefit of mankind [2]. Maslow (1943) further proposed a theory in order to give more contextual meaning to his definition of a self-actualizing entrepreneur. He called it a theory of the need hierarchy of motivation. In this theory, he has defined individual needs in terms of hierarchy. According to this world famous theory, he has defined an individual's need in terms of lower order and higher order needs. An individual will gain satisfaction by fulfilling lower order needs first and then he will gradually move toward fulfilling higher order needs. This process continues up till he reaches the highest order of need which Maslow (1943) refers to as "Self Actualization". At this point, he attends highest satisfaction and a sense of fulfillment as well as accomplishment [2]. Bernheim [1], in her research paper, indicates that microfinance is a mechanism, for providing financial services, to the poor as well as financially excluded people. Further, the services provided are very small amount, which generates high level of transaction as well as operations costs. Therefore, in order to serve this segment, it becomes imperative that innovative way of doing the business be developed [1]

Parikh [3–5] has emphasized on the Maslow's Need theory in his published research papers. In this context, he has pointed the fact, such that a purchasing power of a consumer changes with the change in income and standard of living over a period of time. This has a direct impact on the demand for financial services which he requires for consumption and growth. According to his opinion, this change phenomenon as defined by the Motivation theory requires IT interventions, in the form of more analytical, robust and IT based system, which he calls as, "Microfinance Information Processing Centers" (MIPCs) [5], as one solution for dealing with the change aspect of the microfinance industry.

3 Discussion and Policy Implications

As discussed in the literature review section of this paper, it becomes apparent that the data analytics and the demand forecasting plays a very important role, in efficient delivery of financial services, in the microfinance industry. In this context, it becomes important to study the change in consumers demand and requirements in real time as their purchasing power increases over a period of time. There is a need for developing a client responsive technological solution for the microfinance industry and the MFIs in particular, which could help them to take informed investment decisions based on the real-time data and thus provide better financial products and services to the customer of the microfinance industry.

As explained in Fig. 1, we have constant interaction of various components which impacts the growth and development of the microfinance industry. On one hand, you have big chunk of data which is available from the consumers. This data has to be put in use in real time, analyzed in real time and actions such as policies and programs need to be implemented based on such a study, that too in real time.

Second and third aspects which we could see in Fig. 1 are related to Maslow's Need Hierarchy Theory of Motivation and a need for sustainable rural employment and entrepreneurship for financial inclusion. Enough has been explained in previous sections as to how this theory is important and affects every individual's livelihood. Also, the system such as MIPCs which could provide a robust solution for the MFIs to leverage on the growth potentials of the ICT enabled system for the benefit of its

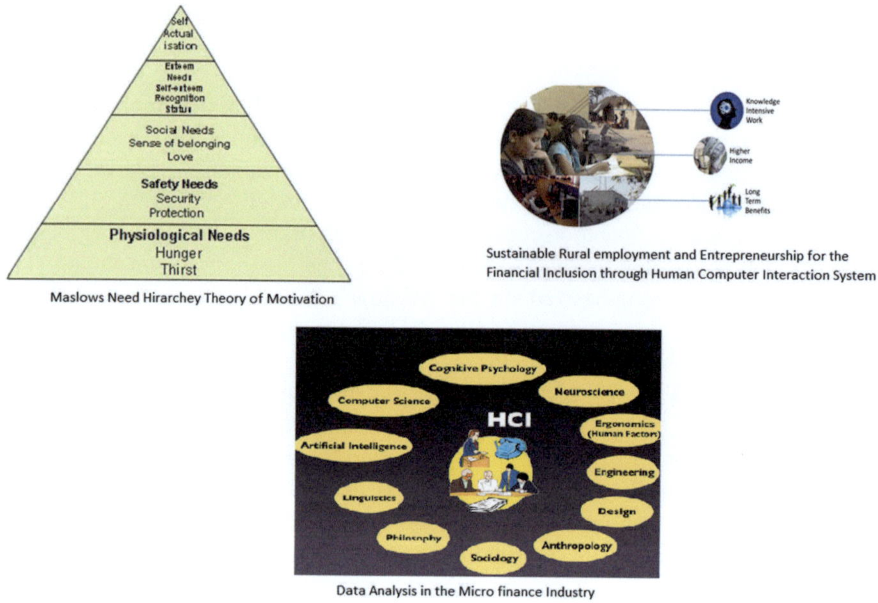

Fig. 1 Multi-dimensional perspective for the micro finance industry

customer has been well covered. These two aspects are the cornerstones while developing an ICT enabled system for human and computer interactions with the customers of microfinance industry.

4 Conclusion and Future Research

An attempt was made through this research paper, to present a theory of Maslow's need hierarchy (1943) and show its relevance in the microfinance industry, particularly at MFI level. The present literature review indicates the gap, which is that, it is difficult for the MFIs to study and keep track of the change in customer demands in relation to the microfinance products and services in real time, using the traditional framework. In this context, it provides with a perspective model such as, "Multi-dimensional perspective for the Microfinance Industry" (see Fig. 1).

Acknowledgements I would like to acknowledge the funding received from Ministry of Human Resource Development, Government of India in terms of Junior Research Fellowship (JRF) towards my PhD research work at IIIT Allahabad.

References

1. Bernheim, E.: Microfinance and micro entrepreneurship: case studies in social entrepreneurship and social innovation. CEB Working Paper. Solvay Brussels School of Economics and Management Center, Universite Libre de Bruxelles (2013)
2. Mui, A.: Entrepreneurship: the act of enhancing one's reality (ERSA). Erasmus School of Economics, Erasmus University, Rotterdam (2010)
3. Parikh, P.: Building of an ecosystem of applications for efficient delivery of financial services: a case for MIPC. In: IEEE Xplore. International Conference on IT in Business, Industry and Government (CSIBIG) 2014, Sri Aurbido Institute of Technology, March, 2014, pp. 218–220, India (2014)
4. Parikh, P.: Cloud computing based open source information technology infrastructure for financial inclusion. In: 12th Thinkers and Writers Forum. 28th Skoch Summit on Mainstreaming the Marginalized, New Delhi, India, 28 March 2012
5. Parikh, P.: Mobile based intelligent computing model for MFIs through MIPC. In: Computer Society of India, ICIS-2014, International Conference on Information Science July, 2014, Kochi, India (2014)
6. Augsburg, B., Schmidt, J.P., Krishnaswamy, K.: Free and open source software for microfinance: increasing efficiency and extending benefits to the poor. In: Business Science References (Ch. 2). New York (2011). http://en.wikipedia.org/wiki?curid=26364383
7. Assadi, D., Hudson, M.: Marketing analysis of emerging peer-to-peer microlending websites. Bus. Sci. Ref. **30**(4) (2005)
8. Das, P.: A case study of Mifos implementation at Asomi. In: Business Science References (Ch. 5). New York (2011)
9. Khan, S.: Automating MFIs: how far should we go? In: Business Science References (Ch. 4). New York (2011)
10. Jawadi, F., Jawadi, N., Ziane, Y.: Can information and communication technologies improve the performance of microfinance programs? Further Evidence from developing and emerging financial markets. In: Business Science References (Ch. 10). New York (2011)
11. Nyapati, K.: Stakeholder analysis of IT applications for microfinance. Business Science References (Ch. 1). New York (2011)
12. Musa, A.S.M., Khan, M.S.R.: Implementing point of sale technology in microfinance: an evaluation of come to save (CTS) cooperatives, Bangladesh. Business Science References (Ch. 6). New York (2011)
13. Makhijani, N.: Non banking finance companies—time to introspect! ANALYTIQUE **9–10**(2) (2014)
14. Quadri, S.M.N., Singh, V.K., Iyenger, K.P.: IT and MIS in microfinance institution: effectiveness and sustainability issues. In: Business Science References (Ch. 3). New York (2011)
15. Sairam, M.S.: Information asymmetry and trust: a framework for studying microfinance in India. Vikalpa **30**(4) (2005)

Unified Resource Descriptor over KAAS Framework

Refining Cloud Dynamics

Subhajit Bhattacharya

Abstract With the advent of information digitization, virtual social networking, and other means of information sharing protocols, today billions of data are available on the World Wide Web from heterogeneous sources. All these data further contribute to the emergence of Big Data gamut. When these data are processed further, we get a glimpse of information which gives some level of understanding on the subject or the matter (person, place, enterprise, etc.). Knowledge is cohesively logically processed related information with the intellect to give us multidimensional information spectrum for decision-making in real time. In today's global environment, data plays crucial role to understand the social, cultural, behavioral, and demographic attributes of a subject. Knowledge-as-a-Service (KAAS) is a pioneering cloud framework inheriting the "Internet of Things" principles that extract data from various sources in a seamless manner and can further decouple–couple logically processed information based on the "matching chromosome" algorithm. Unified Resource Descriptor (URD) is an innovative information modeling technique that operates over KAAS framework to further publish knowledge on the subject on need basis. Based on this concept, every resource or subject is assigned a unique identifier that can perform multilayered search in the KAAS Database to extract relevant knowledge frames. Considering India's context, second most populated country in the world, URD can play an indispensable role to tighten information dynamics holistically and accumulate a broader spectrum of knowledge of the resource to address adverse situations (natural calamity, medication, insurance, etc.), business process solution (Banking, BPOs, KPOs, etc.), and research practices.

Keywords Big data · KAAS · Cloud computing · Knowledgebase · BI

S. Bhattacharya (✉)
Accenture, New Delhi, India
e-mail: Subhajit.bhattacharya07@gmail.com

V.B. Aggarwal et al. (eds.), *Big Data Analytics*, Advances in Intelligent Systems and Computing 654, https://doi.org/10.1007/978-981-10-6620-7_2

1 Introduction

Today, Information Technology has spread its wings wide and social sites have become the boon for social connectivity, every day the World Wide Web is getting cluttered with billions of data from heterogeneous sources. These structured, semi-structured, and unstructured data hubs form the big data gamut. Today, the biggest challenge is the utilization and proper processing of these data to derive adequate information.

Knowledge-As-A-Service is one of the pioneering initiatives to redefine cloud dynamics which enables multi-tier filtering and processing of data over "matching chromosome" algorithm to form information cuboids that are further filtered through analytical engine to get intelligently sliced, diced, and re-clustered to build information pool for a particular resource/subject. Matching chromosome is an AI-based algorithm to compare and then couple, decouple, and recouple the relevant data about the resource and thus formalize knowledge framework that further gets processed through KAAS engine to form knowledge warehouses. The ultimate idea is to bring "Information Neutrality" across the globe.

Here, the primary objective is to optimize and convert huge abandon data in the form of knowledge that can provide significant level of information for decision making and further knowledge transition.

Unified Resource Descriptor (URD) is an innovative information modeling technique that operates over KAAS framework to further publish knowledge on the subject/resource comparing behavioral, demographic, social, political, economic, and other aspects. URD ID operates as a primary key assigned to every resource/subject for which significant volume of knowledge is presented to the end user. It can be further associated as "Social Resource Planning (SRP)".

Considering India's context, URD can play a central role to tighten information dynamics holistically and accumulate a broader spectrum of knowledge of the resources to address adverse situations (war, natural calamity, medication, insurance, etc.), business process solutions (BFSI/FMCG/BPOs/KPOs, etc.), and education/research institutions resulting to cost efficiencies, productivity, and innovation. Most importantly, it can prove one of the significant and indispensable technologies for rural India for education and other vital facilities.

The URD ID is assigned to a subject/resource; the information about that resource will be available to the end user for knowledge and decision purpose. This URD ID works as cohesive meta-knowledge. Under KAAS framework, URD ID is explicitly associated with the resource for unified information representation.

In the KAAS framework, resources are scanned as an image or by data attributes or by videos/audios to get an in-depth insight. Therefore, when a medical firm scans an image of a patient so it can get the patient's past medical reports saving time and cost, an insurance institution scans through person details to get his past insurance details, bank can assess the credibility of the resource or company to save itself from bad debts, defense personnel can scan suspect to see his past history, a villager can scan the ground to understand its fertility, a common person can scan a logo or news headlines to get respective details in fraction of seconds, BPOs/KPOs can get benefits by getting the details of intended clients information in a simplified structured manner, education will be more informative and interactive. E-commerce and commercial firms can get wider information about their existing and prospective consumers and to make the right decision for sales promotions and offer positioning.

2 Technical Insight

2.1 Why KAAS and URD

Due to emergence of new technologies and social media boom, today we are observing global data warming in the huge datacenters across the globe. Global data warming is a gradual increase of unstructured and unproductive data resulting monstrous data space in the World Wide Web with no significant usage.

Cloud technology has certainly brought a number of pioneering initiatives in the IT sector, and mainly in IT-enabled services. Knowledge-As-A-Service has been introduced as another arm of cloud technology to redefine the information dynamics acting as a scavenger to segregate and unite coherent interrelated data from the global databases and form unique information clusters and further process them to generate knowledge warehouses. This will lay foundation for "Information Neutrality".

Highly processed information so produced can be accessed by required subscription and the knowledge on the resource can be obtained as dynamically as just a glance on it. Unlike search engines (Google, Bing, or Yahoo, etc.), it will give an in-depth knowledge about a resource along with URD ID associated with it.

The overall concept works on the below modules:

- Intellibot Crawlers
- Matching chromosome algorithm
- Information integrator
- Test-tube information marts
- Knowledge warehouses.

The world is driven by information. Any technology, innovation, business, government policies, defense strategies, financial, agricultural, and education plans, etc., are dependent on the information that in turn form knowledge hubs to enable optimized decision-making capabilities.

Today, undoubtedly the whole world is facing challenges due to limited amount of relevant information. Until today, Europe could not come out of Euro-Crisis occurred due to bad debts years ago, most of the developed and developing nations are facing security issues, no centralized patients' record repository, monotonous non-interactive education; farmers are handicapped due to limited visibility and non-decision-making capabilities to judge the soil and climate conditions.

To overcome all these constraints, KAAS framework has been introduced working on seven principles:

- Capturing and indexing the heterogeneous data from big data clusters
- Data so collected are parsed and run through matching chromosome algorithm to get coupled/decoupled on match basis
- Information collector further collects and collaborates information iteratively to form processed information hubs
- Related information hubs are clubbed together and further segregated and coupled together to form knowledge test-tube marts
- The knowledge test-tube marts are channelized and fused together to form knowledgebase
- URD ID is assigned to every individual resource/subject to uniquely describe a resource
- This URD ID basically makes foundation of meta-knowledge.

Strategically KAAS framework formulates technology endeavor that will enable a person or an institution to have in-depth knowledge about other resources just by a glance either by keyed in the details or scanned through device camera, so explicitly the system will hit the KAAS server and fetch the details onto the screen with all relevant information. This can be well used in the process of pre-job background checking of a candidate or credibility checking of an organization.

KAAS framework iterates the information processing so many times under the information collector and test-tube marts that finally it harvests quality knowledgebases. This knowledgebase is continuously updated on real-time basis.

KAAS framework can further be tuned-up to keep continuous scanning on the global satellite maps for real-time information collaboration to combat natural calamities, crimes, and terrorism.

In Fig. 1, it is shown that in KAAS framework, data are collected from the heterogeneous sources and then went through various levels of ETL processes to get stored into various staging databases. Matching chromosome algorithm and information integrator modules are the heart of KAAS that plugs-in and plugs-out data source connections to perform various permutation/combination for generating highly processed information by coupling/decoupling the processed data.

This behavior enables the KAAS to generate the most relevant information for optimal decision-making.

In Fig. 2, it is shown that in the below KAAS framework, we can see there are six major layers. Data are extracted, processed, transformed, and loaded at every layer. At every layer, different manifestation of information is available until it gets purified at the extreme level to generate knowledge for decision-making. At every staging databases, BI tools are integrated for further segregation, purification,

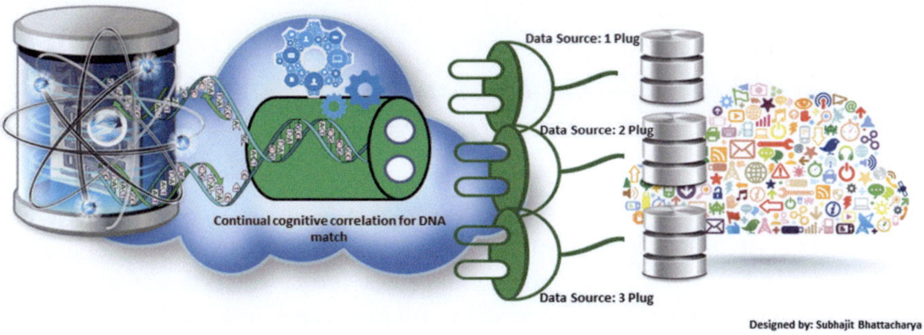

Fig. 1 Data collection mechanism in KAAS

processing, integration, and analytics. Once the knowledge information is collected into the centralized knowledgebase, URD ID is tagged with every resource/subject to provide unified resource description. All these are catered together into global KAAS datacenter to simulate Social Resource Planning for information neutrality and just-in-time decision-making capabilities.

KAAS provides the highest level of abstraction, scalability, and visualization along with security to maintain confidentiality and segregation of knowledge usage.

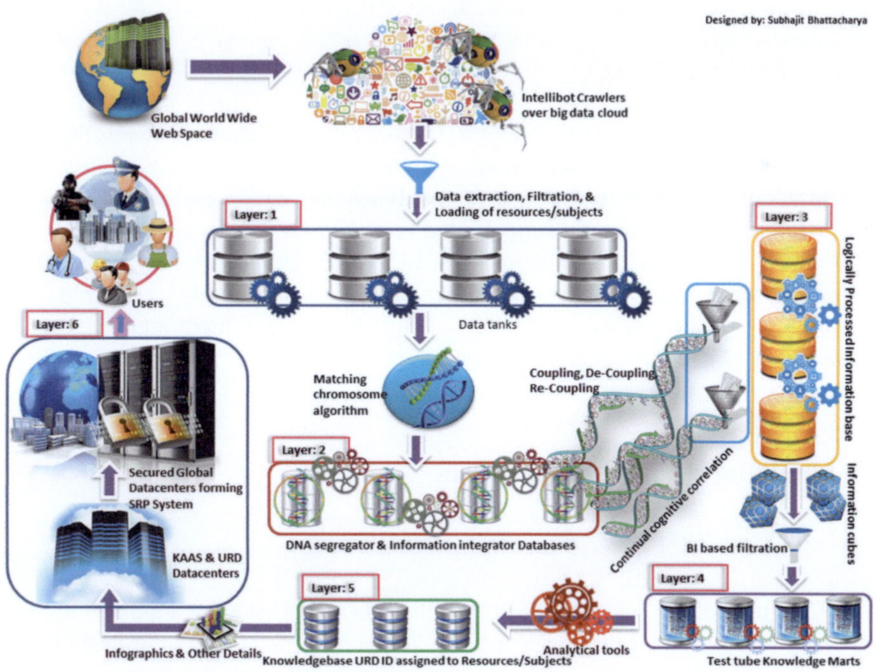

Fig. 2 Working model of KAAS framework

3 Case Study

3.1 A Well-Known Medical Insurance Company Was Being Cheated by Its Customer for over a Decade—A Case Study

In 2009, one of India's top consulting firms was in discussion with one of the well-known Indian medical insurance companies for IT solution. As of now, the insurance company was doing decent job and they made a deal with the consultancy firm to device a long-term solution to monitor insurance subscribers' annual medical claims and other background checks. Till the date, the insurance company used to take medical papers and fair background checks for the claims, however, post-solution automation it was realized that few of the subscribers were allegedly cheating the company by showing fake claims and medical reports. The customer actually never had such decreases for which he was claiming the benefits for the past several years.

It was identified not only by customer background reports and other channels of database integration but a critical assessment of past data by the application to conclude some probabilistic reports that were undergone further manual investigations. The application so devised was WHO compliant.

Until today many insurance and other financial institutions claim that their processes are too robust to be cheated, however it was found that around 30–35% of the financial or insurance institutions being cheated and vicé versa despite all possible legitimate checks.

Similar cases are happening with the corporates that perform pre-job background checking and by the time it realizes the fakeness of candidature it is too late.

The bottom line is that despite all hypothetical claims of having holistic and well-protocolled system for information analytics and tracking, till date organizations and end consumers are being cheated in various ways due to lack of relevant information bases that add to knowledge to induce decision-making capabilities. This is because many of the companies were failed miserably, either due to bankruptcy or other means, and on the other hand, consumers and loaners are becoming prey to the fraudulent companies.

4 Challenges and Impediments

4.1 Key Challenges

Although most of the organizations claim that they have opted secured and holistic approach to assess their resources and clients but unfortunately it is irrelevant fact. Also when individuals claim that they have significant knowledge about firm or another person or a place, it is not absolutely correct because at any given instance, he will be having limited information due to limited source of data.

In Indian context, we have often seen that due to limited infrastructure and IT enablement, most of the crucial operations are still being performed manually which is in itself error prone and on top of it, there is no mechanism currently available to set up unified information system working centrally on a distributed cohesive platform providing real-time knowledgebase.

Key challenges to capture relevant and authentic information for knowledge building and decision-making:

- Improper thought process: Every innovation comes through an in-depth thought process and brainstorming. Due to lack of holistic approach, India as a potential country has failed to devise strategic knowledgebase server.
- Inappropriate development framework: Concept alone cannot play a role, but there should always be a development framework that accommodates the concept to model a working solution to address the challenges.
- Lack of infrastructure: Like any complicated long term project, this also needs a promising infrastructure and strong IT process enablement otherwise it will be just like dreaming of castle in the air.
- Lack of data collection and integration mechanisms: Although big data has fantasized IT industries for quite some time, however, due to lack of data exploration, extraction, comparison, integration, and restoration mechanisms, a robust system could never come into existence.
- Inadequate test plan: Test plans and cases to check system readiness are always advisable. Often systems failed due to vulnerabilities and risks areas that could not have been detected proactively.
- All at one go: Planning to develop and onboard the application in single instance without measuring the complexities and challenges can lead to a major mishap.
- Weak project management: There must be a well thought-out project management plan from initiation till closure keeping close eye on every phase otherwise any dodge can turn the table upside down. Lag in proper project plan and flaw in risk mitigation plan can lead the business into disastrous situations. Despite nitty-gritty checks and followed automation principles, improper plan and solution model could not yield successful result.
- Level of information access authority: It has to be made mandatory to segregate information access authority and confidentiality for the company and individuals as per the approval from government body depending case to case basis.
- An integrated collaboration channel should be set up among government, nongovernment organizations, and solution providers to address social resource planning holistically with the help of URD.

5 Solution Ahead

5.1 Methodology and Process Framework

In the above case study, we have found a number of key challenges and dependencies behind the failure of insurance company to detect the fraudulent practices. If we try to frame the above scenario under KAAS model and perform information scrutiny more holistically, it might have brought some quantifiable results.

Here, we may figure out below five major road blocks:

(1) Lack of information integration
(2) Lack of fraudulent check processes
(3) No standard application in place for information binding
(4) Lag in resource identification mechanism
(5) No or little due diligence done on the process quality and test plans.

KAAS framework, on contrary, could have played an important role to deal with the above scenario:

- Intellibot crawlers are the artificial agents based crawlers that crawl through the World Wide Web containing heterogeneous data around and capture all the raw data to store them into data tank
- Matching chromosome algorithm further interprets data sequence and performs coupling, decoupling, and recoupling to form structured information of the resource
- Information integrator is a tool which holistically maps all the relevant information crushed through n-tier filter mechanism to build processed information base built on demographic, behavioral, social, economic, etc. parameters
- These high-end information microbes are further fused together to form test-tube knowledge marts
- Multiple test-tube knowledge marts collaborated and channeled together to form knowledge warehouse
- Although there could be various staging knowledgebases in between before being stored into the knowledge warehouse
- Every resource that has entry in the knowledgebase is assigned a URD ID
- URD plays primary role to identify the resource, based on the scanned image or information attributes and displays infographics onto the screen
- Post go-live, government, and nongovernment users can subscribe to the KAAS to get relevant information of the resource/subject. Knowledgebase keeps getting updated on a regular interval to furnish latest information
- SRP and information neutrality can help various organizations to have a 360° view on the resource/subject
- This hybrid model can further be used for processed information recycling and fix the knowledge gap.

In Fig. 3, it is shown that how KAAS framework can be used by various types of users on subscription basis in real time. Knowledge about a resource can be searched by taking or scanning an image (including live image), videos/audios, and plain search data. Knowledgebase is continuously getting refreshed; therefore likelihood of getting real-time data on just-in-time basis is too high with least latency. Knowledgebase is secured and optimally encapsulated to maintain high degree of confidentiality and at the same time maintains degree of information segregation for business and government benefits.

5.2 *Quantified Benefits to Business*

- SMART information processing and sharing in terms of knowledge on contrary to the traditional approach
- Information availability and neutrality can bring a major radical leap in industrial development and performance, especially in the case of India and other developing nations

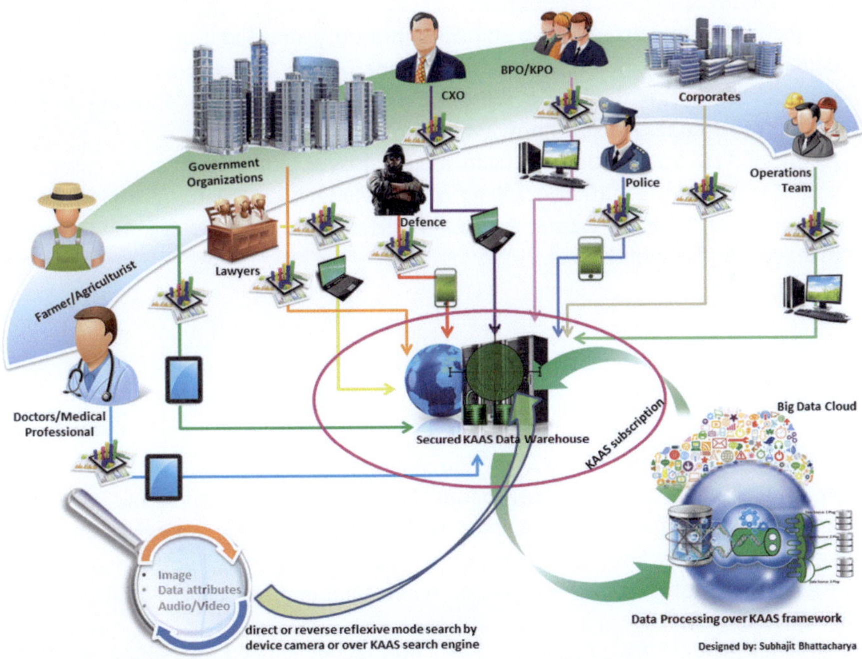

Fig. 3 Operational dynamics of KAAS framework

- Inclusion of KAAS framework can produce better result even though there is no in-house data or information warehouse or repository
- With the strategic alliance along with KAAS, companies can yield higher ROIs and meet challenging KPIs
- Authentic and the most up-to-date information will be available at all time, only a click away
- URD with the capability of direct or reverse reflexive search will change the outlook of data analysis to information analysis
- Infographics will give added advantage for graphical information presentation
- Social Resource Planning (SRP) and URD together may bring a new edge of socio-technology trend giving a new generation to the knowledge harvesting
- Inclusion of information security will make sure of confidentiality and integrity
- Organization can keep focusing on its major line of businesses while the business-related and sensitive information and other information will rest on cloud servers
- Defense, income tax, excise/custom, agriculture commodities, BFSI, hospitality, BPOs/KPOs, health care, etc., organizations will get tremendous benefits out of KAAS
- Forecasting business strategies, risks, budgets, and preparing respective plans will become easier as information is articulated in a highly structured manner topped with analytical capabilities
- As the matching chromosome algorithm not only slices and dices the processed data and coupling/decoupling information, further repositioning the original subject/resource will yield a set of related knowledge sets forming a wider spectrum of cohesive sub-knowledgebase
- As the KAAS framework has been modeled over cloud, it gives an essence of scalability assuring further scale-up of knowledgebase, enabling a platform for virtualization wherein we get a virtual interface to interact with knowledgebase managed at the cloud level.

6 Conclusion

Knowledge-As-A-Service is one of the pioneering initiatives to redefine cloud dynamics to process all the heterogeneous data from big data gamut and channelize them through serialized AI processes and forms a holistic knowledgebase for business growth and knowledge awareness across the globe. The idea is to bring information neutrality for all the people while maintaining security and confidentiality at all levels.

Unified Resource Descriptor has been introduced as an information modeling technique that operates over KAAS framework to further publish knowledge on the subject/resource comparing behavioral, demographic, social, political, economic, and financial aspects. URD acts as a unique key assigned to every resource/subject for which significant volume of knowledge can be presented to the end user from the knowledgebase.

With the growth of information technology and social network, foundation for "Social Resource Planning" has been laid for collaboration and information sharing.

Objective of this framework is to basically enable government and non-government sectors to process their operations more strategic protocolled manner.

Figure 1: In KAAS framework, data are collected from the heterogeneous sources and then went through various levels of ETL processes to get stored into various staging databases. Matching chromosome algorithm and information integrator modules are the heart of KAAS that plugs-in and plugs-out data source connections to perform various permutation/combination for generating highly processed information by coupling/decoupling the processed data.

This behavior enables the KAAS to generate most relevant information for optimal decision-making.

Figure 2: In the KAAS framework, we can see there are six major layers. Data are extracted, processed, transformed, and loaded at every layer. At every layer, different manifestation of information is available until it gets purified at the extreme level to generate knowledge for decision-making. At every staging databases, BI tools are integrated for further segregation, purification, processing, integration, and analytics. Once the knowledge information is collected into the centralized knowledgebase, URD ID is tagged with every resource/subject to provide unified resource description. All these are catered together into global KAAS datacenter to simulate Social Resource Planning for information neutrality and just-in-time decision-making capabilities.

KAAS provides the highest level of abstraction, scalability, and visualization along with security to maintain confidentiality and segregation of knowledge usage.

Figure 3: In the diagram, it is shown that how KAAS framework can be used by various types of users on subscription basis in real time. Knowledge about a resource can be searched by taking or scanning an image (including live image), videos/audios, and plain search data. Knowledgebase is continuously getting refreshed; therefore likelihood of getting real-time data on just-in-time basis is too high with least latency. Knowledgebase is secured and optimally encapsulated to maintain high degree of confidentiality and at the same time maintains degree of information segregation for business and government benefits.

References

1. Minelli, M., Chambers, M., Dhiraj, A.: Big Data, Big Analytics: Emerging Business Intelligence and Analytic Trends for Today's Businesses. O'Reilly (2012)
2. Larman, C.: Agile and iterative development: a manager's guide. Addison-Wesley Professional (2013)
3. Thomas E., Zaigham M., Ricardo P.: Cloud Computing: Concepts, Technology & Architecture. Prentice Hall (2013)

4. Patel, B., Shah, D.: Meta-Search Engine Optimization. LAP Lambert Academic Publishing (2014)
5. Morabito, V.: Big Data and Analytics: Strategic and Organizational Impacts. Springer, Berlin (2014)
6. Hubert, C.: Knowledge Management: A Guide for Your Journey to Best-Practice Processes. APQC (2013)
7. Schlessinger. Infrared Technology Fundamentals. CRC Press (1995)
8. Sabherwal, R., Becerra-Fernandez, I.: Business Intelligence. Wiley (2011)

An Adaptable and Secure Intelligent Smart Card Framework for Internet of Things and Cloud Computing

T. Daisy Premila Bai, A. Vimal Jerald and S. Albert Rabara

Abstract Internet of Things (IoT) and cloud computing paradigm is a next wave in the era of digital life and in the field of Information and Communication Technology. It has been understood from the literature that integration of IoT and cloud is in its infantile phase that has not been extended to all application domains due to its inadequate security architecture. Hence, in this paper, a novel, adaptable, and secure intelligent smart card framework for integrating IoT and cloud computing is proposed. Elliptic Curve Cryptography is used to ensure complete protection against the security risks. This model ensures security and realizes the vision of "one intelligent smart card for any applications and transactions" anywhere, anytime with one unique ID. The performance of the proposed framework is tested in a simulated environment and the results are presented.

Keywords IoT · Cloud · Smart card · Elliptic curve cryptography · Security

1 Introduction

Internet of Things (IoT) and cloud computing play a vital role in the field of Information Technology [1]. IoT is characterized by the real world of smart objects with limited storage and processing power [2]. The vision of the IoT is to enable things to be connected anytime, anyplace, with anything, and anyone ideally using any path or network and any service in heterogeneous environments [3]. In contrast, cloud computing is characterized by virtual world with unlimited capability in terms of storage and processing power [4]. Though the cloud and IoT have emerged as

T. Daisy Premila Bai (✉) · A. Vimal Jerald · S. Albert Rabara
Department of Computer Science, St. Joseph's College, Trichy, Tamil Nadu, India
e-mail: daisypremila@gmail.com

A. Vimal Jerald
e-mail: vimaljerald@gmail.com

S. Albert Rabara
e-mail: a_rabara@yahoo.com

V.B. Aggarwal et al. (eds.), *Big Data Analytics*, Advances in Intelligent Systems and Computing 654, https://doi.org/10.1007/978-981-10-6620-7_3

independent technology, integrating these two will enhance the digital world to reach the heights of availing any services and applications anywhere, any time, any firm, and any device irrespective of any underlying technology. "Anytime, anywhere" paradigm gains its momentum with the development of mobile devices and smart card technologies [5]. Mobile devices and smart cards, the portable devices could complement each other to realize the vision of "Anytime, anywhere" prototype. Smart cards are considered to be the smart solutions to avail any applications and any services since the smart cards could be easily interfaced with the mobile devices and the card readers [6].

Existing smart cards are the most secure devices widely used and adopted in many application domains like telecommunications industry, banking industry, health care services, audiovisual industry, transportation, access control, identification, authentication, pocket gaming, e-commerce, remote working, remote banking, etc., with the adoption of the various smart card standards and specifications [7]. The major drawback is that for each application, a user should have an individual smart card for each application. This will undoubtedly fill the wallet of the users with many numbers of cards and leave them with the difficulty of remembering the personal identification number (PIN) of each application [8].

The literature study reveals that there are various research works that have been carried out to enhance the smart card technology for varied application [9]. But there is no research proposal to report that one smart card can support all application domains invariably. So far the smart cards in use are intra-domain dependent where a card issued for one particular concern has the ability to avail various services and applications provided by the same but not the inter domain services due to security concerns [10]. To mitigate the security risks Elliptic Curve Cryptography is adopted which is suitable for resource constrained devices [11]. In addition, smart cards have only limited storage and processing capacity. This could be surmounted with the adoption of cloud technology where it has unlimited storage and processing power [12, 13]. Hence, in this paper, an IoT-enabled adaptable and secure intelligent smart card framework for integrating IoT and cloud computing is proposed.

This paper is organized as follows. Section 2 describes the proposed framework. Performance analysis and the performance results are illustrated in Sect. 3. Section 4 concludes the paper.

2 Proposed Framework

The proposed adaptable and secure intelligent smart card framework for integrating IoT and cloud is envisaged to offer secure smart services and applications anywhere, anytime, with one IoT-enabled User Adaptable Intelligent Smart Card (UAISC). This framework consists of four key components, namely IoT enabled intelligent system, security gateway, IP/MPLS core, and cloud platform. It is depicted in Fig. 1. IoT-enabled intelligent system comprises of a User Adaptable

Intelligent Smart Card (UAISC), Smart Reader, Mobile Device, and Smart Gateway.

UAISC is an IoT-enabled active card which conforms to the ISO/IEC standard which consists of RFID tag, biometric template, image template, and Unique Identification Number (UID) as special features. It is depicted in Fig. 2. A new application security interface is proposed to communicate with the RFID reader and to mutually authenticate the IoT enabled UAISC using Elliptic Curve Cryptography. Multiapplication can be installed on the same UAISC using MULTOS which ultimately consolidates multiple cards down to a single card with the default feature of Mandatory Access Control (MAC) of the operating system. Users can have control over the choice of applications to be installed on their cards or to be deleted from their card at their convenience with the adoption of MULTOS platform. Multiplications present on the card are separated from one another with firewalls to ensure the privacy of the user at any context. Biometric template stores the encrypted extracted features of the fingerprint and image template stores the encrypted facial image of the person on UAISC. Storing the template on card helps the card holder to have their biometric template on their hands always. It adopts system on card process for matching and ensures the protection of the personal data. UID is a newly defined unique 20 digit number which can be used as a unique ID in any smart environment, to access diversified applications and services anytime and anywhere [14].

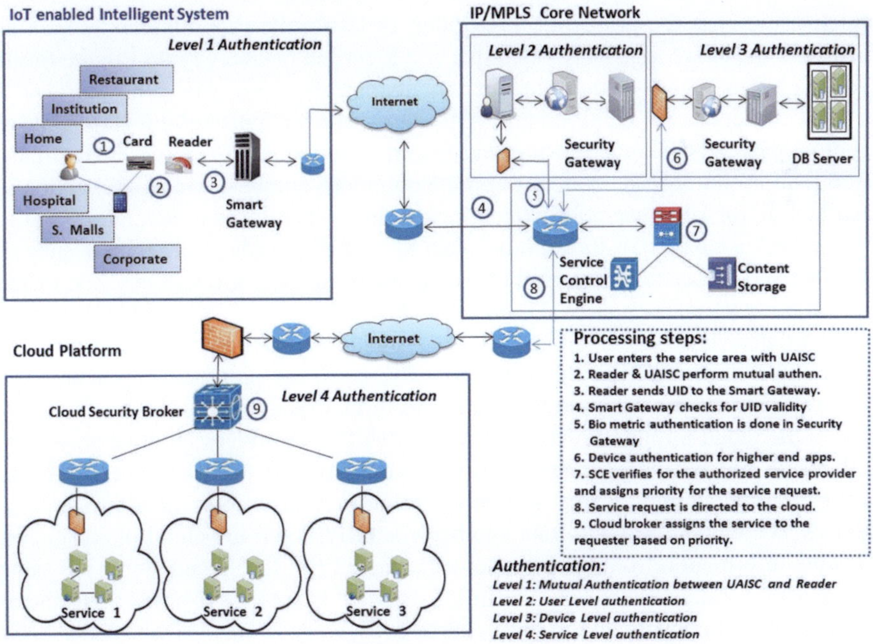

Fig. 1 Smart card framework for IoT and cloud computing

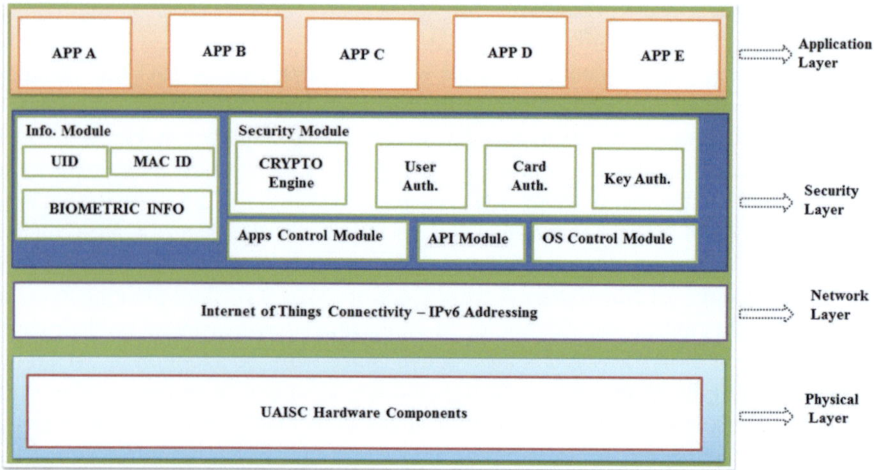

Fig. 2 Smart card components

The UAISC can be the employee ID, student ID, bank ID, patient ID, transport ID, etc. Hence, one User Adaptable Intelligent Smart Card (UAISC) for any applications will reduce the burdensome of carrying so many cards and will reduce the risk of remembering Personal Identification Numbers (PINs) for each application. This helps the user to use the "easy to remember PIN" for all applications which overcomes the problem of forgetting or losing the PIN numbers [14]. This facilitates the entire system to be unique and secure in nature. Crypto Engine of the UAISC has a security controller and microcontroller. Security controller has a crypto coprocessor for cryptographic algorithms which adopts 160-bit elliptic curve cryptography algorithm to ensure end-to-end security. Microcontroller has hardware random number generators to produce random numbers which are needed in smart cards for key generation which makes the system more robust. RFID tag in the UAISC is capable of transmitting data to an RFID reader from the distance of 100 feet and the data are transferred to the smart gateway through any one of the available networks such as WiFi, Ethernet, etc.

Smart gateway is very compatible and adaptable for both IPv4 and IPv6. It collects the data, stores the data temporarily, performs preprocessing, filters the data, reconstructs the data into a more useful form, and uploads only the necessary data to the cloud through IP/MPLS core. IPMPLS core bridges intelligent systems and cloud and provides secure and fast routing of the packets from source to destination by adopting packet switching technology. It enables all heterogeneous devices to communicate with one another via TCP/IP and the cloud platform collects the information from the core network via HTTPs REST and stores the same in the cloud data centers. The security gateway adopts ECC-based multifactor authentication to ensure end-to-end security [15].

2.1 Security Requirements

The security requirements of the proposed work can be defined in terms of mutual authentication, confidentiality, integrity, and availability. Mutual authentication of RFID tag in the UAISC and the RFID reader is very crucial and critical to ensure the identity of the devices involved in communication. Confidentiality is one of the major concerns since the involvement of smart objects in the IoT environment is more and there is no physical path to transmit the data. Integrity also is a challenge to ensure that the information is protected from unauthorized change. To strengthen the security requirements of the proposed model, elliptic curve cryptosystem is adopted [15].

2.2 Security Framework

The proposed ECC-based security framework consists of seven phases, namely initialization phase, registration phase, mutual authentication phase, reregistration phase, user authentication phase, mobile device authentication phase, and service level authentication phase. The security framework is depicted in Fig. 3. The elliptic curve chosen for the proposed framework is

$$Y^2 = X^3 + (-3)x + 1 \mod \left(p > 2^{160}\right) \tag{1}$$

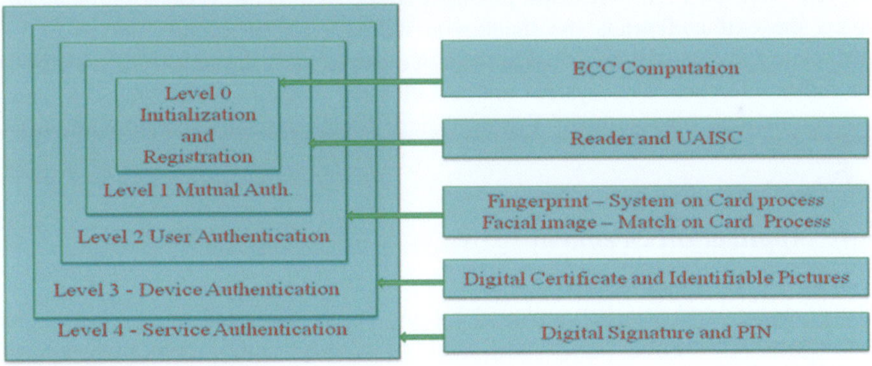

Fig. 3 Security framework

2.3 Use-Case Restaurant

The entry of the customer with UAISC is recognized by the RFID reader mounted at the entrance of the restaurant premises and performs the mutual authentication. Then, the UID of the UAISC is captured by the RFID reader and sent to the smart gateway to check for its validity. Since the smart gateway, i.e., the server of the restaurant is linked with the cloud server of CIRC (Card Issuing and Registration Centre), it is feasible to retrieve the information pertained to UID sent, if it is registered and valid. Smart gateway fetching the information displays the customer information on the digital board at the entrance and instructs the customer to do the biometric authentication. System on card process will be initiated to match the biometric features which are already extracted and stored in an encrypted form in the UAISC. At the same time, the facial image of the user will be captured by CCTV and Match on Card process will be performed. If both biometric and facial images match, the user is affirmed as the legitimate UAISC holder. Then, the door at the restaurant will be opened automatically and the customer can proceed to choose the place at café.

Simultaneously the "Welcome message" is sent to the registered mobile device of the legitimate user and the device is authenticated with digital certificate X.509v3 and identifiable pictures stored on the mobile device and the cloud server of CIRC. If the device and the customer are authenticated, restaurant app will be downloaded to the mobile device where the customer can choose the required service. According to the service requested, the customer will be directed digitally. If the service requested is for ordering edibles, it will be served and the bill will be sent to the mobile device and the customer can make the m-payment (mobile payment) with the UID and the PIN. When the payment is successful, the system automatically opens the exit and sends the thank you message to the mobile device of the customer. The data will be stored in the cloud data centers through IPMPLS plug-in for future reference. This system initiates efficient machine to machine communication, eliminates the number of intermediary personnel, and ensures security.

2.4 Application Scenario

The proposed work can be employed for any applications and transactions under two categories namely on-premise and off-premise applications. On-premise applications are such as availing services from shopping malls, hospitals, universities, etc., which require entry check in and identification of the legitimate user. Off-premise applications are like e-ticketing, e-ordering, accessing cloud resources, etc., which are facilitated through authenticating users' mobile device which acts as the card reader and the smart gateway. The proposed UAISC can be a dynamic Aadhar ID for the citizens of India which could be one of the contributions for Digital India.

3 Experimental Study

The experimental study of the proposed system has been carried out in a lab environment and the results are obtained in a simulated environment. The test bed of the proposed system consists of the security components of the UAISC, Mobile device, smart gateway, security gateway, IPMPLS core, and cloud platform. Servers of varied configuration are used as smart gateway server, security gateway server, and cloud servers. The various performance analyses carried out for the proposed system are mutual authentication between UAISC and the reader, user authentication, and device authentication.

3.1 Performance Analysis Over Mutual Authentication

The security feature involved between the UAISC and the reader is the mutual authentication and key generation. ECC computation is adopted and observed the time taken for both by using virtual smart card emulator. The graph generated is depicted in Fig. 4.

The graph shows that the time taken for mutual authentication and key generation is less than 20 ms. It ensures that it is difficult for the adversaries to read the details on the UAISC and guarantee the privacy of the user.

3.2 Performance Analysis on User Authentication

User authentication is analyzed with biometric matching using system on card process. The virtual smart card architecture emulator is used to observe the time taken to perform biometric capturing, matching, and verification. It is graphically presented in Fig. 5.

The results prove that the time taken to perform user authentication is very less.

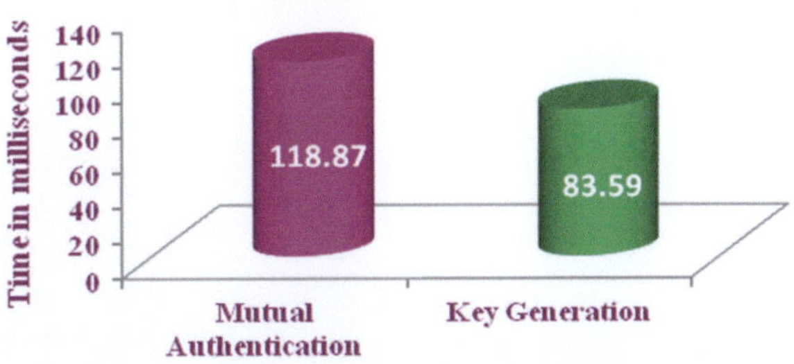

Fig. 4 Performance analysis over mutual authentication

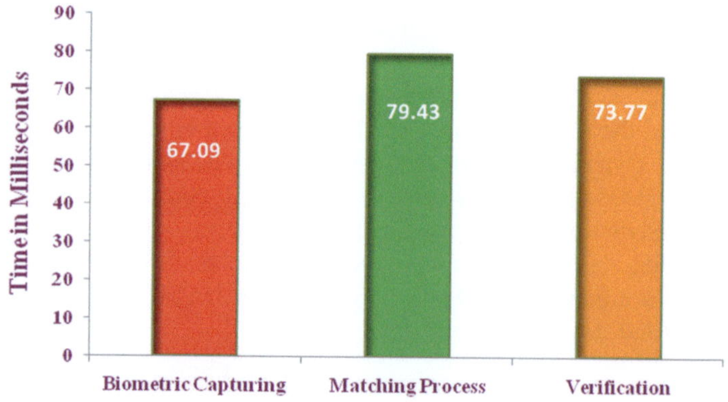

Fig. 5 Performance analysis on user authentication

3.3 *The Performance Analysis on Device Authentication*

The device authentication verifies the identity of the client device using ECC based X.509v3 digital certificate and the unique identifiable pictures. The performance is done with respect to the time taken for the following: 1. Invoke Client Certificate, 2. Client Certificate Verification, 3. Invoke Server Certificate, 4. Fetching Serial Number from Server Certificate, 5. OCSP Protocol Initiation, 6. Server Certificate Validation and Device Authentication, and 7. Matching the identifiable pictures at server and mobile device. The result generated is presented graphically in Fig. 6.

From the results, it is observed that the time taken to perform all the above-mentioned aspects is relatively less. It ensures the unique identification and the authentication of the device.

Fig. 6 Performance analysis on device authentication

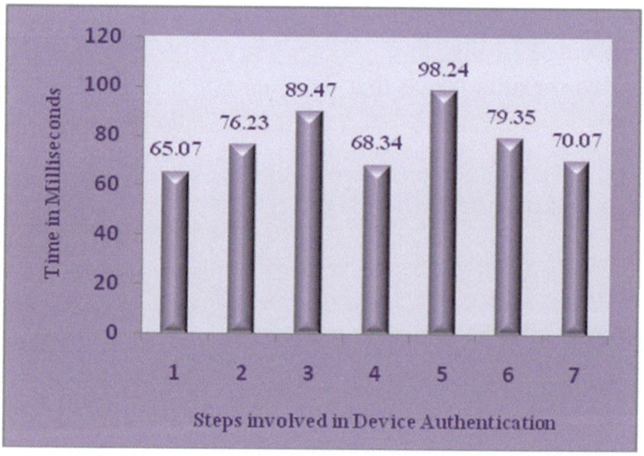

The overall performance analysis of the proposed system ensures that the confidentiality, integrity, privacy, and unique authentication are achieved in relatively less time. It is very adaptable for resource constrained devices such as UAISC and mobile device.

4 Conclusion

The proposed adaptable and secure intelligent smart card framework for Integrating Internet of Things and cloud computing realizes the vision of the future networks to avail any applications and any services irrespective of any underlying technologies anywhere, anytime with one UAISC. This UAISC is unique and the users can carry one smart card for any applications and transactions in a smart environment. By implementing this architecture, the UAISC can connect people and enable automatic machine to machine communication. The simulated results prove that the proposed system eliminates ambiguity and enhances security by providing unique authentication, confidentiality, privacy, and integrity. This guarantees that the users and the service providers can adopt this system, ultimately the government of India to build digital India with its salient features of ease of use and security. Higher level security by incorporating ECC, overall simulation of this architecture and real-time implementation are in progress of this research.

References

1. Gubbi, J., Buyya, R., Marusic, S., Palaniswami, M.: Internet of things (IoT): a vision, architectural elements and future directions. In: Future Generation Computer Systems, vol. 29, pp. 1645–1660. Elsevier (2013)
2. Roman, R., Najera, P., Lopez, J.: Securing the internet of things. In: IEEE Computer, vol. 44, pp. 51–58. IEEE (2011)
3. Vermesan, O., Friess, P.: Internet of Things from Research and Innovation to Market Deployment. River Publishers, Aalborg, Denmark (2013)
4. Buyya, R., Broberg, J., Goscinski, A.: Cloud Computing Principles and Paradigms. WILEY Publications (2011)
5. Cisco Visual Networking Index: Global Mobile Data Traffic Forecast Update, 2014–2019. White Paper, Cisco VNI Mobile (2015)
6. Das, R.: NFC-Enabled phones and contactless smart cards 2008–2018. Card Technol. Today (2008)
7. Wu, X.J., Fang, X.: Developing smart card application with PC/SC. In: International Conference on Internet Computing and Information Services, pp. 286–289. IEEE Computer Society (2011)
8. Mayes, K., Markantonakis, K.: An introduction to smart cards and RFIDs. In: Secure Smart Embedded Devices, 3 Platforms and Applications, pp. 1–25. Springer, New York (2014)
9. Sauveron, D.: Multiapplication smart card: towards an open smart card. In: Information Security Technical Report 14, pp. 70–78. Elsevier (2009)

10. Akram, R.N., Markantonakis, K.: Rethinking the smart card technology. In: Tryfonas, T., Askoxylakis, I. (eds.) HAS 2014. LNCS, vol. 8533, pp. 221–232. Springer, Switzerland (2014)
11. Bafandehkar, M., Yasin, S.M., Mahmod, R., Hanapi, Z.M.: Comparison of ECC and RSA algorithm in resource constraint devices. In: International Conference on IT Convergence and Security, pp. 1–3. IEEE (2013)
12. Botta, A., Donato, W., Persico, Valerio., Pescap, A.: On the integration of cloud computing and internet of things. In: International Conference on Future Internet of Things and Cloud, pp. 23–30. IEEE Computer Society, Washington (2014)
13. Zhou, J., Leppänen, T., Harjula, E., Ylianttila, M., Ojala, T., Yu, C., Jin, H., Yang, L.T.: CloudThings: a common architecture for integrating the internet of things with cloud computing. In: 17th International Conference on Computer Supported Cooperative Work in Design, pp. 651–657. IEEE (2013)
14. Bai, T.D.P., Rabara S.A.: Design and development of integrated, secured and intelligent architecture for internet of things and cloud computing. In: 3rd International Conference on Future Internet of Things and Cloud, pp. 817–822. IEEE Computer Society (2015)
15. Bai, T.D.P., Jerald, A.V., Rabara, S.A.: Elliptic curve cryptography based security framework for internet of things and cloud computing. Int. J. Comput. Sci. Technol. **6**, 223–229 (2015)

A Framework for Ontology Learning from Taxonomic Data

Chandan Kumar Deb, Sudeep Marwaha, Alka Arora and Madhurima Das

Abstract Taxonomy is implemented in myriad areas of biological research and though structured it deals with the problem of information retrieval. Ontology is a very powerful tool for knowledge representation and literature also cites the conversion of taxonomies into ontologies. The automated ontology learning is developed to ward off the knowledge acquisition bottleneck; but thereof the limitation includes text understanding, knowledge extraction, structured labelling and filtering. The system, ASIUM, TEXT TO ONTO, DODDLE II, SYNDIKATE, HASTI, etc., includes some inadequacies and does not exclusively deal with taxonomic texts. The proposed system will deal with the taxonomic text available in agricultural system and will also enhance the algorithms thereby available. We also propose a framework for learning of the taxonomic text which will overcome the loopholes of ontology developed from generalized texts. Finally, a framework of comparison of the manually developed ontology and automatically developed ontology will be ensured.

Keywords Automated ontology learning · Taxonomic texts · Knowledge acquisition

C.K. Deb (✉) · S. Marwaha · A. Arora
Indian Agricultural Statistics Research Institute, New Delhi, India
e-mail: chandan@iasri.res.in

S. Marwaha
e-mail: Sudeep.Marwaha@icar.gov.in

A. Arora
e-mail: Alka.Arora@icar.gov.in

M. Das
Indian Agricultural Research Institute, New Delhi, India
e-mail: madhurima.iari@gmail.com

V.B. Aggarwal et al. (eds.), *Big Data Analytics*, Advances in Intelligent Systems and Computing 654, https://doi.org/10.1007/978-981-10-6620-7_4

1 Introduction

Nowadays, knowledge structuring and knowledge management are the key focuses of the scientific communities. Ontology is a very powerful knowledge representation technique. On the other hand, the taxonomic knowledge has a great correspondence to the ontology. As [1] proposed a methodology for the conversion of taxonomies into ontologies; but manual ontology building is a tremendous labour intensive task. Although unstructured data can be made into structured; it encompasses a very lengthy process and henceforth the automated ontology learning approach is developed to ward off this knowledge acquisition bottleneck, hitherto, it includes some serious limitation in text understanding, knowledge extraction, structured labelling, and filtering [2]. Under conventional condition, the ontology learning deals with the normal text. Ontology learning from normal text is not so efficient. It is also dangerous to extract the concept from the normal text. However, no attempt has been made for ontology learning from taxonomic text. Thus, a novel approach is proposed to engineer the taxonomic text and make it as the input of the ontology learning. In agriculture, this kind of ontology learning has not yet been attempted.

2 Literature Review

Ontology learning is a new field of artificial intelligence and machine learning. A limited number of ontology learning tools and techniques have been developed so far and some of them are listed below:

References [3, 4] developed a system namely ASIUM. ASIUM learns sub-categorization frames of verbs and ontologies from syntactic parsing of technical texts in natural language. It is developed in French language. The ASIUM method is based on conceptual clustering. Reference [5] developed a system to classify nouns in context. It is able to learn categories of nouns from texts, whatever their domain is. Words are learned considering the contextual use of them to avoid mixing their meanings. This system was a preprocessor of ontology learning. References [6, 7] developed a system of ontology learning named TEXT TO ONTO. TEXT TO ONTO learns concepts and relations from unstructured, semi-structured, and structured data, using a multi-strategy method which is a combination of association rules, formal concept analysis, and clustering. But this is based on the shallow natural language processing. This system fails to address complex levels of understanding. Mostly, it identified concepts through regular expression. Reference [8] developed a system namely DODDLE II. DODDLE II is a Domain Ontology Rapid Development Environment. It can construct the hierarchical and nonhierarchical relationship of the domain concepts. For the hierarchical relationship, it uses WordNet. References [9–11] developed a system namely SYNDIKATE. SYNDIKATE is a system for automatically acquiring knowledge from real-world texts. It is available in German language. It has the problem of co-reference resolution. References [12, 13] developed a system namely HASTI. HASTI is an automatic ontology building system, which builds dynamic ontologies from scratch. HASTI learns the lexical and ontological knowledge from natural language texts. This is available in the Persian language.

Reference [14] developed a system that integrates machine learning and text mining algorithms into an efficient user interface; lowering the entry barrier for users who are not professional ontology engineers. The main features of the systems include unsupervised and supervised methods for concept suggestion and concept naming, as well as ontology and concept visualization. Reference [15] developed a system that integrates the external source knowledge like DBPedia and OpenCyc for getting the automatic suggestions for labelling the concepts. Reference [16] discussed how to learn large-scale ontology from Japanese Wikipedia. The large ontology includes IS-A relationship; class–instance relationship; synonym; object and data type properties of domain. However, a big problem of weakness in upper ontology arose against building up higher quality general ontology from Wikipedia. Reference [17] proposed a novel model of an *Ontology Learning Knowledge Support System (OLeKSS)* to keep the Knowledge Support System updated. The proposal applies concepts and methodologies of system modelling as well as a wide selection of ontology learning processes from heterogeneous knowledge sources (ontologies, texts, and databases), in order to improve KSS's semantic product through a process of periodic knowledge updating.

Reference [18] developed a semi-supervised ontology learning based focused (SOF) crawler. This embodies a series of schemas for ontology generation and web information formatting. In this system, the web pages are segregated by Support Vector Machine (SVM). Reference [19] proposed a ontology learning approach that has been used for developing the ontology. They used Linking Open Data (LOD) cloud which is a collection of Resource Description Framework (RDF). They used domain ontology for learning ontology and called Mid-Ontology Learning. Mid-Ontology learning approach that can automatically construct a simple ontology, linking related ontology predicates (class or property) in different data sets. Reference [20] gave an approach of clustering of the web services for efficient clustering. They adopted the ontology learning to generate ontologies via hidden semantic pattern. But they also mentioned the chances of failure of the ontology based discovery of web services. Reference [21] used heterogeneous sources like databases, ontologies, and plain text for ontology learning. Reference [22] generated ontology structure called ontology graph. The ontology graph defines ontology and knowledge conceptualization. The ontology learning process defines the method of semiautomatic learning and generates ontology graphs from Chinese text of different domains.

3 Objectives of the Proposed Work

The proposed system will deal with the taxonomic text available in agricultural system. We also propose a framework for learning of the taxonomic text which will overcome the loopholes of ontology developed from generalized texts. One system has been developed on the basis of the learning frame work. Finally, a framework of comparison of the manually developed ontology and automatically developed ontology will be ensured.

4 Proposed Framework

This proposed framework will mainly differ from the conventional ontology learning process in the input of the ontology learning framework. The conventional ontology learning system claims to have the capability of dealing with a range of texts but these systems are trapped by the inherent hindrance of the ontology learning. On the other hand, this framework is totally focused on the taxonomic text available in agricultural system. The proposed framework will mainly deal with two sub-module—first, how to deal with the taxonomic text and second, how to validate of the result of the first module.

4.1 Algorithmic Framework

This proposed framework subdivides the ontology learning process into well-demarcated category. It neutralizes the complexity of the ontology learning process. Figure 1 shows the schematic diagram of the total framework.

4.1.1 Categorize the Taxonomic Data

The taxonomic texts are available in different forms or categories. The first task of this framework is to find out the category of the taxonomic text on the basis of different sources (e.g. Taxonomic Books in Agriculture). Based on this category, the whole process of the ontology learning will be done.

4.1.2 Preprocess the Text

Preprocessing of the taxonomic data is very important because whatsoever the source of the data and category they have; there exists two basic type of text—

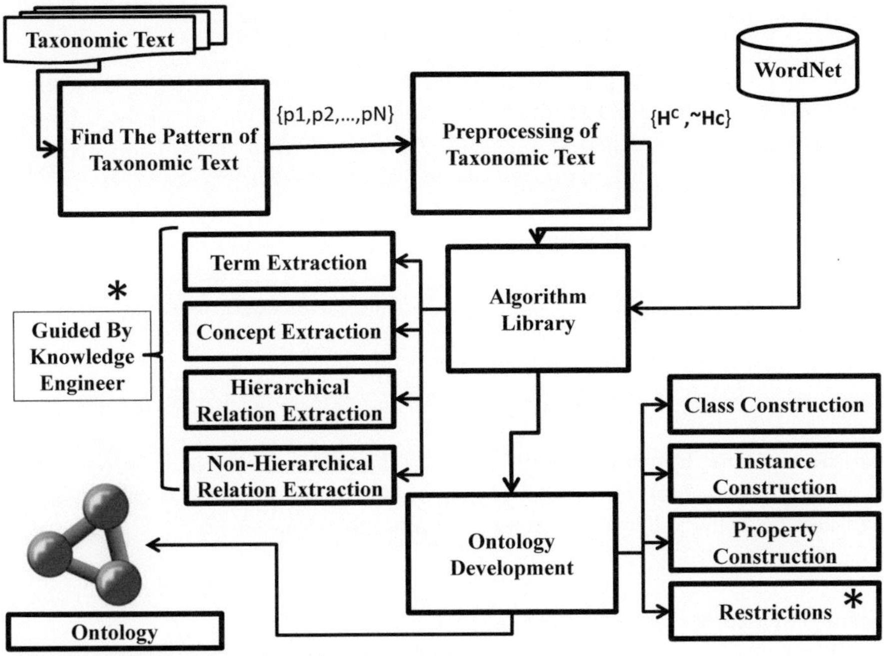

Fig. 1 Schematic task flow of algorithmic framework

hierarchical and nonhierarchical. For this, the ontology engineer can use any algorithm which can be helpful for the partitioning of the data (e.g. SVM).

4.1.3 Development of the Algorithmic Library

First part of the total framework, i.e. Algorithmic Framework wholly deals with the algorithms for the taxonomic text ontology learning; it deals with the following task.

Term Extraction

This sub-module actually commences the ontology learning process; it is from this level that the extraction of the ontology building block is started. The term extracted is used for class and instance construction. A repository will be developed for the extracted term. For extracting the term, the tools and techniques of natural language processing can be used.

Concept Extraction

Next step towards ontology learning is the extraction of the concept. The concept extraction can be done in two ways—the first approach is the use of the taxonomy for the concept labelled and second with the help of WordNet API like JNWL.

4.1.4 Relationship Extraction

In preprocess module, the text is subdivided into two categories:

Hierarchical Relation Extraction

On the basis of the pattern of the data, the hierarchical or ISA relation will be extracted. These algorithms will be based on the taxonomic data so these relations will also be extracted from the basis of taxonomic data.

Nonhierarchical Relation Extraction

Apart from the hierarchical relation or ISA relation, there are many relations like hasA, partOf for construction of the ontology.

4.1.5 Mapping to Ontology

After the extraction process of term and concept; the class and subclasses will be constructed for developing the ontology. The identification of the properties is also a subtask of this task. Restrictions will be imposed on the class by the help of the knowledge engineer.

4.2 Architecture of Proposed System

The given framework has been implemented in MVC architecture. Here, we proposed java-based *N*-tier architecture. Different layer has its individual importance as well as they are important as a whole. The layers are as follows and Fig. 2 depicts the architecture of the software:

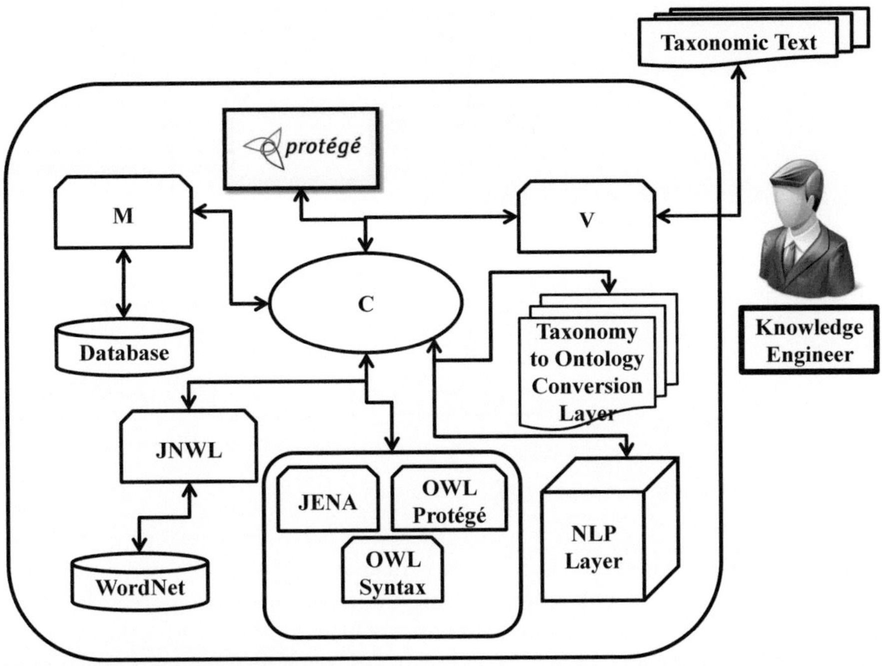

Fig. 2 Architecture of the system

4.2.1 MVC Layer

In this layer, the model, view, and controller are developed. The controller part of MVC interacts with the other part of the software and it works as a central control to the whole system.

4.2.2 Natural Language Processing Layer

The layer of this architecture is important, because all the preprocessing before automatic ontology development, it extracts all the building block of ontology. The term extraction, concept extraction, etc., are given in the framework and have been implemented in this layer.

4.2.3 Tax-to-Onto Layer and Semantic Web Layer

This layer deals with some very important tasks and components of ontology learning. It is connected with protégé which is the knowledge base of the ontology. It has several API's as its components (e.g. JENA, OWLProtege, JNWL and Wordnet).

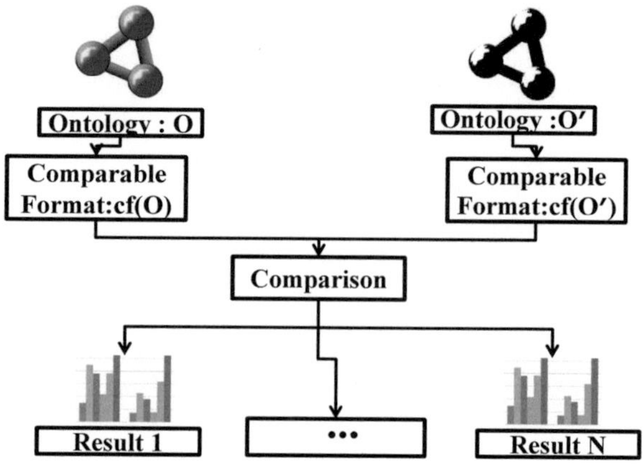

Fig. 3 Comparisons of the ontologies

4.3 Comparison Framework

This framework provides the approach of comparison between the two ontologies. By this approach, we can also evaluate our framework of ontology learning from taxonomic text. For comparing the ontology, we have to convert both the ontology into a single comparable format. The comparable format may be the conversion of ontology to a graph. Then compare both the ontology on the basis of class, instance, and properties. Comparison can also be done on the basis of concept extraction. Figure 3 depicts the comparison framework of ontology.

5 Conclusion

The software developed on the basis of the proposed framework will help in automatic ontology learning from taxonomic texts and also overcome the inherent problems of conventional ontology learning in terms of knowledge acquisition. The proposed methodology may be used in the biological fields, where taxonomy has its own importance. Besides biological field, this methodology is generic enough to be applied in other fields also. Lastly, this framework also provides a more simplistic way of comparison between manually developed and automatically developed ontology.

Acknowledgements The first author gratefully acknowledges the INSPIRE Fellowship provided by Department of Science and Technology, New Delhi.

References

1. Bedi, P., Marwaha, S.: Designing ontologies from traditional taxonomies. In: Proceedings of International Conference on Cognitive Science, Allahabad, India (2004)
2. Zouaq, A., Gasevic, D., Hatala, M.: Unresolved issues in ontology learning. In: Proceedings of Canadian Semantic Web Symposium (2011)
3. Faure, D., Nédellec, C., Rouveirol, C.: Acquisition of semantic knowledge using machine learning methods: The system "ASIUM". In Universite Paris Sud (1998)
4. Faure, D., Thierry, P.: First experiments of using semantic knowledge learned by ASIUM for information extraction task using INTEX. In: Ontology Learning ECAI-2000 Workshop (2000)
5. Chalendar, G., Grau, B.: Knowledge engineering and knowledge management. In: Methods, Models and Tools. Springer, Berlin (2000)
6. Maedche, A., Staab, S.: Discovering conceptual relations from text. In: Proceedings of the 13th European Conference on Artificial Intelligence. IOS Press, Amsterdam (2000)
7. Maedche, A., Volz, R.: The ontology extraction maintenance framework text-to-onto. In: Proceedings of the Workshop on Integrating Data Mining and Knowledge Management (2001)
8. Yamaguchi, T., Izumi, N., Fukuta, N., Sugiura, N., Shigeta, Y., Morita, T.: DOODLE-OWL: OWL-based semi-automatic ontology development environment. In: Proceedings of the 3rd International Workshop on Evaluation of Ontology based Tools (2001)
9. Hahn, U., Schnattinger, K.: Towards text knowledge engineering. In: Proceedings of the 15th National Conference on Artificial Intelligence, Madison, Wisconsin (1998)
10. Hahn, U., Romacker, M.: The SYNDIKATE text Knowledge base generator. In: Proceedings of the 1st International Conference on Human Language Technology Research (2001)
11. Hahn, U., Markó, K.: An integrated dual learner for grammars and ontologies. Data Knowl. Eng. **42**, 273–291 (2002)
12. Mehrnoush, S., Ahmad, B.: An introduction to hasti: an ontology learning system. In: Proceedings of the Iasted International Conference Artificial Intelligence and Soft Computing. Acta Press, Galgary, Canada (2002)
13. Mehrnoush, S., Ahmad, B.: The state of the art in ontology learning: a framework for comparison. Knowl Eng Rev **18**, 293–316 (2003)
14. Fortuna, B., Grobelnik, M., Mladenić, D.: OntoGen: Semi-automatic ontology editor. In: Proceedings of Human Interface, Part II, HCI International, LNCS 4558 (2007)
15. Weichselbraun, A., Wohlgenannt, G., Scharl, A.: Refining non-taxonomic relation labels with external structured data to support ontology learning. Data Knowl. Eng. **69**, 763–778 (2010)
16. Tamagawa, S., Sakurai, S., Tejima, T., Morita, T., Izumiy, N., Yamaguchi, T.: Learning a large scale of ontology from Japanese Wikipedia. In: Proceedings of International Conference on Web Intelligence and Intelligent Agent Technology (2010)
17. Gil, R.J., Martin-Bautista, M.J.: A novel integrated knowledge support system based on ontology learning: model specification and a case study. Knowl. Based Syst. **36**, 340–352 (2012)
18. Dong, H., Hussain, F.K.: SOF: a semi supervised ontology earning based focused crawler. Concurr Comput Pract Experience **25**, 1755–1770 (2013)
19. Lihua, Z.H.A.O., Ichise, R.: Integrating ontologies using ontology learning approach. IEICE Trans Inf Syst **96**, 40–50 (2013)
20. Kumara, B.T., Paik, I., Chen, W., Ryu, K.H.: Web service clustering using a hybrid term-similarity measure with ontology learning. Int. J. Web Serv. Res. **11**, 24–45 (2014)
21. Gil, R., Martin-Bautista, M.J.: SMOL: a systemic methodology for ontology learning from heterogeneous sources. J Intel Inf Syst **42**, 415–455 (2014)
22. Liu, J.N., He, Y.L., Lim, E.H., Wang, X.Z.: Domain ontology graph model and its application in Chinese text classification. Neural Comput. Appl. **24**, 779–798 (2014)

Leveraging MapReduce with Column-Oriented Stores: Study of Solutions and Benefits

Narinder K. Seera and S. Taruna

Abstract The MapReduce framework is a powerful tool to process large volume of data. It is becoming ubiquitous and is generally used with column-oriented stores. It offers high scalability and fault tolerance in large-scale data processing, but still there are certain issues when it comes to access data from columnar stores. In this paper, first, we compare the features of column stores with row stores in terms of storing and accessing the data. The paper is focused on studying the main challenges that arise when column stores are used with MapReduce, such as data co-location, distribution, serialization, and data compression. Effective solutions to overcome these challenges are also discussed.

Keywords MapReduce · Data Co-location · Column stores · Data distribution · Serialization

1 Introduction

In the digital era, there is an emerging discrepancy between the volume of data being generated by a variety of applications and the ability to analyze this huge data. As the size of data is growing day by day, it is getting challenging both to store and process this large-scale data so as to analyze and derive meaning out of it. All recent database systems use B-tree indexes or hashing to speed up the process of data access. These data structures keep data sorted and allow very fast and efficient searching, sequential accessing of data and even insertion and deletion of data from the underlying storage. Modern DBMS also incorporate a query optimizer that optimizes query before execution and may use either an index file or may execute a sequential search for accessing data.

N.K. Seera (✉) · S. Taruna
Banasthali Vidyapeeth, Jaipur, India
e-mail: sk.narinder@gmail.com

S. Taruna
e-mail: staruna71@yahoo.com

V.B. Aggarwal et al. (eds.), *Big Data Analytics*, Advances in Intelligent Systems and Computing 654, https://doi.org/10.1007/978-981-10-6620-7_5

The problem of processing and analyzing huge data sets has been answered by MapReduce, a programming model where users write their programs while concentrating only on program details ignoring the internal architecture of MR. MapReduce has no indexing feature and hence it always performs brute force sequential search. However, most of the column-oriented data storage systems that use MapReduce use index mechanisms in their underlying data storage units. Apart from this, sometimes MapReduce also suffer from a serious performance drawback due to large number of disk seeks. This can be illustrated with the following example.

In MapReduce model, M output files are produced by N map instances. Each of the M output files is received by a different reduce instance. These files are stored on the local machine running the map instance. If N is 500 and M is 100, the map phase will generate 50,000 local files. When the reduce phase begins, each of the 100 reduce instances reads its 500 input files by using FTP protocol to "pull" each of its input files from map nodes. With 100 of reducers operating concurrently, it is expected that multiple reducers will try to access their input files from the same mapper (map nodes) in parallel—producing huge number of disk seeks and bringing down the effective data transfer rate of disk by a factor of 20 or more. Due to this reason, parallel database systems do not materialize their split files and use "push" rather than "pull".

Below, we discuss the motivation behind using column-oriented stores and employing MapReduce techniques with such systems. The rest of the paper is organized as follows: Sect. 3 introduces how the data is stored and read from column-oriented stores. In Sect. 4, we explore the main issues related to the use of column-oriented stores with MapReduce. Finally, in Sect. 5, we conclude the paper (Fig. 1).

2 Motivation

The main features provided by row oriented stores are:

1. The speed at which data is loaded in HDFS blocks is very fast and no additional processing overhead is incurred.

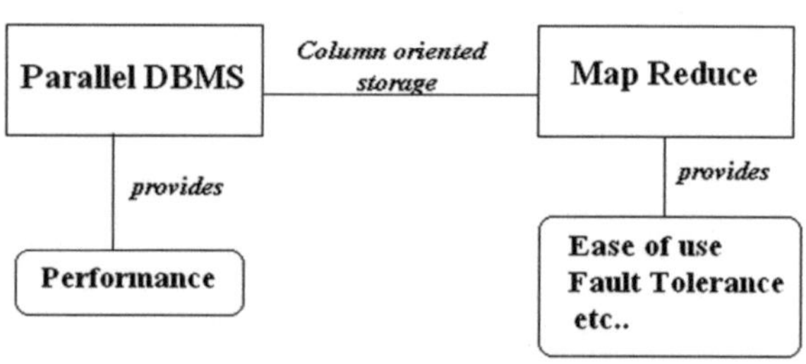

Fig. 1 Parallel DBMS versus MapReduce

2. All columns of the same tuple or row can be accessed from the same HDFS block.

Besides these features, row stores suffer from few serious drawbacks, which are listed below:

1. All columns of the same row are rarely accessed at the same time.
2. Additional processing overhead is added due to compression of different types of columnar data (as data types of different columns are generally different).

Figure 2 depicts how read operations are performed in row stores. The read operation is a two-step process. First, the rows from data nodes are read locally at the same time. Second, the undesired columns are discarded.

To overcome the limitations of row stores, column stores are generally gaining popularity and are believed to be best compatible with MapReduce. In the next section, we discuss how the data is managed in column stores and is used by MapReduce. We also discuss the challenges and solutions of adhering column stores with MapReduce.

3 MapReduce with Column Stores

Compared with row stores, I/O cost in column stores can be reduced to a great extent. The reason for this is that only desired columns are loaded and these columns can be easily compressed individually. Figure 3 illustrates the read operations in column stores. As an example, to access columns A and C, which are available at data node 1 and 3, respectively, first the columns from both the data

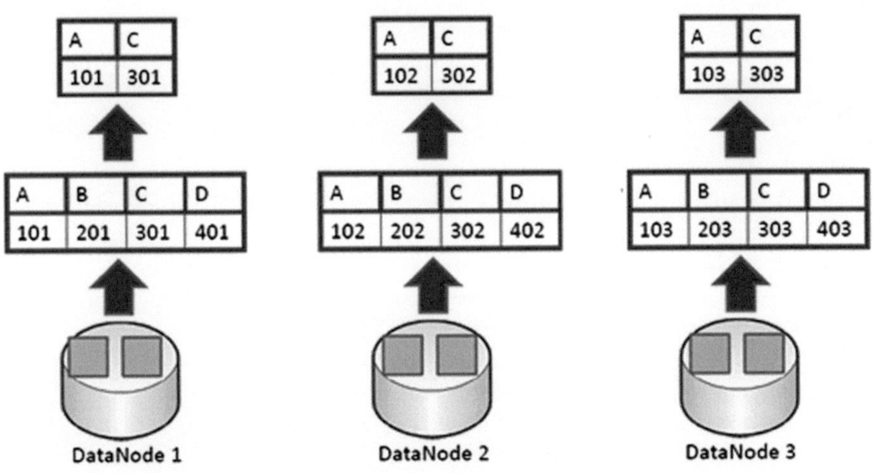

Fig. 2 Read operation in row stores

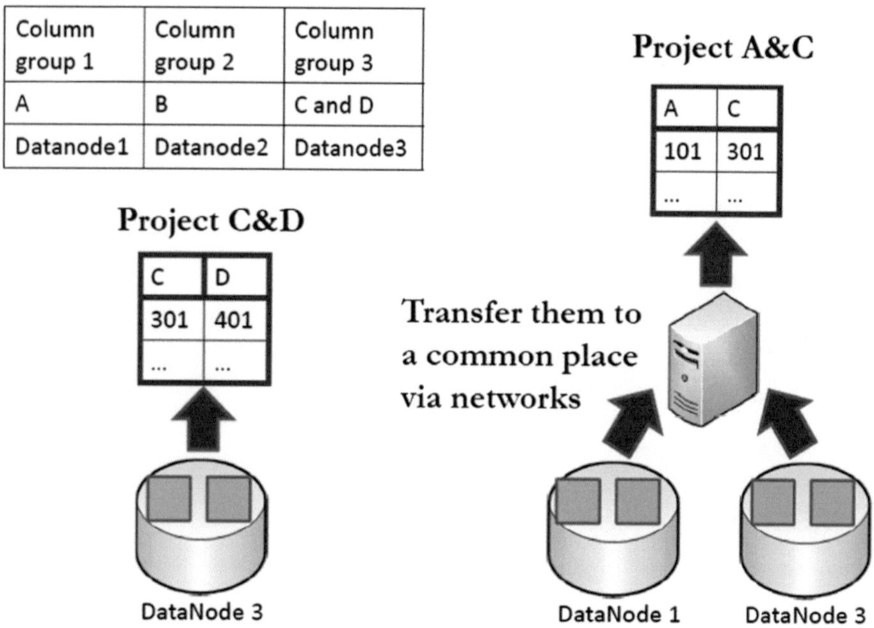

Fig. 3 Read operation in column stores

nodes are fetched at one common place, and then projection is performed over attributes A and C.

The only drawback of column stores is that—accessing columns from different data nodes entail additional data transfers in network.

The biggest motivation behind using column stores is to increase the performance of I/O in two ways [1]:

1. Minimize the data transfer in network by eliminating the need to access unwanted columns
2. Reducing the processing overhead to compress all the columns individually.

Distributed systems and programming model such as MapReduce also prefer column data stores due to the features they offer. HadoopDB [2] also adheres to columnar data store—Cstore [3] as its underlying data storage unit. Dremel [4]—an interactive ad hoc query system also use nested columnar data storage, for processing large data sets of data. It employs column-striped data storage for reading data from large storage space and reducing I/O costs due to inexpensive compression. Bigtable offered column family store for grouping multiple columns as a single basic unit of data access. Hadoop—an open source implementation of Java, also gained popularity because of its underlying column-wise storage, called HFile.

4 Challenges and Solutions

In the above section, we see how the data is stored and accessed in column-oriented stores. In this section, we throw a light on the main issues in concern with the problems of using MapReduce with column-oriented stores and few possible solutions.

a. Generating equal size splits—The problem is—in order to parallelize the job effectively over the nodes of a cluster, the data set must be partitioned into almost equal size splits. This can be done by partitioning the dataset horizontally and placing all partitions in separate sub-directories in Hadoop; where each sub-directory will serve as a separate split.
b. Data Co-location [5]—The default data placement policy of Hadoop randomly allocates the data among nodes for load balancing and simplicity. This data placement policy is fine for those applications which need to access data from a single node. But if any application wants to access data from different nodes concurrently, then this policy shows performance degradation, as:

   - It raises the cost of data shuffling
   - It increases network overhead due to data transfer
   - It decreases the efficiency of data partitioning.

   The problem here is that this data placement policy does not give any data co-location guarantee. So how can we improve the data co-location on the nodes so that the related values among different columns in the dataset are available on the same node executing the map task (or mapper).

   Babu [6] proposed an algorithm to resolve this issue, named dynamic co-location algorithm. This algorithm decreases the average number of nodes which are engaged in processing a query by placing the frequently accessed data sets on the same node, thereby reducing the data transfer cost. This algorithm dynamically verifies the relation between data sets and reshuffles the data sets accordingly. This algorithm has shown significant improvements in the execution time of MapReduce jobs.

   Figure 3 illustrates how two files A and B can be co-located using a locator table. File A has two blocks and file B has three blocks. All the blocks of both the files A and B are replicated on the same data nodes. A locator table is used to keep track of all the co-located files. It stores locator's information along with a list of files on the locator (Fig. 4).
c. Data Distribution [7]—In Hadoop, all the nodes store input and output files related to job currently executing on them. These nodes manage the distribution of file blocks over other nodes of the cluster, as required. When any node needs a file, available on any other node, only the desired file block is copied on it to avoid unnecessary traffic. The method of dividing the data for the map tasks can be defined by the user.

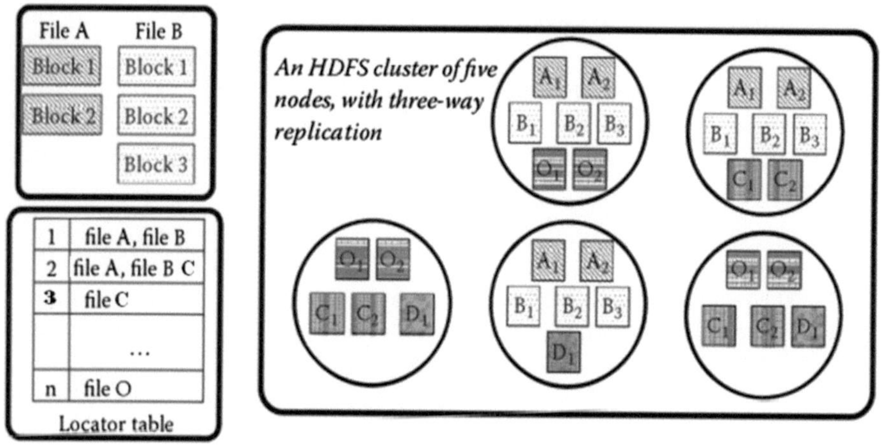

Fig. 4 Data co-location using a common locator table

Hadoop always try to schedule the job execution on the map instance that requires minimal amount of data transfers. In other words, a map instance is provided with a task which can be performed on the files already available on it. In case where a node has all of the required data blocks but is busy in running another task, Hadoop will allot the task to some other node. This may increase file transfer, but it is still more feasible than waiting for the previous job to finish.

d. Serialization and Lazy record Construction [8]—Serialization is the technique of converting structured objects into a byte stream. There are two main objectives of serialization:

- To transmit an object from one node to another over a network for the purpose of inter-process communication.
- To write an object to a persistent storage.

In Hadoop, the inter-process communication among multiple nodes is achieved by means of RPC (Remote Procedure Calls). RPC also uses serialization to convert the original message (to be sent over the network) into a byte stream. The receiver node receives the bye stream and again converts it into the original message. This reverse process is called deserialization.
In Hadoop, the main advantage of this technique is that only those columns are deserialized which are actually retrieved by the map nodes. Hence, it reduces the deserialization overhead as well as unnecessary disk I/O.

e. Columnar Compression [9]—Generally, columnar formats are likely to show fine compression ratios due to the fact that data within a column is expected similar than data across different columns. There are various compression methods which are adopted by column-oriented stores such as ZLIB, LZO, etc. All these methods have some advantages and certain limitations. For example,

ZLIB provides superior compression ratios but puts extra CPU overhead while decompression. LZO is generally employed in Hadoop to give better compression rates with lesser decompression overhead. It is usually adopted in cases where low decompression overhead is more required rather than the compression ratio. These compression methods use a special compression approach called block compression algorithm.
Block Compression: This approach compresses a block of columnar data at once. After compressing multiple blocks of the same column, they are loaded into a single HDFS block. The rate of compression and the overhead of decompression both are affected by using this strategy. Further, the size of compressed blocks, which can be defined at load time, also influences these factors. Each compressed block contains a header that gives information about the number of values in the block and the size of the block. By looking at the header, the system comes to know whether any value has been accessed in it. If there is no value in the block, then it can be skipped easily. And if, the header shows the presence of some values in it, the whole block is accessed and then decompressed.

f. Joins [5]—To easily and efficiently implement the join strategy, the schema and expected workload must be known in advance, as it helps in co-partitioning the data at the loading phase. The fundamental idea is—for given two input data sets, better performance can be achieved by:

   - applying the similar partitioning function on join compatible attributes of both the data sets at loading phase and
   - storing the co-group pairs with same join key on the same node would result in better performance.

   As a result, join operations can be performed locally within each node at query time. Executing joins with this idea do not need any modifications to be made in the current implementation of Hadoop framework. The modifications need to be made only at the internal process of the data splitting.

5 Conclusion

MapReduce programming model was devised by Google to process large data sets. In this paper, we introduced column stores with row stores in terms of reading and accessing data. The paper also explored the features of parallel database systems in contrast with MapReduce systems. The main challenges of using column stores with MapReduce such as data co-location, data distribution, serialization, compression, joins, etc., have been discussed along with some feasible solutions.

References

1. Lin, Y., Agrawal, D., Chen, C., Ooi, B.C., Wu, S.: Llama: leveraging columnar storage for scalable join processing in the MapReduce framework. In: Proceedings of the ACM SIGMOD International Conference on Management of Data (SIGMOD), pp. 961–972 (2011)
2. Abouzeid, A., Bajda-Pawlikowski, K., Abadi, D.J., Rasin, A., Silberschatz, A.: Hadoopdb: an architectural hybrid of mapreduce and Dbms technologies for analytical workloads. PVLDB **2**, 922–933 (2009)
3. Stonebraker, M., Abadi, D.J.. Batkin, D.J., Chen, X., Cherniack, M., Ferreira, M., Lau, E., Lin, A., Madden, S., O'Neil, E., O'Neil, P., Rasin, A., Tran, N., Zdonik, S.: C-store: a column-oriented dbms. In: VLDB (2005)
4. Melnik, S., Gubarev, A., Long, J.J., Romer, G., Shivakumar, S., Tolton, M., Vassilakis, T.: Dremel: interactive analysis of web-scale datasets. PVLDB **3**(1), 330–339 (2010)
5. Kaldewey, T., Shekita, E., Tata, S.: Clydesdale: structured data processing on map-reduce. ACM (2012) (978-1-4503-0790-1/12/03)
6. Babu, S.: Dynamic colocation algorithm for Hadoop. In: Advances in Computing Commmunication and Informatics ICACCI (2014)
7. Peitsa: Map-reduce with columnar storage. Seminar on columnar databases
8. Floratou, A., et al.: Column oriented storage techniques for Map-Reduce. Proc. VLDB Endowment **4**(7) (2011)
9. Chen, S.: Cheetah: a high performance, custom data warehouse on top of MapReduce. Proc. Endowment (PVLDB) **3**(2), 1459–1468 (2010)
10. He, Y., Lee, R., Huai, Y., Shao, Z., Jain, N., Zhang, X., Xu, Z.: RCFile: a fast and space-e_cient data placement structure in MapReduce-based warehouse systems. In: Proceedings of International Conference on Data Engineering (ICDE), pp. 1199–1208 (2011)
11. Dittrich, J., Quian_e-Ruiz, J.-A., Jindal, A., Kargin, Y., Setty, V., Schad, J.: Hadoop++: making a yellow elephant run like a cheetah (without it even noticing). Proc. VLDB Endowment (PVLDB) **3**(1), 518–529 (2010)
12. Dittrich, J., Quian_e-Ruiz, J.-A., Richter, S., Schuh, S., Jindal, A., Schad, J.: Only aggressive elephants are fast elephants. Proc. VLDB Endowment **5**(11), 1591–1602 (2012)
13. Eltabakh, M.Y., Tian, Y., Ozcan, F., Gemulla, R., Krettek, A., McPherson, J.: CoHadoop: exible data placement and its exploitation in Hadoop. Proc. VLDB Endowment (PVLDB) **4** (9), 575–585 (2011)
14. Pavlo, A., et al.: A comparison of approaches to large scale data analysis. In: SIGMOD 2009, June 29–July 2, 2009, USA
15. Dean, J., Ghemawat, S.: Map-reduce: simplified data processing on large clusters. In: OSDI 2004, p. 10 (2004)
16. Dittrich, J., Quian_e-Ruiz, J.-A.: Efficient big data processing in Hadoop MapReduce. Proc. VLDB Endowment (PVLDB), **5**(12), 2014–2015 (2012)
17. Jindal, A., et al.: Trojan data layouts: right shoes for a running elephant. In: SOCC 2011, Portugal (2011)
18. Apache Software Foundation: Hadoop Distributed File System: Architecture and Design (2007)

Hadoop: Solution to Unstructured Data Handling

Aman Madaan, Vishal Sharma, Prince Pahwa, Prasenjit Das and Chetan Sharma

Abstract Data is nothing but information of anything and we know it will continue to grow more and more. Unspecified format of data is unstructured data known as big data. 25% of the data that exist is in specified format, i.e., structured data and other 75% is in unspecified format. Unstructured data can be found anywhere. Generally, most of people and organizations pass out their lives working around unstructured data. In this paper, we have tried to work on how one can store unstructured data.

Keywords Big data · Hadoop · Analytics · Unstructured

1 Introduction

The one thing we know about data is that it will continue its pace. Terabytes are old, now we have petabytes, zetta bytes. Unstructured data can be defined as elements within data have no unique structure. The projects under big data offers the potential

A. Madaan (✉) · V. Sharma · P. Pahwa · P. Das · C. Sharma
Chitkara University, Baddi, Himachal Pradesh, India
e-mail: amanmadaan90@gmail.com

V. Sharma
e-mail: sharmavishal660@gmail.com

P. Pahwa
e-mail: princepahwa35554@gmail.com

P. Das
e-mail: prasenjit.das@chitkarauniversity.edu.in

C. Sharma
e-mail: chetan.sharma@chitkarauniversity.edu.in

V.B. Aggarwal et al. (eds.), *Big Data Analytics*, Advances in Intelligent Systems and Computing 654, https://doi.org/10.1007/978-981-10-6620-7_6

to confront wide range of problems that appear when collecting and working with big data are Variety, Volume, Velocity. Volume (capacity), i.e., Gigabytes to Terabytes to Petabytes. Velocity, i.e., streaming. Variety is texts, images, sounds. Organizations with big data are over 60% more likely than other organizations to have Business Intelligence projects that are driven primarily by the business sector not by IT-sector [1]. According to study, nearly 70–80% of data in a company is unstructured figures which comprise of statistics from docs and different social media technologies. Although it seems difficult to analyze even structured data but Hadoop has made it easy to analyze, store and access unstructured data. According to a study, world is now producing data eight times faster. Analytics-The use of data and related insights developed through applied analytics disciplines. Analytics are of three types: predictive, descriptive or prescriptive. Big firms and business tycoons believe that analytics connected with BD (big data), is going to play a major role in the economy in next 10–20 years. Some suggest today's big data will be the data of future.

Big data is very important nowadays in every sector whether it is scientific, industrial, public or even education sector.

1.1 Few Amazing Statistics

Every minute 121,000 tweets, 671 new websites are created, 3.5 quintillion bytes of data is produced in unstructured format every hour from different data origins like social networking sensors. To handle big data could be easy but it was difficult to handle unstructured large amount of data until Hadoop was developed.

Hadoop: This project was laid by Google and yahoo both. A prime role played by Yahoo for the growth of Hadoop for companies applications.

The success of "Google" is because it always focused on large amount of data, i.e., Big data analytics and social networking sites like Facebook, Twitter are best and successful example of application of big data (as daily there are millions of photos and statuses uploaded daily), so to store that one really needs big data analytics. Hadoop is for situations like clustering and targeting.

1.2 Components that Make up Hadoop

HDFS stands for Hadoop Distributed File System which is expandable as well as genuine storage system which stores each fork in a Hadoop cluster into a unbounded file system [2]. It helps in storing the file in form of big chunks which allows it to store large files on numerous machines efficiently. Chunks of data can be accessed parallely, without scanning complete file into a single computer's memory. By making replica of data on numerous hosts accuracy is achieved; by default, each chunk of data is stored, on three different PCs. If any fork or node fails, the data can be accessed from additional copy of blocks. This approach allows HDFS to dependably store massive amounts of data. For instance, in late 2012, the Apache Hadoop clusters at Yahoo had grown to hold over 350 petabytes (PB) of data across 40,000+ servers. Once data has been loaded into HDFS, we can begin to process it with MapReduce.

1.3 MapReduce

The programming dummy or model by which Hadoop can process great amount of data efficiently is MapReduce and it helps Hadoop to break large data processing troubles into numerous steps, a collection of Maps and Reduce which worked on multiple computers in parallel at the same time.

The purpose of MapReduce is to work with Hadoop. Apache Hadoop automatically optimizes the execution of MapReduce programs so that a given Map or Reduce step runs on HDFS node that contains the blocks of data which is necessary to complete the process. Data processing troubles that once required plenty of time to complete on large and costly computers now can be programmed that can be completed in seconds on machines that are not expensive.

1.4 YARN

As previously noted, Hadoop was initially adopted by many of the large web properties and was designed to meet their needs for large web scale batch type processing. The number of ways to store data in Hadoop expanded clusters and adoption expanded of Hadoop community has broader ecosystem, popular examples being Apache Hive is for querying and Apache Pig for processing of scripted data and Apache HBase for database.

Because of these open source projects, it created door for much richer and wider set of applications and are built on top of Hadoop—but these projects did not address the design limitations inherent in Hadoop; mainly batch-oriented data processing.

YARN is a key piece of Hadoop version 2 which is currently under development in the community. It provides a resource management framework for any processing engine, including MapReduce. It allows new processing frameworks to use the power of the distributed scale of Hadoop. It transforms single application to multi-application data system. This is future of Hadoop.

2 Survey and Motivation

Figure 1 explains that there will be huge increase in data by 2020 and so will be unstructured data. This graph is rising exponentially. According to this rise in graph [3]. Universe will grow from 50-fold up to 2020 and this is need of hour to study how to manage unstructured big data now which will help in future.

Figure 2 depicts that how much amount of unstructured data the world is going to use by 2020 is low as compared to structured data.

BD is defined as unstructured and semi-structured data that can be from all kinds of places, different sources and formats, suitable example would be web content, posts from twitter, contents from Facebook. Insights from these contents were not possible few years back but now it is easy to analyze because of advancement in technology. Decoding the human genome was merely impossible but now it can be achieved in one week only.

3 Architecture of Hadoop

It runs on plenty of machines that do not work on common memory or any storage devices and you can invest on bunch of commodity servers, store them in a structure, and successfully execute the Hadoop software on every one [4]. How you can load Hadoop by your organization's data? Applications break that data into small data

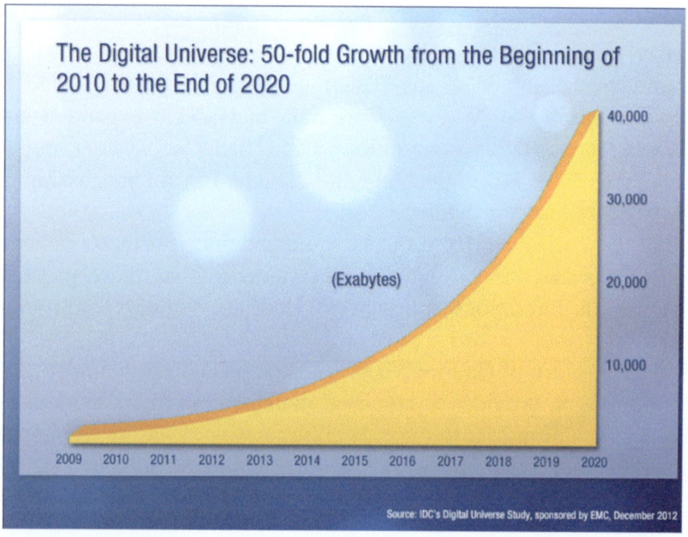

Fig. 1 Digital universe in 2020. 40,000 exabyte's by 2019–2020. 1 exabyte consist of 10^{18} bytes which is similar to 1,000,000 TB

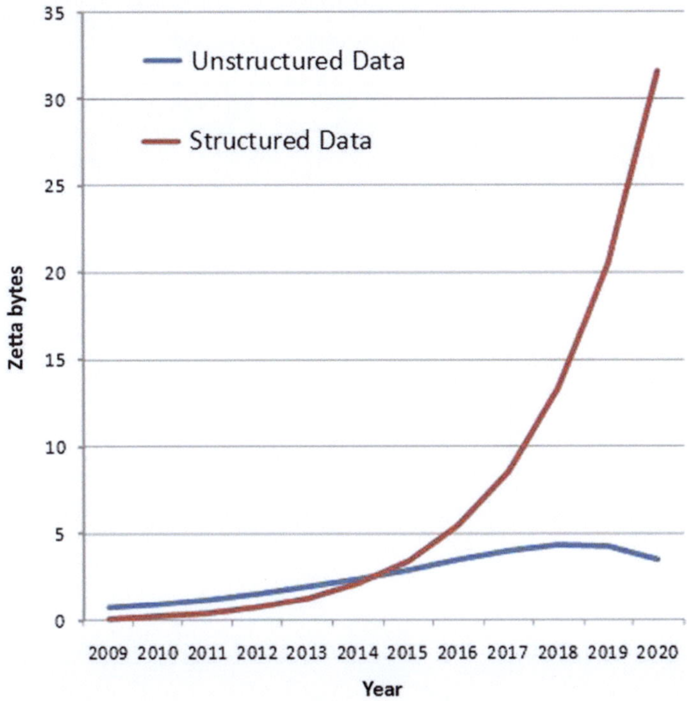

Fig. 2 Unstructured data v/s structured data

and then these data pieces spread across different servers. There is not a single place where you can eye all your data; Hadoop helps to track where your data kept. And as there are numerous copies to single data are stored, data stored on a server can be automatically replaced from a known good copy when it goes offline or dies.

In a unified database system, there are four, eight or big processors are connected to big disks. In a Hadoop cluster, every one of those servers has two or four or eight CPU's. Hadoop breaks the data and stores them in the Hadoop Distributed File System (HDFS), that can go to number of forks on a single cluster and in a single instance can support tens of millions of files. It is then set to be analyzed by the MapReduce framework (Figs. 3 and 4).

4 Proposed Solution

Our only problem is to handle unstructured data and it can be solved by using Hadoop technology. Hadoop acts as a Data warehouse. This helps in getting quality into the data through advanced analytics. It stores data in its native form until we need it. Business analytics and data mining tools are used to retrieve the data required.

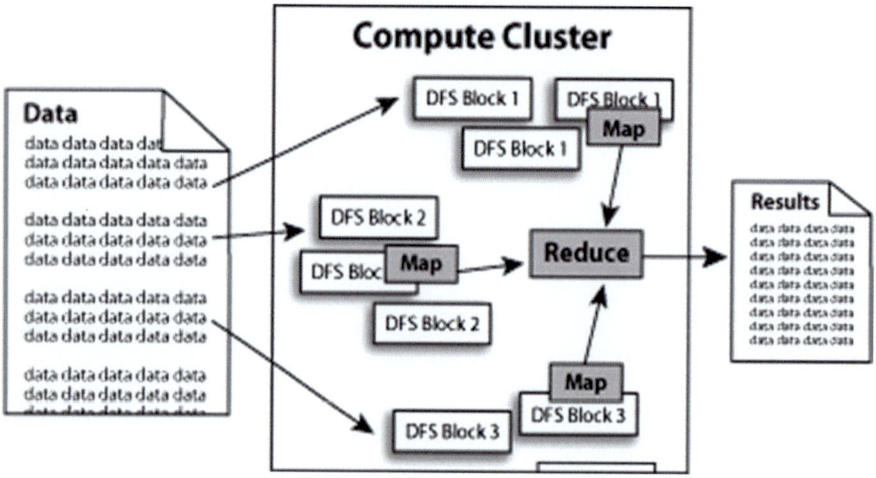

Fig. 3 Hadoop architecture

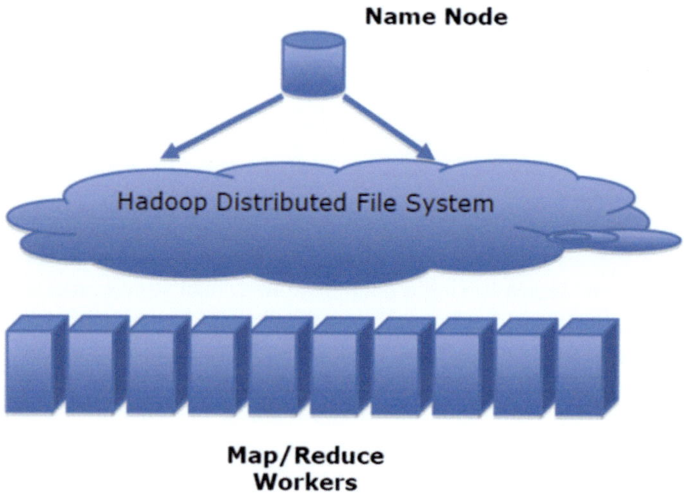

Fig. 4 MapReduce

4.1 Benefits to Use Hadoop

1. Hadoop is open source software so it is very economical to use it.
2. MapReduce is the framework in the Hadoop stack for software programming [5].

3. Existing database and analytics infrastructures are supported by Hadoop. Big data is a big opportunity to those who provides solutions. As an example, $740 million dollars has been invested by Intel into the rising distribution for Hadoop.
4. Quickly processing big data is done through the distributed computing model. As more computing nodes we use, more the processing power we have.
5. Hardware failure does not affect data and application processing.

4.2 Challenges

The most important problem is to collect, combine and analyze the data. Obtaining consent from users is very hard to manage including machine generated sources.

Data integration is time-consuming

In today's world data scientists spend large amount of their time on collecting and moving large amount of data, before it can be explored for useful nuggets. Big data is heterogeneous by nature; as analysts can ask new, different and more instinctive questions of the data, with a focus on mind that what is more profitable.

Real-time analytics is difficult to achieve

Hadoop has been in major use for the exploration of data. Although Hadoop can process large amount of data quickly, it has restrictions. Emerging area for Hadoop is real-time analytics, transferring large amount of data quickly has been a big challenge.

5 Conclusion and Future Work

In this paper, we tried to cover every glimpse of big data, i.e., how unstructured data can be stored and accessed. Hadoop can handle all types of data: structured and unstructured (mixture of data). With no prior need for a schema various kinds of data can be stored in Hadoop. In other words, no need to know how data will be stored. Hadoop reveals hidden relationships and answers many problems which have been hidden from a long time. We can start making decisions based on actual data.

In future we will work on how big data can be used in different fields whether it is educational sector, geosciences, and bio-energy. We will try to use big data analytics in these fields so that these sectors can be uplifted. With the advancement in technology we can perform better in these fields also by knowing some analytics or relationships which were not possible few years ago but now it is need of hour to work on these fields with these technologies.

References

1. http://www.datamation.com/applications/big-data-9-steps-to-extract-insight-from-unstructured-data.html
2. http://www.sas.com/en_us/insights/big-data/hadoop.html
3. http://blog.sqlauthority.com/2013/10/02/big-data-what-is-big-data-3-vs-of-big-data-volume-velocity-and-variety-day-2-of-21/
4. https://beta.oreilly.com/ideas/what-is-hadoop
5. http://www.searchcio.techtarget.com/intelsponsorednews/Five-Things-to-Know-About-Hadoop-for-Managing-Unstructured-Data
6. http://www.digitalreasoning.com/resources/Holistic-Analytics.pdf
7. http://www.dummies.com/how-to/computers-software/Big-Data/Data-Management/Hadoop.html
8. http://www.theglobaljournals.com/gra/file.php?val=February_2013_1360851170_47080_37.pdf
9. http://www.hadoop.apache.org/core/docs/current/api/

Task-Based Load Balancing Algorithm by Efficient Utilization of VMs in Cloud Computing

Ramandeep Kaur and Navtej Singh Ghumman

Abstract Although a lot of fundamental research is being carried out in a field of cloud computing, but still it is in infancy stage. In today's era of computing, it is trending Internet technology, which suffers from various issues and challenges. This research addresses load balancing as one of the major challenges in cloud computing. The paper proposes a dynamic load balancing algorithm for cloud computing environment and compares with the existing algorithm. The results show that proposed algorithm outperforms existing algorithm in terms of average response time, turnaround time, and total cost.

Keywords Cloud computing · Challenges · Load balancing · Utilized power · Load balancer · Datacenter broker (DCB)

1 Introduction

The word, "cloud" is a metaphor for Internet and "computing" means performing computations using computer technology. Therefore, cloud computing means Internet-based computing. Since it is becoming popular day by day, so its challenges and issues are also coming up. As, the number of users is being added, various issues such as load balancing, security issues, interoperability, quality of service (QoS) issues and a much more are coming up [1, 2]. This research focuses on load balancing in cloud computing. As the number of users may increase or decrease at any point of time, so these dynamic changes in the system must be handled quickly and optimally so as to minimize execution/response time and

R. Kaur (✉) · N.S. Ghumman
Department of Computer Science and Engineering, SBSSTC, Ferozepur, Punjab, India
e-mail: ramandipkaur23@gmail.com

N.S. Ghumman
e-mail: navtejghumman@yahoo.com

V.B. Aggarwal et al. (eds.), *Big Data Analytics*, Advances in Intelligent Systems and Computing 654, https://doi.org/10.1007/978-981-10-6620-7_7

achieve higher resource utilization. Load balancing is an optimization technique to balance the work load across the nodes of the system as each node does an equal amount of work.

2 Literature Survey

The paper [3] proposed a task-based load balancing algorithm based on QoS driven in cloud computing. This algorithm considers priority and completion time. The paper [4] proposed a VM-assign load balance algorithm to find out the least loaded VM using the index table and the load is assigned to that VM if it is not the last used VM. The paper [5] proposed a cloud light weight algorithm which not only balances the load but also ensures QoS to the users. The paper [6] proposed an algorithm, which considers only the response time of the incoming request and reduces communication cost and extra computation at the server. The paper [7] proposed a heuristic model for load balancing based on the utilized power of the virtual machine. It considers the heterogeneous nature of the VMs and the cloud computing system.

3 Proposed Algorithm

The definitions and terms used in the algorithm are given in Table 1. The existing algorithm [7] does not take into consideration the actual processing power of each virtual machine in terms of MIPS (millions of instructions per second). Thus, both

Table 1 Definitions and terms used in the algorithm

Average value	It is obtained by sum total of all values divided by total number of values
Avg_length	This is obtained by calculating the average value of the length of all the tasks that are submitted by the user for execution
MI	Millions of instructions. The length of tasks is measured in terms of MI
MIPS	Millions of Instructions Per Second. The processing capacity of a resource (virtual machine) is given in terms of MIPS
Avg_MIPS	This is obtained by calculating the average value of MIPS of all the virtual machines that are created in the system
Cloudlet	It is a user's request/task and is termed as Cloudlet in CloudSim simulator
Upper class group	This is the group of all those tasks/VMs whose length/MIPS is greater than their corresponding average value
Lower class group	This is the group of all those tasks/VMs whose length/MIPS is less than their corresponding average value

utilized power and MIPS should be considered during load distribution. The proposed methodology takes into account the utilized power as well as the actual processing power in terms of MIPS.

3.1 Task-Based Load Balancing Algorithm

- The proposed algorithm is an enhanced form of the existing algorithm. It works in three phases.

Phase 1: **Grouping of Tasks and Virtual Machines**.

- Initially, the algorithm groups the tasks by calculating the average value of the length of all the tasks and compares it with the length of each task.
- The tasks whose length are greater than or equal to the average value, they are added to a group of upper class tasks and the other ones are added to a group of lower class tasks.
- Similarly, the grouping of virtual machines takes place and here the average value of MIPS of all the VMs is taken in comparison with MIPS of each virtual machine.
- Here again, the VMs whose MIPS is greater than or equal to the average value of MIPS are added to a group of upper class VMs otherwise to the group of lower class VMs.

Phase 2: **Sending a group of Tasks to a group of VMs**.

- When grouping is done, then the upper class tasks are submitted to group of upper class VMs.
- The lower tasks are submitted to group of lower class VMs and also they are submitted to group of upper class VMs in case, any of them is available.

Phase 3: **Calculation of Utilized Power and submitting task to VM**

- Before submitting a task of the corresponding group to a VM of corresponding group, the utilized power of each VM is calculated using Eq. (1). The task is allocated to a VM, which is more powerful in terms of utilized power (VM with low value of utilized power is considered more powerful). The utilized power of that VM is updated after each task's execution. In case of ties, FCFS (First Come First Serve) is used.

The execution of the tasks continues until there is no task left for execution. The response time and average response time is calculated using (2) and (3). Unit cost is the addition of processing cost, cost per storage, cost per memory, and cost per bandwidth. Then the total cost is calculated using (4). The turnaround time (TT) of each task r_i and total turnaround time is calculated using (5) and (6).

$$\mathrm{PW}(k) = \mathrm{PW}(k) + \mathrm{CPU}(r_i)^{*}\mathrm{Size}(r_i)/\mathrm{CPU}(k) \tag{1}$$

$$\mathrm{RT}(r_i) = \mathrm{FT}(r_i) - \mathrm{ST}(r_i) \tag{2}$$

$$\mathrm{Total\,Cost}(r_i) = \mathrm{RT}(r_i)^{*}\mathrm{unit\_cost} \tag{3}$$

$$\mathrm{ART} = \sum_{i=1}^{i=n} \mathrm{RT}(r_i)/n \tag{4}$$

$$\mathrm{Turnaround\,Time} = \mathrm{FT}(r_i) - \mathrm{AT}(r_i) \tag{5}$$

$$\mathrm{TAT} = \sum_{i=1}^{i=n} \mathrm{TT}(r_i), \tag{6}$$

where

k	any kth virtual machine.
r_i	any ith task (i = 1 to n).
n	total number of tasks.
Size	task length/number of instructions (in MI).
CPU (r_i)	number of processing elements required by the task.
CPU (k)	number of processing elements required by the virtual machine (VM).
ST	start time of task
FT	finish time of task
AT	arrival time of task

3.2 Performance Parameters

The various performance parameters used in the load balancing algorithm are explained as follows:

- **Response Time**: It is calculated by subtracting the finish time of a task from start time of execution of a task. Lower the value of response time, higher is the performance of a load balancing algorithm.
- **Average Response Time**: It is obtained by taking the average value of response time of all the tasks. It is calculated as the sum total of all response time by the total number of tasks.
- **Turnaround Time**: It is the total taken by a load balancing algorithm between the submissions of a task for execution and return of the output to a user. It is calculated as subtracting arrival time of task from the finish time of a task.

4 Implementation

4.1 Simulation Environment

CloudSim is a cloud simulation toolkit developed in the CLOUDS laboratory at Department of Computer Science and Software Engineering at University of Melbourne [8]. It is a widely used toolkit which consists of following main entities: CIS (Cloud Information Service), Datacenter and Datacenter Broker.

4.2 Experimental Setup and Results

Table 2 gives the characteristics of cloud resources used in the simulation. We have created four virtual machines, namely, VM0, VM1, VM2, and VM3 in the simulator of varying MIPS. We have also created cloudlets (or tasks) of varying lengths (number of instructions) in the cloudlet. Later on, we conducted the experiments using PlanetLab workload.

We have conducted experiments by varying the number of tasks. Figure 1 shows a variation of average response time by taking 500, 5000, 20,000, and 5 lakh cloudlets in case of the existing algorithm and proposed algorithm. Figure 2 shows a variation of total cost and Fig. 3 shows the variation in total turnaround time with increase in workload in case of the existing algorithm and proposed algorithm.

5 Conclusion and Future Work

This paper focuses on the issue of load balancing in cloud computing. This paper proposed a task-based algorithm by efficient utilization of VMs in cloud computing. The results show that proposed algorithm gives better results as compared to the existing algorithm in terms of average response time, the total turnaround time, and total cost. As a future work, we have decided to improve various others

Table 2 Characteristics of cloud resources used in the simulation

VM ID	Processing capacity (MIPS)	Memory (in MB)	No. of processing elements	Bandwidth
VM0	100	256	1	300
VM1	150	256	1	100
VM2	350	256	1	100
VM3	750	256	1	100

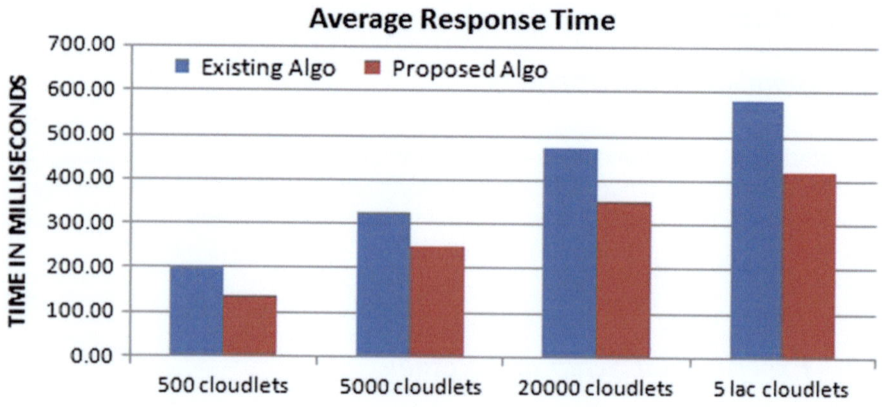

Fig. 1 Compares the average response time with increase in load

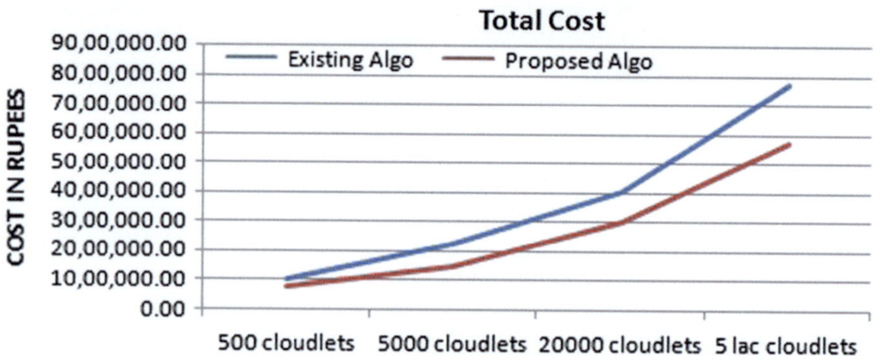

Fig. 2 Compares the processing cost with increase in load

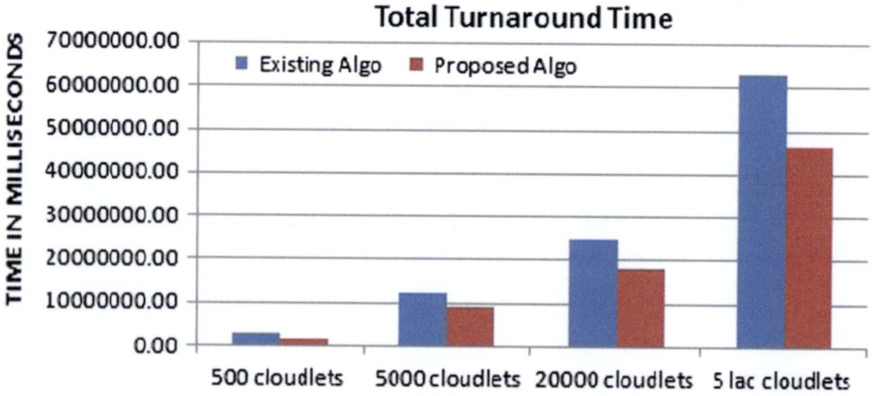

Fig. 3 Compares the total turnaround time with increase in load

performance parameters such as waiting time, throughput. The results of the algorithm can be further improved by taking a real cloud environment and creating dynamic grouping of the tasks and VMs.

References

1. Velte, A.T., Elsenpeter, R., Velte, T.J.: Cloud Computing a Practical Approach. TATA McGraw-HILL Edition, USA (2010)
2. Sonawane, S., Arnikar, P., Fale, A., Aghav, S., Pachouly, S.: Load balancing in cloud computing. J. Inf. Knowl. Res. Comput. Eng. **3**(1):573–576 (2014)
3. Wu, X., et al.: A task scheduling algorithm based on QoS-driven in cloud computing. Procedia Comput. Sci. **17**: 1162–1169 (2013)
4. Domanal, S.G., Reddy, G.R.M.: Optimal load balancing in cloud computing by efficient utilization of virtual machines. In: 2014 Sixth International Conference on Communication Systems and Networks (COMSNETS), IEEE (2014)
5. Mesbahi, M., Rahmani, A.M., Chronopoulos, A.T.: Cloud light weight: a new solution for load balancing in cloud computing. In: 2014 International Conference on Data Science & Engineering (ICDSE), pp. 44–50, 26–28 Aug 2014
6. Sharma, A., Peddoju, S.K.: Response time based load balancing in cloud computing. In: 2014 International Conference on Control, Instrumentation, Communication and Computational Technologies (ICCICCT), pp. 1287–1293, 10–11 July 2014
7. Haidri, R.A., Katti, C.P., Saxena, P.C.: A load balancing strategy for Cloud Computing environment. In: 2014 International Conference on Signal Propagation and Computer Technology (ICSPCT), pp. 636–641. IEEE (2014)
8. Calheiros, R.N., et al.: CloudSim: a toolkit for modeling and simulation of cloud computing environments and evaluation of resource provisioning algorithms. Softw. Pract. Experience **41** (1):23–50 (2011)

A Load Balancing Algorithm Based on Processing Capacities of VMs in Cloud Computing

Ramandeep Kaur and Navtej Singh Ghumman

Abstract Cloud Computing is a computing paradigm which has made high-performance computing accessible even to SMEs (small and medium enterprises). It provides various types of services to the users in the form of hardware, software, application platforms. The cloud computing environment is elastic and heterogeneous in nature. Any number of users may join/leave the system at any point of time; it means the workload of the system increases/decreases randomly. Therefore, there is a requirement for a load balancing system which must ensure that the load of the system is fairly distributed among the nodes of the system and aims to achieve minimum completion time and maximum resource utilization. The paper presents a load balancing algorithm based on processing capacities of virtual machines (VMs) in cloud computing. It analyses the algorithm and finds the research gap. It also proposes the future work overcoming the research gap in this field. The simulation of the algorithm is carried out in the CloudSim simulation toolkit.

Keywords Cloud computing · Challenges · Load balancing · Existing algorithms · Round-robin · Heuristic approach · Processing capacities

1 Introduction

Cloud computing is an emerging technology which permits users to access their stored data, applications and avail various types of cloud services via Internet. The cloud provides users' with various types of services such as physical hardware,

R. Kaur (✉) · N.S. Ghumman
Department of Computer Science and Engineering, SBSSTC,
Ferozepur, Punjab, India
e-mail: ramandipkaur23@gmail.com

N.S. Ghumman
e-mail: navtejghumman@yahoo.com

V.B. Aggarwal et al. (eds.), *Big Data Analytics*, Advances in Intelligent Systems and Computing 654, https://doi.org/10.1007/978-981-10-6620-7_8

programming tools and environments, softwares, business-related applications. These various types of services are as well known by the name, "service models of cloud".

1.1 Open Challenges [1]

- **Load Balancing**: It is a process of balancing the workload among the nodes of the system in order to achieve minimum response time and higher resource utilization.
- **Interoperability and Portability**: Interoperability is the ability to use the same tools and applications across various different cloud service providers' platforms. Portability can be the solution to address this issue. It says that one cloud solution works with various different types of applications, platforms, and other clouds also.
- **Resource Scheduling and Management**: It deals with the resource provisioning and management in order to provide the desired quality of service to a user.
- **Security and Privacy of Users' Data**: The users' data are kept with some third party by the service provider. So, how the cloud service provider addresses the security and privacy concerns is an issue.

2 Related Work

There are various types of load balancing techniques which are classified as static and dynamic.

- **Static Load Balancing Techniques**.

The static load balancing techniques are of static nature, which does not adapt themselves to the changing computing environment. Round-robin algorithm, min-min algorithm, max-min algorithm are static load balancing techniques. Static techniques perform well in a homogeneous and predictable computing environment.

- **Dynamic Load Balancing Techniques**.

The dynamic load balancing techniques are of dynamic nature, which adapts themselves to the changing environment. They follow the various policies for the load distribution in a dynamic heterogeneous computing environment. Honey bee Algorithm, active clustering, random biased sampling is dynamic load balancing algorithms.

2.1 Performance Metrics for Load Balancing Techniques

- **Response Time**: It is the time after which user's task is completed. It is calculated as subtracting total execution time from the start time. It should be minimized for better performance.
- **Fault Tolerance**: It is the ability to recover from failure by shifting the workload to some other remote working node. Thus, the load balancing algorithm should be highly fault tolerant.
- **Scalability**: It is the ability of an algorithm to perform load balancing for a finite number of nodes. In cloud system, number of users may increase or decrease dynamically and correspondingly the load is dynamic. Therefore, the load balancing algorithm should be highly scalable.

2.2 Existing Algorithms

There are various existing load balancing algorithms. The paper [2] proposes a round-robin algorithm, in which the tasks are allocated the virtual machines (VMs) for a fixed time quantum. The paper [3] proposed a min-min algorithm, in which smaller tasks are scheduled before the longer tasks. The paper [4] proposed a dynamic algorithm based on exponential smoothing forecast. It is employed to balance the load of real servers and takes into consideration the unique features of the long connectivity applications.

3 Load Balancing Algorithm

The task is actually a users' request which is independent and computational one. Let k be any virtual machine and "r_i" be any ith task (or cloudlet). As soon as the tasks are submitted, the load balancer first calculates the utilized power PW(k) of each VM using (1). The task is allocated the virtual machine (VM), which is more powerful in terms of processing capacity. Here, VM with lower value of power is more powerful. Then the task, "r_i" is dispatched to the selected VM. After the successful completion of the task, load balancer updates the power PW(k) of that VM using (1). In case of ties, the tasks are scheduled according to first come first serve (FCFS) basis.

The execution of the tasks continues until there is no task left for execution. The response time, average response time is calculated using (2) and (3) and total turnaround time (TAT) is calculated using (4).

$$\mathrm{PW}(k) = \mathrm{PW}(k) + \mathrm{CPU}(r_i)^{*}\mathrm{Size}(r_i)/\mathrm{CPU}(k) \tag{1}$$

$$\mathrm{RT}(r_i) = \mathrm{FT}(r_i) - \mathrm{ST}(r_i) \tag{2}$$

$$\mathrm{ART} = \sum_{i=1}^{i=n} \mathrm{RT}(r_i)/n \tag{3}$$

$$\mathrm{TAT} = \mathrm{FT} - \mathrm{AT}, \tag{4}$$

where,

k any kth virtual machine.
r_i any ith task (i = 1 to n).
n total number of tasks.
Size task length/number of instructions.
CPU (r_i) number of processing elements required by the task.
CPU (k) number of processing elements required by the virtual machine (VM).
ST start time of task
FT finish time of task
AT arrival time of task

3.1 *Illustrative Example*

Here we are going to discuss the working of the load balancing algorithm based on processing capacities of VMs with the help of an illustrative example. Here, we take four virtual machine, namely, VM0, VM1, VM2, VM3 of varying MIPS. Table 1

Table 1 Shows the characteristics of cloudlets during simulation

Cloudlet ID	Cloudlet length	File size	Output size	No. of processing elements (CPU)
C0	1000	1300	300	1
C1	3000	1300	300	1
C2	5000	1300	300	1
C3	7000	1300	300	1
C4	4000	1300	300	1
C5	3500	1300	300	1
C6	8000	1300	300	1
C7	9000	1300	300	1
C8	3000	1300	300	1
C9	4500	1300	300	1

Table 2 Shows the power of VMs before first cloudlet execution

VM ID	VM0	VM1	VM2	VM3
Utilized power PW(*k*)	0	0	0	0

Table 3 Shows the power of VMs during the execution of 10 cloudlets

VM ID	0	1	2	3
PW(*k*)	1000	**0**	**0**	**0**
PW(*k*)	1000	3000	**0**	**0**
PW(*k*)	1000	3000	5000	**0**
PW(*k*)	**1000**	3000	5000	7000
PW(*k*)	5000	**3000**	5000	7000
PW(*k*)	**5000**	6500	**5000**	7000
PW(*k*)	13,000	6500	**5000**	7000
PW(*k*)	13,000	**6500**	14,000	7000
PW(*k*)	13,000	9500	14,000	**7000**
PW(*k*)	13,000	9500	14,000	115,000

shows the characteristics of the cloudlets during simulation in this example. We have taken 10 cloudlets having lengths in a range of 1000–10,000. We have assumed that initially the utilized power of each VM is zero. Also, the virtual machine with low utilized power is more powerful.

Here, we know all the virtual machines have the same power. Therefore, in such cases FCFS is used. Tables 2 and 3 show the execution result.

4 Simulation Framework and Results

We have used CloudSim [5] as a simulation framework with Netbeans IDE. It is a simulation toolkit to model and simulate the Cloud Computing environment. We have employed four Virtual Machines, namely, VM0, VM1, VM2, VM3 having varying MIPS. We have conducted the experiments to observe the change in average response time and total turnaround time and compared it with round-robin algorithm.

We have obtained the following graphical results by conducting the experiments for 500, 2000, 5000, and 20,000 cloudlets (or tasks) using round-robin algorithm and heuristic load balancing algorithm. Figures 1 and 2 shows the variation of average response time and turnaround time in the case of round-robin approach and heuristic approach respectively.

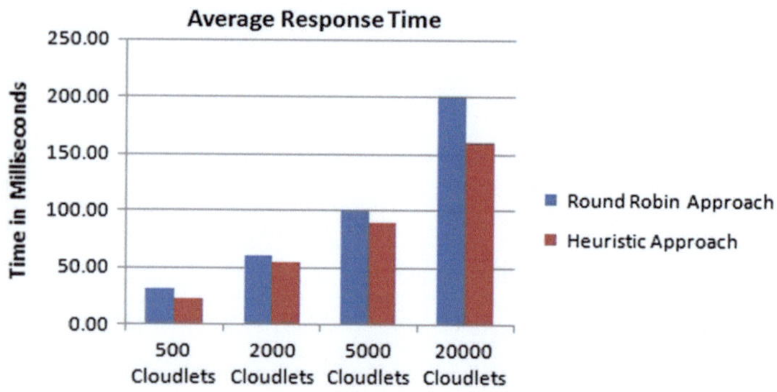

Fig. 1 Shows the variation in average response time in the case of Round-Robin approach and Heuristic approach

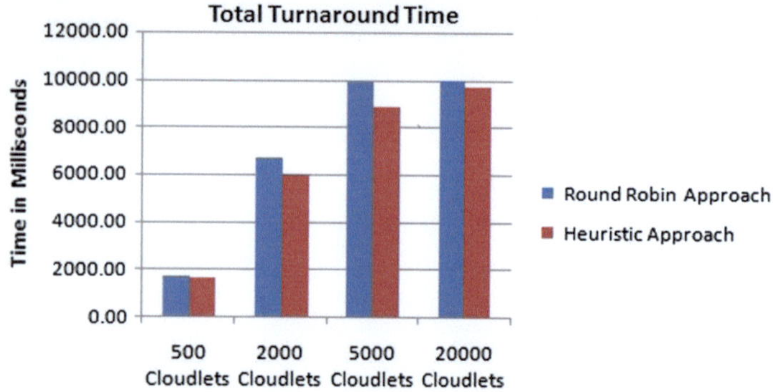

Fig. 2 Shows the variation in average response time in the case of Round-Robin approach and Heuristic approach

5 Research Gap and Proposed Future Work

The heuristic algorithm [6] is based on centralized load balancing strategy. However, the algorithm does not consider the MIPS of the VMs. The actual processing capacities of the VMs in terms of MIPS as well as the utilized power of the VMs would be taken into account in the proposed future work.

The proposed future work would group the tasks as well as the virtual machines into two groups, namely upper class and lower class. The grouping in the tasks would take place on their length as the threshold value and the grouping of the virtual machine would take place in terms their MIPS value as the threshold value. When grouping of the tasks and the virtual machine is done, the tasks of the lower class group are sent to the VMs of the lower class group and vice versa. Then, the task of corresponding group is sent to the virtual machine of corresponding based on their utilization power of the VMs. Thus, proposed work aims to achieve improvement in response time, processing cost of the algorithm, and the total turnaround time.

6 Conclusions

Load balancing is a serious issue in cloud computing. The paper attempts to highlight the issue of load balancing. The paper analyses a heuristic load balancing algorithm and also compares its performance with round-robin algorithm. Finally, this paper highlights the research gap and gives an approach to overcome it.

References

1. Sajid, M., Raza, Z.: Cloud computing: issues & challenges. In: International Conference on Cloud, Big Data and Trust (2013)
2. Mohapatra, S., Rekha, K.S., Mohanty, S.: A comparison of four popular heuristics for load balancing of virtual machines in cloud computing. Int. J. Comput. Appl. **68**(6):33–38 (2013)
3. Elzeki, O.M., Reshad, M.Z., Elsoud, M.A.: Improved max-min algorithm in cloud computing. Int. J. Comput. Appl. **50**(12):22–27 (2012)
4. Ren, X., Lin, R., Zou, H.: A dynamic load balancing strategy for cloud computing platform based on exponential smoothing forecast. In: 2011 IEEE International Conference on Cloud Computing and Intelligence Systems (CCIS), pp. 220–224, 15–17 Sept 2011
5. Calheiros, R.N., et al.: CloudSim: a toolkit for modeling and simulation of cloud computing environments and evaluation of resource provisioning algorithms. Softw. Pract. Experience **41** (1):23–50 (2011)
6. Haidri, R.A., Katti, C.P., Saxena, P.C.: A load balancing strategy for cloud computing environment. In: 2014 International Conference on Signal Propagation and Computer Technology (ICSPCT), pp. 636–641, IEEE (2014)

Package-Based Approach for Load Balancing in Cloud Computing

Amanpreet Chawla and Navtej Singh Ghumman

Abstract Cloud computing is a developing technology in today's Internet world which offers the users with on demand access to resources through different service models. In spite of providing many advantages over the traditional computing, there are some critical issues in cloud computing. Load balancing is a crucial issue in cloud computing that distributes the user's requests to the nodes in such a manner to balance the load on nodes. A proper load balancing algorithm is required to execute the process and manage the resources. The common objective of load balancing algorithm is to achieve the minimum execution time and proper utilization of resources. In this paper, we proposed a new technique to achieve the load balancing called packet-based load balancing algorithm. The motive of this algorithm is to design the concept of load balancing using the grouping of packages and perform the virtual machine replication, if requested package is not available. In this paper, task is achieved with minimum execution time and execution cost which is profitable for the service provider and the user.

Keywords Load balancing · Cloudlets · Task length · Virtual machine (VM)

1 Introduction

Cloud computing is a great revolution in the IT industry and in its development trends. Cloud computing provides heterogeneous services such as application, servers, and storage to different peoples through the Internet. Cloud computing services are used by individuals and businesses to access the application from

A. Chawla (✉) · N.S. Ghumman
Department of Computer Science and Engineering, SBSSTC,
Ferozepur, Punjab, India
e-mail: aman9999preet@gmail.com

N.S. Ghumman
e-mail: navtejghumman@yahoo.com

V.B. Aggarwal et al. (eds.), *Big Data Analytics*, Advances in Intelligent
Systems and Computing 654, https://doi.org/10.1007/978-981-10-6620-7_9

anywhere in the world on demand. Cloud term is used for the cloud service provider that holds the resources for storing and accessing the data [2].

Cloud computing is an Internet-based computing and very successful because of its characteristics like on demand service, pool of resources, ubiquitous network access, measured service, and rapid elasticity. Cloud provides the services such as IaaS, PaaS, SaaS to clients. The IaaS delivers the cloud computing infrastructure storage, server and operating system to users on rent basis for various purposes. In case of platform as a Service (PaaS), it provides the environment for users to develop, test, host, and maintain their applications. In case of software as a service, software is hosted by cloud service provider and made available to clients over the Internet.

Cloud computing is adopted by many industries such as social networking websites and online applications so number of users is increasing to reach cloud. Load balancing is a main requirement for managing the performance of cloud and properly utilizing the resources. Load balancing is an optimization technique that is used to allocate the workload across the different nodes. The load is assigned in an efficient manner to enhance the response time of task and to achieve the efficient resource utilization [2, 3].

In this study, we aim to develop an optimized load balancing algorithm which gives the maximum benefit to the cloud service provider.

2 Literature Survey

Chawla and Bhonsle [7] has developed a technique, which is based on cost-based task scheduling algorithm. The main aim of this algorithm is to map the jobs to resources to achieve the utilization of resources and results of the grouped task is compared with non-grouped task.

Agarwal and Jain [8] presented the generalized priority based algorithm in which it allocates the cloudlets to virtual machine according to processing power. In this paper, the highest length of task gets the highest processing capacity of virtual machine. Authors compare the generalized priority algorithm with existing algorithms like round robin and FCFS algorithm.

Damanal and Reddy [9] have proposed the VM assign load balance algorithm. This algorithm assigns the user requests to VMs according to the status of the VMs.

Shahapure and Jayarekha [10] have proposed the optimal cost scheduling algorithm. In this algorithm, the workload is distributed in a manner to achieve the resource utilization. In this, each virtual machine contains the package and when client request for the package then VM consisting of that package is executed that is beneficial for user and service provider.

Selvarani and Sadhasivam [11] have proposed the improved cost-based scheduling algorithm that efficiently maps the job to resources. In this algorithm, grouping of tasks is based on computational capacity of cloud resources. According to processing power of resource and task length, user task is grouped. This algorithm increases the resource utilization level by sending the group of tasks to resource.

3 Proposed Work

In this paper, we proposed the package-based approach for load balancing. In this proposed algorithm, the workload is divided across all the virtual machines to ensure that no one virtual machine is highly loaded and no one virtual machine is lightly loaded. It is a task scheduling algorithm that optimizes the cost and schedule of the resources.

In the existing algorithm, resources are grouped as package in each VM. Whenever a user requests for the package, the VM consisting of that package is executed. In the existing cost scheduling algorithm, if user required two package, then user have to process two VM's because each VM consist package. This increased the cost of service provider and user [10].

In proposed algorithm, each VM consists of multiple packages and when user requests for two packages then VM consisting of that packages is executed. This algorithm brings down the execution cost of service provider.

Algorithm

Initialize the cost;

s_cost = cost occurred to provider*time taken by client;

Pr = u_cost − s_cost;

$\text{u\_cost} = \sum \text{u\_cost};$

$\text{s\_cost} = \sum \text{s\_cost};$

$$\sum_{k=1,2...k}^{k} \text{Pr} = \sum_{k=1,2..k}^{k} (\text{u\_cost} - \text{s\_cost}),$$

where s_cost is service provider cost, u_cost is user cost, and Pr is profit. The cost occurred to provider is computed by combining the package cost and virtual machine cost and user cost is computed by multiplying the cost fixed by service provider and time taken by the client. The cost fixed by service provider includes the cost occurred to provider and profit.

Steps of our proposed algorithm

1. Create the tasks and VMs. Each virtual machine has multiple packages.
2. Group the VMs that have similar packages and sort the VMs in descending order of processing power.
3. Group the tasks according to VM packages and sort the tasks in descending order of task length.
4. Based on task length, user requests are allocated to VMs according to package. Cloud broker processes these task to virtual machines based on the processing power and package on the virtual machine.
5. If package is not available in VM then cloud broker replicate the VM and dynamically generate a required package.
6. Calculate the cost occurred to service provider and client.

4 Simulation Results

A CloudSim simulator is used to test the algorithm. There are some modules of the CloudSim such as virtual machine, packages, datacenter, host, and cloudlets. Each virtual machine has multiple packages, each package has a fixed price and cloudlets are the tasks.

The user selects the packages and sends the request for the package and if the cloud service provider accepts the request, the user has to pay for the service. The cost to execute service requested by the user at the service provider is reduced by the half. The performance of our algorithm is analyzed by comparing the result of proposed algorithm with existing algorithm. To do this comparison, various experiments are performed with number of tasks 10,000, 20,000, 30,000, 40,000, and 50,000.

Figure 1 shows a log file that is generated when service is given to the user. It gives the details of users and request id and package, etc.

Figure 2 shows the total cost of the cloudlets in existing algorithm and proposed algorithm.

Figure 3 shows the comparison of total waiting time and turnaround time of the existing algorithm and proposed algorithm. It shows that our proposed algorithm decrease the waiting time as compared to existing algorithm.

Figure 4 shows the comparison of total execution time of the cloudlets in existing algorithm and proposed algorithm. We observed that our proposed algorithm gives the better execution time as compare to existing algorithm.

```
Time : 10002.0
Cloudlet id : 28702
Vm Id: 2
Client Cost : 4100820.0
Provider Cost : 2050410.0
Profit : 2050410.0
=========================================================
Time : 10026.0
Cloudlet id : 80714
Vm Id: 0
Client Cost : 4110660.0
Provider Cost : 2055330.0
Profit : 2055330.0
=========================================================
Time : 10000.0
Cloudlet id : 28701
Vm Id: 2
Client Cost : 4100000.0
Provider Cost : 2050000.0
Profit : 2050000.0
=========================================================
```

Fig. 1 Log file

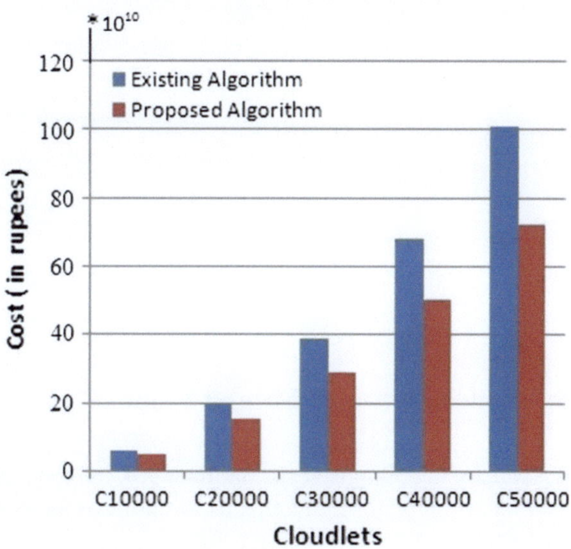

Fig. 2 Comparison of total cost at the provider

Fig. 3 Comparison of total waiting time

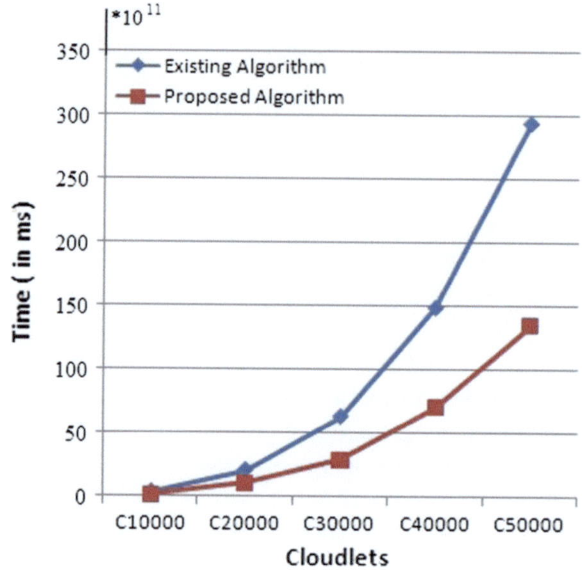

Fig. 4 Comparison of total execution time

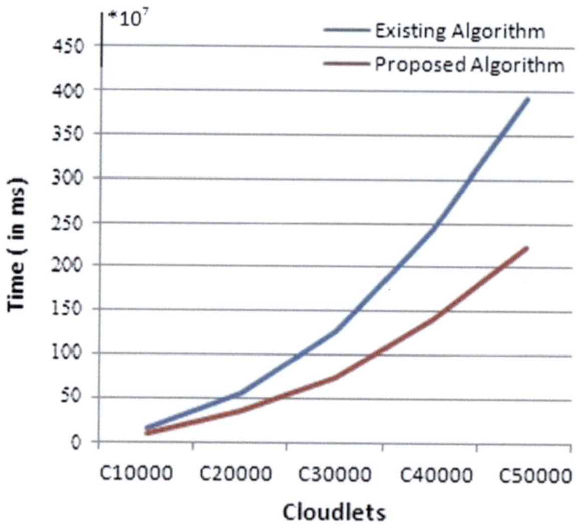

5 Conclusion and Future Scope

Resource scheduling is very important task in cloud computing. The package-based load balancing algorithm helps us to optimize the cost and also helps to minimize the execution time and waiting time.

The proposed algorithm works best when no fault occurs in a VM. In future, an algorithm will be developed which automatically creates the migration of VM. The research work has been tested on a simulator. The results might differ in case of real cloud environment.

References

1. Mell, P., Grance, T.: The NIST Definition of Cloud Computing, vol. 53, p. 50. National Institute of Standards and Technology, USA (2009)
2. Zhang, Q., Cheng, L., Boutaba, R.: Cloud Computing: State of the Art and Research Challenges, pp. 7–18. Springer, Berlin (2010)
3. Priya, S.M., Subramani, B.: A new approach for load balancing in the cloud computing. Int. J. Eng. Comput. Sci. (IJECS) **2**(5):1636–1640 (2013)
4. Khiyaita, A., Zbakh, M., El Bakkali, H., El Kettani, D.: Load balancing cloud computing: state of art. In: 2012 National Days of Network Security and Systems (JNS2), IEEE (2012)
5. Lin, W., Wang, J.Z., Liang, C., Qi, D.: A Threshold Based Dynamic Resource Allocation Scheme for Cloud Computing. Elsevier, The Netherlands (2011)
6. Bagwaiya, V., Raghuwanshi, S.K.: Hybrid approach using the throttled and ESEC load balancing algorithms in cloud computing. In: 2014 International Conference on Green Computing Communication and Electrical Engineering (ICGCCEE), IEEE (2014)
7. Chawla, Y., Bhonsle, M.: Dynamically optimized cost based task scheduling in cloud computing. Int. J. Emerg. Trends Technol. **2**(3):38–42 (2013)
8. Agarwal, A., Jain, S.: Efficient optimal algorithm of task scheduling in cloud computing environment. IJCTT **9**(7):344–349 (2014)
9. Damanal, S.G., Reddy, G.R.M.: Optimal load balancing in cloud computing by efficient utilization of virtual machines. In: 2014 Sixth International Conference on Communication Systems and Networks (COMSNETS), IEEE (2014)
10. Shahapure, N.H., Jayarekha, P.: Load balancing with optimal cost scheduling algorithm. In: 2014 International Conference on Computation of Power and Energy, Information and Communication (ICCPEIC) 2014, IEEE (2014)
11. Selvarani, S., Sadhasivam, G.S.: Improved cost based algorithm for task scheduling in cloud computing. In: 2010 IEEE International Conference on Computational Intelligence and Computing Research (ICCIC), IEEE (2010)
12. Ajit, M., Vidya, G.: VM level load balancing in a cloud environment. In: ICCCNT 2013, IEEE (2013)
13. Ray, S., de Sarkar, A.: Execution analysis of load balancing algorithms in cloud computing environment. Int. J. Cloud Comput. Serv. Archit. (IJCCSA) **2**(5):1–13 (2012)
14. Lamb, D., Randles, M., Taleb-Bendiab, A.: Comparative study into distributed load balancing algorithm for cloud computing. In: Advanced Information Networking and Applications Workshops (WAINA), IEEE (2010)
15. Dillon, T., Wu, C., Chang, E.: Cloud computing: issues and challenges. In: 24th IEEE International Conference on Advanced Information Networking and Applications, IEEE (2010)

Workload Prediction of E-business Websites on Cloud Using Different Methods of ANN

Supreet Kaur Sahi and V.S. Dhaka

Abstract Workload forecasting of cloud-based application depends on the type of application and user behavior. Measurement of workload can be done in terms of loads, data storage, service rate, processing time, etc. In this paper, author has tried to predict workload of e-business website on cloud-based environment. ANN-based approach is used by author to calculate number of cloud instances required to manage workload efficiently. Also different training method of ANN has been applied to perform comparative study. MATLAB neural network toolbox is used for simulation work. An Amazon cloud service is also used for different parameters of data collection.

Keywords Amazon AWS · Simulation · E-Business · IaaS · ANN (Artificial neural network) · MATLAB toolbox · Trainlm · Trainbr · Trainscg

1 Introduction

More and more organizations are using cloud-based environment every year. By 2013, Future of Cloud Computing Survey, out of 855 cloud vendors that includes IT decision makers and business consumers 75% of survey respondents are using the cloud in one way or other [1]. This growth is likely to increase in future. Hybrid computing, big data—cloud computing merger, web-based computing, and security and protections are some of the recent trends of cloud services. The **key features** of cloud computing are as follows [2]:

S.K. Sahi (✉)
Research Scholar, JNU, Jaipur, India
e-mail: Supreet_khurana@yahoo.co.in

V.S. Dhaka
Department of Computer Science and Engineering, JNU, Jaipur, India
e-mail: vijaypal.dhaka@gmail.com

V.B. Aggarwal et al. (eds.), *Big Data Analytics*, Advances in Intelligent Systems and Computing 654, https://doi.org/10.1007/978-981-10-6620-7_10

1. On-demand allocation of resources. The resources are allocated according to requirements and billed accordingly.
2. Scaling. The user is given impression of infinite number of resources.
3. Multitenant environment. Consumers are provided with resources from single cloud implementation resulting in optimization of cost.

Cloud computing workload is application-centric. In this paper, workload estimation of e-business websites is considered which is continuously changing form of workload. Some of the key points that are considered while constructing the model presented in this paper are as follows [2]:

1. Complete understanding of environment in which website is working is very much essential for calculating different metrics involved.
2. On the basis of information like customer behavior, sessions, etc., different workload characteristics are decided.
3. Forecasting the expected workload is critical, as wrong forecasting will lead to customer dissatisfaction. In this paper, proposed model will be able to forecast number of cloud instances required for given workload.
4. Simulation of model is done with help of MATLAB neural network toolbox.
5. Validation of model is essential for calculating errors. Some samples of data will be used for validations and testing.
6. Different graphs and images generated are used to analyze future scenario as well as for comparative study.

In the next session, previous work done in this direction is presented followed by work done by author and conclusion.

2 Background

Almedia [3] has discussed capacity planning steps required for workload forecasting of different websites. Capacity planning is necessary to avoid limitations of inefficient capacity prediction and to meet users' expectations so that cost benefit ratio can be optimized. Scalability and Accessibility plays an essential role for any website hit as discussed by Almeida and Menasce [4]. Author has used case study about an online bookstore to show uncertain customer behavior. In Menasce and Almeida [5] guided about workload management of different e-commerce servers by taking into account different customer activities scenarios. Multilayered architecture of e-business applications is also presented in this paper and it is suggested that workload should be done at each step. The aim of this paper is to provide basic idea of building e-business model on the cloud. The method of reservation by an IaaS provider for long-term contacts in order to optimize profit is presented by Raquel et al. [6]. This paper also gives mathematical model to optimize profit on cloud-based website. Different workload characteristics on which cloud-based applications depend are presented by Fehling [7]. The author in this paper has discussed different types of workload like "static", "once in a lifetime", periodic, etc., with respect to different cloud platforms.

3 Method

Some of the limitations of previous published paper by author are as follows [8]:

- Training sample is less
- Different training methods of ANN are not used to compare the results.

Data collection is done through paper by Raquel et al. [6] and Amazon website [9]. MATLAB neural network toolbox is used for simulation purpose. Performance function used is mean squared error by MATLAB. Neural network used for prediction have 11 input variable and one output variable. Hidden layer of network consist of 10 neurons. Applying different combinations on following input data generates data samples. Total 250 samples of input are used. Out of which 70% are used for training and 15% for validation and testing respectively. The inputs given to model are as follows:

1. Number of instances available
2. Service rate
3. Normal arrival rate
4. Arrival rate during high demands
5. Arrival rate during low demands
6. Service time under low load
7. Service time under high load
8. Service time under normal load
9. Utility gain
10. Threshold
11. Penalty for unsuccessful request.

Output shows how many cloud instances need to be reserved. Figure 1 is generated by MATLAB show internal architecture of neural network used.

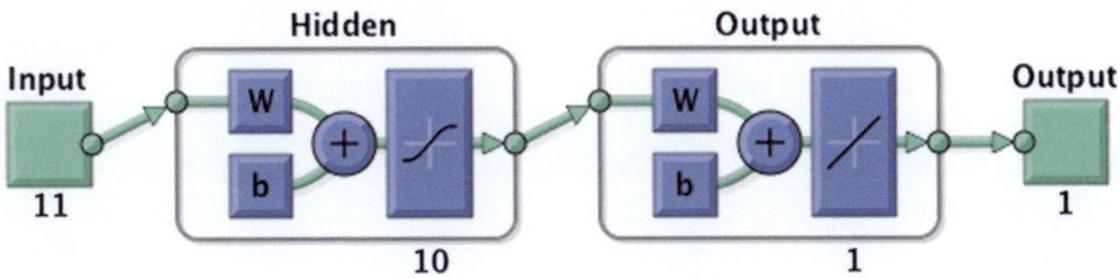

Fig. 1 Structure of neural network

There are different training methods available in MATLAB neural network toolbox. "Trainlm" is typically fastest method, whereas "trainbr" takes more time but may be better option for challenging problems. "Trainscg" utilizes less memory. Some data samples out of 250 as well as result produced with "trainlm" method are presented in Table 1. Author in later sections also presents results by different training methods of MATLAB neural network toolbox.

3.1 Results

Following figures show different results obtained by different training methods.

3.1.1 Results of "trainlm" Method

See Figs. 2 and 3.

3.1.2 Result of "trainbr" Method

See Figs. 4 and 5.

3.1.3 Result of "trainscg" Method

See Figs. 6 and 7.

3.2 Interpretation from Results

Best performance by trainlm is at 8, trainbr required 680 epochs for best performance and trainscg required 48 epochs (Figs. 2, 4 and 6). Best performance of trainlm is 45,819.7162, trainbr is 5469.0499, and trainscg is 43,276.3529. Regression coefficient for trainlm is 0.88579, trainbr = 0.95635, and trainscg is 0.87688 (Figs. 3, 5 and 7). In case of "trainlm", both validation curve and test curve are very much alike. When the test curve had increased significantly before the completion of validation curve, it is the case of over fitting. In case of "trainbr" and "trainscg", some over fitting seems to be done. Also "trainlm" is faster method as compared to others. So in this case "trainlm" is working more efficiently as shown in data presented above.

Table 1 Trainlm results

Max no of instances required	Normal arrival rate	High arrival rate	Low arrival rate	Normal load	Low load	High load	Utility gain	Threshold	Penalty	Service time	Targets	Outcomes
20	220	80	500	5256	1314	2190	0.85	0.9995	15,000	0.2	34	32.5612
20	220	80	500	5256	1314	2190	0.85	0.9995	15,000	0.1	28	30.9985
20.5	220.5	80.5	500.5	5256.5	1314.5	2190.5	0.86	0.9996	15,001	0.5	659	657.5
20	220	80	500	5256	1314	2190	0.85	0.9995	15,000	0.8	258	255
19.5	219.5	79.5	499.5	5255.55	1313.5	2189.5	0.84	0.9994	14,999	1.2	912	910.7265
19.5	219.5	79.5	499.5	5255.55	1313.5	2189.5	0.84	0.9994	14,999	1.3	916	911.5897
19.5	219.5	79.5	499.5	5255.55	1313.5	2189.5	0.84	0.9994	14,999	1.4	915	911.1056
19	221	80.45	499	5256	1315	2190	0.85	0.9996	15,001.25	1.24	906	903.0901
19.1	221.7	80.45	499	5251	1315	2190.1	0.851	0.9996	15,001.25	2.1	209	201.706

Fig. 2 Performance

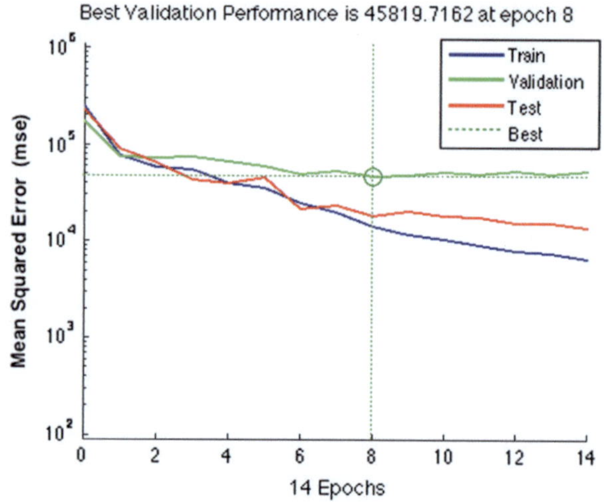

Fig. 3 Regression

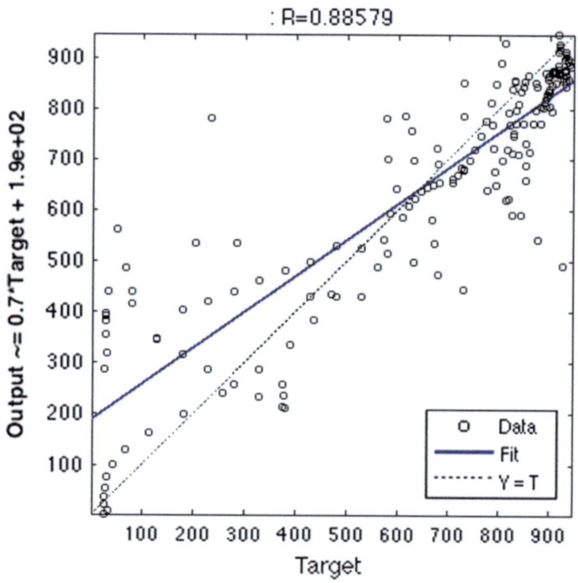

4 Conclusion and Future Work

In this paper, author has increased data samples, so more accurate results are produced. Table 1 shows that expected output and actual output are almost same with minimum error, which can be reduced in future by different error minimization techniques. Also "trainlm" method is working efficiently in this case. Workload prediction on cloud is application specific. In this paper, author has presented

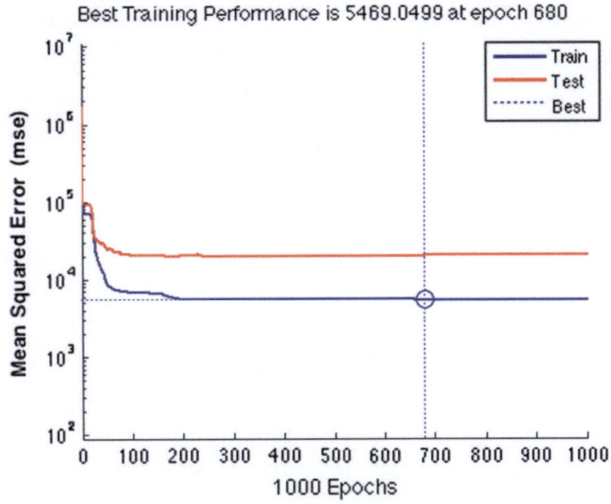

Fig. 4 Performance

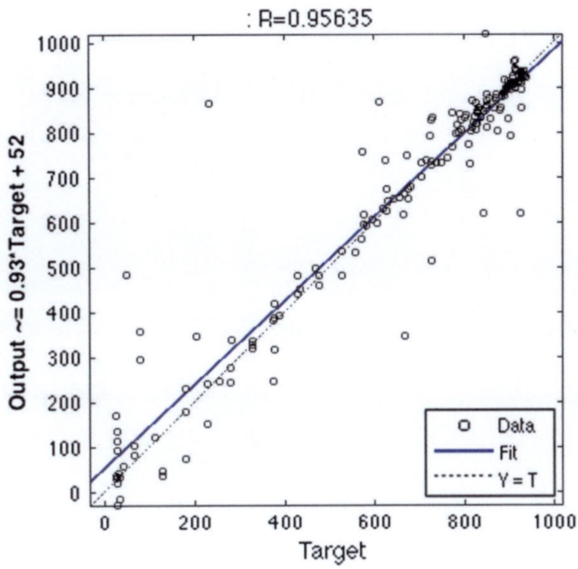

Fig. 5 Regression analysis

workload prediction with respect to e-business websites on cloud. In future, more such kind of work can be done on different applications like finance, security, banking etc., on cloud-based systems.

Fig. 6 Performance

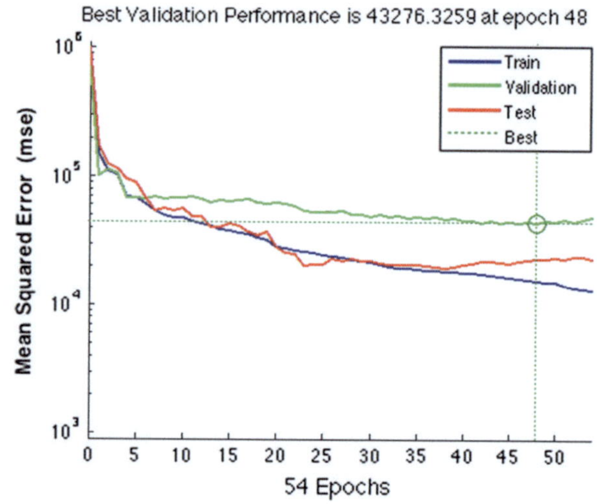

Fig. 7 Regression analysis

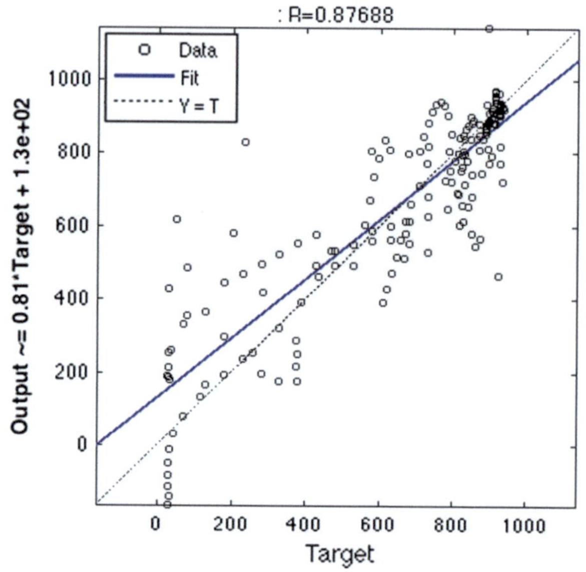

References

1. Cloud computing trends and latest stats. 3 April 2014, SmartDataCollective by Mike Solomonov
2. Cisco cloud computing—Data center strategy, architecture, and solutions. Cisco Systems. (2009)
3. Almeida, V.: Capacity planning for web services. In Performance evaluation of complex systems: techniques and tools, performance, Tutorial lectures, pp. 142–157. London, UK: Springer (2002)

4. Almeida, V.A.F., Menasce, D.A.: Capacity planning: an essential tool for managing web services. IT Prof. **4**(4), 33–38 (2002). doi:10.1109/MITP.2002.1046642
5. Menascé, D.A., Almeida, V.A.F.: Challenges in scaling e-business sites. In: Proceedings of computer measurement group conference, (2000)
6. Lopes, R., Brasileiro, F., Maciel Jr., P.D.: Business-driven capacity planning of a cloud-based IT infrastructure for the execution of web applications. IEEE (2010)
7. Fehling, C., et al.: Cloud computing fundamentals. Cloud computing patterns, 21 doi: 10.1007/978-3-7091-1568-8_2. Springer, Wien (2014)
8. Sahi, S.K., Dhaka, V.S.: Study on predicting for workload of cloud services using artificial neural network. In: Computing for sustainable global development (INDIACom), 2nd International conference IEEE, pp. 331–335 (2015)
9. Amazon Elastic Compute Cloud (EC2). [Online]. Available: http://aws.amazon.com/ec2/
10. Gartner says cloud computing will be as influential as e-business. Gartner. Retrieved 22 Aug 2010

Websites

11. http://in.mathworks.com/products/neural-network/

Data Security in Cloud-Based Analytics

Charru Hasti and Ashema Hasti

Abstract Cloud computing platforms have grown in prominence in last few years, as they have made business applications and information accessible on the move without the need to purchase, set up, and maintain necessary hardware and software. The organizations are churning enormous gains due to scalability, agility, and efficiency achieved through the use of clouds. Data analytics involves voluminous data crunching to determine trends and patterns for business intelligence, scientific studies, and data mining. The incessant outburst of data from multiple sources such as web applications, social media, and other Internet-based sources motivate leveraging cloud technology for data analytics. Different strategies are being studied and incorporated to use the subscription-based cloud for serving analytics systems. The paper focusses on understanding the security threats associated with cloud-based analytics and approaches to cloud security assurance in data analytics systems.

Keywords Analytics as a Service (AaaS) · Multi-tenancy · Cryptography · VMWare · Trusted third-party auditor

1 Introduction

Cloud computing service technology inherently involves pooling and sharing of resources thus helping cut the costs of enterprises in the investment and maintenance of the technology and infrastructure. The delivery models encompass infrastructure as a service, software as a service, application cloud as a service, business process as a service, and now analytics as a service as well. Analytics is one of the areas getting enthused by cloud benefits today.

C. Hasti (✉)
Delhi Institute of Advanced Studies, Delhi, India
e-mail: charru.h1@gmail.com

A. Hasti
Mewar University, Rajasthan, India
e-mail: ashema.hasti@gmail.com

V.B. Aggarwal et al. (eds.), *Big Data Analytics*, Advances in Intelligent Systems and Computing 654, https://doi.org/10.1007/978-981-10-6620-7_11

Multiples of cloud vendors such as AWS and Cloud1010 offer services for a distributed data infrastructure and in-memory accelerating technologies for data access for the data analytics projects. Cloud vendors focus on one or more of the aspects viz. data models, processing applications, data storage, and computing power, to enable demand-based analytics. In-house business intelligence (BI) applications are capable of providing fast solutions to the users yet they require a lot of attention in terms of installation, execution, and maintenance. A cloud-based BI, on the other hand, is useful to the firms which otherwise cannot afford fully owned applications to analyze their data. Moreover, firms can extend the scale of data usage at much less cost. Remote provisioning of the warehousing facilities and sharing of resources through virtualization in areas such as social media analytics further enables focus on monetizing data via data exploration and gaining useful insights without concerning about maintaining and organizing exabytes of data.

2 Cloud Implementation Approaches in Data Analytics

Cloud framework involves three tiers: infrastructure, software, and platform. Infrastructure as a Service (IaaS) lets the companies such as Amazon and Google let the OS, storage, apps, and selected network components managed by the users. This has led to a cut down on server costs that the firms initially invested in a lot. Moreover, the exponential growth in the data has swamped the firms and made them think about diverting focus away from infrastructure through subscription-based IaaS. On the other hand, when an organization simply needs to get instantaneous and synchronized data and figures such as hits on an application, they simply employ a dashboard provided by a cloud vendor through Software as a Service (SaaS). The data dealt with can range from enterprise resource planning systems to inventory systems to customer relationship management systems. For instance, customer actions are captured as potential data to understand and analyze the behaviors and patterns in customers. This looks a bit scary in terms of customer privacy though is quite useful as well in order to make it customer friendly. Another opportunity that comes with cloud SaaS is that multiple users accumulating the data can benefit from each other by aggregating results from multiple sources. Platform as a Service (PaaS) cloud involves plugging in the BI or analytic capabilities into the applications for the customers. Independent software vendors such as Salesforce.com develop improved analytical applications as a software service or analytical engines as a platform service. These are then deployed by the client organizations to get an edge over others in the analytics market. These sources may provide structured forms of data or unstructured forms of data. The functional requirements of drawing useful trends and patterns through these data drive firms toward taking services from cloud vendors who focus on making data farms and warehouses for different needs. Therefore, the firm can build its own data center in the private cloud and follow the best practices of a public cloud environment or

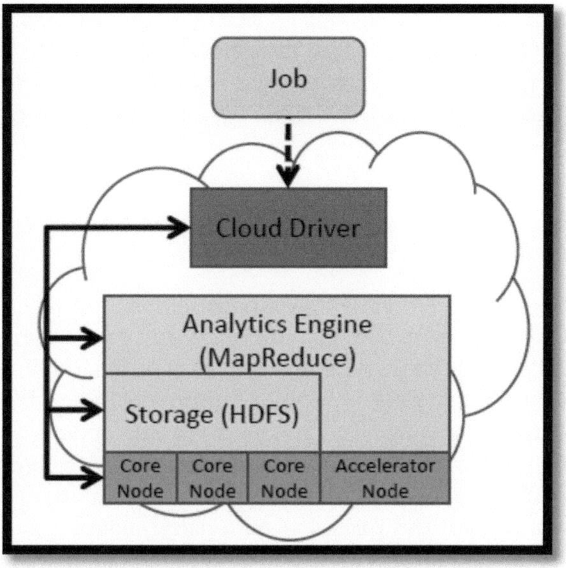

Fig. 1 Data analytic cloud architecture [12]

acquire a private cloud service from a cloud vendor. A cloud analytics service can also encompass organizations facilitating the consumption of analytic applications that have already been created [1] (Fig. 1).

3 Security Issues in Cloud Analytics

Several security risks and vulnerabilities have to be addressed by both the parties: providers as well as subscribers. In general, all information technology assets need to be safeguarded against the privacy threats irrespective of the service delivery model employed. Some of the common security risks that have been identified by researchers are listed below that encompass any cloud application [2, 3].

1. User access control and authentication
2. Data confidentiality conservation during data movement between clouds
3. Business continuity, recovery, and disaster management
4. Data location control
5. Data segregation by encryption
6. Controlled resource allocation
7. Investigative support for any illegal activity
8. Long-term viability of data
9. Virtual machine monitoring and security
10. Regulatory compliance.

These issues encompass but may not only include concerns of cloud service users such as ambiguity in responsibility, loss of governance and trust, switching service provider, data leakage, and concerns of CSPs such as protection inconsistency, un-administered APIs, license risks and so on [4].

4 Current Strategies for Cloud Security Assurance

Several solutions have been under research in lieu of standardizing cloud security assurance protecting against one or a class of security threats. Many CSPs, as well as research organizations, have been working toward achieving the trust of cloud users. Major work is focused toward identifying techniques to ensure data is protected from unwanted access by using appropriately designed encryption and decryption techniques. The areas such as secured browsers, proofs of the location of data, authentication of sensitive information are rigorously studied by researchers worldwide. The role of a third-party auditor has also been found over various studies as essential to maintain dynamic auditing control as well as compliance.

Boyd [5] has explained the role of cryptography in securing data. The techniques reviewed are searchable encryption, homomorphic encryption, proofs of storage, and proofs of location. These methods enable data encryption, integrity, location check. The traditional cryptography algorithms may not be useful to cloud users since the data is entrusted upon, stored, and processed at a distant location. Various cryptographic measures have been reviewed by Boyd to provide data assurance to users without entrusting the cloud provider. Certain improved storage schemes have been researched, for instance in the works of Shacham and Waters [6]. Proofs of location are discussed by Boyd further for achieving assurance of location to the users that compute the total time taken by data to reach the user from the requested site. Cloud Geolocation protocols were also exemplified that determine file locations on clouds using distance bounding protocols, based on the fact that an economically rational provider does not want to incur an additional cost of saving additional copies of the same file in multiple places. Distance Bounding Protocols estimate data transmission delays on the Internet. Proofs of Redundancy have also been shown as significant. These techniques are also based on timing methods and estimate delay in retrieving data. The research has suggested a geographic separation of multiple copies in order to provide assurance of more robust backup. Methods to process encrypted data that have been considered include searchable encryption (enabling server to identify requested file among all stored data without knowing contents of the file), homomorphic encryption (using such an encryption scheme that allows computations to be performed on data without the need of decrypting it), and homomorphic authentication (authenticating the output of computations on encrypted data).

Sharma and Gupta [2] have discussed the need of designing an architecture-independent policy that works well with all delivery models and cater to the underlying requirements of an organization or business purpose. They explained certain security framework policies that ensure the cross-domain accesses. These included Security Assertion Markup Language (SAML) developed by OASIS, designed to solve Single Sign-on problem; eXtensible Access Control Markup Language (XACML), part of XML, used to set up rules according to the policies in order to check the authorization requests; OpenID decentralized authentication protocol used for authenticating a user to access many web applications through a single username and password; and WS-Security, WS-Trust, WS-Secure Conversation, WS-Federation, WS-Security Policy, Privacy and Identity Management for Europe (PRIME) that maintains and protects user information through a single console. Besides these policies in place, it was shown that a trusted third-party security analyst (T2PA) is required to confirm data consistency and integrity during inter-cloud data movement. This mechanism was concluded to be easy to implement by the data owner and reduced computational cost for the customer who cannot afford high-end security mechanism in place. Additionally, the traditional encryption and decryption algorithms were proposed to be deployable such as XML file signature in each file and AES (Advanced Encryption Standard) keys. AES algorithm has been found to be the most efficient in terms of speed, time, and throughput for cloud services. The trusted third-party analyst is used to resolve any kind of inconsistency between cloud service provider and client.

Syam Kumar and Subramanian [7] had proposed a protocol for dynamic data verification and remote data integrity checking in which a consumer generates some metadata which can be used later by the user to challenge the server for integrity of certain file blocks through challenge–response protocol.

Sasireka and Raja [8] explained an efficient approach to prevent data mining attacks and hence ensure data security. The suggested approach involves three steps: classification of data as sensitive, fragmentation of data into chunks, and distribution of data to different CSPs depending upon the reliability of cloud provider and data sensitivity.

Numerous authentications, as well as encryption policies, are undergoing study that needs an improvement to balance different risks associated with multiple delivery models. The CloudTrust Protocol (CTP) specified by Cloud Security Alliance [9] is a step in the direction of formalizing the assurance policies. It entrusts the responsibility of data security onto the CSPs and it is meant to create transparency between the providers and users to gain digital trust on the cloud.

5 Mapping Security Techniques to Cloud Analytics

There is a trade-off between on-premise analytics software or self-maintained warehouses versus cloud empowered analytics. It is concerned about privacy and latency versus total cost of ownership, ease of use versus less functionality, and private cloud within versus user's firewall versus highly scalable pool of cloud data centers. The efficacy of cloud-based analytics increases if the security concerns are addressed well. Many techniques and strategies have been recently proposed by researchers in enhancing security in cloud analytics.

In the initial efforts, data have been stored in a layered set of servers which classified data depending upon their security restrictions and functions or categorization such as structured or unstructured. Therefore, mechanisms were put in place to secure the data stored in these silos. However, the inherent characteristic of data analytics on cloud is an efficient aggregation of data and results from across multiple sources for carrying out analysis. So the traditional approaches are not able to work well with cloud analytics since these segregated locations with varying access controls make it infeasible to access and collect data together at once. A workaround is to allow access between these layers for data sharing but this too becomes difficult as well as expensive to manage when scale of databases increases. Access management also becomes a challenge since source of data reads and updates is unrecorded most of the times.

The privacy-preserving analysis technique, proposed by Naganuma et al. [10], can be used to analyze data in encrypted form to provide data security when performing big data analysis on third-party cloud servers. The core of the proposed method is a searchable encryption technique that permits searching of data in encrypted form and can be used for statistical or correlation rule analysis of encrypted data. Because this privacy-preserving analysis technique only requires encrypted data and encrypted queries, it reduces the risk in the event of unauthorized access or a data leak (Fig. 2).

Conceived by Booz Allen Hamilton and the US government, the Cloud Analytics Reference Architecture [11] tags the data with security metadata once it enters the data lake repository. This framework aims at securely storing, analyzing, and maintaining data on the cloud. Firms can perform tagging using off-the-shelf tools in order to attach metadata to data on the cloud. Still, there can be challenges related to legal and political policies of sharing and aggregating data. Such issues need to be handled by the parties involved along with the decision makers corroborating with them. Hence, all firms subscribing to cloud analytics can establish their practices and then use the security metadata tagged to each of the data as per their mutually agreed rules for managing security in terms of compliance, authentication, and configuration (Fig. 3).

The cloud service vendors are constantly finding ways to keep their customer's trust and ensuring no information leaks by adopting standard cloud security techniques. Still, a lot of effort is required to make analytics as a foolproof service addressing all the security risks.

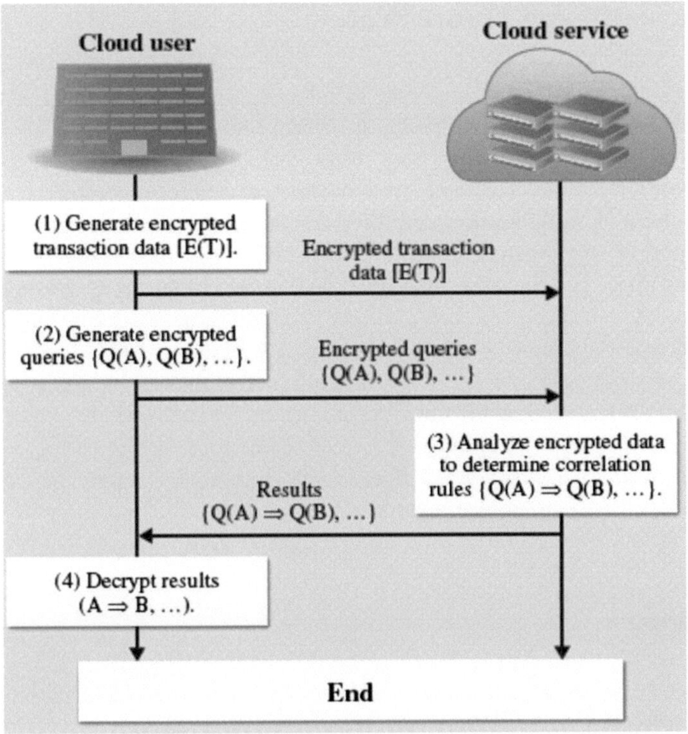

Fig. 2 Flowchart for correlation rule analysis of encrypted transaction data [10]

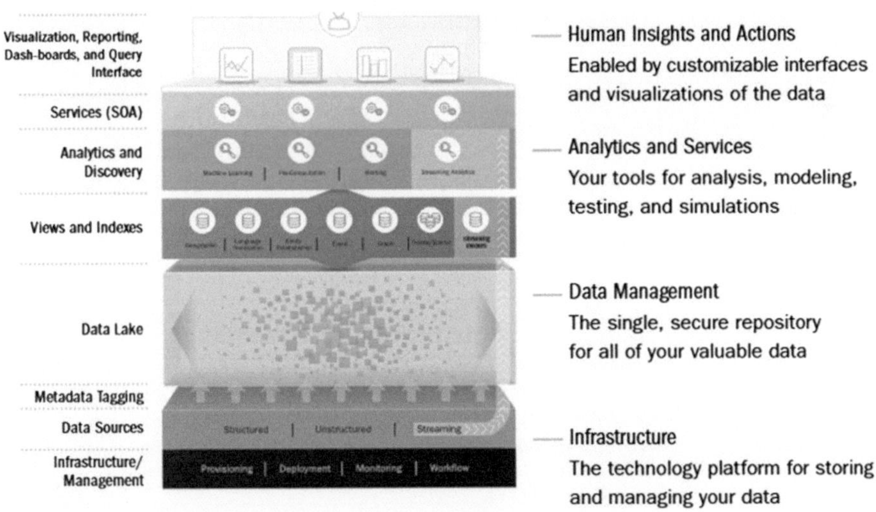

Fig. 3 Primary elements of the cloud analytics reference architecture [11]

6 Conclusion and Future Scope

Unification of analytics services and cloud computing has become a significant game changer. It is not only reshaping how firms deal with data number crunching, but also has started influencing how users make use of information technology. With numerous technical as well as monetary advantages associated with cloud analytics, there is an unquestionable need for meeting all security concerns due to relinquishing of data control as well as cross sharing of data lakes.

Efficient risk management systems need to be in place to ensure constant monitoring of data accesses and controls. The privacy-preserving analysis technique [10] and the Cloud Analytics Reference Architecture [11] are a few of the efforts in this direction. Yet there are multiple constraints to be addressed such as transparency, shifting away from more secure and expensive owned legacy systems. Any firm wanting to employ or provide cloud analytics must first analyze the benefits as well as security level that can be provided through the adoption of cloud-based security assurance techniques.

References

1. Schlegel, K., Sallam, R.L., Yuen, D., Tapadinhas, J.: Magic quadrant for business intelligence and analytics platforms. Gartner, 5 Feb 2013, G00239854
2. Sharma, P.D., Gupta, H.: An implementation for conserving privacy based on encryption process to secured cloud computing environment. Int. J. Eng. Sci. Res. Technol. (2014)
3. Hashizume, et al.: An analysis of security issues for cloud computing. J. Internet Serv. Appl. **4**, 5 (2013)
4. Jain, R., Singh, R.: A survey on current cloud computing trends and related security issues. Int. J. Res. Appl. Sci. Eng. Technol. **2**(I) 2014
5. Boyd, C.: Cryptography in the cloud: advances and challenges. J. Inf. Commun. Converg. Eng. (2013)
6. Shacham, H., Waters, B.: Compact proofs of retrievability. Advances in cryptology—ASIACRYPT 2008. Lecture notes in computer science, vol. 5350, (2008)
7. Syam Kumar, P., Subramanian, R.: An efficient and secure protocol for ensuring data storage security in cloud computing. Int. J. Comput. Sci. Issues **8**(6) (2011)
8. Sasireka, K., Raja, K.: An approach to improve cloud data privacy by preventing from data mining attacks. Int. J. Sci. Res. Publ. **4**(2) 2014
9. Cloud Security Alliance: https://cloudsecurityalliance.org/research/ctp/
10. Naganuma, K., Yoshino, M., Sato, H., Sato, Y.: Privacy-preserving analysis technique for secure, cloud-based big data analytics
11. http://www.boozallen.com/media/file/Enabling_Cloud_Analytics_with_Data-Level_Security.pdf
12. Leey, G., Chunz, B.-G., Katzy, R.H.: Heterogeneity-aware resource allocation and scheduling in the cloud. In: Proceedings of HotCloud, pp. 1–5 (2011)

Ontology-Based Ranking in Search Engine

Rahul Bansal, Jyoti and Komal Kumar Bhatia

Abstract Today's web is human readable where information cannot be easily processed by machines. The current existing Keyword-Based Search Engines provides an efficient way to browse the web content. But they do not consider the context of the user query or the web page and return a large result set, out of which very few are relevant to the user. Therefore, users are often confronted with the daunting task of shifting through multiple pages, to find the exact match. In addition, the Ranking factors employed by these search engines do not take into account the context or the domain of the web page. In this paper, to rank a context sensitive web page, a ranking factor is developed which uses the underlying ontology of the particular domain in which it lies. The value of this factor is computed by calculating the number of data properties present in the web page.

Keywords Ontology · Search engine · Ranking · Data properties

1 Introduction

Ranking is the process by which a search engine shows most relevant pages at the top. Ranking plays a major role in the success of a search engine because every user wants information urgently and it is possible only when the relevant results exist on the first page of the search engine. The Keyword-Based Search Engines employ ranking factors such as PageRank, Domain Age, No. of keywords matched, keywords present in the URLs, etc., but they do not consider the context of the user

R. Bansal (✉) · Jyoti · K.K. Bhatia
Department of Computer Engineering, YMCA University of Science & Technology, Faridabad, India
e-mail: rahul.bansal3927@gmail.com

Jyoti
e-mail: justjyoti.verma@gmail.com

K.K. Bhatia
e-mail: komal_bhatia1@rediffmail.com

V.B. Aggarwal et al. (eds.), *Big Data Analytics*, Advances in Intelligent Systems and Computing 654, https://doi.org/10.1007/978-981-10-6620-7_12

query or domain of the web page in which the web page lies. Suppose if the query is ambiguous (having different senses in a different context) it generally returns a large result set, out of which very few are relevant to the user. Therefore, users have to go through multiple pages to find the exact match.

Approximately 75% [1] of the user never goes beyond the 1st page of the Google. In addition, out of these, 35% clicks on the first 3 links only [2]. Surveys also indicate that almost 25% of the web searchers are unable to find useful results in the first set of URLs that are returned [3]. So, if a user does not find "The most relevant links" on the 1st page, it will hamper the reputation of the Search engine.

This paper deals with ranking of context sensitive documents according to their relevancy by using Ontology [5–8]. After employing the proposed technique, the user receives only those pages that exactly match with his context and in the order of his preference when he searches for ambiguous queries like apple, jaguar, etc., which have different meaning in different contexts (like jaguar can be classified under animal and as well as vehicle class).

2 Literature Review

Ontology-Based Search Engine [9, 10] is a kind of search engine that prompt the user to select a proper class for the query if the query is found to be an ambiguous one. And then returns a set of documents that belongs to a specific class. So in this way the size of the result set is quite small as compared general search results. Main construct of this search engine are as follows.

2.1 Ontology

Ontology has been described as a "formal, explicit specification of a shared conceptualization". They are used to capture or represent knowledge about a particular domain. Ontology describes the concepts in the domain and also the relationships that hold/exists between those concepts (or classes). Different Ontology languages provide different facilities. The most recent development in standard Ontology languages is OWL [11] from the World Wide Web Consortium (W3C). Various tools Like Protégé [12] are freely available to construct an Ontology. Every Ontology consists of some classes, individuals, data properties, object properties and some restrictions. It allows large amount of data to be related in a logical fashion. Various Ontologies on wide ranges of domain is freely available for use. For this paper brief Ontologies on Fruit, Manufacture, Animals and Operating System domains have been created by using Protégé 4.3 [12] and successfully utilized for ranking. A sample Ontology on Animal domain has been shown in Fig. 1.

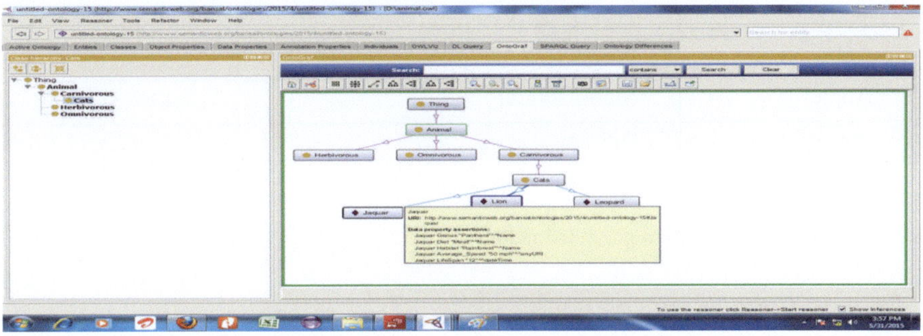

Fig. 1 A sample ontology on animal domain using Protégé 4.3

The Ontologies developed using Protégé can also be reused and combined with existing Ontologies. The main components of the above Ontology are Classes, Properties and Individuals that are described below.

Classes

Classes are sets that contain individuals. For, e.g., Animal class would contain all individuals that are animals like jaguar, dog, cat, etc. A class may have sub classes as well.

Properties

Object Properties: Object Properties are binary relations on individuals. They link two individuals together. For example, the Object property like "hasSibling" links the individual Matthew to the individual Gemma.

Data Properties: Data properties link an Individual/Object to some literal values. For example, CEO is a Data property that links the company Apple Incorporation to the name "Tim Cook". As shown in Fig. 1 various Data properties related to Animal class are Habitat, Genus, Average Speed, Lifespan, etc. The literal value for the property "Habitat" corresponding to the individual Jaguar is Rainforest.

Individuals

Individuals represent objects in the domain/class. Like jaguar can be an individual in Animal class.

2.2 *Ontological Grounded Index*

Ontology grounded index is an extension to earlier existing index structure named 'Inverted Index'. This new structure is added with the concept of **Ontological class** and a relative modification in the existing arrangement of its contents as shown in Fig. 2.

Term	Ontological Classes	Posting
Apple	Fruit	1,5,6,7,109
Apple	Manufacturer	3,4,67,872,33
Jaguar	Animal	2, 56,822,33,35
jaguar	Vehicle	45,4,56,77,324

Fig. 2 A sample ontological grounded index

Here Ontological Grounded Index is used in place of inverted index to extract context/class of the user query and the related document ids. If a user types query, the system will look for the context of the query. For, e.g., if a user types apple in his or her query what happens in simple inverted index-based system is the first system will look for the apple in the index and finds its corresponding documents. Here the result set will be quiet large as it will contain pages from fruit and as well as manufacture domains. But Ontology-Based Search Engine will first check in the ontology the possible classes of the term apple and ask user to select a proper class for apple. Here the result set will be quite small.

3 Related Work

Gurdeep et al. [13] proposed an approach to rank web pages according to the underlying ontology. They first created an ontological Sub-Graph for the query and every page that exist in a particular domain. After that, they calculated the relational probability of query Sub-Graph w.r.t. to ontology and similarly the relational probability of web page Sub-graph w.r.t. ontology. Finally, they calculated Joint Probability of query and web page w.r.t. ontology and rank the pages in decreasing order of the similarity.

Kim et al. [14] proposed an approach to improve the rank of documents if they contain query words in the same sentence by using ontology.

Haveliwala [15] proposed a Topic-Sensitive PageRank, in which each page is supposed to be consist of many topics/category and a specific weight for each topic is given to a document. At the query, time it finds the best topic for the query and rank document by just considering the weight of the best topic of the query. Its complexity is quite high as it first calculates the topic wise weight of each document by examining all the content of the page. On the other hand, proposed approach in this paper is very simple and cheap to calculate the rank of a web page by using ontology.

4 Proposed Work

Most of the documents of WWW deal with a single Context. For example, most probably a document about "apple" contains information either about apple as a fruit, or apple as a brand (Apple Incorporation). Means the theme of a document is always about a single context. So in the proposed architecture, domain Ontology is utilized to find the exact context of the user query and it has been supplied to the ranking module as an input to rank the document.

4.1 Proposed Architecture of the Ranking System

The architecture of the ranking system is shown in Fig. 3.

The following are the inputs to this ranking module:

User Query: For the ranking purpose, this query must be passed to the ranking module. So here, Query Interface will pass the query to the ranking module.

Unsorted Documents: It is the set of documents that comes as the result of a user query before ranking.

Class: Query classifier will supply the exact class of the "user query" to the ranking module.

Ontology Store: It is the ontology about a particular domain. It is a file which has the extension.owl. This ontology can be constructed using various tools like Protégé, etc.

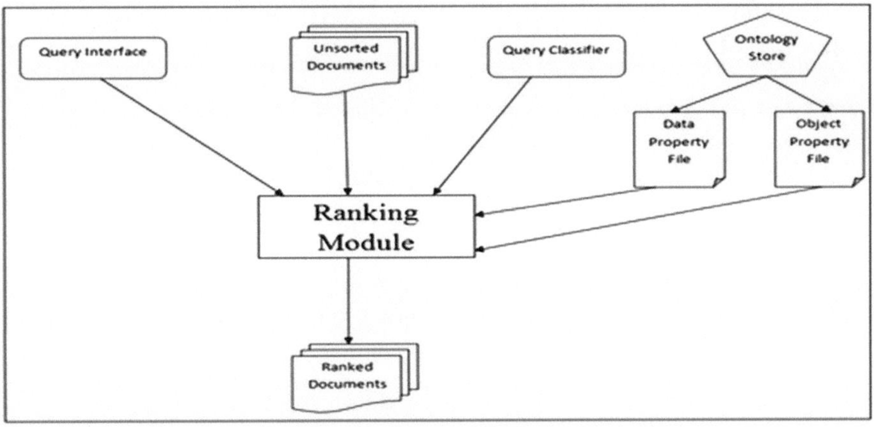

Fig. 3 Simplified diagram illustrating the proposed ranking system

Data Property File: This file is the outcome of the ontology store. It contains two columns one for the "Class name" and other for the List of data properties present in the corresponding class as shown in Table 1.

Object Property File: It is also the outcome of the ontology store. It contains 5 columns as shown in Table 2.

Output of the Ranking Module

Sorted Documents: These are the outcome of the ranking technique. They are sorted in decreasing order of their relevancy.

4.2 Working of the Proposed System

User Interface will provide the user query and the Query Classifier after evaluating the exact context of the query, either by using ONTOLOGICAL GROUNDED INDEX or by using user profile, browser's history, etc., gives the class name to the ranking module. To calculate the rank of the all the unsorted pages that are passed to ranking module data properties of the supplied class is extracted from the Data property File. Suppose if the class is found to be Animal then all the data properties like habitat, breed, etc., will be used in calculating the exact weight of the document. The data properties may be partially or fully present in the web pages so java string functions like equals(), contains() are used. For example, breed is the data property, and document contains a token like breeding then contains() function returns true in this case because both have the same meaning and should be considered as the same.

The query fired by the user can be a single word or multi-word, the below-mentioned technique is used to calculate weight of each document.

Table 1 Contents of the data property file extracted from the ontology store

Class name	Data properties
Fruit	Taste, color, weight, origin, smell
Manufacturer	Revenue, CEO, headquarters, city
Animal	Breed, eyes, speed, legs, tail, habitat
Vehicle	Mileage, speed, weight
Fruit	Taste, color, weight, origin, smell, etc.

Table 2 Contents of the object property file extracted from the ontology

Term 1	Class of term 1	Term 2	Class of term 2	Object property
Apple	Manufacturer	IOS	Operating Sys	"Uses"
ITunes	Apps	IOS	Operating Sys	"UsedIn"

For single word query

Suppose if the user query consist of a single word like "apple" and the class supplied by the Query Classifier is Fruit. The data properties belonging to Fruit class are origin, taste, color, size, etc. The Ranking Module will parse the unsorted documents one by one and calculate the weight of each document by using the formula as given below.

$$\mathrm{Weight}(d) = \sum_{t=1}^{n} (\mathrm{Score(t)}) \tag{1}$$

Here d is the document number; n is the number of data properties present in the supplied class and t is used to denote a data property-term. For example, t can be color, taste, size, cost, etc., when Fruit class is considered. Score(t) means a score of the data property-term in a web page and it can be calculated as.

$$\mathrm{Score(t)} = \begin{matrix} \{1 + \log(\mathrm{tf}), & \text{if tf} > 0 \\ 0, & \text{otherwise}\} \end{matrix} \tag{2}$$

Here a positive weight of 1 is assigned for each data property of the class. A number of times a property present in a web page that is term frequency(tf), also add some positive weight. If tf of any property is zero then its Score(t) will become be zero.

After calculating weights of all unsorted documents. Documents are then arranged in decreasing order of weights to provide the desired results.

For Multi-Word Query

For multi-word queries like "taste of apple" or "cost of apple", etc. The data property-terms like cost and taste which are also present in the user query is given more weight and score for such term is calculated as shown below. Here qt is the term that is present in the query and acts as a data property also.

$$\mathrm{Score(qt)} = \begin{matrix} \{2 + \log\left(\mathrm{tf_{qt}}\right), & \text{if Npq} > 0) \\ 0, & \text{otherwise}\} \end{matrix} \tag{3}$$

Here $\mathrm{tf_{qt}}$ is the term Frequency of the data property that is present in the query. Npq is the no. of data properties present in the query.

4.3 Algorithm of the Proposed Approach

```
   RankingAlgorithm(Docs[], C , Query)
Step 1: Get Data Properties of class C
        Let P[]
```

```
is the array containing all the Data Properties corresponding to class C
        T = P.Length; \\T is the no. of data properties
        D = Docs.Length; \\ D is the no. of Docs
```

Step 2: For every property term calculate the term frequency tf_j for each document.

Step 3: Tokenize the Query and find the property terms present in the Query

```
          PropQ[] = Split(Query);\\ where PropQ is array that
                    contains data property present in the query
             Npq = PropQ.Length;\\where Npq is the No. of data
                                      property present in the query
```

Step 4: Initialize Weight of all the Documents for all corresponding data properties to be Zero.

```
        for ( n = 1 to n = D ) do
                for( j = 1 to j = T) do
                        W [n, j] = 0;
                end for
        end for
```

Step 5:

```
Step 5: for ( n = 1 to n = D ) do
            for( j = 1 to j = T ) do
             for( k = 1 to k = Npq ) do
              if(P[j] == PropQ[k]) then
                 if (tf_j > 0 )//tf_j is term frequency in n^th Doc
                  W[n,j] = 2 + log(tf_j);
                  else
                  W[n,j] = 0;
              else
                 if (tf_j > 0 )
                  W[n,j] = 1 + log(tf_j);
                 else
                  W[n,j] = 0;
              end for
            end for
          end for
```

```
Step 6: Calculate the total weight of each document
        for( n = 1 to n = D )
               for( j = 1 to j = T )
                      Weight[n] = Weight[n] + W[n,j];
               end for
        end for
```

```
Step 7: Sorts Documents according to the total weight.
```

Unsorted Document, Query's Class and User query act as input parameters to the Ranking Module. The ranking module then finds out the data properties corresponding to the given query class. It then parses each unsorted document and calculates the term frequency of each property-term in that document. If the query is multi-word query then it split the query and find out each token in the query. Here the token can be a data property and this data property is given extra weight because it lies in the user query as well as shown in formula (3). By using step 5 it calculates the weight of each property present in the document. After that, it calculates the total weight of each document and arranged the documents in decreasing order to show the results.

5 Implementation and Results

Suppose user fires a query "jaguar" on a Keyword-based search engine like (Google). It will show the results as shown in Fig. 4. Clearly, it does not take into account the exact context of the query. User might be searching for jaguar fittings or Jaguar animal. So here, users have to shift multiple pages to find the exact match.

5.1 Experimental Setup

In this paper, top 40 document are taken from Google when user fires the query "jaguar" such that 20 belongs to Animal class and rest 20 belongs to vehicle class. There were documents relating to jaguar fittings as well but as far as the Ontology store as concerned only Animal and vehicle classes documents are taken for the experiment.

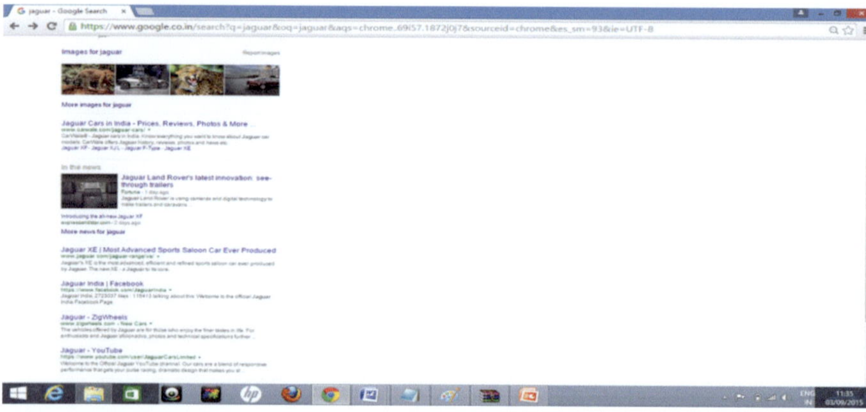

Fig. 4 Result page of google when "Jaguar" query is fired

5.2 *Output of the Ontology Store*

An ontology extractor program has been used to extract following files from the ontology store.

Class file: It contains class name and its associated terms (individuals). It has been extracted using Jena API from the Ontology Store (Fig. 5).

Data Property file: This file is the outcome of the ontology store. It contains two columns one for the "Class name" and other for the List of data properties present in the corresponding class.

User Interface:

It is designed user interface where the user can enter queries to search any information, shown below.

class	terms
fruit	apple, banana, orange, pineapple, watermelon, guava, papaya, grapes
manufacturer	apple, nokia, samsung, karbonn, intex, iphone, lava, micromax, asus
OS	android, IOS, windows, linux, unix, solaris, macintosh, symbian
app	itune, mxplayer, whatsapp, hike, viber, line, candycrush, truecaller
Vehicle	audi, maruti, jaguar, landcruiser,alto, lamborgini, duster, bolero
animal	jaguar, rabbit, deer, wolf, monkey, dog, cat, rat, elephant, lion, fox
university	iit, du, mdu, ymcaust, dcrust, mriu, mmu, jmiu, jnu, nit, ignou, lu

Fig. 5 Class file

Class	Data Properties
Fruit	Shape, Taste, Color, Origin, Cost, Size
Manufacturer	Revenue, CEO, HeadOffice, Cost
Animal	Habitat, Genus, Lifespan, AverageSpeed, Diet
Vehicle	Mileage, Cost, MaxSpeed, Brand, CubicCapacity

Fig. 6 Data property file

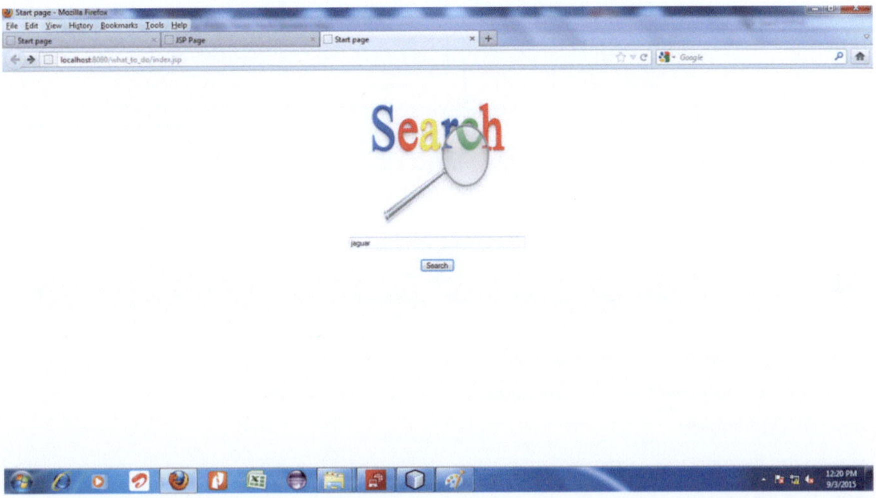

Fig. 7 User interface

Query Classifier can provide the Class as Animal or Vehicle. The ranking module then calculates the weight of each unsorted document. The Calculated weights are shown in Figs. 6 and 7.

From Fig. 8, it has been found that Documents weight is different in different domains. If vehicle class is taken into account relevancy/weight of Doc14 > Doc11 > Doc16 … > DOC4. If Animal class is taken into account relevancy of Doc3 > Doc1 > Doc7 … > Doc18. It has also been found that the documents that have the maximum importance in one domain can have least importance in other domain, e.g., Doc14 have maximum importance when domain being selected is Vehicle and have least importance when Animal domain is selected. This is in accordance with our hypothesis that a document is always centered about a particular domain.

After sorting the documents in decreasing order of their weights the output is as shown in Fig. 9.

Weights of Docs when vehicle class's data properties are taken	
Docs No.	Weight
Doc1	1.4771212547196624
Doc2	0.0
Doc3	2.6020599913279625
Doc4	0.0
Doc5	1.0
Doc6	1.0
Doc7	1.3010299956639813
Doc8	0.0
Doc9	1.0
Doc10	1.4771212547196624
Doc11	10.220944476323414
Doc12	4.243038048686294
Doc13	6.922206277439017
Doc14	10.738431714820287
Doc15	7.193124598354462
Doc16	7.292256071356476
Doc17	5.431363764158988
Doc18	5.301029995663981

Weights of Docs when animal class's data properties are taken	
Docs No.	Weight
Doc1	5.982271233039569
Doc2	3.0
Doc3	7.602059991327962
Doc4	1.477121254719662
Doc5	3.477121254719662
Doc6	4.698970004336019
Doc7	5.447158031342219
Doc8	1.477121254719662
Doc9	2.0
Doc10	0.0
Doc11	0.0
Doc12	0.0
Doc13	0.0
Doc14	0.0
Doc15	0.0
Doc16	0.0
Doc17	0.0
Doc18	0.0

Fig. 8 Weights of the documents computed by ranking module

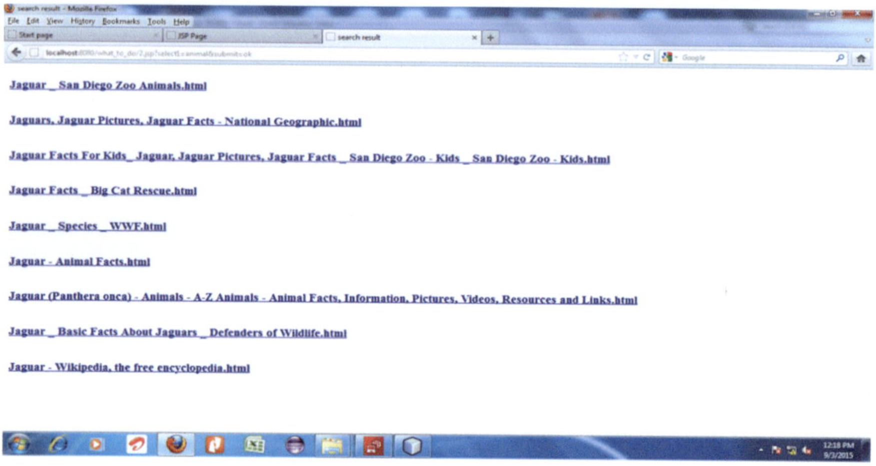

Fig. 9 Showing results page when animal class is chosen as the required domain

6 Conclusion and Future Work

To determine the correct order or to rank the result pages, a ranking factor is developed in this paper. This factor uses the underlying ontology to determine the weight of each resulted page and then sorts the pages in decreasing order of their weight. This technique is very impressive and makes the context of the web page the real king in deciding the relevancy of a web page. One of the main advantages of this method is that it can act as an offline factor in deciding the overall rank of a web page and can be used in Keyword-Based Search Engines. One can easily find the data properties from an ontology using Jena (JAVA API) and can calculate the overall weight of the document.

Data properties can be given different weights according to their significance.

References

1. http://www.searchenginegeneral.com
2. A study from http://slingshot.com
3. Roush, W.: Search Beyond Google. Technology Review, Mar 2004
4. http://www.en.m.wikipedia.org/wiki/Context-Sensitive_help
5. http://w3.org/onotologies
6. Noy, N.F., McGuinness, D.L.: A Guide for Creating Your First Ontology. Stanford U. Report
7. Gruber, T.R.: A translation approach to portable ontologies. Knowl. Acquis. **5**(2), 199–220 (1993)
8. Uschold, M. Gruninger, M.: Ontologies principles methods and applications. AIAI-TR-191, Feb 1996
9. Gupta, P.N. et al.: A novel architecture of ontology based semantic search engine. Int. J. Sci. Technol. **1**(12) (2012)
10. Mukhopadhyay, D. et al.: Domain specific ontology based semantic web search engine
11. Heflin, J: An Introduction to the Owl Web Ontology Language. Lehigh University
12. Knublauch, H. et al.: A practical guide to building OWL ontologies using protege 4 and CO-ODE tools
13. Kaur, G. Nandal, P.: Ranking algorithm of web documents using ontology
14. Kim, J., McLeod, D.: A 3 tuple information retrieval query interface with ontology based ranking
15. Haveliwala, T.H.: Topic-sensitive pagerank: a context-sensitive ranking algorithm for web search

Hidden Data Extraction Using URL Templates Processing

Babita Ahuja, Anuradha and Dimple Juneja

Abstract A lot of work has been carried out in the deep web. Deep web is like a golden apple in the eyes of the researchers. Most of the deep web search engines extract the data from the deep web, store them in the database, and index them. So, such kind of techniques have the disadvantage of less freshness, large repository requirement and need of frequent updating of the deep web database to give accurate and correct results. In order to overcome these drawbacks, we propose a new technique "Hidden Data Extraction using URL Template processing" where the fresh results from the website server database are fetched dynamically and are served to the users.

Keywords Search engines · Surface web · Hidden web · Query interfaces

1 Introduction

Most of the websites store their data in the databases. These databases contain high quality and a large amount of data [1]. The data in the databases are not accessible directly by the traditional search engines. The user has to fill the query interfaces in order to retrieve the data in the databases. These query interfaces act as a blockage

11th International Conference on Wirtschaftsinformatik, 27th February–01st March 2013, Leipzig, Germany.

B. Ahuja (✉)
MRU, Faridabad, India
e-mail: babitaspark@mru.edu.in

Anuradha
YMCAUST, Faridabad, India
e-mail: anuangra@yahoo.com

D. Juneja
DIMT Kurukshetra, Faridabad, India
e-mail: dimplejunejagupta@gmail.com

V.B. Aggarwal et al. (eds.), *Big Data Analytics*, Advances in Intelligent Systems and Computing 654, https://doi.org/10.1007/978-981-10-6620-7_13

in accessing the deep web data [2]. A major part of the hidden web data is behind the query interfaces. Many researchers have worked on it. However, major of the techniques suffer from the problem of freshness, bulk database requirement and frequently crawling the web for hidden data. When users issue the query in these techniques, the deep web data residing in the local database repository of search engines are displayed to the user. The deep web local database loses its freshness in a few minutes and even in few seconds.

1.1 Traditional Method to Uncover Deep Web

When user wants to access the deep web, he has to fill multiple query interfaces as shown in Fig. 1. Steps taken by user to access deep web in traditional search engines are:

Step 1. User fills the single search text field query interface of search engine.

Step 2. The result web pages from deep web and surface web are displayed to user. The deep web data contains the stale web pages stored in search engine local repository and the query interfaces which act as an entry point for accessing deep web.

Step 3. In order to access the fresh data, user opens the query interfaces. User fills all the text fields of the query interface and submits the page. The result is displayed to user.

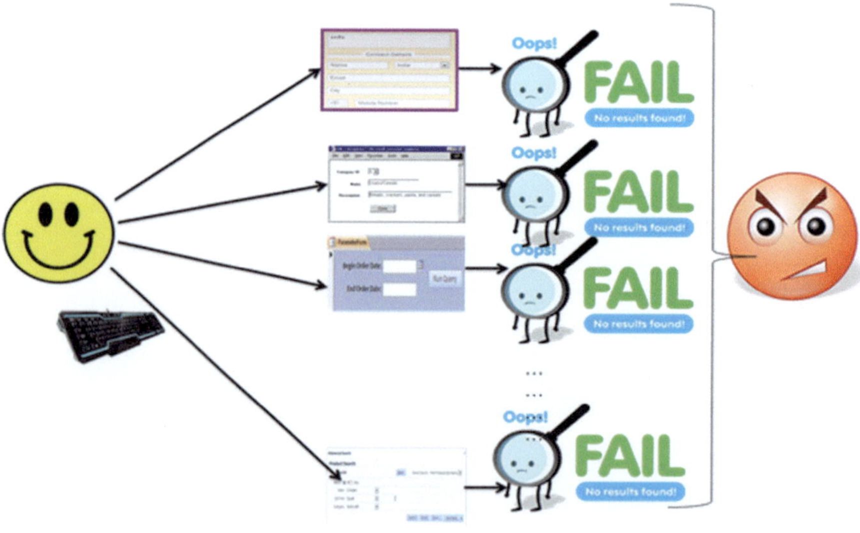

Fig. 1 Traditional way to see deep web

Step 4. User recursively repeats the same step 3 until desired results are retrieved. Filling the same values in thousands of query form is tedious and monotonous. Therefore, user finally quits and is unsatisfied with the results.

1.2 Steps of Proposed Technique to Uncover Deep Web

In the proposed technique, the user is not required to fill all the query interfaces. User will fill a single search text field for his query as shown in Fig. 2. The steps taken by user in proposed technique to access deep web are:

Step 1. User fills the single search text field query interface of search engine.
Step 2. The user query is processed.
Step 3. User keywords are placed in the URL templates and dynamic URL is generated.
Step 4. For post methods of form, the user keywords are embedded in the source code of the page and are submitted.
Step 5. The results are fetched on the fly from the website servers. These fresh results are displayed to the user.

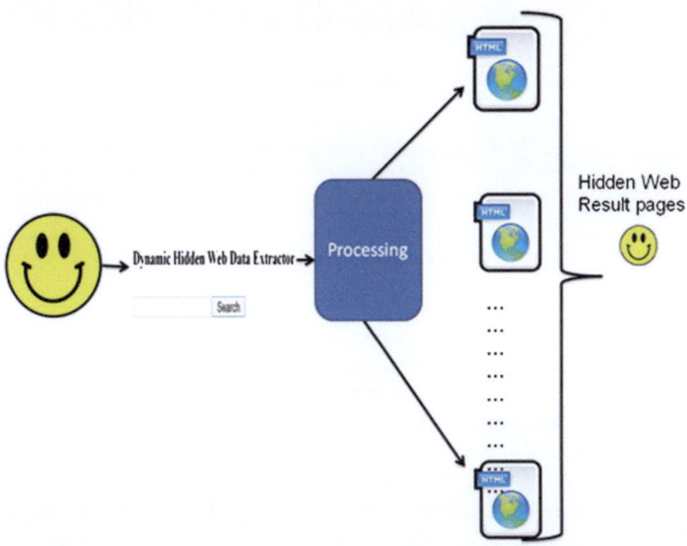

Fig. 2 Steps taken by user in proposed technique to fetch deep web pages

2 Related Work

Manuel Alvarez developed a hidden web crawler called DeepBot [4] to access Deep web. DeepBot has a "mini-web browser" to handle client-side scripts and session. Maintaining mechanism. Sriram has created a Hidden web crawler called HiWE [5]. HiWE stands for Hidden Web Exposer. HiWE is a task-specific hidden web crawler. HiWE extracts the data hidden behind the web query interfaces. Dr. Komal Kumar Bhatia proposed an incremental web crawler [6]. The incremental web crawler continuously refreshes the Web Repository. Ntaulas developed a search engine called HiddenSeek [7]. HiddenSeek works on the single-attribute database. It also detects the spam websites and ranks the pages also. Dr. Anuradha has created a Hidden Web Search Engine [8]. The hidden web search engine auto-fills the web query interfaces, extracts the result records, store them in a repository for later searching. Mining data records (MDR) [9] proposed by Chen. MDR searches for relevant data by looking for the form and the table tag in the web page. The "Layout-Based Data Region Finding" is a wrapper technique proposed by Chen [10]. The advantages and disadvantages of different techniques are given below in Table 1.

Table 1 Comparison of different hidden web extraction tools

	Type of tool	Method	Advantages	Disadvantages
1	Hidden web crawlers	DeepBot	It deals with both client-side scripting code and server side deep web data	Domain definitions are required, need mass storage
2	Hidden web crawlers	HIWE	It extracts the data from hidden databases	Need human assistance to fill the forms, need mass storage
3	Hidden web crawlers	Incremental web Crawler	It calculates the time to revisit and hence no unnecessary crawl is required	The page repository needs to be updated very frequently for few pages
4	Hidden web search engine	HiddenSeek	Uses different query selection policies, handles spam websites	Work on single-attribute databases, mass storage required
5	Hidden web search engine	Hidden web search engine	It works on multi-attribute interfaces, data is compiled and service is given to user	Millions of queries and Mass storage is required
6	Wrapper technique	Mining data records	It can mine the data records in a table automatically	Some advertisement and irrelevant records are also fetched
7	Wrapper technique	Layout-based data region finding	Constructs tree for getting data	The tags like <div>, <span> are not considered

3 Proposed Work

We propose a new technique “Hidden Data Extraction behind Query Interfaces” shown in Fig. 3. In the proposed system on the system side, the query interfaces are extracted and categorized on the basis of domain and the form submission method. The URL of these query interfaces are analyzed thoroughly. After analyzing, the query interfaces the URL templates are created and are stored in the URL templates repository.

For query interfaces having the Post method of form submission, the source code of the query interfaces is updated in order to fetch the fresh results from web servers. On the end user side when user will issue the query. The user query will be processed and keywords will be extracted. These keywords are placed in the URL templates of query forms having GET method of submission. In the case of POST method of submission, the keywords are placed in the source code of the query forms. After that, the results behind the query interfaces are pulled out. These results pages are then displaced to the user. Modules of the proposed.

Algorithm:

1. Query Interface Extraction.
2. URL Template Extraction of Query Interfaces having “GET” method of form submission.

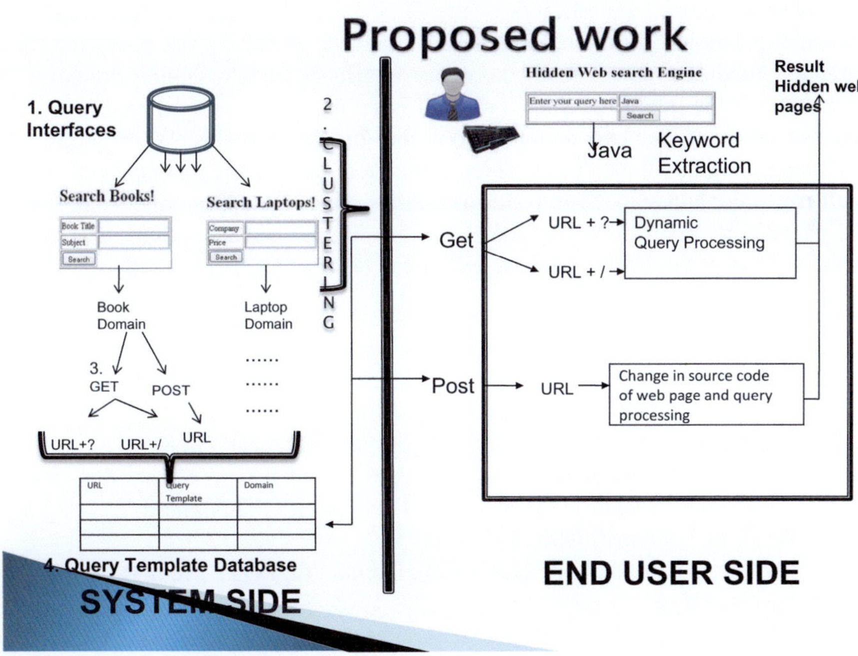

Fig. 3 Proposed architecture of hidden data extraction behind query interfaces

3. For POST method of submission extract the result page URL.
   3.1. Extract the query form of the page.
   3.2. Change the source code of the page.
4. Process the user query.
5. Create the dynamic URL of GET method Query Interfaces and fetch the results.
6. Set the values of user query in the source code of the post query interface and auto submit the page. Fetch the results.
7. Show 10 pages having maximum page rank. For these web pages and the other web pages calculate the fresh page rank. The pages are then ordered on the basis of the page rank and displayed to the users.

3.1 *Query Interface Extraction*

The data behind the query interfaces forms a lion's share of the data on the hidden web. The query interfaces act as a very significant channel to access the databases residing on the server machines databases. These query interfaces are created on computer machines but the irony is that the computer machines are not able to understand them. So fetching the query interfaces is a major task. The query interfaces can have two form processing techniques GET and POST. Most of the techniques developed consider only the GET method of form submission. The proposed technique works on both the GET and the POST. In the query interface extraction module we will fetch the query interfaces of few sample domains. In order to fetch the query interfaces, we will issue the query using the Google API. Here we will consider two domains book and the car domains. When a query is fired using google API ex: "book" then results of book domain are displayed. These result pages contain static web pages as well as pages containing query interfaces. The pages containing the query interfaces are filtered and are stored. The stored query interfaces are further categorized on the basis of GET and POST.

```
Algorithm:
1. Initializing an array Domains which can be of n size i.e. Domains d[n]
2. for each  di  send request to google using API
3.    for each result page pj returned from google API repeat 4 to 8
4.      if (pj .contains( method="GET") )
5.        Add to Database db1: PageURL pj, Domain di, GET Method
6.      else if (pj .contains( method="POST") )
7.        Add to Database db1: PageURL pj, Domain di, POST Method
8.      else discard pj
```

3.2 URL Template Creation

The URL filtered above contains the query interfaces. The query interfaces having GET method of form submission will be handled in this module. When these query interfaces are submitted to servers the result pages are shown. In GET as the input field data changes so does the result page's URL changes. The URL template of these result pages will be fetched and will be stored in the database. In order to accomplish this task the form tag of the query interfaces will be extracted. A temporary web page will be created which will contain the code of form tag extracted in the previous step. The websites provide the relative path of the result pages. Therefore, these relative paths will be converted into the absolute path. The initial input field will be filled with any value. The temporary web page will be created in such a way that it will automatically be redirected to the result page. The URL of the result page will be extracted. The URL will be analyzed and a generic template of the URL will be created and stored in the URL template database.

Algorithm:
URL Template Creation (DB_URL pages [ ])
// extracting the URL pattern of GET method web pages

1. for each Page^{i} in DB1 where method= "GET" repeat 2 to 8
2. Extract the form tag in the web page
3. Get the action attribute of <form> tag
4. Change the relative URL to the absolute URL
5. Fill any value in the first input field of the form only.
6. write to updated form in a file "temp.html"
7. resultUrl=autosubmit(temp.html)
8. Analyze resultUrl and create Url Template
9. Add to DBTemplete : Url Template, domain, method

3.3 Template Extraction

The query interfaces extracted in the first step contains web pages having both GET and POST methods of form submission. In GET as the input field data changes so does the result page's URL changes. In GET URL template is stored. However, in the POST method, the result page's URL does not change on the change of the input field data. For every query interface having POST method of form submission, a separate html page will be created. This html page contains only the form tag data of the original query interface. The page will be created in such a way that the input field values will be filled atomically by the value that is provided by the user while issuing the query in a single search textbox. The values will be filled automatically and the submission too will be done automatically. The fresh results from the actual website's servers will be presented to the user.

Algorithm:
1. for each Page^i in DB where method= "POST" repeat 2 to 5
2. Extract the form tag in the page
3. The values of text field in the form are replaced by a dynamic value.
4. The updated form tag is written to a HTML file "formpage^i .html".
5. Add to DBTemplate: formpage^i .html, domain, method.

3.4 User Query Processing

The user will issue the query in a single search text field. The user query will be processed. The tokens or keywords will be extracted from the user query. The punctuation symbols, etc., will be removed from the user query. The lemmatization or stemming of user query will be done to formulate the final list of user query keywords. The keywords will be processed to identify the domain of the user query.

Algorithm:
1. Keywords [] =split ("query"," ")
2. Remove stop words from keywords
3. Stemming of keywords
4. Identify domain of user query

3.5 Query Interfaces Having GET Method of Submission

All the URL templates of user query domain will be picked from URL template database. The user keywords will be placed in the URL templates and the form input data fields. The URL's will be created and will be displayed to the user. When user will click on the URL then the result pages from the actual website will be fetched and will be displayed to the user.

Algorithm:
1. URLs extracted from URL template database
2. for every URL^i repeat 3 to 6
3. if(URL^i .method="GET")
4. { // Generate dynamic query string
5. add keywords in URL template
6. Result_set1= dynamic URL's created }

3.6 *Query Interfaces Having POST Method of Submission*

The web pages having POST method of submission will be handled here. The web pages created in module 3 template extraction, will be updated and the values from the user query keywords will be placed in the text field of the web page.

Algorithm:
1. if (URL^i .method="POST")
2. { // open the files created
3. open $formpage^i$ .html
4. $formpage^i$.setValues(form_fields, keywords[])
5. autosubmit($formpage^i$.html)
6. Result_set2= fetch result pages
7. Display pages (result_set1, result_set2)}

4 Experimental Results

The admin on the system side will extract the URLs of the query interfaces of particular domain. The generic query templates of these URL have been created and are stored in the database as shown in Fig. 4. After the query interface extraction, the generic templates of the result pages will be created as shown in Fig. 5. These generic templates are stored in the local repository of the system. When user query in the single search text field the query is processed and the results are displayed to the user as shown in Figs. 6 and 7.

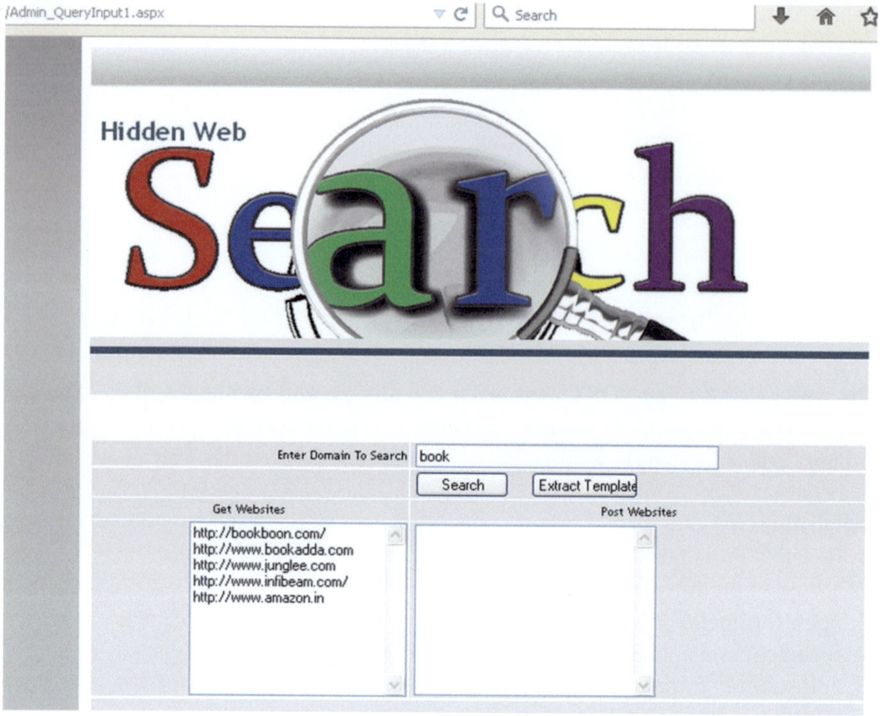

Fig. 4 Query interface extraction

5 Comparison with Other Search Engines

The parameters on which the comparison is done are relevancy and optimized results. Relevancy means how much relevant result pages according to the user query are fetched from deep web servers. The implementation results show that deep web pages fetched by the proposed work are highly relevant as compared to other search engines as shown in Figs. 8, 9 and 10.

Another factor taken into consideration for comparison is the optimum result. The results shown by another search engine in terms of price of the book or any other item are not optimum as shown in Figs. 11, 12, 13 and 14.

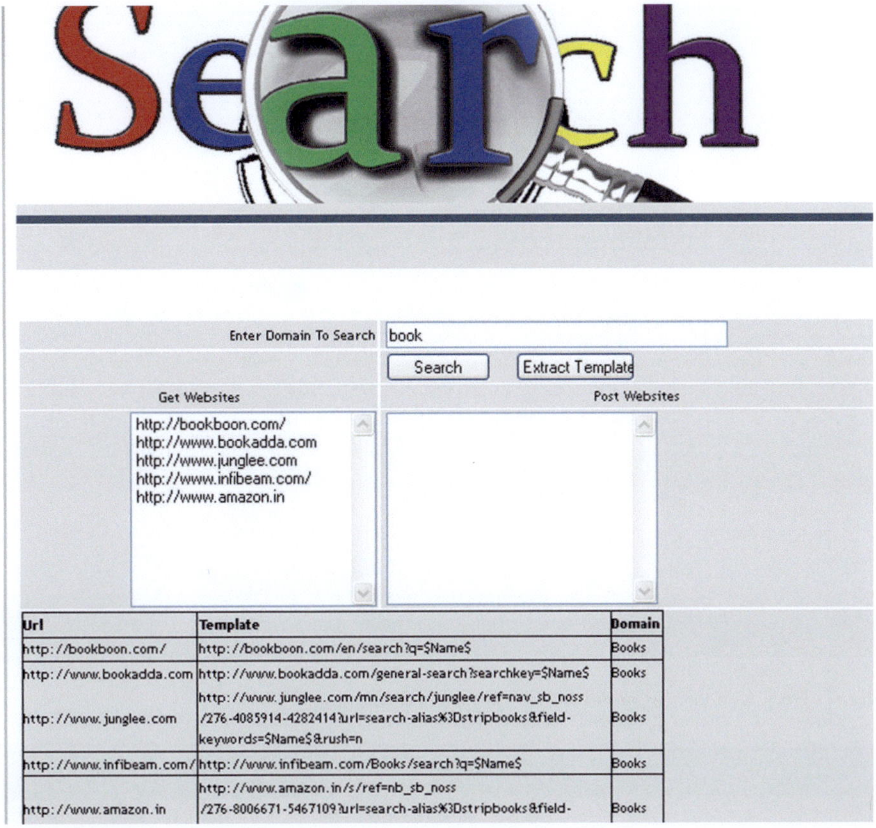

Fig. 5 Template extraction

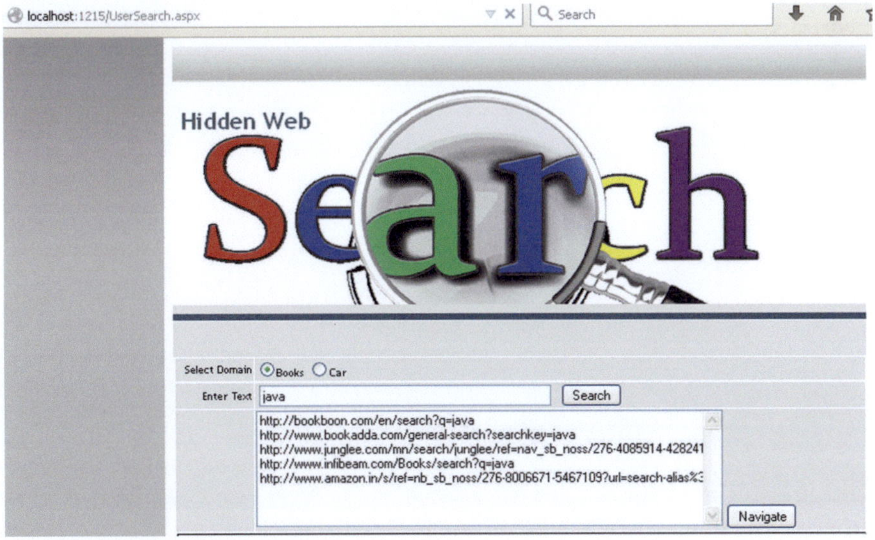

Fig. 6 Result page displayed to user

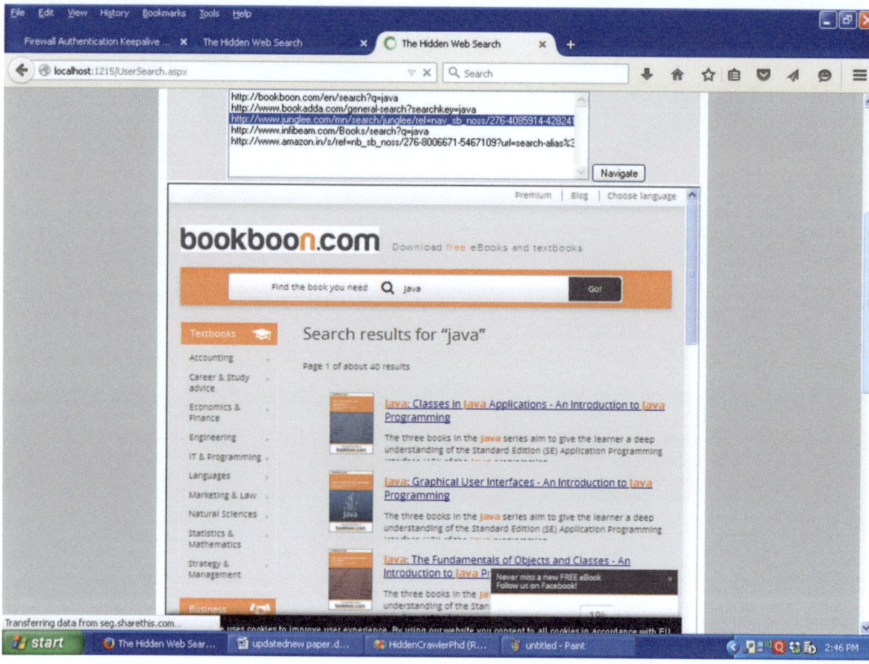

Fig. 7 Deep web data from the website presented to the user

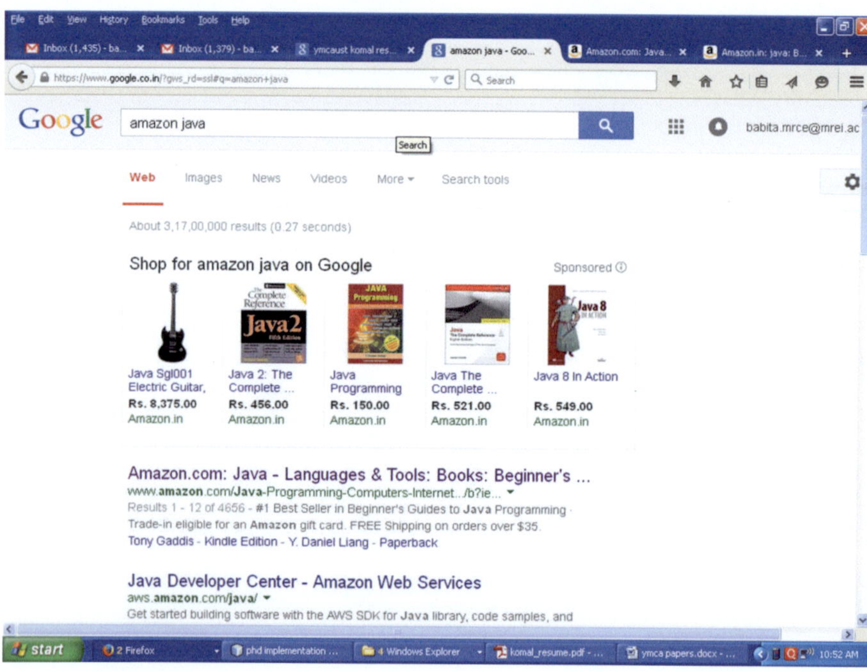

Fig. 8 Query fired on other search engine

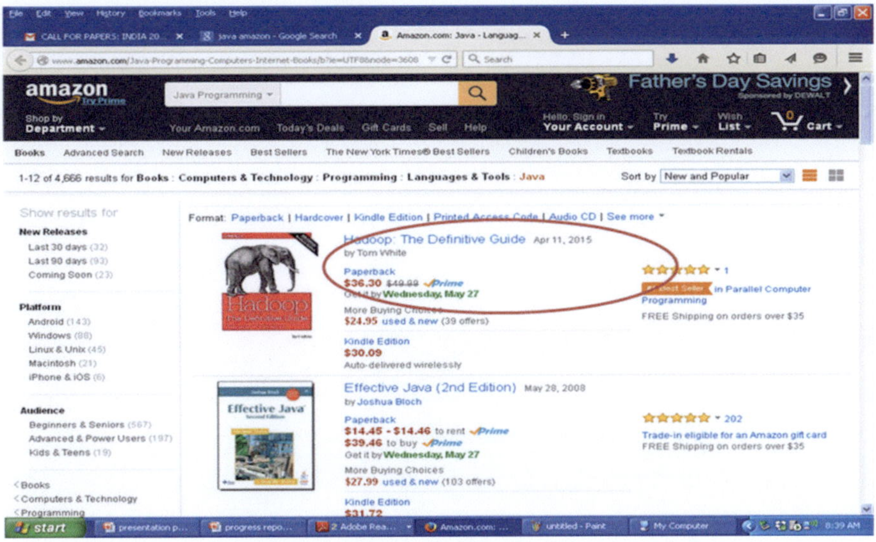

Fig. 9 Irrelevant result shown by other search engine

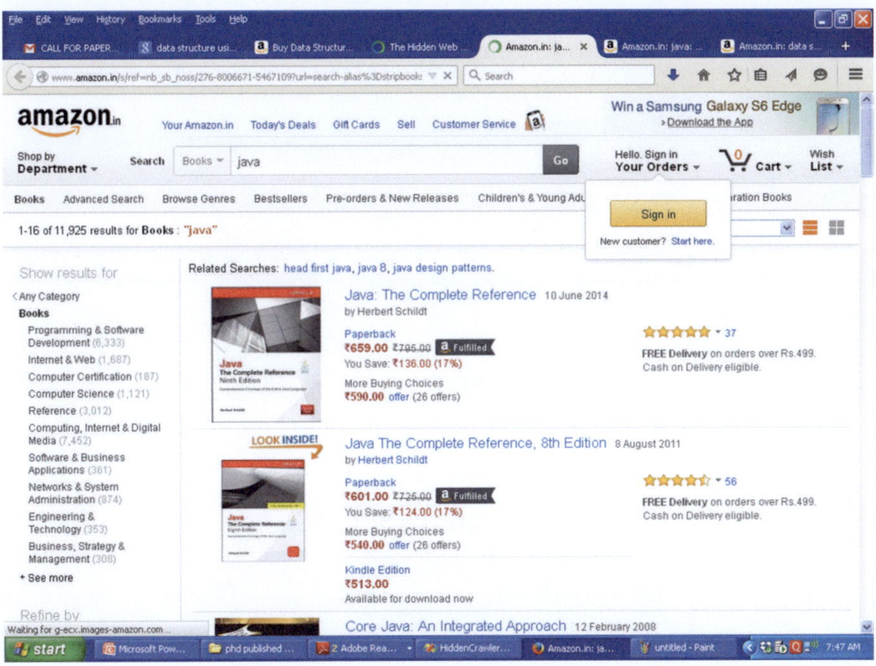

Fig. 10 Relevant data shown when query issued by proposed work

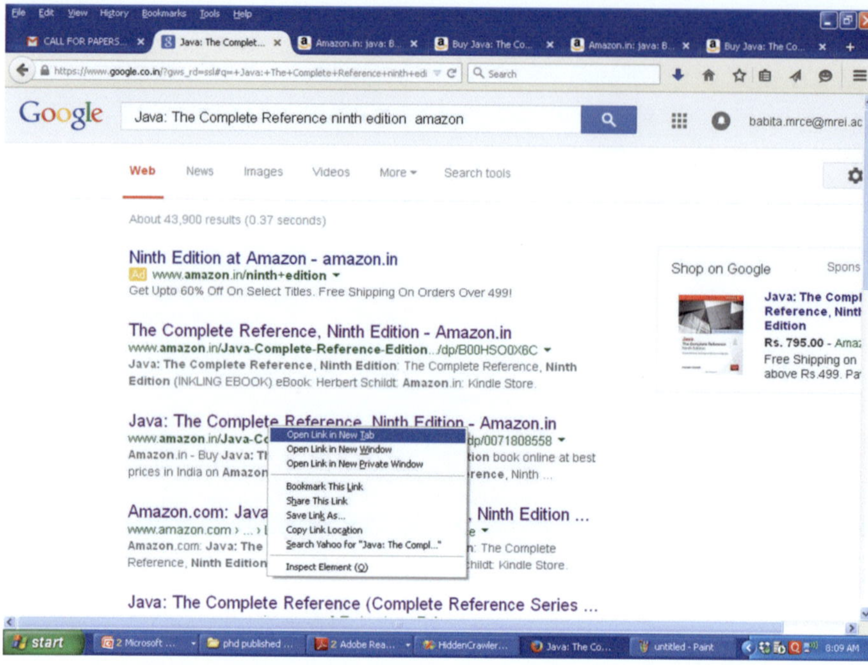

Fig. 11 Query fired on other search engine

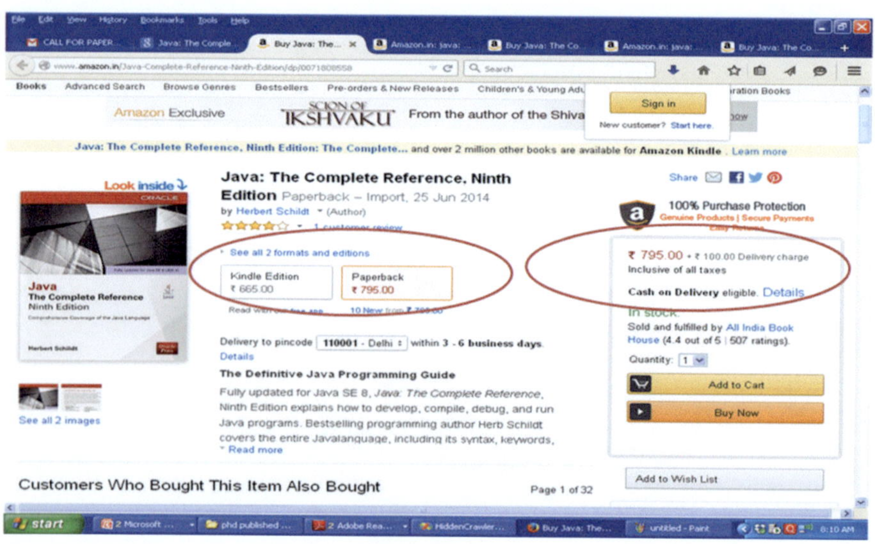

Fig. 12 High price book shown by other search engine

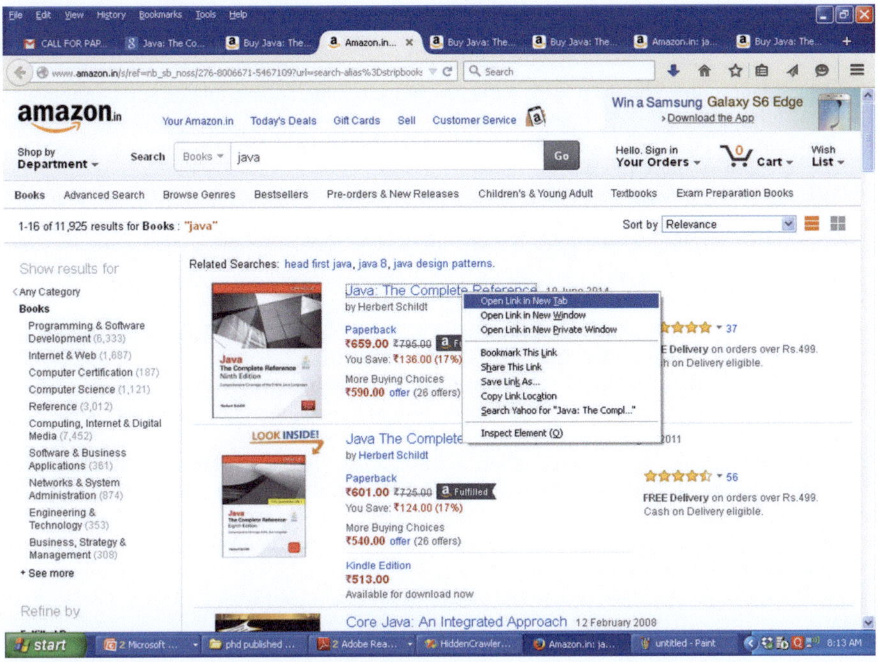

Fig. 13 The result shown by proposed work

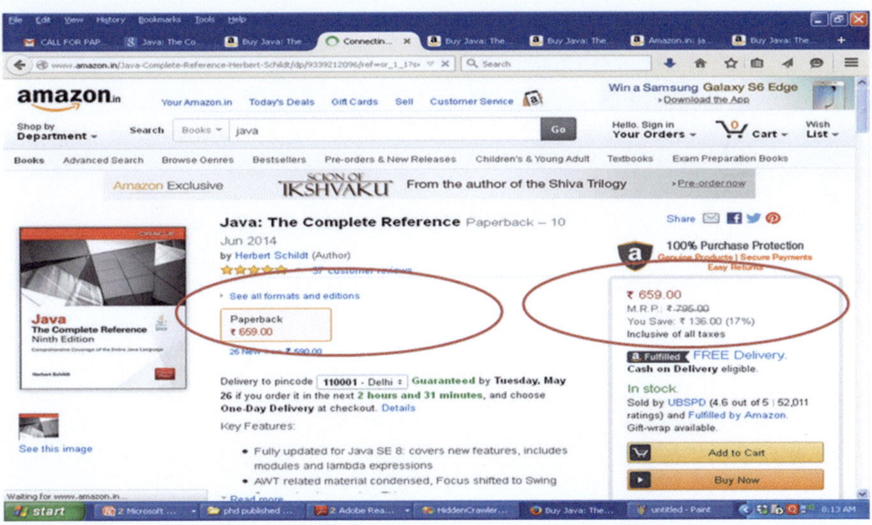

Fig. 14 The low price book shown by proposed work

References

1. BrightPlanet.com. The deep web: surfacing hidden value. Accessible at http://brightplanet.com, July 2000
2. Sherman, C., Price, G.: Hidden Web. Uncovering Information Sources Search Engines Can't See. CyberAge Book (2001)
3. Bergman, M.K.: White paper. The deep web: surfacing hidden value. J. Electron. Publ. **7**(1) (2001)
4. Álvarez, M., Raposo, J., Cacheda, F., Pan, A.: A task-specific approach for crawling the deep web. Eng. Lett. **13**(2), EL_13_2_19 (Advance online publication: 4 Aug 2006)
5. Raghavan, S., Garcia-Molina, H.: Crawling the hidden web. VLDB, (2001)
6. Madaan, R., Dixit, A., Sharma, A.K., Bhatia, K.K.: A framework for incremental hidden web crawler. Int. J. Comput. Sci. Eng. **02**(03), 753–758 (2010)
7. Ntoulas A., Zerfos, P., Cho, J.: Downloading hidden web content. Technical Report, UCLA
8. Anuradha, Sharma, A.K.: Design of hidden web search engine. Int. J. Comput. Appl. **30**(9) (2011) (0975-8887)
9. Chen, H.-P., Fang, W., Yang, Z., Zhuo, L., Cui, Z.-M.: Automatic Data Records Extraction from List Page in Deep Web Sources; 978–0-7695-3699-6/09 c, pp. 370–373. IEEE (2009)
10. Liu, B., Grossman, R., Zhai, Y.: Mining data records in web pages. In: KDD'03: Proceedings of the Ninth ACM SIGKDD International Conference on Knowledge Discovery and Data Mining, pp. 601–606, New York

Automatic Generation of Ontology for Extracting Hidden Web Pages

Manvi, Komal Kumar Bhatia and Ashutosh Dixit

Abstract WWW consists of thousands of web pages which are hidden behind search interfaces. To retrieve those hidden web pages user fills in the details manually in various fields of form pages. To automatically extract all this hidden information the crawler (hidden web crawler) must be so intelligent that it understands the interface and fill the required information accurately. This process of understanding and filling forms automatically can be easily and efficiently done with the help of ontology. A database that stores semantic information about objects and their relations may solve this purpose. In this work, a novel technique for creation of ontology with the help of form pages is proposed and implemented.

Keywords Hidden web · Ontology · Database · Semantic · OWL

1 Introduction

A huge amount of information on the WWW is available only when the user input values in the fields present at the interface of different websites. These pages that we get as a result of inputting various values are often referred as Hidden Web. The hidden web crawler is specially designed to automatically fill these interfaces and downloads the resultant pages. For filling these types of interfaces precisely and getting the desired information, a database of values is required. A database that

Manvi (✉) · K.K. Bhatia · A. Dixit
Computer Engineering Department, YMCA University of Science & Technology, Faridabad, India
e-mail: manvi.siwach@gmail.com

K.K. Bhatia
e-mail: komal_bhatia1@rediffmail.com

A. Dixit
e-mail: dixit_ashutosh@rediffmail.com

V.B. Aggarwal et al. (eds.), *Big Data Analytics*, Advances in Intelligent Systems and Computing 654, https://doi.org/10.1007/978-981-10-6620-7_14

stores semantic information about objects and their relations may solve this purpose. This database can be defined with the help of Ontology which defines a common vocabulary for each term [3].

In this paper, a novel technique to generate Ontology, using hidden web form interfaces is derived. This technique is novel in the sense that it is using the information present on the search interface itself to create the ontology. The ontology thus created is stored in the semantic database in Oracle 10 g in the form of triples <Subject, Predicate, Object>. This ontology will be used in future to make hidden web crawler which will fill the form interfaces and get the hidden web pages as result.

2 Related Work

The size of this hidden web has been estimated around 500 times the size Surface Web [4]. As the volume of hidden information is on a fast pace, researchers have increased their interest to work in this field, hence constant work to find out techniques that allow users and applications to leverage this information is going on. To address the problem of crawling and retrieving the contents from hidden web many works have to be done in this area. Few among them are discussed below:

Raghavan and Garcia-Molina *proposed* HiWE [5], a task-specific hidden web crawler. The main focus of this work was to learn hidden web query interface. **Ntoulas et al.** provided a theoretical framework for analyzing the process of generating queries in *Framework for Downloading Hidden Web Conten*t [6]. The Crawler has to come up with meaningful queries to issue to the query interface. This body of work was often referred to as query selection problem over the Hidden Web. Disadvantage of this work was that it focuses on single attribute queries rather than multi attribute or structural queries. **Okasha et al.** *In Exploiting Ontology for Retrieving Data Behind Searchable Web Forms* [7] classified each searchable form to its relevant domain then exploit the suitable ontology to automatically fill out these forms. **Hao Liang et al.** in *Extracting Attributes from Deep Web Interface Using Instances* al [8] designed a new method to automatically extract the attributes and instances of hidden web pages. They added the semantics to attributes using the WordNet. Also, a hierarchy tree has been generated by an ontology for the same.

3 Proposed Work

As WWW is growing tremendously and people are relying on it for finding study materials including Academics and non-Academic books. Also for doing research, a person downloads the material from Internet. For Example if a user wants to access an ebook he/she has to specify book's name along with other information like author's name, ISSN number, etc., or if a user wants to access some research work he has to specify the paper name or journal name, issue number, conference name, etc. After specifying all these fields and after inputting values for all the fields user will be brought to various links which further contain the URL's for various websites which contain the relevant data. Hence there is a huge requirement for developing a common framework (interface) where a user can enter a single query and get the desired result.

For generating and responding to user query in hidden web environment, we need a database that is populated knowledge base which satisfies the user's need of information. This database will be helpful to deal with the search interface means the values that are stored in database will be used to fill the form that lies behind the hidden web. As user specify queries using different keywords but having same meaning, Ontology is one of the best ways for creating Domain knowledge that has common understanding of the structure of information among people.

The Proposed Architecture along with the Components is shown in Fig. 1:

1. Form Downloader
2. Search Interface Repository
3. Ontology Converter
4. Database in Oracle

The detailed description of each component is given below:

(a) **Form Downloader**

This is a special downloader which starts from a given seed URL, downloads the content of the form pages and sends the downloaded page to the next component *Search Interface Repository*. This is special in the sense that only

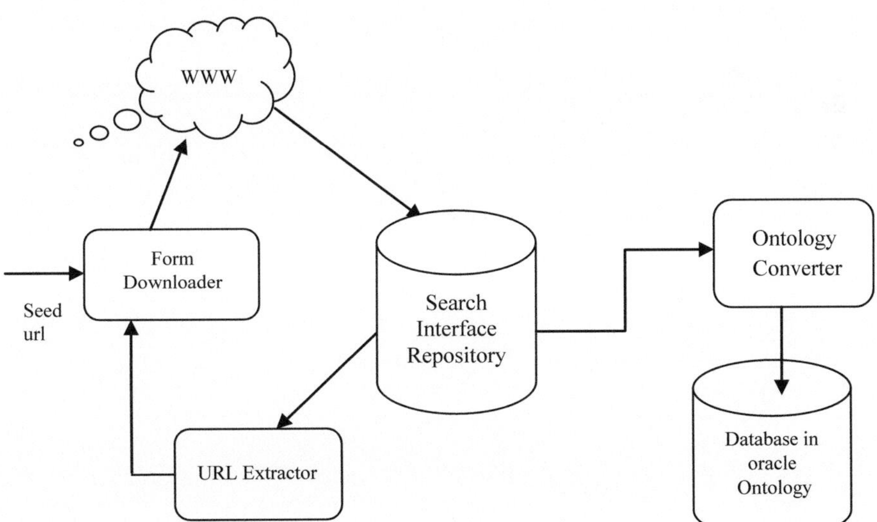

Fig. 1 Ontology construction from hidden web pages

those web pages which are having an entry point for hidden web documents are downloaded and stored. The downloader checks from the source code of the web page, whether the page contains the **<form>** element or not. If the source code of page contains the <form> tag, i.e., this page is actually the entry point for hidden web is taken to the next step. Hence those pages that contain fields to be filled by the user are considered only rest are discarded essential that all illustrations are as clear and as legible as possible.

(b) **Search Interface repository**
This repository contains the source code of form pages which will be processed in next step for creating ontology with the help of information present within the tags and also the information present between a pair of tags.

(c) **Ontology Converter**
This is the most important component of the system. This component will take the source code of hidden web pages stored in the repository, parse them and extract the meaningful information from various tags present in the page and then convert this information into ontology. Different form pages are having different formats like RDF, XML, HTML, OWL, etc., so to create a generic and well-populated ontology, according to the type of web pages they are sent to different parsing modules where each different module extracts all the information in form of RDF triples <Subject, Predicate, Object> and store these triples into database which may be defined as ontology-based semantic database.

(d) **URL Extractor**
If in any page stored in interface repository there exists, new URL the URL Extractor will take that URL and further sends to the Form downloader to download the required page.

(e) **Database in Oracle**
The ontology converter after extracting all the values from various hidden web form pages stores them in the form of triples of <S, P, O> in semantic database in Oracle 10 g.

This work emphasizes on automatic generation of ontology as semantic database in Oracle, with the help of hidden web interface pages. Hence leaving the description of all the components as in Sect. 3, the ontology converter is described in detail in Sect. 4. This database will contain values/instances that will be used to fill in the hidden web interfaces to extract hidden web data.

4 Ontology Converter

As shown in Fig. 2 following are the subcomponents of Ontology converter

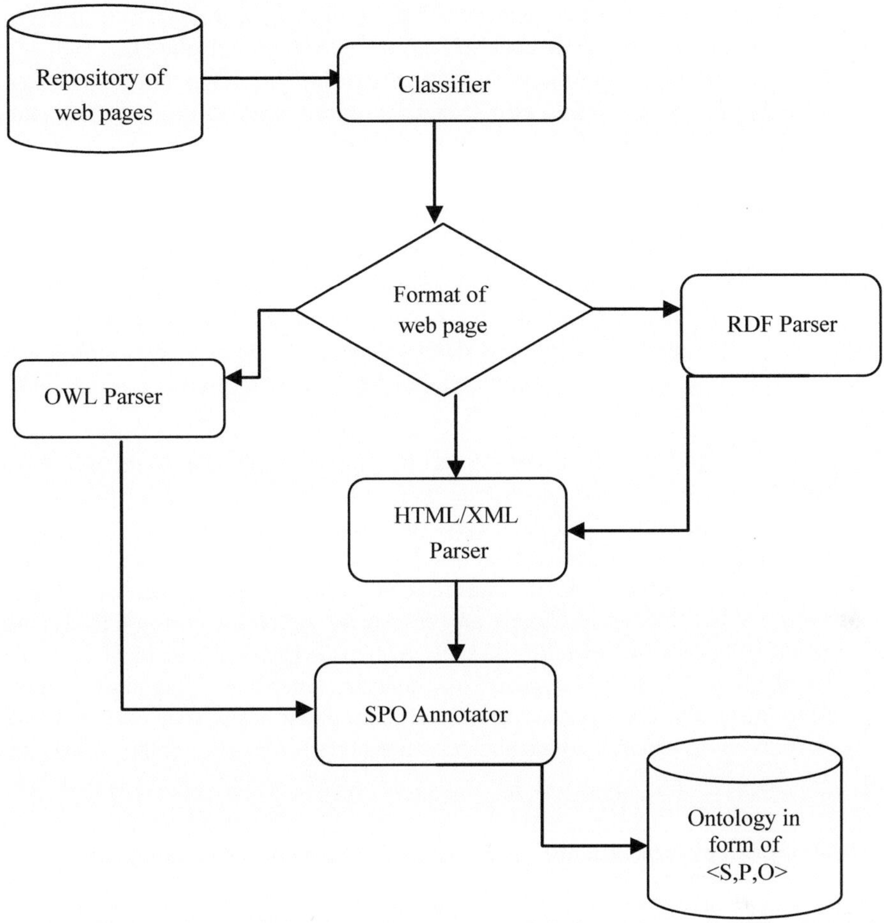

Fig. 2 Components of ontology converter

1. Classifier
2. RDF Parser
3. OWL Parsed
4. HTML/XML parser
5. SPO Annotator

Detailed description of each component of Ontology Converter

4.1 **Classifier**: This component after getting the form pages from repository reads the tags present in the page and classifies them according to the type of tags present. The different classification may be as follows: (i) OWL/RDFS (ii) RDF/XML (iii) XML/HTML (iv) HTML.

4.2 **OWL Parser**: The parser here first find the OWL tag, then RDF/RDFS tags enclosed within the source code of web page. It then finds the class, subclass and property tags from the web page. Also there are range and domain tags available in the code itself. However, there is not much information available online in OWL format, i.e., there is not any form page available in OWL format online, e.g. The URL "http://ebiquity.umbc.edu/ontology/publication.owl" taken from SWOOGLE [11] search engine is in OWL format, but it is not a form page in Fig. 3.

The algorithm/procedure to extract SPO information form OWL tags is defined in Fig. 4. As there is not much information available in the form of web pages for OWL format, the above algorithm is designed so as to cover as many things as possible. In future new tags may come upon hence, the algorithm can be extended for the same.

4.3 **RDF Parser**: This component after getting the attached RDF of the web page parses the content and convert the data into <SPO> triple according to the following procedure. RDF is a standard for describing resources. It is similar to conceptual models such as entity-relationship model. It is based upon idea of making statements about resources in form of subject–predicate–object expressions. These expressions are known as triples in terms of RDF. For example "Book on operating system" can be represented in RDF as triple where "book" denoting subject, "on" denoting predicate, "operating system" denoting object. The subject of an RDF statement is either a URI or blank node, both of which denote resources. Resources indicated by blank nodes are

```
<owl:Ontology rdf:about="http://ebiquity.umbc.edu/ontology/
  publication.owl#publication">
<owl:versionInfo>0.1</owl:versionInfo>
  <owl:Class         rdf:about=         "http://swrc.ontoware.org
/ontology#InBook">
  *1 <rdfs:subClassOf>
<owl:Class
rdf:about="http://swrc.ontoware.org/ontology#Publication"/>
  </rdfs:subClassOf>

*2<rdfs:subClassOf>
  <owl:Restriction>
  <owl:onProperty
rdf:resource="http://swrc.ontoware.org/ontology#publisher"/>
      <owl:allValuesFrom>
      <owl:Class
rdf:about="http://swrc.ontoware.org/ontology#Organization"/>
      </owl:allValuesFrom>
      </owl:Restriction>
  </rdfs:subClassOf>*2
```

Fig. 3 Example of web page in OWL

Algorithm/Procedure:

Step 1. For Finding **SUBJECT**: Find the **rdf:about** tag, this contains the root of the page i.e. the main class .This specifies the URL of the page we are going to consider for parsing. This is stored as **Subject** of <S,P,O> for which next predicate and object will be discovered and is added to a set U.

Step 2: For Finding **SUBJECT** Find the **rdf:class** tags which define the parent of all children nodes and itself is the child of root node. The required information attached with class tag may be a URI or an ID as specified in figure 3 above. Class specifies the element about which we are talking currently. An OWL page may contain more than one class tags. Hence all becomes the **Subject** in triples. All these attributes extracted as subject are added to a set ***S*** of subjects.

Step 3: For Finding **Object:** The **subclassof** tag in between <owl:class> tells about two things in an OWL code. i) If the subclassof tag contains <Owl:class> tag then this specifies that the above said class in <rdf:about> tag is the subclass of resource specified in <Owl:class> tag*1. It means the **about resource** is having an is-a relation with the **Owl:class**. All the above said < rdf:about> elements are treated as **Object** and <Owl:class> are taken as subject with is_a relation. They further are treated as subject in case ii.

ii)The number of subclass tags enclosed in a class tag having property as <owl:restriction> tag defines the number of children and the name of each child node can be extracted from the **onproperty/label** tag. These will be treated as OBJECT in SPO having has relationship with <rdf:about> in Owl:class.

The attributes extracted above are stored in a set O of objects.

Step 4: For finding Predicate: Two relations have been derived from step 3 is-a.For deriving more relations the data found in various other tags like <owl:dataproperty> <rdfs:**domain/range/label/id etc.>** is parsed and required meaningful information is extracted and used. The relations extracted are also stored in a set P of predicates.

Fig. 4 Algorithm for OWL parser

called anonymous resources. The predicate is a URI which also represents a resource relationship. The object can also be a URI, blank node or string literal. For example given below are the two ways to specify RDF. Where Fig. 5a represent RDF/XML format and Fig. 4b represents the pure RDF format.

(a) RDF/XML format	(b) Pure RDF format
<rdf:RDF xmlns:rdf="http://www.w3.org/1999/02/22-rdf-syntax-ns#" xmlns:dc="http://purl.org/dc/elements/1.1/"> ***<rdf:Description*** rdf:about="http://www.w3.org/"> <dc:title>World Wide Web Consortium</dc:title> </rdf:Description></rdf:RDF>	<rdf:Property rdf:about="isbn" rdfs:label= "ISBN Number" rdfs:comment="The ISBN number of the book."> </rdf:Property> <rdf:Property rdf:about="authoredBy" rdfs:label="AuthoredBy" rdfs:comment="An author of this book.">

Fig. 5 **a** RDF/XML format, **b** pure RDF format

In Fig. 5a the description tag is associated with www.w3.org having title as World wide web Consortium hence www.w3.org is treated as Subject and title will be treated as object. The dc or property tag may contain a label and/or a comment associated with the corresponding attribute, e.g., title and label tags in above figures, respectively.
In Fig. 5b in the property tag we have label as ISBN treated as object of rdf: about this rdf property is associated with some rdf:class which is book. Hence book is subject and isbn is object here.

As it is difficult to find out relation/predicate from RDF document **dc/property** tag value is useful for the same, i.e., to find out the Predicate of <SPO>. In case of dc tag contains two things **1.** Attribute after: **2.** text between <dc> and </dc> which after reading and processing can be helpful in finding the relation between element in <rdf:description> and attribute in <dc> (Fig. 6).

4.4 **XML Parser**: To parse XML document DOM parser which parses the entire XML document and loads it into memory, then models it in form of a" Tree structure" for easy traversal or manipulation is used. According to DOM, everything in XML document is in form of node be it document element or attribute (Fig. 7).

Portion of source code is taken of Book domain from the website named www.cheapesttestbooks.com and used for extraction of data from various tags and meta tags defined in XML/HTML file in. Only relevant values which required to be filled in search interface form fields are retrieved and stored in form of <SPO> triples.

4.5 **HTML Parser**: Every HTML page contains elements like <LABEL>, <SELECT>, and <OPTION> that occur in pairs as shown in Figure. To find

Algorithm for RDF Parser
Step 1:Find <**rdf:Description**> tag element in <rdf:RDF> tag.
Step 2: Extract <**rdf:about**> tag in <rdf:Description> Tag to define Resource of information and assigns it as root node, The first element of Subject Set **S.**
Step 3: Next find other tags like <**dc**>, <**rdf:property**>,<**vCard:FN**> tag to describe property of Resource as Predicate where <dc:> and <rdf: property> specifies instance or attribute property, FN is property Name in vCard namespace. These tags contain information that will help to find the relationship between S and O.
Step 4: Extract </dc> or </rdf:property>or <vCard:FN> information enclosed in between these tags and treat them as **object v**alue for defined property. Here dc tag contain the value after : which is treated as object and property tag contain other tags like comment and label, label is treated as **objec**t and comment can be used to find the predicate. The values find are added to set O and P correspondingly.
Step 5: Repeat this process for all meta tags until </**rdf:Description**> tag is not null.
Step 6: Repeat steps 3 to 6 until retrieves </rdf:RDF> as end of file

Fig. 6 Algorithm for RDF parser

Algorithm for XML file
Step 1: Find root element by *getnodename()* function already defined in DOM model.
Step 2: Create variable ***nlist*** of type nodelist and intialise it with count of all ***<dl>*** tags found in XML file by method name *getelementsbytagname(dl)*.Where nlist value may be considered as no of children of root node. However label of children nodes is not assigned yet .
Step 3: Repeat steps 4 to 6 for each children node while ***nlist*** length not equal to null.
Step 4: Create variable of type ***Node*** and ***empty node*** got created each time loop is executed. However label is extracted further in next step.
Step 5:Extract a node label L with help of method calling ***getelementsbytagname(dt)*** by <dt> Tag.
Step 6: Label value (instance value) v is extracted with help of method called ***getelementsbytagname(dd)*** by <dd> tag.
Step 7: If required any attribute for more info related to <dt> tag can be extracted with function named getattribute().

*****where Label L*** of children node is retrieved with help of ***<dt>*** tag and can be classified as ***subclass***, whereas ***Label value*** v may be found in form of ***<dd>*** tag in conjuction with ***<dt>*** tag and can be classified ***as instances*** of subclasses

Fig. 7 Algorithm for XML parser

the attributes required for creating <SPO> of ontology, these tags are identified and the information present between these tags after processing is stored. Here it can be easily seen that the information is present in two ways (i) in between the angular brackets <> of the particular tag, e.g., **<label for="-search by">** and **<option value="key">** and (ii) in between the opening and closing of tag, e.g., <option value="titl"> **By Title </**option>. Both type of information is extracted and used to found Subject and Object. One thing to be noted here is that the predicate or relation from pure HTML form page is difficult to extract so to find out the relation between attributes Wordnet is used (Fig. 8).

4.6 **SPO Annotator**: This module after getting the attribute values from the classifier processes them before storing because the values cannot be directly used (Fig. 9).

The attributes values found above are specific to particular web page they should be converted into more general forms, e.g., some attributes may contain some special symbols like "leaving_from", some may contain plural form like "adults" and others may contain some abbreviation, e.g., dept_date for departure date, etc. Keeping these things in mind algorithm to annotate various terms is designed and applied to each element of both sets S and O.

(a)

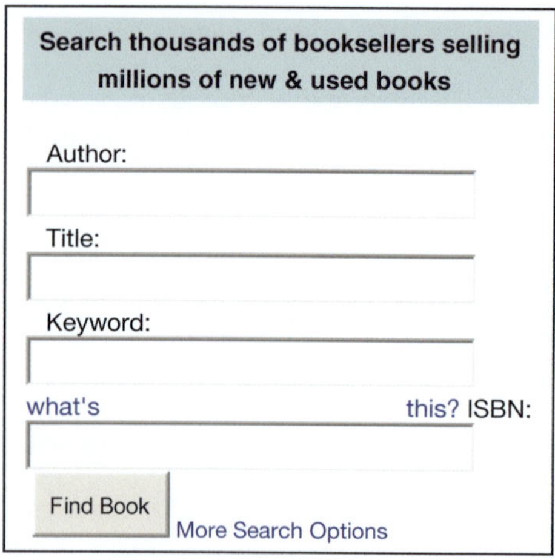

(b)

```
<FORM action= "..." method= "...">
<label for="searchBy">Search Books:</label>
<select id="searchBy" name="sby">
<option value="key">By Keyword</option>
<option value="tit">By Title</option>
<option value="aut">By Author</option>
<option value="isbn">By ISBN</option>
<option value="pub">By Publisher</option>
</select>
<input class="search-ln-
en" id="searchText" type="text" name="stext
maxlength="100" aria-label="Search Abe
Books"/>
<button id="site-search-
btn" type="submit"><span>Find
Book</span></button>
```

Fig. 8 **a** HTML of query form from www.abebooks.com. **b** Source code of the same page

Algorithm SPO _Annotator
Step 1: Get the set S and O of Subject and Object respectively from classifier
Step 2: For each S_i€ **S** and O_i €**O** do
- i) Remove special symbols like: (, -, _, @, $, &,#, ?, !, *,etc.) and make two elements connected by special symbols.
- ii) Remove duplicated in S and O.
- iii) Expand abbreviations if any.

Step 3: Extend the synonym values above of both sets by utilizing WordNet and expand the sets.
Step 4: Find Relation/Predicate if not present and store in P.
Step 5: Send to database for storage.

Fig. 9 Algorithm of SPO annotator

The data extracted from all steps above have been stored in sets S, O and P. These sets individually are given for further processing to SPO annotator like removing duplicates stemming, lemmatization, etc.

E.g., one interface may contain "leaving_from" and other may contain "departure from". Firstly all the values are stored as elements of the set "leaving_from and departure, from". The special symbols like underscore from leaving_from is removed and leaving and from are disconnected as two elements in step 2(i). As from comes two times hence duplicate term is removed in step 2(ii). One thing here to be noted is that simple syntactic comparison is done at this step. The values after all this processing are stored in database.

5 Implementation and Snapshots

Form pages of two domains (i) Airline and (ii) Book domain are taken and information retrieved form various interfaces is stored in semantic database Oracle 10 g. For implementing the code for OWL and RDF files JENA is used. JENA is a java API which can be used to create and manipulate RDF graphs. JENA has object classes to represent graphs, resources, properties and literals. In JENA graph is called model. RDF model is represented as set of statements. JENA model interface defines a liststatements() method which return an StmtIterator(a subtype of java iterator over all statements in model). It has method nextstatement() which returns the next statement from the iterator. Statement interface provides methods for subject, Predicate and Object named getSubject(), getPredicate(), and getObject().

The following methods are imported to use JENA for Owl/RDF files

```
import com.hp.hpl.jena.util.FileManager;
import com.hp.hpl.jena.vocabulary.*;
import java.io.*;
```

DOM parser is used for XML/HTML documents, The methods used are (Figs. 10 and 11):

```
import org.w3c.dom.NodeList;
import org.w3c.dom.Node;
import org.w3c.dom.Element;
 import java.io.*;
 import java.sql.*;
```

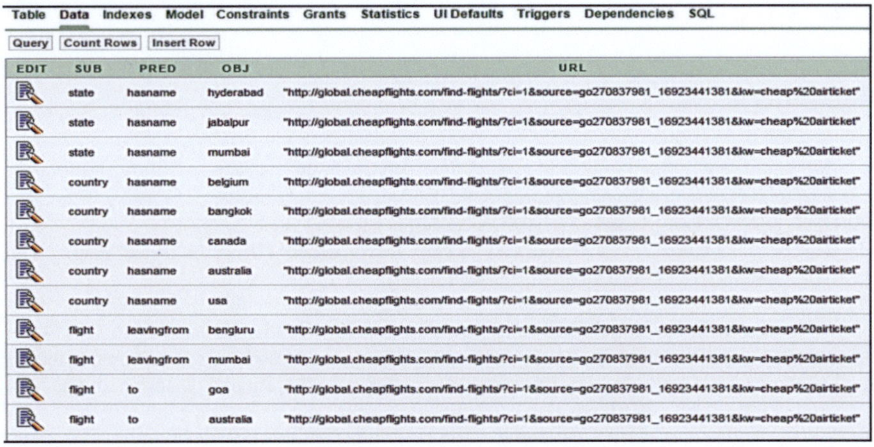
Table Data Indexes Model Constraints Grants Statistics UI Defaults Triggers Dependencies SQL

Query | Count Rows | Insert Row

EDIT	SUB	PRED	OBJ	URL
	state	hasname	hyderabad	"http://global.cheapflights.com/find-flights/?ci=1&source=go270837981_16923441381&kw=cheap%20airticket"
	state	hasname	jabalpur	"http://global.cheapflights.com/find-flights/?ci=1&source=go270837981_16923441381&kw=cheap%20airticket"
	state	hasname	mumbai	"http://global.cheapflights.com/find-flights/?ci=1&source=go270837981_16923441381&kw=cheap%20airticket"
	country	hasname	belgium	"http://global.cheapflights.com/find-flights/?ci=1&source=go270837981_16923441381&kw=cheap%20airticket"
	country	hasname	bangkok	"http://global.cheapflights.com/find-flights/?ci=1&source=go270837981_16923441381&kw=cheap%20airticket"
	country	hasname	canada	"http://global.cheapflights.com/find-flights/?ci=1&source=go270837981_16923441381&kw=cheap%20airticket"
	country	hasname	australia	"http://global.cheapflights.com/find-flights/?ci=1&source=go270837981_16923441381&kw=cheap%20airticket"
	country	hasname	usa	"http://global.cheapflights.com/find-flights/?ci=1&source=go270837981_16923441381&kw=cheap%20airticket"
	flight	leavingfrom	bengluru	"http://global.cheapflights.com/find-flights/?ci=1&source=go270837981_16923441381&kw=cheap%20airticket"
	flight	leavingfrom	mumbai	"http://global.cheapflights.com/find-flights/?ci=1&source=go270837981_16923441381&kw=cheap%20airticket"
	flight	to	goa	"http://global.cheapflights.com/find-flights/?ci=1&source=go270837981_16923441381&kw=cheap%20airticket"
	flight	to	australia	"http://global.cheapflights.com/find-flights/?ci=1&source=go270837981_16923441381&kw=cheap%20airticket"

Fig. 10 Snapshot of semantic database in Oracle 10 g in form of <SPO> for airline domain

Query Count Rows Insert Row

EDIT	SUB	PRED	OBJ
	OperatingSystems:InternalsandDesignPrinciples(0133805913)	published in	December 2012
	OperatingSystems:InternalsandDesignPrinciples(0133805913)	has ISBN	0133805913
	OperatingSystems:InternalsandDesignPrinciples(0133805913)	written by	AbrahamSilberschatz
	AbrahamSilberschatz	haswritten	OperatingSystems:InternalsandDesignPrinciples(0133805913)
	GregGagne	haswritten	OperatingSystems:InternalsandDesignPrinciples(0133805913)
	Peter Galvin	haswritten	OperatingSystems:InternalsandDesignPrinciples(0133805913)
	Thomas Anderson	haswritten	Operating Systems: Principles and Practice 0985673516
	Michael Dahlin	haswritten	Operating Systems: Principles and Practice 0985673516
	Andrew S. Tanenbaum	haswritten	Operating Systems Design and Implementation 8120329554
	Albert Woodhull	haswritten	Operating Systems Design and Implementation 8120329554
	Tom Carpenter	haswritten	Microsoft Windows Operating System Essentials 1118195523
	Lee Rainie	haswritten	Networked: The New Social Operating System 0262526166
	Wiley	has published	OperatingSystems:InternalsandDesignPrinciples(8thEdition)0133805913
	OperatingSystems:InternalsandDesignPrinciples(0133805913)	published in	December 2012
	OperatingSystems:InternalsandDesignPrinciples(0133805913)	has ISBN	0133805913

Fig. 11 Snapshot of semantic database in Oracle 10 g in form of <SPO> for Book domain

6 Conclusion and Future Scope

Many systems have been developed to store information of a particular domain in relational database. But with the help of ontology one can successfully create semantic database in Oracle. The work discussed above mainly focused on storing in the form of RDF triples. And in future work the instance values stored in database will be used to fill the Hidden Web form interfaces. This database can also be used in future to map two ontologies. A hidden Web crawler will be implemented based upon above work which will download the form interfaces and those interfaces will be filled with the help of above ontology database. Then after getting the resultant pages they will be filtered and shown to user.

References

1. Bergman, M.K. The Deep Web: Surfacing Hidden Value September 2001, http://www.brightplanet.com/deepcontent/tutorials/DeepWeb/deepwebwhitepaper.pdf (2001)
2. OWL Web Ontology Language Reference. http://www.w3.org
3. Noy, N.F., Deborah, L.: McGuinness: Ontology Development 101. A Guide to Creating Your First Ontology Stanford University, Stanford, CA
4. Manvi et al.: Design of an Ontology based Adaptive Crawler for Hidden Web. In: IEEE International Conference, CSNT 2013, http://dx.doi.org/10.1109/CSNT.2013.14 (2013)
5. Bhatia, K.K., Sharma, A.K., Madaan, R.: AKSHR: a novel framework for a domain-specific hidden web crawler. In: 1st International Conference On Parallel Distributed and Grid Computing (PDGC 2010)
6. Sriram, R., Garcia, M.H.: Crawling the Hidden Web. Stanford University

7. Ntoulas, A.: Downloading Textual Hidden-Web Content Through Keyword Querie. University of California, Los Angeles
8. El-desoky, A.I.: Exploiting ontology for retrieving data behind searchable web forms. In: International Conference on Networking and Media Convergence (2009)
9. Liang et. al.: Extracting Attributes from Deep Web Interface Using Instances, World Congress on Computer Science and Information Engineering, IEEE (2009).
10. Jung, et al.: Semantic Deep Web: Automatic Attribute Extraction from the Deep Web Data Sources. Department of Computer Science, New Jersey Institute of Technology, SAC'07, 11–15 Mar 2007 (2007)
11. Swoogle, Semantic Web Search Engine, Swoogle.umbc.edu
12. Manvi, et. al.: Generating domain specific ontology for hidden web, 01–02 March 2014. In: IEEE International Conference at GLA Mathura, ISCON (2014)

Importance of SLA in Cloud Computing

Angira Ghosh Chowdhury and Ajanta Das

Abstract Cloud computing can be thought of as service provider that involves delivering hosted services over the Internet. It does not mean handling of the application using local or personal resources nor using the dedicated network to provide service like office or home network. Consumers and providers both need to face some challenges in spite of accessing many utilities as a process in cloud computing. Service level agreement (SLA) is a common legal document where both the party needs to agree to the terms and conditions for provisioning and consuming the service. Hence, SLA plays a major role in cloud computing in order to access service as expected with a few realistic limitations. The objective of this paper is to explain briefly the importance of SLA in cloud computing along with phases of its lifecycle, template, and parameters. This paper also proposes sample SLA template on which basis service provisioning and monitoring being carried out successfully.

Keywords Cloud computing · Service level agreement (SLA) · Service monitoring

1 Introduction

Cloud Computing has brought a revolution in providing service. Service is a self-containing and self-describing piece of code which can be discovered. Every utility starting from infrastructure or hardware, platform or operating system and software or application can be provided as service through the cloud. Provider use

A.G. Chowdhury (✉)
Department of Electronics and Information Technology, National Informatics Centre, West Bengal State Centre, Kolkata 700091, India
e-mail: angira.chowdhury@nic.in

A. Das
Department of Computer Science & Engineering Kolkata Campus, Birla Institute of Technology, Mesra, Kolkata 700107, India
e-mail: ajantadas@bitmesra.ac.in

V.B. Aggarwal et al. (eds.), *Big Data Analytics*, Advances in Intelligent Systems and Computing 654, https://doi.org/10.1007/978-981-10-6620-7_15

"Multi-Tenancy", where the pool of resources are shared among multiple clients. Services in cloud is provided on pay-as-you-use basis, i.e., with proper terms and conditions consumers can access the service and need to pay according to usage. Permanent hardware, software buying is no longer required at consumer side. Hence, cloud computing is cost effective and becoming more popular. A piece of formal agreement will be very helpful in doing the business such a way that nobody suffers. There will be penalties for wrong access or incurred losses.

Service Level Agreement or SLA is a very important part of contract note between cloud provider and consumer. As providers are selling cloud service on shared mode, also they have different resource provisioning plans and consumers are paying for their usage. It is essential to create an agreement based on specific criteria metric for demand by consumers and duration of usage and price, penalties for non-fulfillment of promises made or over usage. The SLA is "the formal legal document" which gives a target to the provider for service provision and to consumers SLA gives metric to monitor and assess the usage of resources. Provider or consumer can only set target or challenge against non-fulfillment of promises with the help of formal legal document. A standard, clear unambiguous SLA helps both parties involved in provisioning and monitoring services.

Objective of this paper is to explain briefly the importance of SLA in cloud computing along with phases of its lifecycle, template, and parameters. This paper also proposes sample SLA template on which basis service provisioning and monitoring being carried out successfully. SLA provides a basic foundation for provisioning of services in future. Organization of the paper as follows: Sect. 2 presents related work and overview of cloud computing is presented in Sect. 3. Details of service level agreement with its different phases of lifecycle, template definition and parameters are studied and discussed in Sect. 4. Service monitoring is carried out at a regular interval based on sample SLA template definition. This has been explained in Sects. 5 and 6 concludes the paper.

2 Related Work

This section presents the study of related work in the SLA-based cloud computing research and finalizes its motivation. According to Chouhan et al. [2], SLA is not only a piece of document it provides the necessary parameters to compare different service provider. This paper proposes an algorithm for parameter matching in the cloud by comparing different SLAs. Alhamad et al. in [1] provided a conceptual SLA framework and detailed listing of the parameter for different service models.

Patel et al. [7] discussed how to use Web Service Level Agreement (WSLA) in cloud computing architecture as cloud also works on service mode. In Keller et al. [6] proposed a WSLA framework in order to define and monitor SLAs related to dynamic e-business. In [8], the research is a detailed technical report for monitoring quality of service in web service presented by Zegnis and Plexousakis. It also contains discussion on SLA framework. This research work studies the phases of

SLA lifecycle, template, and parameters. Finally, this paper proposes a non-functional or general xml schema and standard SLA template with some service level metric for SaaS.

3 Overview of Cloud Computing

Cloud enables access to information from any web-enabled hardware and provides the facility to run the service from many devices at the same time. Though resources are distributed in nature but essential difference between distributed computing and cloud is dedicated network Vs internet or web. Cloud Service is essentially distributed in nature comprising of main three service models, i.e., "IaaS", "PaaS", "SaaS" and four deployment model, i.e., "Private", "Public", "Community" and "Hybrid" clouds [4].

In spite of accessing many utilities as a process, some of the challenging issues in cloud computing are Security, Terms, and Condition of Service Usage, Technical Difficulties and Downtime and Lack of control and flexibility. To overcome the challenges of hosting the service in cloud nowadays SLA-based provisioning, as well as monitoring of services, are required. As promises are meant to be broken so a legal formal document is needed to be verified for any claim.

4 Service Level Agreement

Service level agreement (SLA) is the formal contract between provider and consumers of service which formally states the objective of the services and quality of output. Role and responsibilities of provider and consumers are also defined in this agreement. It is desirable that based on customers expectation and service limitations a realistic target is defined in SLA. SLA sets the standardized expectations and obligations of both parties and acts as a roadmap to the successful implementation of service. SLA acts as a future foundation for provisioning and monitoring of services in cloud computing.

Consumers need SLAs to specify their requirements regarding quality of service, security, and a backup plan for performance failure. SLA also includes the list of parameters which cloud provider wants to be excluded from the contract signed with consumers. However, consumers are free to choose between different service providers. As proposed in Cloud Standardization Guidelines [3] SLA should be platform independent, business neutral, technology independent, worldwide applicable. It is possible to define different types of SLA related to the same service. As the consumers (single user, medium business consumer and corporate users) vary, the expectations and terms and conditions will be changed. Service-Based SLA emphasizes on providers restrictions while Customer-Based SLA prioritizes consumers need or requirement.

4.1 SLA Life Cycle

General awareness of all the phases of SLA life cycle is essential for both the parties before making the agreement. Different phases proposed by Zegnis and Plexousakis [8] are described below:

(a) *Service and SLA Template Development*: This phase identifies SLA parameters and its measurement metrics according to consumer requirement.
(b) *Negotiation*: Maximum and minimum values to be set for each SLA parameter identified in earlier phase, price for service provisioning, penalty of violation of terms, termination or renewal conditions are negotiated in this phase.
(c) *Preparation*: Configuring runtime environment of service, i.e., resource allocation as per the SLA and final deployment.
(d) *Execution*: Execution phase includes two sub phases service execution and service monitoring based on collection of SLA parameter at runtime.
(e) *Assessment*: Each SLA parameter is assessed against monitored value and defined formulas for specified metric related to this parameter.
(f) *Renewal or termination*: It defines the validity period for each contract. On completion of this period, SLA will be renewed or terminated.

4.2 SLA Template

First and foremost task for SLA-based management is to formalize an SLA template. Standard SLA template will bring clarity and understanding on how the target will be achieved by the service. Comparable SLA can be prepared using a standard template. A standard SLA template consists of the following characteristics:

(a) *Purpose*: It establishes the goal of this agreement.
(b) *Stakeholders*: It includes participants in the agreement establishment process and their role.
(c) *Validity Period*: The period up to which the agreement will be valid.
(d) *Review Period*: Interval after which service will be assessed or reviewed.
(e) *SLA Parameter*: It includes non-functional objectives of the service through different parameters. These parameters, values are computed and verified through the metric using formula.
(f) *Penalties*: It is a boost for the reputation of the service provider. The penalty for non-fulfillment of the target by the provider or over usage by the consumer may be stated here.
(g) *Exclusion Terms*: Provider or consumer may put some exclusion term (e.g., Network provider's speed) which will not be covered by SLA.

4.3 Parameters

According to SLA life cycle and SLA template discussed so far it is found that to implement SLA-based monitoring and assessment, identification of service level parameter and objective of each parameter (SLO) is a very important factor. Key performances indicators (KPI) are measurable metric with threshold/boundary value (Maximum-Minimum value). KPI is used to decide whether SLOs are fulfilled are not. KPI are different for different cloud services.

Some important SLA parameters are Availability, Response time, Cost/Billing, Reliability, Usability, Customizability, and Scalability. To monitor these parameters KPI metrics need to be identified. For example, Uptime and Percentage of the successful request are KPIs for Availability parameter.

5 Service Monitoring Based on SLA

In cloud computing, service needs to be monitored based on signed SLA. SLA or KPI defined in SLA plays a critical role in determining whether SLOs are achieved or violated. SLOs can be achieved only when all the KPIs are within the range of agreed or negotiated values for each SLA parameter. KPIs are metric for data collection which generally contains raw data. KPI constraints are generally minimum, maximum values, but it also includes average value. State of SLA parameters can be calculated through KPI data. If for each SLA parameter, calculated value from each KPI metrics are within their limit of defined constraints then only SLO for that parameter is achieved. This paper proposes SLA template and presented in Fig. 1.

Although services could be scalable in large scale cost effectively some challenges exist with SLA parameters. According to [7], three common web-based SLA level services exist which can be adapted to cloud context. These services are briefly mentioned in the following:

(i) *Measurement Service*: Measures the runtime parameters (response time, throughput, duration of usage and price per usage) which dynamically changes with clients' or consumers' demand.
(ii) *Condition Evaluation Service*: It considers input as obtained from *Measurement Service* and evaluates SLO and check whether any violation happens.
(iii) *Management Service*: considers remedial steps (financial penalties, restoration support, etc.) in case of non-fulfillment of service level objectives.

Private clouds afford consumers direct access to monitoring the computing, network, and storage elements. However, in public cloud, they lose direct control of —and visibility over—the assets comprising the services.

```
<xs:element name="sla_preparation">
    <xs:complexType>
        <xs:sequence>
            <xs:element name="purpose" type="xs:string"/>
            <xs:element name="Stakeholders" type="xs:string"/>
                <xs:complexType>
                    <xs:sequence>
                        <xs:element name="provider_name" type="xs:string"/>
                        <xs:element name="consumer_name" type="xs:string"/>
                    </xs:sequence>
                </xs:complexType>
            <xs:element name="validity_period" type="xs:string"/>
            <xs:element name="review_period" type="xs:string"/>
            <xs:element name="parameter_name">
                <xs:complexType>
                    <xs:sequence>
                        <xs:element name="id" type="xs:string"/>
                        <xs:element name="description" type="xs:string"/>
                        <xs:element name="measure_metric">
                            <xs:complexType>
                                <xs:sequence>
                                    <xs:element name="metric_id" type="xs:string"/>
                                    <xs:element name="metric_name" type="xs:string"/>
                                    <xs:element name="agreed_value" type="xs:string"/>
                                    <xs:element name="start_time" type="xs:string"/>
                                    <xs:element name="end_time" type="xs:string"/>
                                </xs:sequence>
                            </xs:complexType>
                        </xs:element>
                    </xs:sequence>
                </xs:complexType>
            </xs:element>
            <xs:element name="penalty" type="xs:string"/>
            <xs:element name="exclusion_term" type="xs:string"/>
        </xs:sequence>
    </xs:complexType>
</xs:element>
```

Fig. 1 SLA Template

6 Conclusion

This paper presents the overall importance of SLA in cloud computing. Quality of service (QoS) is inevitable in the cloud as everything in cloud computing is delivered as service. The ability to deliver QoS guaranteed services and to retain QoS are crucial in cloud computing. SLA plays an important role in this scenario. This paper studies the phases of SLA lifecycle, template and parameters from various existing research work. Then it also proposes a non-functional and standard SLA template with some service level metrics for evaluation. As clearly defined targets reduce the chances of customer disappointments. These targets also help provider to stay focused on customer requirements and ensures that the internal processes remain in right track.

References

1. Alhamad, M., Dillon, T., Chang, E.: Conceptual SLA framework for cloud computing. In: Network-Based Information Systems (NBiS), 2010 13th International Conference, Sep 2010, pp. 321–324 (2010)

2. Chouhan, T., Chaudhary, S., Kumar, V., Minal, V.: Service Level Agreement Parameter Matching in cloud computing. In: Information and Communication Technologies (WICT), 2011 World Congress on 2011 (2011)
3. C-SIG, Brussels: Cloud service level agreement standardization guidelines. In: Digital Agenda for Europe Newsroom Editor on 26 June 2014 (2014)
4. Dillon, T., Wu, C., Chang, E.: Cloud computing: issues and challenges. In: 24th International Conference on Advanced Information Networking and Applications (2010)
5. Frey, S., Luthje, C., Reich, C.: Key performance indicators for cloud computing SLAs. In: Emerging 2013: The Fifth International Conference on Emerging Network Intelligence (2013)
6. Keller, A., Ludwig, H.: Defining and monitoring service level agreements for dynamic e-business. In: Proceedings of the 16th System Administration Conference (2002)
7. Patel, P., Ranabahu, A., Sheth, A.: Service Level Agreement in Cloud Computing. In: 2009-corescholar.librarie.wright.edu (2009)
8. Zegnis, C., Plexousakis, D.: Monitoring the QoS of Web Services using SLAs. In: ICS-FORTH Technical Report, 2010

A Survey on Cloud Computing

Mohammad Ubaidullah Bokhari, Qahtan Makki and Yahya Kord Tamandani

Abstract Cloud computing technology is the way to provide everything to clients as services through internet connection. Using this technology the clients would be able to rent the required services via web browsers. This study gives a proper definition to cloud computing, highlighted the related technologies, the essential characteristics, cloud architecture and components. Comparison among three service models (SaaS, PaaS, and IaaS) as well as deployment models: private, public, and community cloud has been given. Furthermore, the chapter includes information security requirements of public and private cloud according to different service models. The aim of this chapter is to giving the researchers a clear vision about this technology and the information security requirements for private and public cloud as well as the main security issues for future researches.

Keywords Cloud computing · Service models · Cloud architecture · Security requirements · Deployment models

1 Introduction

According to US NIST (National Institute of Standards and Technology), Cloud computing is a style of providing unlimited shared pool resources such as (Hardware/Software) to client as soon as requested through the internet, these resources can be automatically scaled up and down according to the client's demand [1–3].

M.U. Bokhari · Q. Makki (✉) · Y.K. Tamandani
Department of Computer Science, Aligarh Muslim University, Aligarh, India
e-mail: qahtan.mekki@yahoo.com

M.U. Bokhari
e-mail: mubokhari.cs@amu.ac.in

Y.K. Tamandani
e-mail: Yahya.kord@gmail.com

V.B. Aggarwal et al. (eds.), *Big Data Analytics*, Advances in Intelligent Systems and Computing 654, https://doi.org/10.1007/978-981-10-6620-7_16

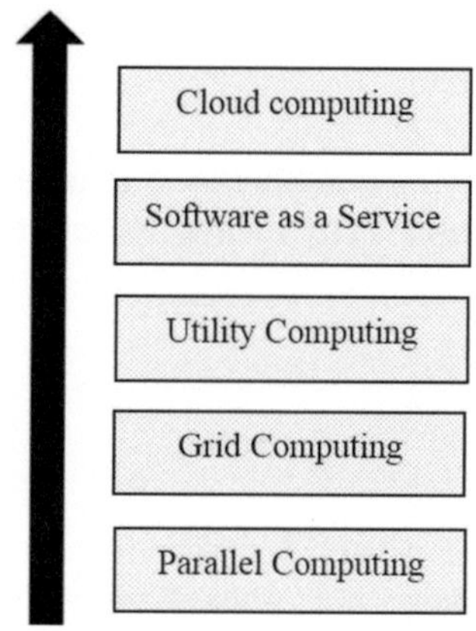

Fig. 1 Cloud computing evolution

Leonard Kleinrock which is the chief scientists of the original Advanced Research Projects Agency Network (ARPANET) made a prediction on 1969 by saying that "At this moment, computer networks still are in their early stages, however as they grow up and turn to be sophisticated, we will most likely notice the spread of 'computer utilities' including present electric and telephone utilities, which would service individual homes and offices throughout the country" [4, 5]. In 1990 the grid computing has been issued to allow the user to have computing power on request [6–8]. The cloud computing became famous and gained increasing attention when Google and IBM have cooperated to promote it in October 2007 [9–11]. Figure 1 depicts the cloud computing evolution.

The current chapter proceeds as follows: in Sect. 2 we have given a brief detail about some related technologies to cloud. Section 3 explains the five essential characteristics. Section 4 explains the components of cloud computing. Section 5 describes the Cloud computing architecture. Section 6 describes the different deployment models. Section 7 explained the security challenges in cloud computing. Finally, we conclude this chapter in Sect. 8.

2 Related Technologies

The paradigm of cloud computing has contribution of many technologies such as parallel computing, grid computing, utility computing, virtualization, Autonomic computing, Ubiquitous computing, Software as a service, web 2.0, distributed computing, and web 2.0. We will explain some of the technologies which related to cloud computing.

2.1 Parallel Computing

The concept of parallel computing is to divide the computing problem which is scientific into many small tasks, and run them at the same time on a parallel computer [12]. Usually, the parallel computing is used whenever need of high computing performance, such as in the field of energy exploration, military, medicine, and biotechnology. A parallel computer is a set of many homogeneous processing units, which are able to solve large computational problems faster through collaboration and communication [13, 14].

2.2 Grid

Grid is the technique which is used to shift the workload to the place which requires the computing resources that are remote and immediately available to be used. It is split the one main task into many subtasks to be executed in parallel, applications are also required by the grid to verify grid software interfaces [15].

2.3 Utility Computing

It provides the resources based on the client's demand and charging them according to the usage [16]. It uses a fully utility-based pricing scheme for making reasonable charges to clients. With the ability of providing the resources on-demand and fully based pricing scheme, the utility computing maximizes the use of resources and minimizes the cost of providing resources [5, 17].

2.4 Virtualization

The virtualization technology is presented since 40 years back but there was a limitation for the application of virtualization by the technologies, the limitation has been exposed to be depended by cloud computing as a major technology [6]. Virtualization is a technology that separates the underlying physical hardware and provides virtualized resources to the applications [5]. A typical server is capable of hosting a number of virtual machine instances, consequently giving the ability to customize the software on-demand. So this is the technology of providing the virtual server to the client-based on-demand such as VMware, vCloud, Amazon EC2, and others [6]. Virtualization is the basis of cloud computing, as it enables the pooling of computing resources from a group of server which is clusters and dynamically assigns the virtual resources to the client as required and reassigns once unrequired [5]. The virtualization is attractive technology due to the ability of isolation and customization environments with little impact on performance [5, 18, 19].

2.5 Autonomic Computing

Presented in 2001 by IBM, it is constructed of many computing systems to make them able to do self-management such as automatic observations to external and internal and acting without any human interaction [20]. The main purpose of autonomic computing is to control over the complexity of computer systems. Also cloud computing has another powerful feature which is automatic resource provisioning in order to reduce the cost of resources rather than decreasing the complexity of the system [5, 21].

2.6 Ubiquitous Computing

The idea of Ubiquitous computing has been presented by Mark Weiser in 1988 as well as predicted that this method would be pervasive. In 1990, people got an extensive attention to the concept of pervasive computing and they started step by step exciting to Ubiquitous computing idea. Officially the concept has been proposed by IBM in 1999. In 1999, the first session has been held by IBM. In 2000, the first International Conference on Pervasive Computing has been held. Furthermore, the IEEE Pervasive Computing journal is founded in 2002 [22]. One of many significant goals in ubiquitous computing is to enable the computer equipment to feel the changes in surrounding environment and to modify the behaviors according to those changes. Radio network technology has been used in Pervasive computing in order to make users able to access the information without any limitations of place and time [13, 22].

2.7 Software as a Service

It is a web-based software application which is providing a software to subscribers, SaaS is a model of software attribution in which the applications have designed to be delivered through the network. This model almost priced in a package format such as monthly paying, this monthly paying will be cover the maintenance cost of applications, license fee and the cost of technical support. SaaS model can be considered as the best option to use the advanced technologies for the small and medium companies [13, 23].

3 Cloud Computing Characteristics

According to National Institute of Standard Technology (NIST, U.S. Department of Commerce), there are five essential characteristics of cloud computing mentioned below [24].

3.1 On-Demand Self-service

On-demand means that the clients can access to resources immediately as requested. Self-service means that the provision of resources will be automatically and without any human interaction [9, 25].

3.2 Broad Network Access

The resources of cloud computing are accessible and deliverable through the network and used by many client applications with a different type of platforms (such as mobile phone and PDAs) [2, 8, 24, 25].

3.3 Resource Pooling

The provider's resources are collected to be used by multiple clients using a multi-tenant type, with different resources which are assigned and reassigned dynamically according to client's order [2, 25].

3.4 Elasticity

The cloud computing has a unlimited number of resources, these resources can be provided from provider to clients at any time and quantity. The provided resource can be increased automatically when application load increase and vice versa [9, 25].

3.5 Measured Service

Although the resources of computing are shared and pooled by many different clients (such as multitenancy), the infrastructure of the cloud is having the ability to use suitable mechanisms to measure what each individual client has used the resources [25]. The rate of hire is different from a cloud provider to another [8].

4 Cloud Computing Components

The three major components of cloud computing are: Clients, Data center, and distributed servers as shown in Fig. 2. Each component has a specific purpose and role. We will illustrate each of them as below [24].

4.1 Clients

It is the devices which are used by end-user to manage his resources in cloud, these devices could be desktop, laptop, smartphone, iPad, and so on. Thin client does not need to have a high-speed processor and big data storage, it needs to be able to run a web browser such as (Google Chrome, Firefox, and so on). The categories of clients could be divided into three types (thin clients, mobile, thick clients) [15, 24].

4.2 Data Center

The applications which are used by the clients of cloud computing are hosted in many numbers of servers, it could be a building or a room which it is not necessary to be in your place but must be accessible by the Internet. Multiple Virtual Machine (VM) can be run together on a single physical server known as a host, the number of VM will be limited to many factors such as type of the applications that are run on virtual server, speed, and size of physical server [15, 26].

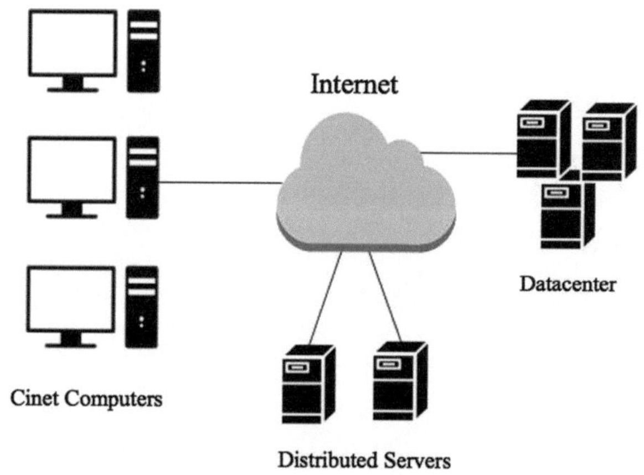

Fig. 2 Main components of a cloud computing solution

4.3 Distributed Servers

In order to provide the reliability and availability to servers, the cloud has distributed the servers in the different geographic area. In the case of failure in the specific server, then the other server will take the action, on the other hand, to increase the scalability when an extra server is needed then simply the new one will be added to the existing one [27].

5 Cloud Computing Architecture

5.1 A Layered Model of Cloud Computing

As Fig. 3 shows, the cloud computing contains a four layer of architecture design, each layer in cloud architecture having the flexibility to cooperate with above and below layers. We will illustrate all of them as below:

1. Application layer:
   The application layer is responsible for running the applications of cloud on the client's PC [15]. The applications in this layer can achieve the automatic-scaling to do a maximum performance [28]. The provider examples are force.com, Microsoft and IBM [29].
2. Platform layer:
   It refers to OS and software. By this service, the client can ensure that he can get an appropriate platform for his application to do his purpose like deployment, development, hosting of web application,and testing. The main goal of platform layer is to decrease the burden of deployment of the application to VM containers directly [29, 30].
3. Infrastructure layer:
   It is responsible for providing the user with hardware and software such as hard disk capacity, the size of RAM, CPU and so on. By the help of virtualization

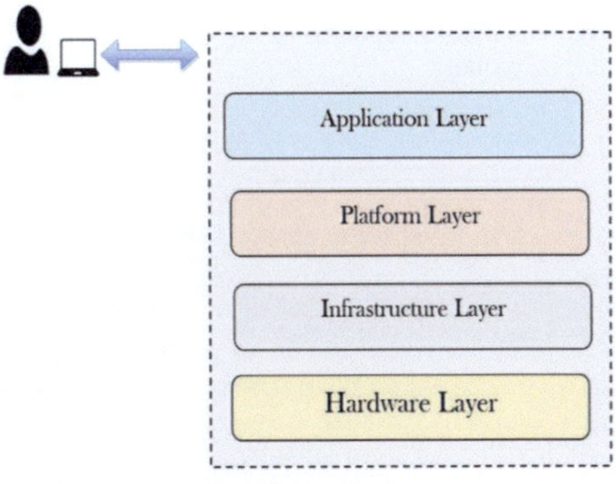

Fig. 3 Cloud computing architecture layers

technology, the infrastructure layer can be divided the physical resources to create the storage pool and computing resources like Xen, KVM, and VMware. Examples of these service providers are GoGrid, Layered technologies Joyent and Flexiscale [29, 30].

4. Hardware layer:
   the purpose of this layer is to do the management for physical resources. The physical resources of the cloud are routers, cooling system, servers, switched, power equipment and so on. This layer is working for the servers of data centers which are connected together by a set of routers, switches, and many other equipment. So the main issues of hardware layer are traffic management, fault tolerance, cooling, and power management and hardware configuration [29, 30].

Each layer of above is able to evolve independently. This architectural modularity enables cloud computing to provide a huge number of application requirements whereas decreasing the maintenance and management overhead.

5.2 *Business Models*

Conceptually, every layer of the architecture described in the previous section can be implemented to the layer above as a service, conversely each layer can be acted as a customer for the below layer. As Fig. 4 shown the service models of cloud computing are consist of three services which are SaaS, PaaS, and IaaS.

1. The Software-As-a-Service Model: The provider allows the user to use provider's software, the software reacts with the user's interface [8, 9, 31]. By using cloud technology, client only has to rent the software via the internet connection, every client in the cloud which using the same software feel that it independently belongs to him only but in the fact it is shared on the same infrastructures [32]. By the technology of cloud, the user can use the software by either participation way or pay per use model. Preliminary statement is needed to find organization particular data for the service to be completely utilized and

Fig. 4 Cloud computing service model

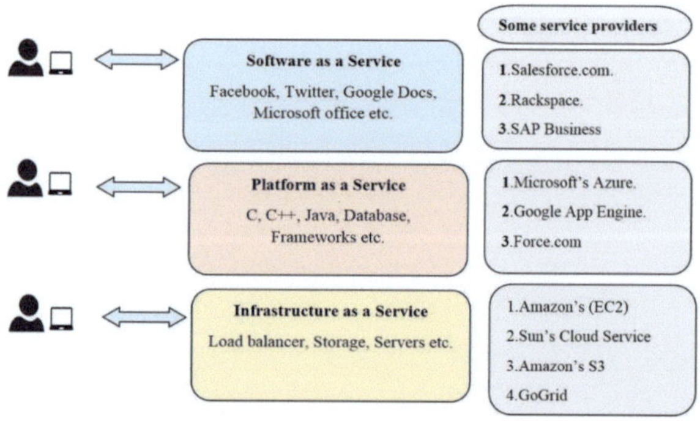

combine with other applications that are not part of the platform of SaaS. The application is handed over through internet to the organization's firewall [11].
2. The Platform-As-a-Service Model: It is used by the clients who are interested to develop the application because the providers are providing the development environment and toolkit [9, 11]. The development toolkits are hosted in the cloud and being used by the clients through web browser [11]. Developers will make the development of applications without taking care of the processor's ability and the size of memory which going to be used by the applications [9, 11]. PaaS is allowing the clients to use platform resources such as operating system support and software frameworks [8].
3. The Infrastructure-As-a-Service Model: As the name refers, it is providing the infrastructure as a service to clients, IT service or data center usage will be measured according to the usage time of CPU per hour, Storage usage and Data transfer per gigabyte [1, 28, 32]. It is provide virtualized resources on request [9]. In IaaS the client has a privilege to do many things like changing firewall rules, install a virtual disk on it, install a software package, on and off the server, and set access license [9, 32].

There are a lot of resources of cloud which cannot classify into IaaS, SaaS or PaaS such as Apple's App Store, online games, and Electric books on Amazon [28]. According to different factors such as service type, user control on, provider control in, flexibility/generality, difficulty level, scale and vendors the comparison among three service models SaaS, PaaS and IaaS has been done as shown in Table 1 [13, 33, 34]:

6 Cloud Computing Deployment Models

There are four types of cloud computing which are public, private, hybrid, and community, each type has different security risk and IT management. We are going to explain each of them as below.

6.1 Public Cloud

It can be reached by public people [8], the services are given by specific provider and mostly being used in the basis of pay per use, or might be offered as free services to clients [1, 9]. The resources are located in the physical location of service provider. It is maintained, owned, managed and operated by third-party vendor [1, 11]. The public cloud providers are: Amazon's AWS (EC2, S3 etc.), Rackspace Cloud Suite, and Microsoft's Azure Service Platform [1, 9].

Table 1 Comparison between SaaS, PaaS and IaaS

Classification	Service type	User control on	Provider control on	Flexibility/generality	Difficulty level	Scale	Level	Vendors
SaaS	Application with specific function	No thing	Application, data, runtime, middleware, O/S, virtualizations, servers, storage, network	Low	Easy	Small	User level	SalesForce.com, Google documents, Facebook.com, Gmail, Hotmail, Quicken Online, IBM®, WebSphere, Oracle on-demand, SAP, Netsuite
PaaS	Application hosting environment	Application, data	Runtime, middleware, O/S, virtualizations, servers, storage, network	Middle	Middle	Middle	Developer level	Google AppEngine, Microsoft Azure, Manjrasoft Aneka, Coghead, Force.com, Yahoo Developer Network, **MSFT,** Heroku, Mosso, Engine Yard
IaaS	Basic computing, storage, network resource	Application, data, runtime, middleware, O/S	Virtualizations, servers, storage, network	High	Difficult	Large	IT level	Amazon EC2 and S3, Nirvanix, Op source, Gogrid, RACKSPACE, IBM BlueHouse, Linode, VMWare

6.2 Private Cloud

The infrastructure of provider is supplied to the organization within its border and is used only by the members of the same organization, also it is not accessible by the other organization [11]. These enable to deliver some advantage of cloud computing like data security, flexibility, scalability, and reliability [9, 11]. The service should be provided behind the firewall to a limit number of people. The organization network and the administrator of data center must be a service provider because of the advance of virtualization and the distributed computing to provide their member in the organization [1]. It could operate, maintain and owned by the same organization [1, 8, 24].

6.3 Community Clouds

It is a set of above different types (private, public), It is used by a group of users which belong to different organizations or group of organizations for special purposes [24], by using Hybrid cloud will give the cloud users the ability to make a new cloud with new attached services. Community cloud could be located either on premise or off premise. For instance is Open Cirrus formed by HP, Intel, Yahoo, and others [9]. The responsibility to build, manage and operate the community cloud could be by one organization, a group of organizations, third-party or gathering of the three [24].

6.4 Hybrid Clouds

Hybrid is an assembly of two clouds or more of above three models (private, public or community) which are stay unique structure, but are limited to each other by standardized or proprietary technology that will make the data and application able to be mobility [9]. Due to a combination of private and public cloud, it allows the organizations to execute both non-core applications and core applications. It has more flexibility and power than public cloud and private cloud itself [8]. Comparison of deployment models: private, public and community cloud according to theoretical chapters based on their advantages and attributes have been given in Table 2. Additionally, the mandatory and optional requirement of security information for public and private cloud according to three service models (SaaS, PaaS, and IaaS) also illustrated in Table 3 [28, 32, 35–38].

Table 2 Comparison of deployment models

	Public	Private	Community
Description	• It is not dedicated to any specific organizations or client • Public clouds are less secure than other types • Reduce cost and risk by flexibly extending the IT infrastructure of consumers	• It is dedicated for a specific organizations or client • Usually the private clouds are installed and constructed by the third parties	• It is dedicated for many organizations that means the infrastructure will be shared among several organizations • It provides higher level of security, policy compliances and privacy
Attributes	• Location of infrastructure is located on the site of provider • Anyone can be consumer of public cloud and without any limitations • Provider is external	• Location of infrastructure is located on the site of consumer • Part or whole of enterprise is consumer of private cloud due to the purpose of confidentiality and security of their personal data • Provider is external or consumer's IT	• Location of infrastructure is located on-premises or off-premises • Members of community are the consumers of community cloud • Provider is external provider or community member
Advantage	• Not difficult to be used and not expensive as all application, storage capacity and bandwidth will be service provider responsibility • It is maintained, owned, managed and operated by third-party vendor • Scalable as the users are required • Only pay whenever we use, so that will not allow the resource to be wasted • Technical expertise is available 24/7	• A private cloud gives the organization high control over the infrastructure and computing resources • It is optimize and maximize the utilization of resources which are available in-house • Saving the cost of transfer the data from the organization's infrastructure to public cloud • It is more secure than public	• The Cost of install a community cloud is cheaper than individual private cloud, because of the division of costs between all participants • It can be constructed and managed either by one organization, a group of organizations, third-party or gathering of the three • Tools existing in community cloud can take the advantage of the information which stored to serve clients and the supply chain

Table 3 Information security requirements for public and private cloud according to three service models

			SaaS	PaaS	IaaS
Information security requirements	Private cloud	Identification and authentication	Mandatory	Optional	Mandatory
		Authorization	Mandatory	Optional	Optional
		Confidentiality	Mandatory	Mandatory	Optional
		Integrity	Mandatory	Mandatory	Optional
		Non-repudiation	Mandatory	Optional	Optional
		Availability	Mandatory	Mandatory	Mandatory
	Public cloud	Identification and authentication	Mandatory	Optional	Mandatory
		Authorization	Mandatory	Mandatory	Mandatory
		Confidentiality	Mandatory	Optional	Optional
		Integrity	Mandatory	Optional	Mandatory
		Non-repudiation	Mandatory	Optional	Optional
		Availability	Optional	Mandatory	Mandatory

7 Security Challenges in Cloud Computing

There are so many advantages of using cloud technology such as unlimited scalability, High performance, reduced upfront investment, Great availability, excellent fault tolerance capacity, and pay per use. On the other hand, the cloud has many disadvantage or risks attached with it. While the cloud is used by many different users and they are sharing the resources, then every user does not know who else is working in same server [39]. Usually, the cloud is located outside of organization's or company's firewall. This will lead to a significant effect on organization's decision toward migrating to cloud [40]. When client decides to migrate his work to the cloud, he must be aware of the challenges in cloud, there are many challenges in the cloud such as below [41–43]:

- Privileged User Access: The data leak risk is increased whenever the client's data got accessed outside the enterprise and the client unable to buy a new membership for verification.
- Data Location: When the user stored his data in cloud that means he might unable to know where the data are stored as well as unable to know from where the data are hosted.
- Investigative Support: If any illegal and inappropriate activity occurred in cloud computing along with client data, in that case, it is impossible to do a proper investigation regarding it.
- Data segregation: The client data exist in the same infrastructure which contain the other clients' data, which are using the services in parallel.

- Recovery: Because of some natural disasters or problems the data center or server will become ruined, the provider of the cloud will inform each client about his data condition.
- Availability: Many users willing to get the services of cloud but the company rang is not always available.
- Regulatory Compliance: The provider of cloud does not ever permits any audits from external and refuses to setup new security certificates to the network.

8 Conclusion

In this chapter, a proper definition has been given to cloud computing technology and various cloud architecture layers. Additionally, cloud service and deployment models are briefly discussed. Comparison of different models of cloud computing services, deployment models: private, public, and community cloud as well as information security requirements of public and private cloud according to different service models have been given. However, cloud computing has many characteristics such as on-demand self-service, broad network access, resource pooling, elasticity and measured service but it cannot be completely trusted. Finally, the main challenges and issues of cloud computing with regards to the security for further researches have been discussed in the chapter.

References

1. Computing, M., Thakral, D., Singh, M.: Virtualization in cloud computing. Int. J. Comput. Sci. Mob. Comput. **3**(5), 1262–1273 (2014)
2. Mell, P., Grance, T.: The NIST definition of cloud computing recommendations of the National Institute of Standards and Technology. NIST Spec. Publ. **145**, 7 (2011)
3. Armbrust, M., Fox, A., Griffith, R., Joseph, A.D., Katz, R.H., Konwinski, A., Lee, G., Patterson, D.A., Rabkin, A.: Above the clouds: A Berkeley View of cloud computing, (2009)
4. Kleinrock, L.: A vision for the internet. ST J. Res. **2**(1), 4–5 (2005)
5. Kim, W.: Cloud computing: today and tomorrow. J. Object Technol. **8**(1) (2009)
6. Foster, I., Zhao, Y., Raicu, I., Lu, S.: Cloud computing and grid computing 360-degree compared. Grid Comput. Environ. Work 1–10 (2008)
7. Buyya, R., Sulistio, A.: Service and utility oriented distributed computing systems : challenges and opportunities for modeling and simulation communities utility-oriented computing systems. Symp. A.Q. J. Mod. For. Lit. 68–81 (2008)
8. Grids, M.C. Computing and global grids: an introduction, pp. 3–27 (1801)
9. IBM: Google and IBM announced university initiative to address internet-scale computing challenges, 8 Oct 2007
10. Vouk, M.: Cloud computing—Issues, research and implementations. In: 30th International Conference on Information Technology Interfaces, pp. 235–246 (2008)
11. Hashemi, S.M.S.M.S.M., Bardsiri, A.K.: Cloud computing vs. grid computing. ARPN J. Syst. Softw. **2**(5), 188–194 (2012)

12. Ye, S.J., Min, Z.L.: Research on MPI based on cloud computing. J. Converg. Inf. Technol. **8**, 8 (2013)
13. Doukas, C.: An introduction to cloud computing. Build. Internet Things Arduino **2**, 42–59 (2012)
14. Golub, G.H., Ortega, J.M.: Scientific Computing: An Introduction with Parallel Computing. Elsevier, Amsterdam (2014)
15. Jadeja, Y.: Cloud computing—concepts, architecture and challenges. In: International Conference on Computing, Electronics and Electrical Technologies (2012)
16. Espadas, J., Molina, A., Jimenez, G., Molina, M., Ramirez, R., Concha, D.: A tenant-based resource allocation model for scaling software-as-a-service applications over cloud computing infrastructures. Futur. Gener. Comput. Syst. **29**(1), 273–286 (2013)
17. Ben-Yehuda, O.A., et al.: The rise of RaaS: the resource-as-a-service cloud. Commun. ACM, **57**(7) (2014)
18. Xavier, M.G., et al.: Performance evaluation of container-based virtualization for high performance computing environments. 2013 21st Euromicro International Conference on Parallel, Distributed and Network-Based Processing (PDP). IEEE (2013)
19. Jain, R., Paul, S.: Network virtualization and software defined networking for cloud computing: a survey. IEEE Commun. Mag. **51**(11), 24–31 (2013)
20. Frei, R., McWilliam, R., Derrick, B., Purvis, A., Tiwari, A., Di Marzo Serugendo, G.: Self-healing and self-repairing technologies. Int. J. Adv. Manuf. Technol. **69**(5–8), 1033–1061 (2013)
21. Lalanda, P., McCann, J.A., Diaconescu, A.: Autonomic Computing: Principles, Design and Implementation. Springer, Berlin (2013)
22. Baecker, R.M. (ed.).: Readings in Human-Computer Interaction: Toward the Year 2000. Morgan Kaufmann, Burlington (2014)
23. Tiwari, S.D., Mahesh, Ku., Preeti, M.: Cloud computing: implementation of software as a service (SaaS) multitenancy. Ed. Cloud Distrib. Comput. Adv. Appl. **2** (2013)
24. Sun and Sun.: Cloud Computing at a Higher Level, pp. 1–22 (2009)
25. Gong, Y., Ying, Z., Lin, M.: A survey of cloud computing. In: Proceedings of the 2nd International Conference on Green Communications and Networks 2012 (GCN 2012), vol. 3. Springer, Berlin (2013)
26. Rountree, D., Ileana, C.: The Basics of Cloud Computing: Understanding the Fundamentals of Cloud Computing in Theory and Practice. Newnes (2013)
27. Zhang, Q., Zhu, Q., Zhani, M., Boutaba, R.: Dynamic service placement in geographically distributed clouds. In: Proceedings of the 32nd IEEE International Conference on Distributed Computing Systems (ICDCS 2012)
28. Zhang, Q., Cheng, L., Boutaba, R.: Cloud computing: state-of-the-art and research challenges. J. Internet Serv. Appl. **1**(1), 7–18 (2010)
29. Dinh, H., Lee, C., Niyato, D., Wang, P.: A survey of mobile cloud computing: architecture, applications, and approaches. In: Wireless Communications and Mobile Computing (2011)
30. Kavis, M.J.: Architecting the cloud: design decisions for cloud computing service models (SaaS, PaaS, AND IaaS). Wiley, New York (2014)
31. MirMirashe, S.P., Kalyankar, N.V.: Cloud computing. Commun. ACM **51**(7), 9 (2010). doi:10.1145/358438.349303ashe
32. Buyya, R., Broberg, J., Goscinski, A. (eds.) Cloud Computing: Principles and Paradigms. Wiley, New York. ISBN-13: 978-0470887998, Feb 2011
33. Khurana, S., Verma, A.G.: Comparison of cloud computing service models: SaaS, PaaS, IaaS. Int. J. Electron. Commun. Technol. **7109**, 29–32 (2013)
34. Wyld, D.C.: The utility of cloud computing as a new pricing and consumption - model for information technology. Int.J. Database Manage. Syst. **1**(1) (2009)
35. Hemamalini, B.H., Suresh, L., Radhika, K.R.: A survey on cloud computing. Int. J. Math. Comput. Res. **1**(11), 303–305 (2013)

36. Branch, R., Tjeerdsma, H., Wilson, C., Hurley, R., Mcconnell, S.: Cloud computing and big data: a review of current service models and hardware perspectives. J. Softw. Eng. Appl. **7**(7), 686–693 (2014)
37. Lecznar, M., Patig, S.: Cloud computing providers: characteristics and recommendations. Lect. Notes Bus. Inf. Process **78**, 32–45 (2011)
38. Ramgovind, S., Eloff, M., Smith, E.: The management of security in cloud computing. Inf. Secur. South Afr. 1–7 (2010)
39. Zhao, L., et al.: Cloud Data Management. Springer, Berlin (2014)
40. Modi, C., Patel, D., Borisaniya, B., Patel, A., Rajarajan, M.: A survey on security issues and solutions at different layers of Cloud computing, pp. 1–32 (2012)
41. Tana, X., Aib, B.: The issues of cloud computing security in high-speed railway. In: IEEE International Conference on Electronic & Mechanical Engineering and Information Technology, vol. 8, pp. 4358–4363, Aug 2011
42. Dogra, N., Kaur, H.: Cloud computing security: issues and concerns. Int. J. Emerg. Technol. Adv. Eng. **3**(3) (2013)
43. Grover J., Sharma, M.: Cloud computing and its security issues—a review (2014)

Adapting and Reducing Cost in Cloud Paradigm (ARCCP)

Khushboo Tripathi and Dharmender Singh Kushwaha

Abstract Cloud computing paradigm has been gaining popularity day by day. This is because of the enormous benefits it offers to the user or provider. The upfront cost of setting up a business is greatly reduced by adopting the required delivery models such as platform, software or application as service. In terms of storage, it provides formidable redundancy and guarantees at much lower prices as compared to setting up own data centers. These enormous benefits come at cost and ways and means have to be adopted in order to reduce the recurring and non-recurring cost involved in embracing this technology. Numerous researchers have proposed various solutions for reducing the Cloud Application Development and Deployment cost reduction strategies and techniques. Few authors have proposed efficient service discovery techniques. Others have studied the impact of data transfer from one Virtual machine (VM) to other VM, when both these are on one physical machine or two different machines. Yet, few authors have worked on Multitenant databases for cost reduction. In those situations, where returns on investment fall into high-risk category, Ad Hoc Cloud paradigm has been proposed.

Keywords Cloud security · Multi-tenant database · High availability · Load balancing · DML queries

1 Introduction

The enormous benefits of adopting cloud paradigm come at cost and ways and means have to be adopted in order to reduce the recurring and non-recurring cost involved in embracing this technology. Numerous researchers have proposed

K. Tripathi (✉)
CSE Department, ASET, AUH, Allahabad, India
e-mail: Khushboo83@live.com

D.S. Kushwaha
MNNIT Allahabad, Allahabad, India
e-mail: dsk@mnnit.ac.in

V.B. Aggarwal et al. (eds.), *Big Data Analytics*, Advances in Intelligent Systems and Computing 654, https://doi.org/10.1007/978-981-10-6620-7_17

various solutions for reducing the Cloud Application Development and Deployment cost reduction strategies and techniques. Few authors have proposed efficient service discovery techniques. Others have studied the impact of data transfer from one Virtual machine (VM) to other VM, when both these are on one physical machine or two different machines. Yet, few authors have worked on Multitenant databases for cost reduction. In those situations, where returns on investment fall into high-risk category, Ad Hoc Cloud paradigm has been proposed.

The trust in the cloud delivery model has to be established. Threats and vulnerabilities to data and application security exist [1]. These vulnerabilities include hazards such as disruption of various services, attack on privacy and Information leakage [2–4]. More number of Enterprises are in race to shift to cloud computing paradigm so as to reduce their cost of operations. The upfront cost of setting up a business is greatly reduced by adopting the required delivery models such as platform, software or application as service. In terms of storage, it provides formidable redundancy and guarantees at much lower prices as compared to setting up own data centers'. These enormous benefits come at cost and ways and means have to be adopted in order to reduce the recurring and non-recurring cost involved in embracing this technology. This again involves a host of hidden costs. These costs are stipulated to be stated by the provider in the SLA's (Service-Level Agreements), but are poorly understood by the users. These costs can be avoided with a bit of planning [5–7].

Many kinds cloud delivery models exist today such as Application as a Service (AaaS), Infrastructure as a Service (IaaS), Platform as a Service (PaaS), Software as a Service (SaaS) or for that matter Anything as a Service (AaaS). Physical machine resource allocation also plays an important role in achieving load balancing in order to guarantee proper response time. Few of the parameters in each of the delivery paradigms have been chosen by various researchers in order to reduce the cost either for setting up the cloud architecture or developing an efficient cloud application.

Depending on the delivery paradigm chosen, the consumer either subscribes to certain application on the basis of Pay-as You-Use model or may completely outsource the application to the cloud vendor. With each additional layer that is outsourced, the consumer can potentially reduce costs by leveraging the service provider's economies of scale while sacrificing control and flexibility.

This rest of the chapter is organized into three sections. Section 2 is about the measuring cost factors, whereas Sect. 3 proposes and establishes some of the mechanisms by which cost-cutting can be achieved. The last section concludes the chapter.

2 General Factors Considered for Measuring Cost of Cloud

The cost involved in setting up a cloud delivery model or infrastructure comprises of Data Centre cost, floor space cost, land, building and construction activity cost. The procurement cost of hardware resources such as servers, mirror servers, switches, wiring and cabling, airconditioning is also to be considered. Various support and administrative staff along with software engineers are also an integral part.

3 Where Cost Can Be Reduced

Figure 2 illustrates few of the important techniques of reducing the architectural and operational cost of the cloud as proposed by various leading researches in the recent past. The techniques include:

- Usage of Shared databases
- Fine Tuning the Physical Machine Parameters such as VM and RAM
- Using Multitenant Databases
- Linguistic Semantics for Service Discovery
- Consolidation and Virtualization
- Outsourcing and managed Services

These cost reduction techniques are elaborated in Fig. 1.

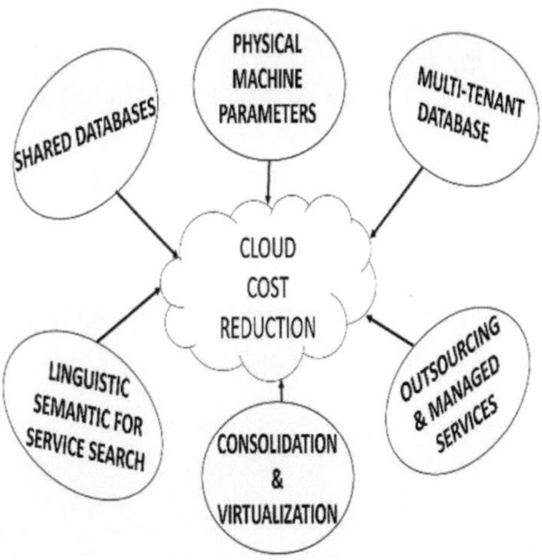

Fig. 1 Factors that contribute to reduction of cost in cloud computing

(a) **Physical Machine Parameters**

Pippal et al. [8] claim that efficient performance of a cloud computing application depends on a lot on how the dynamic and elastic resource provisioning has been made. The basis of this deduction is based and analyzed by studying the allocation and provisioning through virtual machines versus provisioning through stand-alone physical machines. Their results show that the time of data transfers between two machines either virtual or physical increases linearly as the size of data being transferred increases. They also claim that minimum data transfer time is required when the two VMs involved in the process are located on same Physical Machine. Performance for a virtual machine also gets elevated RAM available for the said virtual machine is at least 50% of total available RAM available in the machine. It is claimed by the authors that these parameters if incorporated in the cloud architecture, shall help in greatly reducing the running cost.

(b) **Costs Computation and Analysis Models**

Numerous researchers have worked on the problem of estimating the cost of adopting the cloud technology in the past. One such aggregation of various costs is illustrated in Fig. 2. Researchers have proposed various models [9, 10] for verifying various proposals and arriving at an optimal solution. These optimal solutions may also carry certain limitations as a plethora of constituent elements may contribute to varying degree of influence.

(c) **Consolidation and Virtualization**

Various applications can be shifted onto one workstation or server thereby reducing the number of physical machines required leading to physical resource consolidation. This reduces cost and resources required by the organization, leading to overall cost reduction in terms of land, air conditioning, backup and other related

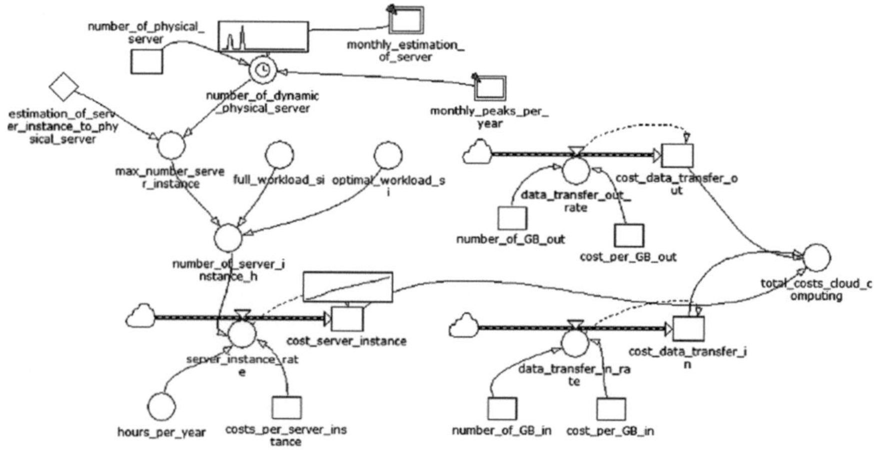

Fig. 2 Cost module for cloud computing

issues thus leading to increased efficiency. The virtualization of storage, servers and networks also presents an opportunity for cloud users to reduce their overall IT cost.

(d) **Linguistic Semantics for Service Search**

Cloud applications consist of Services. Shrabani and Kushwaha [11] propose that a service consumer can be a user, an application, service or some other software module that is in need of that particular service. To access any service, it has to do lookup operation in the service registry. Later it can bind the service over a transport link protocol and carry out the required execution. They also propose that by harnessing the linguistic semantics instead of plain keywords for required Service Search will make the selection of web services more efficient. Their proposed cache-based approach enables feasible time binding for a fresh web search. They also establish that service type information shall assist the requester to select a suitable and trustworthy web service for future lookup operations. The open-source tool SharpNLP is used by the authors to extract parts of speech of the service request query.

(e) **Multi-Tenant Databases**

Pippal et al. [12] propose that in the SaaS cloud architecture, to minimize the cost of the cloud a multi-tenant database may play an important role. By using the multi-tenant databases for cloud, one may face the performance issues but the overall cost is reduced. In the multi-tenant database, to store the data extension tables are used. Extension tables contain lots of metadata so the overall performance may degrade. So the authors propose the modified extension tables for the multi-tenant database. In modified extension tables, the XML Objects are used to store the data of rows. The cost of SaaS cloud reduces by using the multi-tenant database having modified extension tables for storing the data, it also increases the performance of the cloud.

Pippal and Kushwaha [13] also propose that the multi-tenant database may reduce the overall cost of the cloud development as it shares the single database instance with multiple tenants. They also propose the multi-tenant database for shared database and shared schema. In this architecture, the data consistency, replica management and the transaction management are implemented on the application level. In the proposed technique, the replica management is also based on the types of nodes. So the multi-tenant database architecture based on shared database reduces the overall cost of the ad hoc cloud.

(f) **High Availability of Databases**

Many researchers are focusing on increasing the availability of Cloud databases. This results in substantial cost reduction of lookup and query operations. Pippal et al. [2] propose that for faster access to application data, High availability of databases plays a critical role in increasing the efficiency of the services provided to users over the cloud. This availability of database is intrinsically a complex task that demands considerable cost. The authors propose that in case of an unprecedented failure, high availability systems achieve automatic failover and this has become easier with the emergence of virtualization technology. One way proposed to achieve this is through replication of databases. This replication should be based on the number of requests and load on the database servers. Possible security issues during replication need to be properly addressed [14]. The proposed results proposed by the authors claim that asynchronous writes have a better query response time than synchronous write and the improvement is of the order of 97%.

Impact of few of these parameters is analyzed in the next section.

4 Proposed Work

In order to propose and establish the mechanism by which the impact of changing physical resources of the machine like CPU and RAM through virtual machines versus physical machine could be evaluated is described here.

Physical Machine Parameters: We do a simulation for analyzing the impact of changing physical resources of the machine like CPU and RAM through the virtual machines versusphysical machine and evaluated the effect of different parameters on data transfer between two different virtual machines (VMs) that may exist on one physical machine or two different physical machines. The configuration for this set up is Intel(R) Core™ i5 CPU M480 @2.67 GHz, Installed RAM size of 3 GB, 64-bit machine architecture and operating system, Host Operating system: Windows 7 VM as VMware Workstation ver 7 and Guest operating system as Ubuntu 11.10.

A plot for the same is shown in Fig. 3.

Fig. 3 Data transfer rate for 3 scenarios

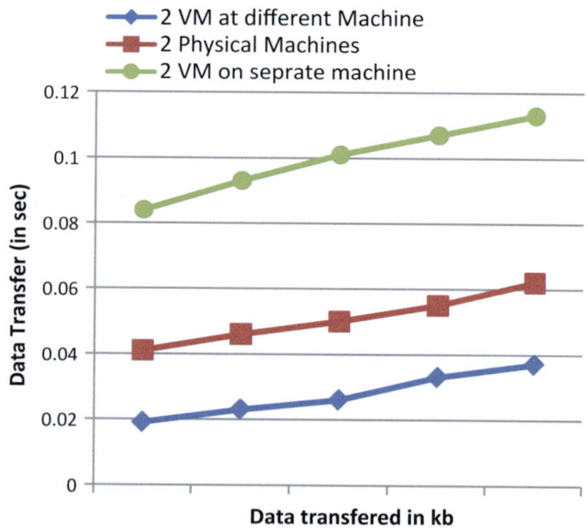

It can be observed from Table 1 and Fig. 3 that for applications that have two communicating processes, it is optimal to run each of these on different VM on the same physical machine as compared to running them on different machines. An average reduction of about 61% in data transfer time is achieved.

Multi-Tenant Databases: Multi-Tenant databases offer operational efficiency in terms of sharing the same table for different users. The Proposed approach for the multi-tenant database is designed over the shared database shared schema paradigm. This uses MySQL database in Ubuntu installed over VMware. To test the proposed architecture, Python has been. The proposed experimental scenario consists of few nodes for the distributed multi-tenant database organization with processing speed of the machines ranging from 500 MHz to 2.4 GHz for the processor, 500 MB to 3 GB of RAM. Data Manipulation Language (DML) Queries like selection, insertion and deletion are run. With more and more attributes added in a table, the performance improves further and requires lesser memory space as compared to the traditional SQL table approach. This advantage is derived by the use of XML in the attributes. Testbed Configurations: Table 2 illustrates a number of queries executed per second for operations such as insertion, deletion, updation and selection queries. The same is depicted in Fig. 4.

The results of the proposed work are able to establish an improvement of 29% to 82% for executing insertion, deletion and updation queries.

Now, the impact of addition of attributes on execution time is computed as shown in Table 3.

Table 1 Data transfer rate for physical machines and virtual machines

S. No.	Data size (kbs)	Time (in seconds)		
		Two VMs on same system (30% RAM size)	Two physical machines	Two VMs on different machines (30% RAM size)
1	1	0.019	0.041	0.084
2	2	0.023	0.046	0.093
3	3	0.026	0.050	0.101
4	4	0.033	0.055	0.107
5	5	0.037	0.062	0.113

Table 2 Number of DML queries executed per second

Type of DML query	Multitenant approach	Traditional approach
Insertion	703	581
Deletion	703	208
Updation	554	164
Selection	854	1172

Fig. 4 Number of queries executed per second

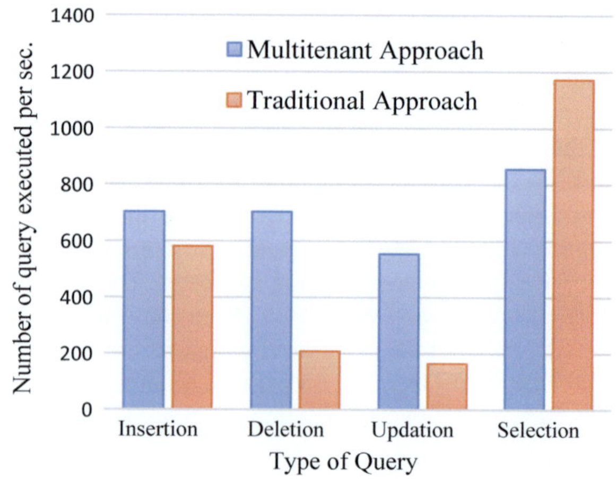

Table 3 Average time taken for added attributes in database

Number of added attributes	Multitenant approach (ms)	Traditional approach (ms)
10	3.127	3.052
20	3.234	4.060
30	3.322	6.151
40	3.524	10.127
50	3.777	18.290

The execution time of the proposed approach remains stable with an increase in a number of attributes but for traditional approach, it deteriorates by about 84% for increased number of attributes up to 50 as can be seen from Fig. 5.

Impact of addition of attributes on execution time is computed as shown in Table 4.

Fig. 5 Average performance for added attributes

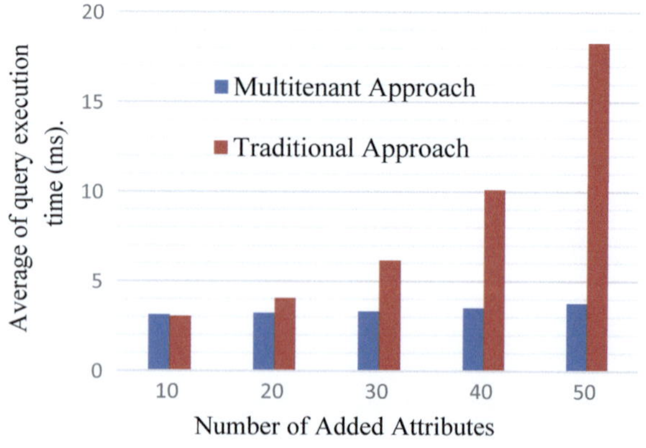

Table 4 Comparison for space requirements (bytes) for added attributes

Number of added attributes	Multitenant approach (bytes)	Traditional approach (bytes)
0	1920	14,400
2	1920	15,360
4	2466	16,768
8	3028	19,177
16	4032	23,184

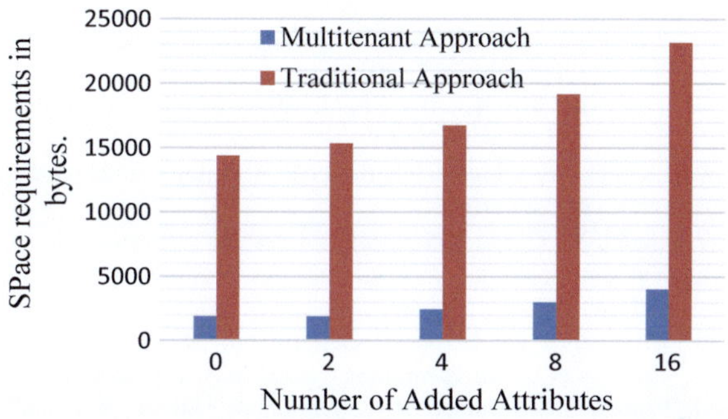

Fig. 6 Space requirements with increase in attributes

The proposed approach also saves memory efficiently by an average of 85% when attributes are increased by 16 (Fig. 6).

5 Conclusions

Cloud computing paradigm can be a cost-effective delivery model that effectively reduces costs and complexity while increasing flexibility and service delivery. In order to reduce cost, we need to adapt to dynamic and elastic physical resource provisioning like CPU share and RAM size. An attempt has been made to analyze impact of resource allocation by VM's versus physical machines and its impact on data transfer between virtual machines (VMs). It is observed that for applications that have two communicating processes, it is optimal to run each of these on different VM on the same physical machine as compared to running them on different machines. An average reduction of about 61% in data transfer time is achieved. For Mult-Tenant database, a number of queries executed per second for DML operations such as insertion, deletion, updation and selection queries is computed. The results of the proposed work show 29–82% improvement. The execution time of the proposed approach remains stable with an increase in number of attributes but for traditional approach, it deteriorates by about 84% when the number of attributes is by up to 50. This proposed approach also saves memory required for execution on an average by 85% when attributes are increased by 16.

References

1. Tripathi, A., Tripathi, K.: Cloudy cloud: security challenges & mitigation. In: International Conference on Control, Instrumentation, Communication and Computational Technologies (ICCICCT-2014), Kanyakumari, India
2. Pippal, S., Singh, S., Kumar, Sachan, R.K., Kushwaha, D.S.: High availability of databases for cloud. In: 2nd International Conference on Computing for Sustainable Global Development, INDIACom-2015. IEEE, New Delhi, Mar 2015
3. CSA: Security guidance for critical areas of focus in cloud computing V2.1. Cloud Security Alliance (2009)
4. Mathisen, E.: Security challenges and solutions in cloud computing. In: Proceedings of the 5th IEEE International Conference on Digital Ecosystems and Technologies Conference (DEST), pp. 208–212 (2011)
5. Trope, R., Ray, C.: The Real Realities of Cloud Computing: Ethical Issues for Lawyers, Law Firms, and Judges (2009)
6. Golden, B.: Cloud CIO: the cost advantage controversy of cloud computing (2011). http://www.cio.com/article
7. Gadia, S.: Cloud computing: an auditor's perspective. ISACA J. **6** (2009)
8. National Institute of Standards and Technology, The NIST definition of cloud computing (2011)
9. Kristekova, Z., Brion, J., Schermann, M., Krcmar, H.: Simulation model for cost-benefit analysis of cloud computing versus in-house datacenters (2012)
10. Pippal, S.K., Dubey, R.K., Malik, A., Singh, N., Jain, P., Bharti, R.K., Kushwaha, D.S.: Performance analysis of resource provisioning for cloud computing frameworks. In: Fifth International Conference on Advances in Communication, Network, and Computing (CNC 2014). Elsevier Procedia Technology, Chennai, 21–22 Feb 2014
11. Mallick, S., Kushwaha, D.S.: LWSDM: a layered web service discovery mechanism. In: Int. J. Adv. Inf. Sci. Serv. Sci. (AISS) **2**(3) (2010)
12. Pippal, S., Kushwaha, D.S.: A simple, adaptable and efficient heterogeneous multi-tenant database architecture for ad hoc cloud. Springer J. Cloud Comput. Adv. Syst. Appl. (JoCCASA) **2**(5) (2013)
13. Pippal, S., Sharma, V., Mishra, S., Kushwaha, D.S.: An efficient schema shared approach for multitenant database with authentication & authorization framework. In: 3PGCIC 2011, 6th International Conference on P2P, Parallel, Grid, Cloud and Internet Computing, Barcelona, Spain, 26–28 Oct 2011
14. Bajpai, D., Vardhan, M., Kushwaha, D.S.: Ensuring security in on-demand file replication system. In: 3rd IEEE Conference on Computer and Communication Technology (ICCCT-2012), Allahabad, India, Nov 2012
15. Hosseini, A., Sommerville, I., Sriram, I.: Research challenges for enterprise cloud computing. In: 1st ACM Symposium on Cloud Computing (SOCC 2010)
16. Subashini, S., Kavitha, V.: A survey on security issues in service delivery models of cloud computing. Elsevier J. Netw. Comput. Appl. **34**, 1–11 (2011)
17. Tsakalozos, K., Kllapi, H., Sitaridi, E., Roussopoulos, M., Paparas, D., Delis, A.: Flexible use of cloud resources through profit maximization and price discrimination. In: Proceedings of 27th IEEE International Conference on Data Engineering (ICDE 2011), pp. 75–86, April 2011

Power Aware-Based Workflow Model of Grid Computing Using Ant-Based Heuristic Approach

T. Sunil Kumar Reddy, Dasari Naga Raju, P. Ravi Kumar and S.R. Raj Kumar

Abstract Grid computing is treated as one of the emerging fields in distributed computing; it exploits the services like sharing of resources and scheduling of workflows. One of the major issues in grid computing is resource scheduling, this can be handled using the ant colony optimization algorithm, and it can be implemented in PERMA-G framework and it is an extended version of our previous work. The ant colony optimization is used to reduce the energy consumption and execution time of the tasks. It follows the nature of ant colony mechanism to compute the total execution time and power consumption of the tasks scheduled dynamically, the experimental results show the performance of the proposed model.

Keywords Power estimation · Power reduction · Grid scheduling · Pheromone

Nomenclature

$\mu_l(t)$	is the updated computation power.
$\mu_l(0)$	is the initial computing power.
ρ	is the pheromone decay parameter i.e. the parameter specifies the decay in computation power after executing the task, the value lies between 0 and 1.
σ	is the pheromone variance.
ϑ	is the index of the overload in task successful execution and under load in fail.
K	is the computing complexity of the task.

T. Sunil Kumar Reddy (✉) · P.R. Kumar
Department of CSE, SVCET, Chittoor, Andhra Pradesh, India
e-mail: sunilreddy.vit@gmail.com

P.R. Kumar
e-mail: ravi.poluru@outlook.com

D. Naga Raju
School of CSE, VIT University, Vellore, Tamilnadu, India
e-mail: raj2dasari@gmail.com

S.R. Raj Kumar
Department of IT, SVCET, Chittoor, Andhra Pradesh, India

V.B. Aggarwal et al. (eds.), *Big Data Analytics*, Advances in Intelligent Systems and Computing 654, https://doi.org/10.1007/978-981-10-6620-7_18

1 Introduction

Grid computing is one of the emerging fields of distributed computing which follows the behavior by providing services to users by distributing resources with multiple supports [1]. Grid computing supports both heterogeneous and parallel computing and it manages sharing of resources to the virtualization environment [2]. The major issue in grid computing is power utilization, to meet the demand of resources, optimization of scheduling workflows is required and the reduction of the total execution time of the tasks plays a major role in optimization. The total execution time will be reduced in the tasks by increasing the clock frequencies, but it leads to the heat dissipation and power utilization [3]. There must be a common interest in between performance and power utilization. Power aware models need not to reduce the power but there may be an option to decrease the power consumption in the processor with the delays. The DVS (Dynamic Voltage Scaling) is the mechanism which reduces the CPU voltage by minimizing the power utilization. The DVS controls the CPU speed with minimal loss in the performance. The DVS algorithm is suggested for the High-level language, but it is different from language to language. In [1], the PERMA framework is executed by using DVS, this algorithm is applied for regions, which is having a single entry and the single exit for controlling execution time and cost. These are the most important QoS factors for heterogeneous and grid computing. For minimizing the completion time, Optimizing Probabilistic Load Balancing Algorithm [4] is used to choose the best resources by analyzing the past status and load balancing is applied to choose the best response time.

Task Load Balancing Strategy [5] is applied for Grid Computing, which provides a hierarchical load balancing strategy associated based on neighborhood property. This strategy privileges local balancing in first and then the upper hierarchical balancing.

Ant colony optimization is a heuristic approach treated as one of the best optimization techniques. The ACO inspired by the ant foraging mechanism in the real environment. This gives a solution for the numerous optimization techniques like telecommunications load balancing and routing problems [6].

Ant colony optimization is applied for the PERMA-G framework, which is to address the energy consumption issues and the overall execution time of the tasks in VMs. The algorithm reduces power consumption and minimizes the total execution time in VMs by the efficient scheduling of tasks over VMs. Our research mainly concentrates in the optimization of power and finding the extent of voltage without compromising the execution time. The model also focuses on the distribution of tasks and load balancing based on the resources.

The paper is organized as follows: Sect. 2 explains the related work. Section 3 discusses the framework of our proposed method Ant Colony Optimization in PERMA-G (ACO-P). Section 4 provides the model for the heuristic mechanism in PERMA-G. The ACO-P is proposed in Sect. 5. Section 6 shows the results and discussion, and finally the conclusion will be drawn in Sect. 7.

2 Literature Survey

Worflow scheduling among the resources is one of the key research areas since decades. The workload distribution is done in both dynamically and statically. The load balancing is the major issue in grid computing which is classified as inter-cluster and intra-cluster mechanisms [7]. In [8], it presents the comparative study on task scheduling algorithms with different conditions like scalability, workload, performance, and adaptability. In [9], an improved ant colony mechanism is proposed to reduce the total cost of the task execution by updating the local and global pheromone. In [10], a new approach is introduced for improving the ACO algorithm by considering the current status of the resource when tasks are scheduled. The heuristic approach for ant colony mechanism is proposed in [11] by adding the additional component as load balancing mechanism. The Meta ant colony approach is proposed in [12] by enhancing the performance of the algorithm with efficient search solutions. The Meta ant colony mechanism uses positive and negative acknowledgments from the ants and shares the search information. Based on the resource capacity and job principles, an ant-based load balancing algorithm is proposed in [13]. There are a small number of scheduling algorithms available for scheduling, shared input data-based listing (SIL) is one of the efficient algorithms and the multiple queues with duplication (MQD) for bag of tasks (BOT) application is proposed for grid environment in [14]. The Metaheuristic algorithms are gaining momentum in scheduling process; exploration and exploitation are the components which are important in Metaheuristics algorithms. These components are explicitly implemented by ACO algorithm. It uses strategic oscillation rate to control the exploration and exploitation in ACO algorithm [15]. In [16], the author uses ACO algorithm to manage the resources in peer to peer grid environment. It uses load balancing process to converge the resources to the VMs. Lu et al. [17], proposed Collection path ant colony optimization model. This model reduced the processing time of tasks and achieves the global solution to the optimization problem. This model overcomes the problems by modifying the heuristic function and the update strategy in the ant-cycle model and established three-dimensional path pheromone storage spaces. The author in [18] proposed an enhanced ACO algorithm for jobs and resource scheduling in grid computing. The proposed model combines both min-max and ACO system and focus on local pheromone trail and updating the grid resource table.

The proposed ant-based heuristic model discovers the optimal resource for the tasks by considering the computing power and total execution time. In this process, the grid maintains the task queue to manage the tasks. Each task is allocated to the idle resource over the grid. If the task fails to execute on the resource, the failed task is moved to the failed task queue and again reallocate the idle resource.

3 Ant Colony Optimization in PERMA-G Framework (ACO-P)

The major role of the grid is to distribute the applications over the VMs for managing and parallelizing. The responsibilities of the grid are to arrange the VMs based on the application properties, detecting and recovering the VMs failures. With respective of power consumption improvement, we proposed a model called as the PERMA-G framework with the combination of effective optimization technique called as ant colony optimization, which is shown in Fig. 1. The PERMA-G presents the new model that figures the energy consumption for tasks to the host which is scheduled in the multi-core grid systems. The proposed model portrays the computing resources in the grid framework using four parameters:

(i) The computing power of a resource, i.e., the number of operations that the resource is able to compute is μ
(ii) The total number of VMs which integrates the processor is 'λ' (VMs)
(iii) The utilization of energy when the resource in idle state is 'η'
(iv) The utilization of energy when the resource is fully loaded is 'ε'

The PERMA-G framework [19] calculates the power μ, energy consumption (η, ε) to schedule the tasks over the VMs. The ACO-P algorithm is used to optimize power and energy consumption. This algorithm evaluates the total execution time of the tasks by verifying the voltages at different levels among the devices.

Figure 1 shows the PERMA-G framework which is a deployment of PERMA over the grid environment.

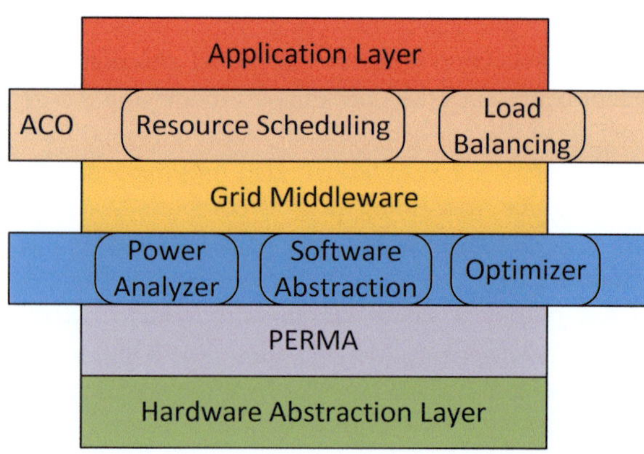

Fig. 1 PERMA-G framework optimized by ant colony optimisation model. Adopted from [19]

4 The Heuristic Approach of PERMA-G Framework

The PERMA-G utilizes the ant colony mechanism for scheduling the tasks into VMs. On allocating the tasks to the resource, the tasks are subdivided and allocated to the VMs based on their computing power (based on MIPS). The respective VMs computes the subtasks through processing elements (called as Processors) and gives the results to the respective VMs where it is combined and return to the resource. Let us consider that total number of resources present in the grid is given as α, each resource contains λ the number of VMs and each VM has β the number of processors. The task allocation based on the PERMA-G model is shown in Fig. 2. Here, the tasks of different sizes are submitted to three VMs which are present in the single host.

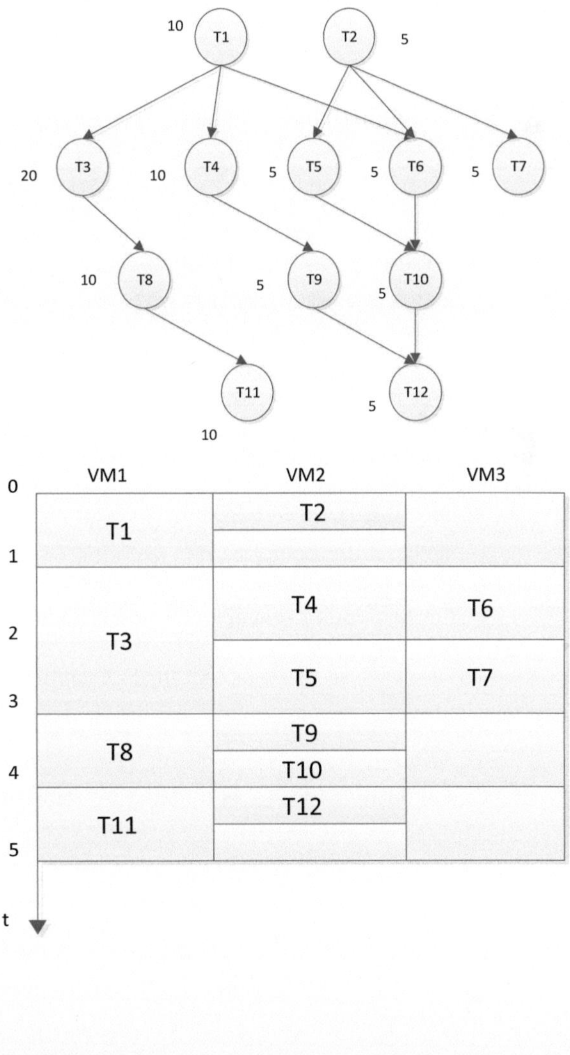

Fig. 2 The workflow model of the tasks over VMs in single host

5 Algorithm for Ant Colony Optimization

In the proposed model, we are considering that the total number of tasks (ants) waiting for the allocation in the queue '*Q*' is denoted as δ. The number of resources available in the grid is given as α.

In ACO-P, the pheromone trail is related to the computational power of the resource. At the initial state, the pheromone trial of the resource is at the starting level (α_l). For each virtual machine m, MIPS for all processors are at the equal rating.

Algorithm: Ant Colony Optimization for PERMA-G
Begin

Step 1 Intial computing power ($\mu_m(0)$) of a Virtual machine 'm' is given as

$$\mu_m(0) = \beta \times (\text{single processor MIPS rating}) \text{for every } m, \quad \text{where } 1 \leq m \leq \lambda \tag{1}$$

Step 2 Intial computing power ($\mu_l(0)$) of a resource '*l*' is given as the sum of the virtual machines computing power ($\mu_m(0)$) compromised by it. Hence,

$$\mu_l(0) = \sum_{\alpha} \mu_m(0) \quad \text{for every } l, \text{ where } 1 \leq l \leq \alpha \tag{2}$$

Step 3 for the resource α_l the allocation if the task '*q*' is assigned, the transaction probability $\rho_l(t)$ is given as:

$$\rho_l(t) = \frac{|\mu_l(t)|^{\varepsilon} \times |\mu_l(0)|^{\eta}}{\sum_l |\mu_l(t)|^{\varepsilon} \times |\mu_l(0)|^{\eta}} \quad \text{for every } l, \text{ where } 1 \leq l \leq \alpha \tag{3}$$

Step 4 The resource which has the maximum value of $\rho_l(t)$ is eligible for executing the task.

Step 5 The task q $(1 \leq q \leq \delta)$ is allocated to the resource α_l, the task may successfully complete its execution or may fail.

Step 6 If the task q $(1 \leq q \leq \delta)$ is successfully executed on the resource α_l, then the computing power (pheromone value) is updated as

$$\mu_l(t) = \rho\mu_l(0) - \sigma \tag{4}$$

$$\sigma = \vartheta \times -\kappa \tag{5}$$

Step 7 The task queue '*Q*' is updated by removing task q

$$Q = Q - \{1\} \tag{6}$$

Step 8 While the task q $(1 \leq q \leq \delta)$ is under execution on the resource, then Update the computing power (pheromone value) of the resource after execution.

Step 9 If the task q $(1 \leq q \leq \delta)$ is failed to execute on the resource α_1, then the computing power (pheromone value) is updated as

$$\mu_l(t) = \rho\mu_l(0) + \sigma \tag{7}$$

Update the computing power (pheromone value) of the resource and add the failed task to the task queue Q.

6 Results and Discussion

The performance of the proposed algorithm (ACO-P) is evaluated by using the Cloudsim toolkit. The cloudsim contains the environment which is similar to the grid and it is an extended version of gridsim toolkit. The makespan and cost of the NPA (Non-Power Aware), DVFS (Dynamic Voltage and Frequency Scaling), Round Robin and ACO-P is evaluated in terms of VMs, the type of Host, MIPS and power utilization is shown in Tables 1 and 2. The proposed ACO-P algorithm provides minimal completion time and cost of the scheduling tasks when compared to the existing algorithms.

The simulation setup to evaluate the performance of ACO-P is shown in Table 3. The total execution time of the resources is tested with the ACO-P algorithm and the tested results are shown in Fig. 3.

The performance of the ACO-P algorithm is tested with different resources having different parameters and the test results by considering resource utilization is shown in Fig. 4.

The overall computing power of the ACO-P is compared with the existing algorithms such as NPA, RR, DVFS, and FCFS. The results are shown in Fig. 5.

Table 1 The simulation setup

Total simulation time	80,100
Hosts	50–100
VMs	100–250
RAM	512
Bandwidth	1000–1,000,000

Table 2 Parameters for Virtual Machines Setup

VMs	VM1	VM2	VM3	VM4
MIPS	750	1000	1500	2000
Cores	2	2	4	4
RAM	512	512	512	512
Bandwidth	1000	1000	1000	1000
Storage	25,000	50,000	50,000	25,000

Table 3 Parameters for Host Setup

Host type	Host0	Host1	Host2	Host3	Host4
MIPS	2000	2500	3500	4500	5000
Cores	2	4	4	4	4
RAM	1024	2048	2048	2048	2048
Bandwidth	10^5	10^5	10^5	10^5	10^5
Storage	10^8	10^8	10^8	10^8	10^8

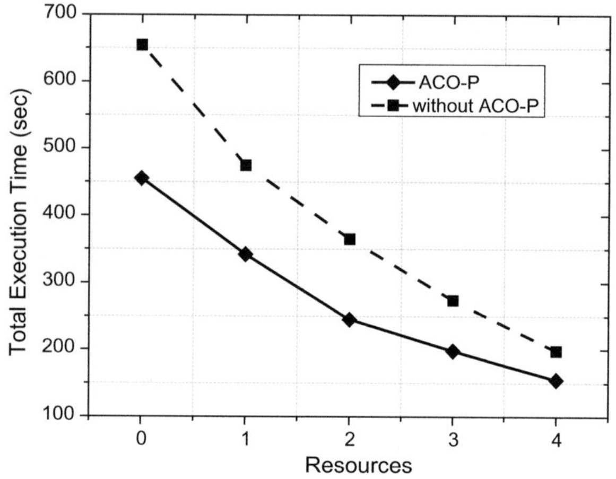

Fig. 3 Total execution time of the resources when tasks = 50

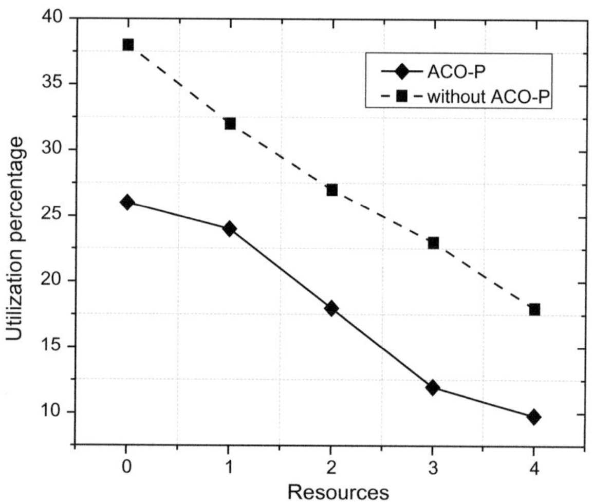

Fig. 4 Utilization percentage of the resources when tasks = 50

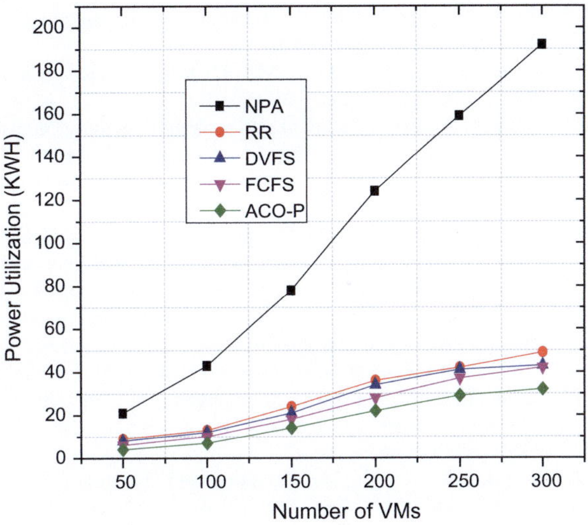

Fig. 5 Overall computing power calculation based on the number of VMs

7 Conclusions

The paper proposed a framework for optimizing PERMA-G using the ant colony mechanism, which is used to reduce the power consumption and total execution time for the grid. The ant colony optimisation addressed the issues of energy consumption, resource utilization, and execution time of the tasks in VMs. The framework balanced the load with the task queue by allocating the task to the resource with total execution time and allocating time taken into consideration using the ant colony mechanism. This methodology optimizes the performance of PERMA-G framework and the results conclude the efficiency of the algorithm.

References

1. Buyya, R., Pandey, S., Vecchiola, C.: Cloudbus toolkit for market-oriented cloud computing. In: Proceeding of the 1st International Conference on Cloud Computing (CloudCom) (2009)
2. Pandey, S., Karunamoorthy, D., Buyya, R.: Workflow engine for clouds. In: Buyya, R., Broberg, J., Goscinski, A. (eds.) Cloud Computing: Principles and Paradigms, pp. 321–344 (2011). Wiley, New York. ISBN-13:978-0470887998
3. Rajasekhara Babu, M., Venkata Krishna, P., Khalid, M.: A framework for power estimation and reduction in multi-core architectures using basic block approach. Int. J. Commun. Netw. Distrib. Syst. **10**(1), 40–51 (2013)
4. Dhinesh Babu, L.D., Venkata Krishna, P.: Versatile time–cost algorithm (VTCA) for scheduling non–pre-emptive tasks of time critical workflows in cloud computing systems. Int. J. Commun. Netw. Distrib. Syst. **11**(4), 390–411
5. Moradi, M., Dezfuli, M.A., Safavi, M.H.: A new time optimizing probabilistic load balancing algorithm in grid computing. Department of Computer and IT, Engineering, Amirkabir University of Technology, Tehran, Iran (2010). IEEE 978-1-4244-6349-7/10/©2010

6. Blum, C.: Ant colony optimization: introduction and recent trends. In: Physics of Life, pp. 271–350. Science Direct
7. Yagoubi, B., Meddeber, M.: Distributed load balancing model for grid computing. Revue ARIMA J. **12**, 43–60 (2010)
8. Mamani-Aliaga, A.H., et al.: A comparative study on task dependent scheduling algorithms for grid computing. In: 13th Symposium on Computing Systems (2012)
9. Chang, R.-S., Chang, J.-S., Lin, P.-S.: An ant algorithm for balanced job scheduling in grids. In: Future Generation Computer Systems, pp. 20–27 (2009)
10. Ku-Mahamud, R., Abdul Nasir, H.J., Din, A.M.: Grid load balancing using enhanced ant colony optimization. In: Proceedings of the 3rd International Conference on Computing and Informatics (ICOCI 2011), Bandung, Indonesia, pp. 37–42, 8–9 June 2011
11. Suryadevera, S., Chourasia, J., Rathore, S., Jhummarwala, A.: Load balancing in computational grids using ant colony optimization algorithm. Int. J. Comput. Commun. Technol. (IJCCT) **3**(3) (2012). ISSN (ONLINE):2231-0371. ISSN (PRINT):0975-7449
12. Umarani, S, Nithya, L.M., Shanmugam, A.: Efficient multiple ant colony algorithm for job scheduling in grid environment. Int. J. Comput. Sci. Inf. Technol. **3**(2), 3388–3393 (2012). ISSN: 0975-9646
13. Goyal, S.K., Singh, M.: Adaptive and dynamic load balancing in grid using ant colony optimization. Int. J. Eng. Technol. **4**(4), 167–174 (2012). ISSN: 0975-4024
14. Abdelsalam, H., Abdelaziz, A., Mukherjee, V., et al.: Trust-based ant colony optimization for grid resource scheduling. In: 13th Symposium on Computing Systems, vol. 22(1), pp. 29–43 (2014)
15. Mustafa Muwafak, A.., Ku Ruhana, K.-M.: Strategic oscillation for exploitation and exploration of ACS algorithm for job scheduling in static grid computing. In: Second International Conference on Computing Technology and Information Management (ICCTIM), pp. 87–92 (2015), 21–23 April 2015. doi:10.1109/ICCTIM.2015.7224598
16. Jain, A., Singh, R.: An innovative approach of Ant Colony optimization for load balancing in peer to peer grid environment. In: International Conference on Issues and Challenges in Intelligent Computing Techniques (ICICT), pp. 1–5 (2014), 7–8 Feb 2014. doi:10.1109/ICICICT.2014.6781242
17. Lu, W., Wang, Z., Hu, S., Liu, L.: Ant colony optimization for task allocation in multi-agent systems. China Commun. **10**(3), 125–132, Mar 2013. doi:10.1109/CC.2013.6488841
18. Nasir, H.J.A., Ku-Mahamud, K.R.: Grid load balancing using ant colony optimization. In: Second International Conference on Computer and Network Technology (ICCNT), pp. 207–211 (2010), 23–25 April 2010. doi:10.1109/ICCNT.2010.10
19. Sunil Kumar Reddy, T., Krishna, P.V, Reddy, P.C.: Power aware framework for scheduling tasks in grid based workflows. Int. J. Commun. Netw. Distrib. Syst. **14**(1) (2015)
20. Yagoubi, B., Slimani, Y.: Task load balancing strategy for grid computing. J. Comput. Sci. **3** (3), 186–194 (2007)
21. Yagoubi, B., Medebber, M.: A load balancing model for grid environment. In: 22nd International Symposium on Computer and Information Sciences (ISCIS 2007), pp. 1–7, 7–9 Nov 2007
22. Randles, M., Taleb-Bendiab, A., Lamb, D.: Scalable self governance using service communities as ambients. In: Proceedings of the IEEE Workshop on Software and Services Maintenance and Management (SSMM 2009) within the 4th IEEE Congress on Services, IEEE SERVICES-I 2009, Los Angeles, CA, 6–10 July 2009
23. Mukherjee, K., Sahoo, G.: Mathematical model of cloud computing framework using fuzzy bee colony optimization technique. In: Proceedings of the 2009 International Conference on Advances in Computing, Control, and Telecommunication Technologies, pp. 664–668, 28–29 Dec 2009
24. Dhinesh Babu, L.D., Venkata Krishna, P.: Honey bee behavior inspired load balancing of tasks in cloud computing environments. Appl. Soft Comput. **13**, 2292–2303 (2013)

Image Categorization Using Improved Data Mining Technique

Pinki Solanki and Girdhar Gopal

Abstract Image categorization is one of the important branches of artificial intelligence. Categorization of images is a way of grouping images according to their similarity. Image categorization uses various features of images like texture, color component, shape, edge, etc. Categorization process has various steps like image preprocessing, object detection, object segmentation, feature extraction, and object classification. For the past few years, researchers have been contributing different algorithms in the two most common machine learning categories to either cluster or classify images. The goal of this paper is to discuss two of the most popular machine learning algorithms: Nearest Neighbor (k-NN) for image classification and Means clustering algorithm. After that, a Hybrid model of both the above algorithms is proposed. These algorithms are implemented in MATLAB; finally, the experimental results of each algorithm are presented and discussed.

Keywords Image categorization · means algorithm · nearest neighbor (NN) algorithm

1 Introduction

The term image categorization refers to the tagging of images into one of a number of predefined categories. Image categorization is an easy task for human beings but it is a difficult problem for machines. There are several techniques for categorization of images depending on the representation of local features and the distance metric to calculate the similarity between images [1]. The local feature technique has been getting a huge attention for the past more than a decade [2]. Recently, many studies

P. Solanki (✉) · G. Gopal
Department of Computer Science and Applications,
Kurukshetra University, Kurukshetra, India
e-mail: solanki.pinki@gmail.com

G. Gopal
e-mail: girdhar.gopal@gmail.com

V.B. Aggarwal et al. (eds.), *Big Data Analytics*, Advances in Intelligent Systems and Computing 654, https://doi.org/10.1007/978-981-10-6620-7_19

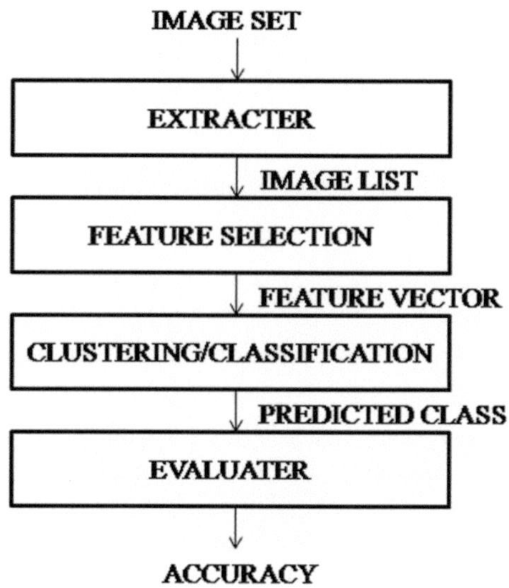

Fig. 1 Image categorization process

are showing interest in learning a metric rather than using a simple metric given a priori (e.g., Euclidean distance) [3]. Image categorization is an important and challenging task in various application domains including web searching, biomedical imaging, biometry, video surveillance, vehicle navigation, industrial visual inspection, robot navigation, remote sensing, etc. Image categorization is a step-by-step process which is shown in Fig. 1. Initially, features are selected from extracted image list. After that clustering or classifying technique is applied on these features to predict the class of image. Finally, evaluation is done to calculate accuracy. After this brief introduction, Sect. 2 of this paper describes previous work which has been done on image categorization. In Sect. 3 proposed work of this paper is discussed in detail and then Sect. 4 contains experimental results. Finally, conclusion and future work of this paper are discussed in Sect. 5.

2 Literature Review

This section describes the previous work which has been done in image classification using Nearest Neighbor and its improvements.

An improved k-NN classification algorithm has been proposed by Li et al. [4]. They applied the proposed algorithm to the object-oriented classification of high-resolution remote sensing image. Firstly, as sample points, image objects are obtained through image segmentation. Secondly, original k-NN, clipping-k-NN, and the improved k-NN are introduced and used to classify those sample points, respectively. Finally, results of classification are compared, which shows that in the same training set and testing set, the improved k-NN algorithm achieves better accuracy in the classification of high-resolution remote sensing image.

An improved version of k-NN to overcome the limitations of it, named as Genetic k-NN (GKNN) was proposed by Suguna and Thanushkodi [5]. k-NN is combined with Genetic Algorithms to form it. In this method, *k* number of samples is selected first and fitness is calculated based on the accuracy of classification. Better fitness is recorded time to time. So to calculate the similarities between all samples are not needed in this method. The performance of proposed method was compared with k-NN which shows that complexity of proposed method is reduced and the accuracy of classification also improved.

A modified classification method based on k-NN algorithm to improve the performance by Alizadeh et al. [6]. It is called Nearest Cluster approach (NC). The samples of neighbors are automatically determined. After training set, the labels are also determined. For specifying the class label of a new test sample, the class label of the nearest cluster prototype is used. Computationally, proposed NC method is faster than previously k-NN. It also leads to the best solution based on feature space. Two data sets are taken to compare the proposed method SAHeart and Monk. Results show that better improvements in accuracy as well as time complexity in comparison with the k-NN method.

Iankiev et al. [7] proposed an "Improved K Nearest Neighbour Classification". The speed of k-NN is improved in this approach while the accuracy level is maintained. It works based on two building techniques. One is model condensing in which all classes with same probability are chosen, then training set of size Q is created by extracting the vector elements from a set of images. This set is refined on iteration basis. Then in second technique, called preprocessing an pattern is compared to the prototype in stages.

The simplicity of K-Means and good accuracy of k-NN algorithm is the prime motivation behind proposed work of this paper.

3 Proposed Work

To achieve the objective of image categorization using improved data mining technique; K-Means clustering algorithm, k-NN classification algorithm and proposed hybrid approach are used. K-Means clustering and k-NN classification are common approaches for image categorization. So in this paper, a hybrid approach is proposed to improve image categorization accuracy. The step-by-step procedure for Image categorization of the proposed work is shown in Fig. 2.

Various Steps used in the proposed work are:

Step 1 First of all, the entire image dataset is extracted and it is converted into grayscale image list through various functions given in MATLAB.

Step 2 For feature selection from the image list Texture analysis and DWT2 using db10, level-3 technique is used. Using DWT2 horizontal, vertical,

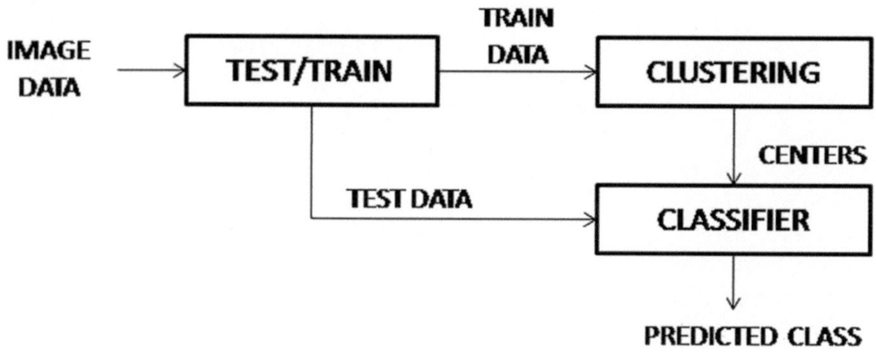

Fig. 2 Block diagram of proposed image categorization

and diagonal features of image list are extracted and through texture analysis, Correlation has been gathered, Energy and Homogeneity features.

Step 3 After feature extraction, testing and training of data are done. Initially, k-means algorithm is used to calculate the centers from trained data. After that, centers calculated by K-Means and test data is passed to k-NN classifier to predict the actual class of the image to which it belongs.

Step 4 Finally, evaluation metrics is calculated to check the relevancy of the output with the input data.

Block Diagram of the proposed work for image Categorization is shown in Fig. 2.

Now the second step of proposed hybrid approach is discussed in detail here.

3.1 Hybrid Approach

1. Apply K-Means algorithm on trained data to calculate centers from the feature vector of the image data.
2. If ‘n’ number of elements are there in feature vector and ‘m’ in each category, mean of ‘m’ elements is calculated and store corresponding center location as shown below.
3. Apply k-NN on these centers and test data to predict the actual class of image to which it belongs.

3.2 Accuracy Metrics Used for Mentioned Methodology

Precision is the probability that (randomly selected) retrieved information is relevant.
Recall is the probability that (randomly selected) relevant information is retrieved in a search.
F-measure A measure that combines precision and recall is the harmonic mean of precision and recall, the traditional F-measure or balanced F-score by $F = 2*[(\text{precision} * \text{recall})/(\text{precision} + \text{recall})]$.

4 Experimental Results and Discussion

As discussed earlier, the basic objective of this paper was to improve accuracy rate and to reduce time complexity in our hybrid model of image categorization.

4.1 Experimental Results

Experimental work was designed to compare the accuracy of K-Means algorithm, k-NN algorithm, and proposed hybrid model. The hybrid model is efficient because instead of passing the trained classes directly to the classifier, centers gathered by K-Means algorithm are passed which make this model hybrid. In the experiment for each run same dataset is entered, to observe the accuracy of all algorithms. These algorithms are applied many times on 'user-defined' dataset in MATLAB. This small data set is constructed by taking various images of human beings with different facial expressions from other datasets like yalefaces [8], etc. The dataset containing images of four persons and ten images of each person, with their classes they actually belong is shown in Fig. 3.

Image categorization is first done with K-Means algorithm on the dataset described above. The accuracy metrics obtained using K-Means only are shown in Fig. 4.

After that k-NN algorithm is applied on the dataset and then the accuracy metrics obtained using k-NN only are shown in Fig. 5.

Now in proposed hybrid approach, initially K-Means algorithm is used to calculate the centers from trained data. After that centers calculated by K-Means and test data is passed to k-NN classifier to predict the actual class of the image to which it belongs. The actual images of the persons and their predicted images given by proposed hybrid approach are shown in Fig. 6.

Table 1 shows the classes of images to which they actually belong and their predicted classes given by hybrid method based on the above results are shown in

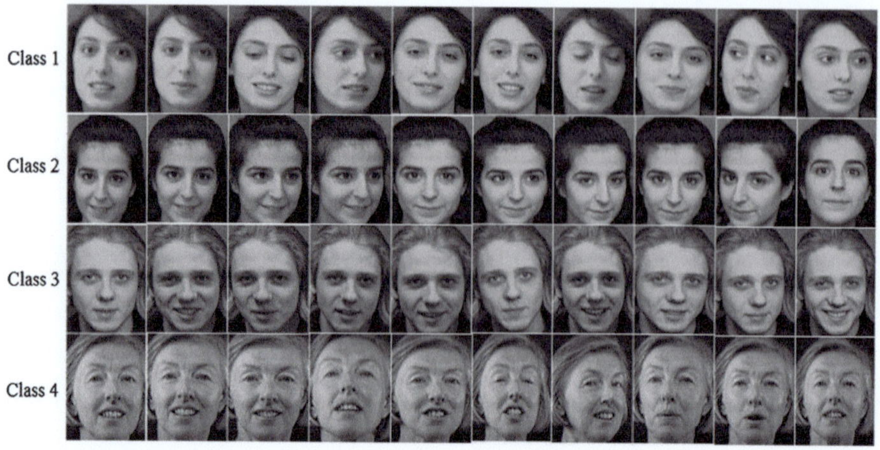

Fig. 3 User defined Data set containing images of four persons and ten images of each (4 * 10)

Fig. 4 Output of K-means algorithm

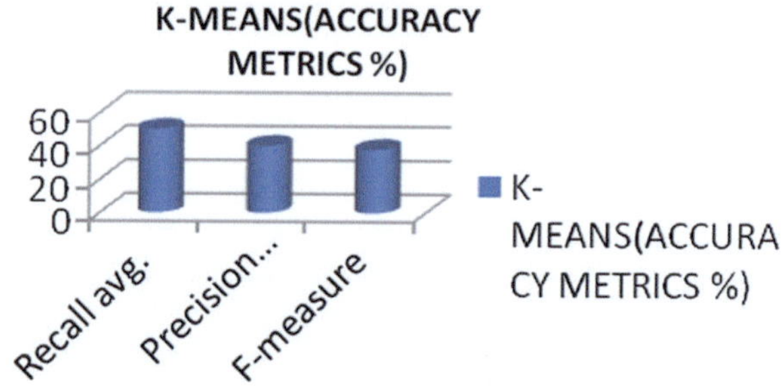

Fig. 5 Output of k-NN algorithm

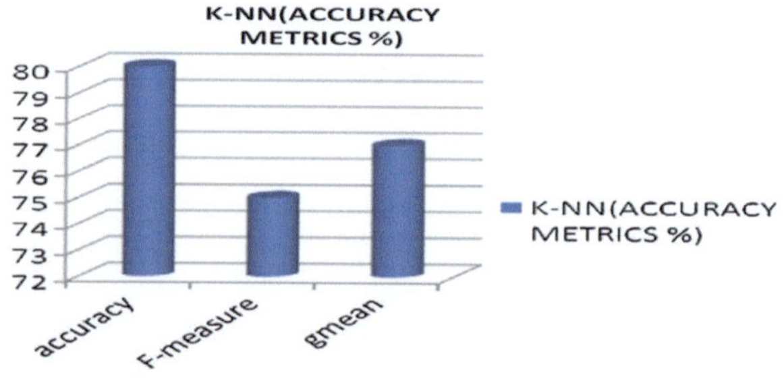

Fig. 6. From the table, it can be concluded that the accuracy achieved by proposed method is higher than the previous methods discussed.

From the above discussions, accuracy metrics for the hybrid method can be drawn. Figure 7 shows the accuracy metrics achieved by the Hybrid method.

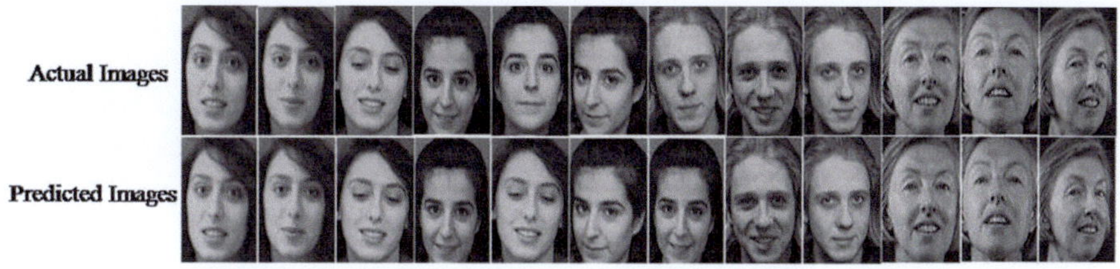

Fig. 6 Actual images and their respective predicted images using hybrid method

Table 1 Actual class of images and their predicted classes

Actual class	Predicted class
1	1
1	1
1	1
2	2
2	1
2	2
3	2
3	3
3	3
4	4
4	4
4	4

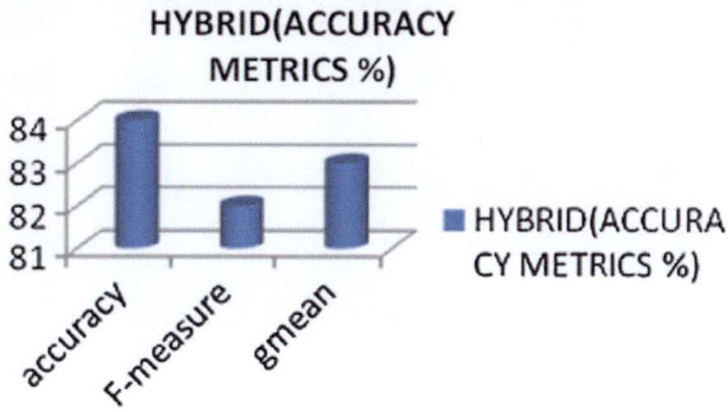

Fig. 7 Output of hybrid algorithm

Experiments were performed one by one with different algorithms on the dataset described. Now from the acquired results, it can be concluded that the accuracy of hybrid model is more than the other two algorithms as shown in Fig. 8.

The second objective of this paper was to reduce time complexity. Various experiments with K-Means, k-NN and proposed hybrid algorithms were performed on the dataset in MATLAB. The time taken by Hybrid method (improved nearest neighbor) or iNN is less than the k-NN algorithm as shown in Fig. 9.

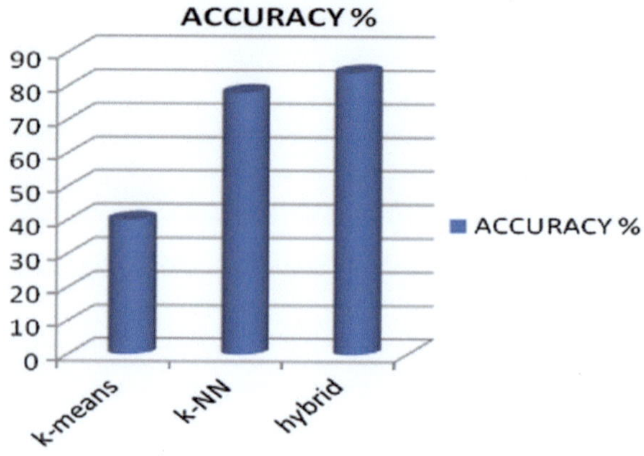

Fig. 8 Accuracy comparison of various algorithms

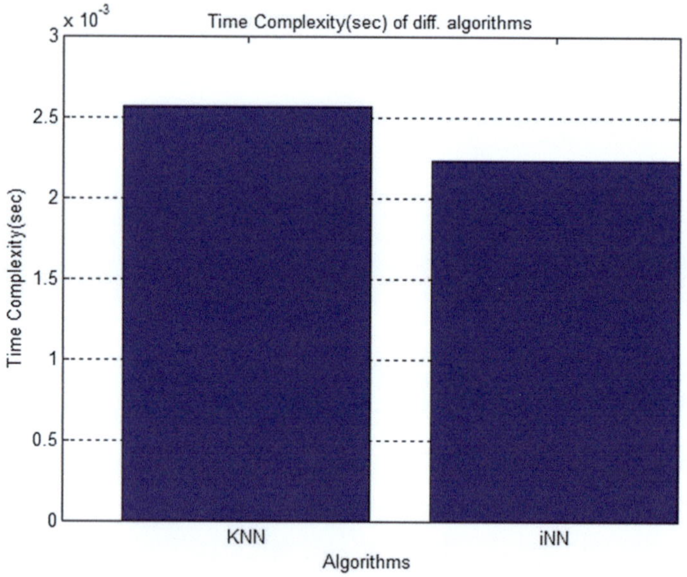

Fig. 9 Time complexity of different algorithm

5 Conclusion and Future Work

In this work, K-means clustering, k-NN algorithm, and their hybrid model are discussed to reduce time complexity and improve accuracy. A new hybrid method of image categorization is discussed in which a dataset is taken and then testing and training of that dataset is done. After that instead of passing the trained classes to the classifier, centers gathered by k-means algorithm are passed. K-mean clustering, k-NN algorithm and hybrid model are compared in terms of the same dataset. K-means clustering algorithm alone does not give good accuracy and time complexity is also high. k-NN algorithm alone gives better results than k-means but the hybrid model introduced in this paper give better results than the other two algorithms and results were given are very satisfactory.

In future, using better algorithms than DWT2 and texture analysis for feature selection; accuracy can be improved and time complexity can be reduced. This technique has been applied to a dataset which has a small number of images but this technique can further be improved for large datasets in future.

References

1. Van De Sande, K.E.A., Gevers, T., Snoek, C.G.M.: Evaluating color descriptors for object and scene recognition. IEEE Trans. Pattern Anal. Mach. Intell. **32**, 1582–1596
2. Ping Tian, D.: A review on image feature extraction and representation techniques. Int. J. Multimedia Ubiquitous Eng. **8**, 385–395 (2013)
3. Bellet, Al, Habrard, A., Sebban, M.: Good edit similarity learning by loss minimization. Mach. Learn. **89**, 5–35 (2012)
4. Li, Y., et al.: An improved k-nearest Neighbour algorithm and its application to high resolution remote sensing image classification. In: 17th International Conference on Geo informatics, pp. 1–4, 12–14 Aug 2009
5. Suguna, N., Thanushkodi, K.: An improved k-nearest Neighbour classification using genetic algorithm. Int. J. Comput. Sci. Issues **7**, 18–21 (2010)
6. Alizadeh, H., et al.: A new method for improving the performance of K nearest neighbour using clustering technique. J. Convergence Inf. Technol. **4**(2) (2009)
7. Iankiev, K.G., Wu, Y., Govindaraju, V.: Improved k-nearest Neighbour classification. Pattern Recogn. **35**, 2311–2318 (2002)
8. http://vision.ucsd.edu/~leekc/ExtYaleDatabase/ExtYaleB.html

An Effective Hybrid Encryption Algorithm for Ensuring Cloud Data Security

Vikas Goyal and Chander Kant

Abstract Cloud computing is one of the most research hot topics in IT industry nowadays. A lot of startup organizations are adopting cloud eagerly due to massive cloud facilities available with minimal investment; but as every coin has two sides, so with cloud. In the cloud, the user data is stored at some off-site location. So cloud data security is one of the main concerns of any organizations, before shifting to the cloud. The data owners can ensure the data security at its premises using firewalls, VPN (Virtual Private Network) like most used security options. But as data owner stores their sensitive data to remote servers and users access required data from these remote cloud servers, which is not under their control. So storing data outside client premises, raises the issue of data security. Thus, one of the primary research areas in cloud computing is cloud data protection. In this research paper, strategies followed include categorization of the data on the basis of their sensitivity and importance, followed by the various cryptography techniques such as the AES (a Symmetric Cryptography technique), SHA-1 (a Hashing technique), and ECC (Elliptic curve Cryptography (an Asymmetric Cryptography technique). Till date, most of the authors were using a single key for both encryption and decryption which is a weak target of various identified malicious attacks. Hence, in the designed hybrid algorithm, two separate keys are used for each encryption and decryption. The cloud user who wants to access cloud data, need to first register with CSP and cloud owner. After registration, user login id, password and OTP (One Time Password) sent to the user registered mobile number, are required to access the encrypted cloud data.

Keywords Cloud · Data security · ECC · AES · SHA-1 · Hybrid algorithm for cloud data security

---

V. Goyal (✉)
NIT, Kurukshetra, India
e-mail: vikas.goyal_85@yahoo.co.in

C. Kant
Department of Computer Science and Application, Kurukshetra University, Kurukshetra, India
e-mail: ckverma@rediffmail.con

V.B. Aggarwal et al. (eds.), *Big Data Analytics*, Advances in Intelligent Systems and Computing 654, https://doi.org/10.1007/978-981-10-6620-7_20

1 Introduction

Cloud storage mainly maintains user's data on an off-site cloud storage system that is maintained by third-party CSP. Nowadays, owner prefers to store their data on cloud due to facilities provided by cloud vendors instead of storing data on users' system hard disk or other memory devices at their own premises. After storing the owner data on a remote database, it will be accessible later through just an internet link between user and cloud databases. In cloud model, customers are associated with cloud through an internet link to access cloud information and resources are priced and provided, on-demand. Mainly, cloud resources are shared among multiple users as office, apartments or storage places as shared among tenants. The cloud facilities are primarily delivered through an internet link, thus the cloud user is free from the worry of maintaining own data center or servers (as shown in Fig. 1). Nowadays, mostly adopted cloud computing services are offered and maintained by big IT giants Amazon and Google for the startup companies.

There are mainly three components of cloud computing model as listed below.

Cloud service provider (CSP)—The third-party vendor which manages all the cloud services, i.e., infrastructure, platform, and the software's offered to cloud users with his technical team. He is completely responsible for providing safe and uninterrupted services to the cloud users.

Client/Owner: An entity, which is generally, an individual or startup organizations, who want to store their large data files either at own premises or in the cloud.

User: An entity enrolled with the data owner and access owners' cloud data after proper authentication from CSP.

Since data is one of the crucial outsourced entity in cloud computing, thus it may suffer from various threats or attacks by exploring the vulnerabilities present in the outsourcing cloud module. The attackers can be an Insider (CSP or CSP employee itself) or Outsider (some mischievous hacker) who desires to access the owner data, which can be utilized for some gain thereafter.

As the data is one of the most critical assets for any company or data owner, thus, whatever sort of threats to the security and integrity of data can lead to horrific consequences for organizations. So as discussed, cloud data security is the main hurdle in adopting cloud services for most of the organizations. If the data security,

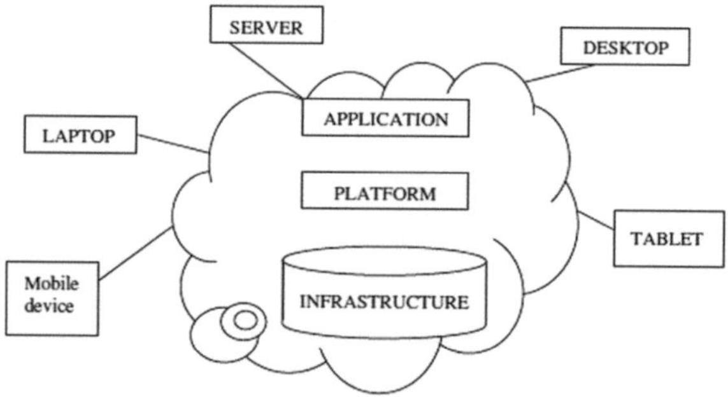

Fig. 1 The cloud

integrity issues will be properly addressed and audited, more data owners, and organizations will switch to cloud storage. One more issue which is to properly address is, resource sharing, such as storage, with other cloud users and CSP (Cloud Service Provider). Thus, if the rival cloud users are sharing the same cloud storage space from same CSP, then their data may be under threat from each other. Thus, it is also the CSP responsibility to isolate one users' data from some other.

The proposed hybrid model comprises of different well-known cryptographic techniques and applying them together to achieve cloud data protection. The paper's propose a hybrid algorithm comprising of three different encryption techniques which efficiently protect the three categories of data throughout the data life cycle, i.e., from the owner to the cloud and then to the end cloud user. As the cloud is combinations of dissimilar resources placed together to offer the services, and so a bunch of vulnerabilities may exist in cloud setup, whose exploration may be horrific for the cloud data storage. The proposed hybrid algorithm uses encryption as a primary security policy. Encoding is the technique for alteration of plain text data in an encrypted form called cipher text that can be deciphered and read by the legitimate person having a valid decryption key only. The illegitimate or mischievous person cannot easily decrypt and interpret the ciphertext in the absence of the decryption key.

This rest of the paper is designed as follows: Sect. 2 highlights the various authors' related work regarding cloud data protection in the last years. In Sect. 3, effective hybrid model is designed to address and solve cloud data storage security issue effectively. Section 4 provides the proposed algorithm. Section 5 provides the security investigation of the proposed hybrid model against various identified attacks so far. Section 6 provides the conclusion and future scope of this paper.

2 Related Work

We have gone through some research papers to identify security issues with existing cloud data storage models and the presented solutions so far. Among them, few research efforts are handled directly with the topics of security and privacy-aware data stored in cloud computing.

The Cloud Security Alliance (CSA) [1] and Louai et al. [2] has risen seven security threats to cloud data storage, those are, exploitation of cloud Computing, vulnerable Application Programming Interfaces (APIs), malicious entity insider, shared technology security issues, information leakage, account or service accessing by an illegitimate user, etc.

Louai et al. [2], Singh et al. [3] and Yu et al. [4] has identified many issues, loopholes and attacks to data's security, integrity, and confidentially over the cloud data storage. The attacks studied include Denial of Service (DOS) attack, cloud malware injection attack, side channel attacks due to shared infrastructure, authentication attack, and man-in-the-middle attack. Yu et al. [4] have concluded that data integrity can be ascertained by the simply SSL protocol during transmission.

Karthik et al. [5] have suggested a new hybrid algorithm using some well-known cryptographic algorithms in a definite array, to enhance and optimize cloud data protection.

Li et al. [6] have presented a hybrid encryption algorithm contains a simple encryption algorithm, which improved to the Vigenere encryption algorithm; and finally, came out with a hybrid encryption algorithm with a Base64 encoding algorithm. The proposed hybrid encryption algorithm significantly improved the data protection.

Tweney et al. [7] have mentioned an incident, back in 2007, from the end of CSP Salesforce.com which sent a letter to all its millions of subscribers demonstrating about how the customer emails, addresses, and rest particulars had been stolen by cybercriminals.

Tang et al. [8], Rong et al. [9], Grobauer et al. [10], Waleed et al. [11], Lin [12] have highlighted the vulnerability of the data security in the cloud, one of the important factors restricting the growth of cloud computing and reviewed the threats to security and privacy of cloud data warehousing.

Divya et al. [13] have proposed a secure cloud storage algorithm using elliptic curve cryptography. The proposed work also concentrates on Online Alert methodology which shows the data owner when an aggressor attempts to alter the data or any malpractice happens during data forwarding.

Kumar et al. [14] have researched elliptic curve cryptography (ECC) encryption technique in particular used for protecting cloud data files which authenticate the legitimate user and refuse the data accessing by mischievous hacker or cloud storage provider.

Fu et al. [15] have focused on safe data deletion on the file systems. The report proposed a file system which supports secure deletion of data. This paper proposed the idea of secret code text-policy trait-based encryption technique (CP-ABE) which supports fine-grained access policy to encrypt files.

Tan et al. [16] have proposed a cloud data security algorithm using fully homomorphic encryption to ensure data protection during both during transmission and storage. The full homomorphic encryption algorithm can process the encrypted data as well.

Sinha et al. [17] has compared the functioning of two asymmetric key encryption algorithm between RSA and ECC experimentally; and concluded that ECC performs better in many respects required key sizes, bandwidth saving, encryption time, small device's efficiency, as well as security as compared to RSA algorithm.

Abdul et al. [18], Pavithra et al. [19] have implemented six most used symmetric key encryption algorithms: DES, 3DES, AES (Rijndael), Blowfish, RC2, and RC6 and comparison was conducted based on several parameters. The report concluded that the AES algorithm is competitive with the rest of algorithm on being fast and flexible.

Marshall et al. [20] have designed a hybrid encryption model by using RSA and AES algorithms to ensure cloud data protection. Since the private key is exclusively in user hold and therefore the user's most sensitive will not be useful to anyone except the legitimate user not even the CSP.

Tripathi et al. [21] have given a comparative work between two well-known asymmetric encryption algorithms between elliptic curve cryptography and the RSA cryptography algorithm in respect of the cloud data security parameter. The paper flared up with experimental results which prove the superiority of elliptic curve-based public key cryptography compared to RSA public key cryptography.

Mohamed et al. [22] have suggested Amazon EC2 cloud users, to must use an AES symmetric algorithm which ensures the highest security with minimum time to code.

Dinadayalan1 et al. [23] have proposed all the principal data security issues and their solutions.

3 Proposed Model

The main focus of this algorithm is to maximize the data owner's control of data during transit as well as storing. Since more locks, we will apply the more time it will take to fetch the data back. So it would be better to categorize the data first. Since all data is not of the same importance, so we can categorize the data initially on the basis of their sensitivity and importance. To achieve the above-defined objective, the data is split into three different protection layers for each privacy categorized data that has different privacy aspects according to the need of sensitive data. For this, a Three-Tier Privacy-Aware Cloud Computing Model is proposed for the three categories of the data described as below

- No Privacy (NP)
- Privacy with Trusted Provider (PTP)
- Privacy with non-trusted provider (PNTP)

There are no encryption and decryption used for the storage and accessing of No Privacy (NP) category data, whereas in Privacy with trusted provider (PTP) security scheme the CSP is responsible and trusted to maintain the data security. CSP uses the AES encryption and decryption technique which automatically generate the public key which is known to everyone. Now in the third case, i.e., Privacy with non-trusted provider (PNTP) for the most sensitive data to work upon, a security scheme is proposed. In this security scheme, both data owners (user) and CSP are responsible to ensure cloud data protection. User encrypts the information using AES algorithm before sending to CSP, then CSP again uses the ECC encryption and decryption technique for complete data protection. In this paper, we have described a security scheme for PNTP module only.

The proposed hybrid algorithm comprises of different coding techniques such as AES (Symmetric Cryptography technique), SHA-1 (Hashing technique), and ECC

(Elliptic curve Cryptography, Asymmetric Cryptography technique) for the categorized sensitive data.

The proposed hybrid algorithm is designed to offer complete data security to the data throughout the data life cycle, such as to data in transit, data in storage, etc. To reach this level of assurance, multiple combinations of the encryption techniques are taken to protect vital and sensitive data from mischievous users. The proposed algorithm is categorized into five phases. The data owner who wants to store data in the cloud is first registered with CSP in the first phase of the algorithm. The data is categorized on the basis of its sensitivity and stored in cloud storage in the second phase. The user who wants to recover the data from cloud undergoes the authentication process in the third phase. The auditors at CSP can verify the data integrity of cloud data in the fourth phase. It is required for SLA assurance and archived information. After passing valid authentication process, the user is allowed to retrieve the cloud data and verify the integrity of the fetched data, to provide proper feedback to the CSP about fetching data in the fifth phase.

3.1 Phase 1 (Registration of Data Owner to CSP)

Foremost of all, the user who wants to get the services of cloud storage, will have to register with the cloud service provider. The user requires to enter his particulars, valid username, password, and mobile number. The particulars and username are stored as such at CSP end. But the password is concatenated by the SALT, which increases password security by concatenating a random string to the password entered by the registered users. After Salting password is hashed using SHA–1 hashing technique and output hash code (512 bits) will be sent to the CSP. The concatenation of the SALT will prevent the dictionary attacks, SQL injection attacks and hash code of the salted password will prevent the CSP or unauthorized individual to steal user credentials from cloud storage (as shown in Fig. 2).

After verifying user's credentials and password, the CSP generates an OTP and send it to the user registered mobile number supplied during the registration procedure. The user is supposed to enter sent OTP to the CSP for completing the certification process; CSP matches it with the OTP generated and thus verify the mobile number if matched else refuse the registration procedure.

3.2 Phase 2 (Storing of Data in Cloud Storage)

After successfully completing the registration process, the data is categorized on the basis of its importance and sensitivity. The data are transmitted to the CSP through various steps in a data storing process described in subsections from 3.2.1 to 3.2.4 which provide a stepwise description of all activities done on the data (as shown in Fig. 3).

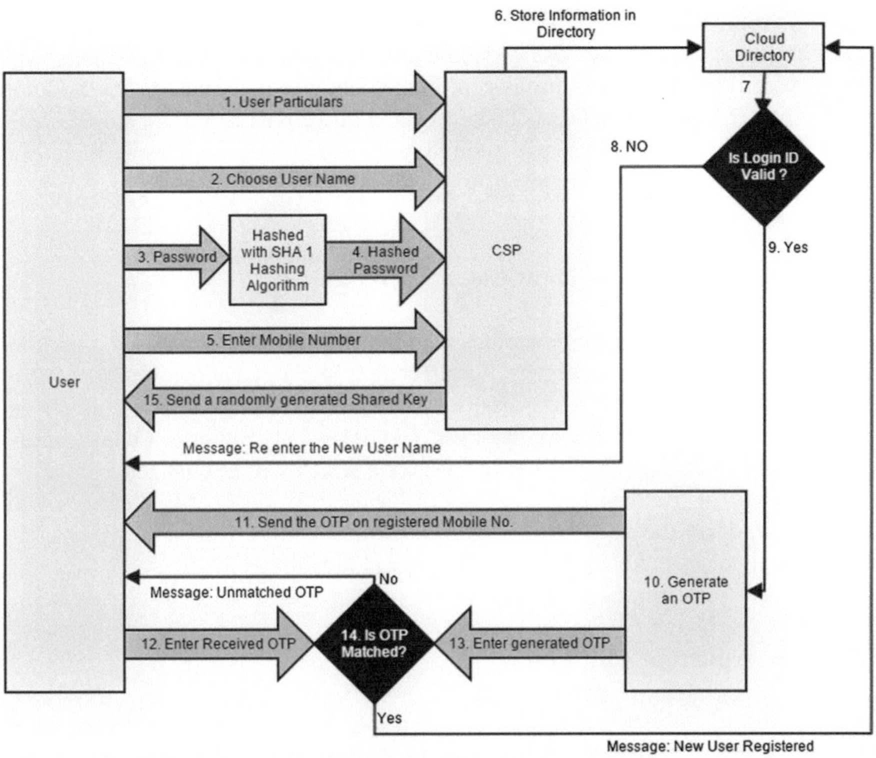

Fig. 2 Registration of cloud user to cloud service provider

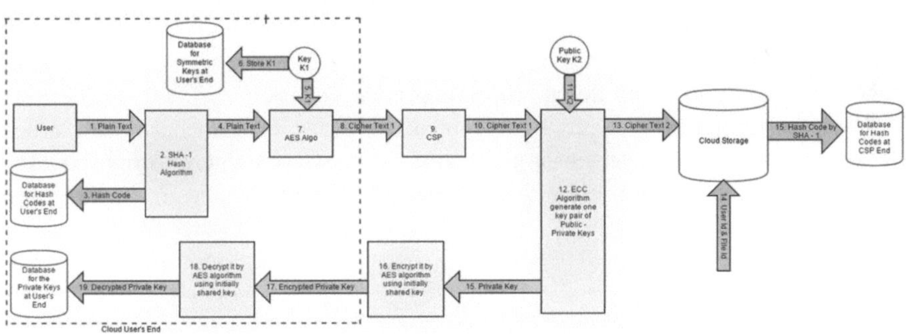

Fig. 3 Storing of data in cloud storage

3.2.1 Encryption at Cloud User (Owner) End

As soon as the user is registered with CSP, he is allowed to store the data in cloud storage. Only instead of sending plain text of PNTP category data directly to CSP, it is first encrypted with a symmetric encryption algorithm AES (advanced encryption algorithm) to avoid the man-in-the-middle attack, insider job attack, etc. The single key generated by AES algorithm is kept in the data owner's database for the future decryption. Thus, the plain text is first encrypted into cipher text 1, for storage to the CSP. The AES algorithm is secure enough in the today scenario because there is no known attack on the AES algorithm till date.

3.2.2 Hash Key Generation at Cloud User's End

The data integrity assurance is another required feature of the proposed algorithm. Thus to ensure user's data integrity, a hash code is generated at the user's end using a SHA-1 hashing algorithm. The hash code generated is kept up at the user's end database for integrity verification later on. The SHA-1 algorithm is a unidirectional cryptographic technique, which gets a hash code which will be changed even after a minor change in the data and then it will be used to verify the integrity of the information. Then the user will be ascertained that neither CSP nor any unauthorized individual has altered the data stored in cloud storage.

3.2.3 Encryption at CSP End

On receiving the cipher text 1 from the user, the CSP applies another very strong asymmetric key cryptographic technique ECC (Elliptic Curve cryptography). In this cryptographic asymmetric algorithm, a pair of public and private key is generated.

The received cipher text 1 is again encrypted with the generated public key and the paired private key is sent back to the legitimate user by encrypting it with the AES encryption algorithm through initially shared a key which is maintained by the user in its database in a secured way. That's how the data can be only unlocked by the authenticated user with the appropriate private key.

Since the information stored is encrypted two times back to back with strong algorithms which eliminate the loopholes of the past researchers' proposals. The double encryption is must since the data are always vulnerable to the unethical CSPs.

3.2.4 Hash Key Generation at CSP End

To maintain the integrity of the user's data, the CSP also generates a hash code at the CSP end using a SHA-1 hashing algorithm and maintain it in its database. Thus, it can be used later during routine auditing at the CSP end by matching the generated hash code. Then that user will be ascertained that neither CSP nor any unauthorized individual has altered the data in cloud storage stored for a long time.

3.3 *Phase 3 (User Authentication on Data Retrieval Request)*

This phase deal with the user authentication process for data retrieval from cloud storage. The user enters his login ID and password to CSP who in turn verify the entered credentials. After verifying the user credentials and password, the CSP generates an OTP, and send it to the user registered mobile number supplied during the enrollment procedure. The user is supposed to enter sent OTP to the CSP for completing the certification process; CSP matches it with the OTP generated, and thus verify the mobile number if matched else refuse the data recovery requests (as indicated in Fig. 4).

3.4 *Phase 4 (Auditing at Cloud End)*

This phase is mainly concerned with the auditing at the CSP end. Since the information stored by the user may not be required of him for a long time, so that to avoid the tempering of the data, one hash code of cipher text 2 is also maintained at the CSP end by SHA–1 hash algorithm. So that during regular auditing the CSP end, the tempering of the data can be distinguished and the proper message will be given to cloud user or data owner. This phase also ensures the SLA (service level agreement) between user and CSP.

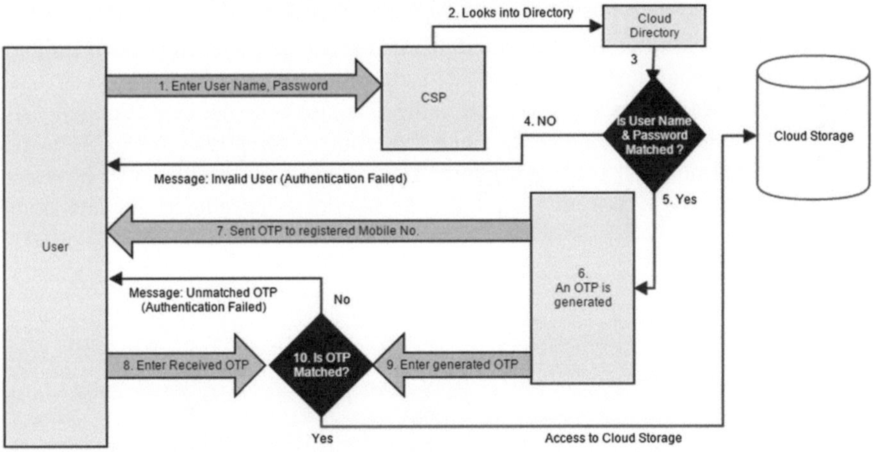

Fig. 4 User's authentication on data retrieval request

3.5 *Phase 5 (Retrieval of Data and Integrity Verification)*

In this phase, the authenticated user retrieves, convert to plain text, and verify the integrity of data. As shortly as the user is authenticated, he is permitted to access the cloud storage and brings in the required data present in cipher text 2 forms and carries it to its own premises to convert plain text mode (as indicated in Fig. 5).

This phase is further categorized into three Sects. 3.5.1 to 3.5.3 providing stepwise actions performed on data. Since all these steps performed on user's premises, then there will be no security breaches.

3.5.1 Private Key Decryption

First, the cipher text 2 is decrypted with the private key generated by ECC algorithm and stored in the user database to convert the retrieved data in cipher text 1 form.

3.5.2 Public Key Decryption

Second, the received cipher text 1 is further decrypted with the public key of the AES algorithm stored in the user database to change the data from cipher text 1 form in plain text configuration.

3.5.3 Hash Code Verification

To verify the integrity of the retrieved data, the user again generates a hash code for the transformed plain text using the SHA-1 algorithm. The generated hash key will be compared with the hash value stored in the database at owner end. If matches the integrity of the information is verified else the problem is reported to be CSP which can result into and legal process against CSP. That's how the user will be ascertained that neither CSP nor any unauthorized individual has altered the data stored in cloud storage.

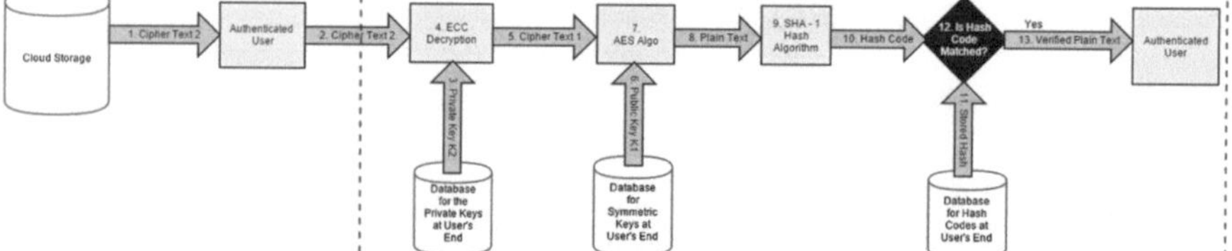

Fig. 5 Retrieval of data and integrity verification

4 Algorithm

Step 1: Registration of the user with CSP
- (a) Enter User Particulars,
- (b) Choose USER_Name, PWD
- (c) Enter M_Number

Step 2: if (USER_Name is valid) then
- (a) Generate a random key Rkey at CSP end and send it to user
- (b) Generate an OTP at CSP end
- (c) UserOTP ⟵ CSPOTP
- (d) Enter the User OTP received on user registered mobile
- (e) if (Entered OTP == CSPOTP) then
  - (i) Message: New User is registered
  - (ii) go to step 3

  else
  - (i) Message: Unmatched OTP & registration is canceled
  - (ii) go to step 10

else
- (i) Message: Invalid USER_Name, Choose some other USER_Name
- (ii) Go to step 2

Step 3: Selecting the category of the data
- (a) Based on the sensitivity of the data FPFID, categorize it into following categories
  - (i) NP (No Privacy) – Mainly Public Data so no encryption is required
  - (ii) PTP (Privacy with Trusted Provider) – Data with little importance and the trusted CSP is allowed to store it into encrypted mode
  - (iii) PNTP (Privacy with NON Trusted Provider) – Data with more sensitivity and importance and the encrypted data is sent to non trusted CSP which again store it into encrypted mode

Step 4: Uploading of user file to CSP
- (a) Select file FP in Plain text mode & assign a unique file ID FID
- (b) δ_{pc} = Privacy Category of file FPFID

Step 5: if δ_{pc} = NP then
- (a) Send (FPFID, NP, USER_ID) to CSP via SSL
- (b) Store in CSP storage with replication factor 3 in plain text form.

Step 6: if δ_{pc} = PTP then
- (a) Send (FPFID, PTP, USER_ID) to CSP via SSL
- (b) Generate a symmetric key CSPpub1 at CSP end
- (c) CSP_FCFID ⟵ Encrpt_AES (FPFID, FID, CSPpub1)
- (d) Store CSPpub1 at CSP end database.
- (e) Store CSP_FCFID at CSP storage with replication factor 3

Step 6: if δ_{pc} = PNTP then
- (a) Generate a Hash code for the file

  HCFID ⟵ HASH CODE_SHA1 (FPFID, FID)
- (b) Generate a symmetric key USERPub for FID by AES algorithm

  FC1FID ⟵ Encrpt_AES (FPFID, FID, USERPub)
- (c) Store HCFID and USERPub in User's Database
- (d) Send (FC1FID, User_ID) to CSP via SSL
- (e) Generate a Public – Private key pair CSPPr and CSPPub2by ECC asymmetric algorithm
  - (i) FC2FID ⟵ Encrypt_ECC(CSPPub2, FC1FID, User_ID)
  - (ii) Generate a Hash code for the file FC2FID

    CSP_HC_FC2FID ⟵ HASH CODE_ SHA1 (FC2FID, FID)
  - (iii) Store CSP_HC_FC2FID at CSP end for Auditing
  - (iv) Store FC2FID and δ_{pc} at CSP storage with replication factor 3
  - (v) Send ECC private key back to the user

    ECSPPR ⟵ Encrpt_AES(CSPPr, Rkey)

(vi) CSPPr ⟵ Decrpt_AES (ECSPPr ,Rkey)
(vii) Store CSPPr in User's Database

Step 7: User's Authentication Request to CSP
- (a) Enter USER_Name, PWD
- (b) if (USER_NAME is valid? && Password matched?) then
  - (i) Generate an OTP at CSP end
  - (ii) UserOTP ⟵ CSPOTP
  - (iii) Enter the User OTP received on the user registered mobile
  - (iv) if (Entered OTP == CSPOTP) then
    1. Message: Cloud access is allowed
    2. Send USER_ID to CSP
    3. go to step 8

    else
    1. Message: Unmatched OTP & login is canceled
    2. Exit

  else
  - (i) Message: Invalid User Credentials, Re enter the correct credentials
  - (ii) go to step 7

Step 8: Data retrieval and verification Process
- (a) CSP will list all users' file against that USER_ID
- (b)The user will opt FC2FID with its privacy category δ_{pc} from the list
- (c) if (δ_{pc} == NP) then
  - (i) CSP will send the file (FPFID, USER_ID) to user via SSL
- (d) if (δ_{pc} == PTP) then.
  - (i) At CSP end, the encypted file is decypted
    FPFID ⟵ Decrpt_AES
    (CSP_FCFID, FID, CSPpub1)
  - (ii) CSP will send the file (FPFID, USER_ID) to user via SSL
- (e) if (δ_{pc} == PNTP) then
  - (i) (FC2FID, USER_ID) will be sent back to user via SSL
  - (ii) FC1FID ⟵ Decrypt_ECC(CSPPr, FC2FID, User_ID)
  - (iii) FP FID ⟵ Decrpt_AES (FC1FID, USERPub, FID)
  - (iv) NEW_HCFID ⟵ HASH CODE_ SHA1 (FPFID, FID)
  - (v) if (NEW_HCFID == HCFID) then
    1. Message: File is retrieved successflly
    2. Send ACK to CSP
    3. go to step 10

    else
    1. Message: File is Corrupt
    2. Send NAK to CSP and start legal procedure
    3. go to step 10

Step 9: Auditing at CSP End
- (a) Generate a New Hash code for the file FC2FID
  - (i) NEW_CSP_HC_FC2FID ⟵ HASH CODE_SHA1(FC2FID, FID)
  - (ii) if (NEW_CSP_HC_FC2FID == CSP_HC_FC2FID) then
    1. Message: File is verified
    2. Send Positive Report to User else
    1. Message: File is Corrupt
    2. Send Negative Report to User and start a legal procedure

Step 10: EXIT

5 Security Analysis of Proposed Model

Designed and implemented algorithm is secure enough against most of the identified attacks, so that the data owner or organizations can store their data to the cloud storage with no worries at all. The proposed hybrid solution can prevent all these attacks described as:

5.1 Brute Force Attack

This attack is mainly concerned about using every possible combination of the key to crack the actual key.

In the proposed algorithm, the introduction of the AES encryption algorithm will fail this attack because only the cracking of AES—256 require about 2^{255} combination, which is not feasible in real time even by using fastest super computer available in today's scenario.

5.2 Authentication Attacks

This attack is mainly concerned about using the credentials of the authorized user to log into his cloud account.

In the proposed algorithm the introduction of the OTP (one-time password) will fail this attack because only the user with credentials and registered mobile number can access the cloud account.

5.3 Dictionary Attacks

This attack is mainly concerned about using all the possible dictionary words to crack the password of the authorized user to log into his cloud account.

In the proposed algorithm the introduction of the saltiest, the concatenation of an arbitrary string in the user password secures it from being error-prone to a dictionary attack.

5.4 Man-in-the-Middle Attack

This attack is mainly concerned about being a forged authenticated user for the data retrieval from cloud storage.

In the proposed algorithm even if an unauthorized user will be able to retrieve the data from cloud storage, it will be in the form of cipher text 2, which will be of no use in the absence of the private key and public key stored within the authorized user's secure premises.

5.5 Cloud Malware Injection

This attack is mainly concerned with introduction of a suspicious malware in the cloud itself so that cloud data can be retrieved from cloud storage without the permission of cloud user and CSP.

In the proposed algorithm even if an unauthorized user will be able to retrieve the data from cloud storage, it will be in the form of cipher text 2, which will be of no use in the absence of the private key and public key stored within the authorized user's secure premises.

5.6 Side Channel Attack

Since the data from various users share same cloud storage in an isolated environment. This attack is mainly concerned of intentional crossing the boundaries of the own cloud storage to penetrate into some other cloud storage.

In the proposed algorithm even if an unauthorized user will be able to retrieve the data from side cloud storage, it will be in the form of cipher text 2, which will be of no use in the absence of the private key and public key stored within the authorized user's secure premises.

5.7 Inside-Job Attack

Since the data is stored in cloud storage in cloud owner control. This attack is mainly concerned of intentional stealing the user's information by CSPs itself for some more profit making purpose.

In the proposed algorithm even if CSP will steal the data from cloud storage, it will be in the form of at least cipher text 1, which will be of no use in the absence of the public key stored within the authorized user's secure premises.

5.8 SQL Injection Attack

This attack is one of the many web attack mechanisms used by hackers to steal data from organizations by using simple SQL commands.

In the proposed algorithm, salting to the password and adding hashing to the salt as well as the OTP concept makes SQL injection attack nearly impossible.

So the proposed algorithm is enough to secure to handle all the main concerned of a cloud user. So the cloud user now can submit its data to the cloud storage with no issues.

6 Conclusion and Future Scope

As discussed earlier, a lot of the startup organizations are adopting cloud eagerly due to huge cloud facilities with minimal investment. Apart from it, cloud data security is one of the main concerns of the organizations, before adopting cloud.

This paper designed and implemented a new hybrid algorithm for securing cloud data using three different security policies for three different types of sensitive data to maximize control of data owner on storing, processing and accessing on it. The proposed hybrid algorithm is found to be highly secure for all types of sensitive data cloud environment.

In future, the algorithm can be tested against the various security attacks practically, the concept can be checked for efficiency and work can be extended to minimize the required time for all processing, even the concept can be combined with biometric traits those can be used for generating keys for encryption and decryption processes to gain an edge in the field of cloud storage.

References

1. Cloud Security Alliance “Top Threats to Cloud Computing” published in USA: Cloud Security Alliance, (2010)
2. Maghrabi, L.A.: The threats of data security over the cloud as perceived by experts and university students. University of the West of England, Bristol, United Kingdom (2013)
3. Singh, A., Shrivastava, M.: Overview of attacks on cloud computing. Int. J. Eng. Innovative Technol. **1**(4), 321–323 (2012)
4. Yu, H.S., Gelogo, Y.E., Kim, K.J.: Securing data storage in cloud computing. J. Secur. Eng. 251–260 (2012)
5. Nandakumar, K., Jain, A.K., Pankanti, S.: Fingerprint-based fuzzy vault: implementation and performance. In: IEEE Transactions on Information Forensics and Security, Vol. 2, no. 4 (2007)
6. Li, X., Yu, L., Wei, L.: The application of hybrid encryption algorithm in software security. 978-1-4799-2860-6, IEEE, (2013)

7. Tweney, A., Crane, S.: Trust guide: An exploration of privacy preferences in an online world. In: Expanding the Knowledge Economy Applications Case Studies. IOS Press, Amsterdam (2007)
8. Tang, Z., Wang, X., Jia, L., Zhang, X., Man, W.: Study on data security of cloud computing. IEEE Xplore: 978-1-4577-1964-6 © 2012 IEEE, pp. 1–3 (2012)
9. Rong, C., Nguyen, S.T., JaatUN, M.G.: Beyond lightning: A Survey on security challenges in cloud computing. In: Elsevier Computers and Electrical Engineering. pp. 47–54 (2012)
10. Grobauer, B., Walloschek, T., Stöcker Siemens, E.: Understanding cloud computing vulnerabilities. IEEE J. Comput. Reliab. Socities **9**(2), 50–57 (2011)
11. Waleed, Al.W., Li, C., Naji, H.A.H.: The faults of data security and privacy in the cloud computing. J. Netw. **9**(12), pp. 3313–3320 (2014)
12. Lin, G.: Research on electronic Data security strategy based on cloud computing. In: IEEE Xplore: 978-1-4577-1415-3 ©2012 IEEE, pp 1228–1231 (2012)
13. Divya, S.V., Dr.Shaji R.S.: Security in data forwarding through elliptic curve cryptography in cloud. In: 2014 International Conference on Control, Instrumentation, Communication and Computational Technologies (ICCICCT), 978-1-4799-4190-2 ©2014 IEEE, pp. 1083–1088 (2014)
14. Kumar, A., Lee, B.G., Lee, H.J., Kumari, A.: Secure storage and access of data in cloud computing. ICTC 2012, IEEE Xplore: 978-1-4673-4828-7 ©2012 IEEE, pp. 336–339 (2012)
15. Fu, Z., Cao, X., Wang, J., Sun, X.: Secure storage of data in cloud computing. In: 2014 Tenth International Conference on Intelligent Information Hiding and Multimedia Signal Processing, IEEE Xplore: 978-1-4799-5390-5 © 2014 IEEE, pp. 783–786 (2014)
16. Tan, Y., Wang, X.: Research of cloud computing data security technology. In: IEEE Xplore: 978-1-4577-1415-3 © 2012 IEEE, pp. 2781–2783 (2012)
17. Sinha, R., Srivastava, H.K., Gupta, S.: Performance based comparison study of rsa and elliptic curve cryptography. Int. J. Sci. Eng. Res. ISSN 2229–5518, **4**(5), 720–725 (2013)
18. Abdul, D.S.H., Abdul Kader, M., Hadhoud, M.M.: Performance evaluation of symmetric encryption algorithms. J. Commun. IBIMA, ISSN: 1943–7765, **8**, 58–64 (2009)
19. Pavithra, S., Ramadevi, E.: Performance evaluation of symmetric algorithms. J. Global Res. Comput. Sci. ISSN 2229-371X, **3**(8), 43–45 (2012)
20. Mahalle, V.S., Shahade, A.K.: Enhancing the data security in cloud by implementing hybrid (RSA & AES) Encryption Algorithm. IEEE 978-1-4799-7169-5 ©. (2014)
21. Tripathi, A., Yadav, P.: Enhancing security of cloud computing using elliptic curve cryptography. Int. J. Comput. Appl. ISSN: 0975–8887, **57**(1), pp. 26–30 (2012)
22. Mohamed, E.M., Abdelkader, H.S., EI-Etriby, S.: Enhanced data security model for cloud computing. In: 8th International Conference on informatics and Systems (INFOS2012), pp. 12–17 (2012)
23. Dinadayalan1, P., Jegadeeswari, S., Gnanambigai, D.: Data security issues in cloud environment and solutions. In: 2014 World Congress on Computing and Communication Technologies, IEEE Xplore: 978-1-4799-2876-7 © 2013 IEEE, pp. 88–91 (2013)
24. Daemen, J., and Rijmen, V.: Rijndael: the advanced encryption standard. Dr. Dobb's J. 137–139. (2001)

Big Data Analytics: Recent and Emerging Application in Services Industry

Rajesh Math

Abstract The term 'Big Data' initially used by Roger Magoulas [1] from O'Reilly media in 2005 is all modern day large data sets and different stakeholders understand the phenomenon in multiple ways. Knowledge workers view Big Data as huge correlated data sets requiring super large computing powers to analyze the process and derive meaningful conclusions. Big Data is multidimensional data these days ranging from info-bytes from newspapers to online journals, from tweets to YouTube videos, social networking updates and blog discussions, which any business/organization is accumulating thru various information channels. The huge explosion of data and increase in Internet devices has led to the rapid rise of Big Data. Majority of data that contribute to Big Data comes from Internet sources or are Internet of Things. The scale of data set referred as "Big Data can be defined as data that legacy DBMS tools can't load and understand the heterogeneous relationship." With the massive current technological advances the cutoff size of data sets qualifying as Big Data is bound to increase. We look at some of the underlying concepts of Big Data and propose solutions in Service Industry as there the quality of service is a key differentiator as compared traditional manufacturing industry where the quality of finished goods or product is important. The primary advantage of Big Data is by aggregating large amount of data integrated from various sources such as CRM, social media, email, web, mobile and tablet and data acquisition from other technologies. In this paper, we try to review the potential applications of Big Data in Service Industry and understand the source of its decision making data from Internet. We understand that the business is not interested in single data but desires to look at the trend and patterns in the data which might boost the business tremendously, and Internet of things would be creating streams of data needed for this purpose.

R. Math (✉)
Dr. D.Y. Patil Institute of Master of Computer Applications,
Savitribai Phule University, Akurdi, Pune, India

V.B. Aggarwal et al. (eds.), *Big Data Analytics*, Advances in Intelligent
Systems and Computing 654, https://doi.org/10.1007/978-981-10-6620-7_21

Keywords Big data · IT applications · Decision-making · Data analytics · Service-Level agreements · DSS · MIS · CRM · Service industry

1 Literature Survey

We start our research with the focus on the decision-making process which is critical for business. We are all aware that decisions are critical for business and enterprises and workflow analytics system which are a specialized area of information systems with a focus on improving the decision-making. Ackoff [2] researched the development of Management Information Systems[MIS] for managerial decision-making. Alavi et al. [3] argued that the MIS systems developed were large and monolithic and the information generated were hard to use for decision-making, Dearden [4] and Gorry et al. [5] researched "decision support systems" (DSS) in their paper and constructed a framework for improving management information systems using Anthony's [6] managerial activity and Simon's [7] classification of decision types. Simon [8] had proposed a behavioral model of decision-making used in various industries by Managers based on a rational choice among various alternatives. This model was used with the modern decision-making systems but with the explosion of data in the modern era, Big Data is the appropriate data provider for the same. There are various references to the projected growth of 'Big Data'. Janakiraman et al. [9] highlight the impact of the growth of Big Data and how developing nations will have a better service level as compared to emerging nations due to larger and longer amount of data. Math and Sharma [10] have referenced the same building blocks of the Big Data Analytics to drive the service industry.

2 Service Industry and Background of Analytics

From the inception of management science which is an essential study for decision-making, researchers developed data analysis models primarily for Manufacturing Industry and designed solutions for Profit Maximization problem, which was maximizing revenues for minimal cost. In case of the service industry, the analytics study has to be focused on workflow analytics and customer satisfaction level with service level as a key differentiator. The Service Industry has a different product which is service which is not a physical and finite item which can be essentially quality checked. To achieve this better level of service and customer satisfaction becomes a nodal requirement for any workflow analytics systems. In the early days, the technology and storage where not really able to serve this purpose.

3 Big Data Analytics: Trends and Service Industry

The quick surge in Big Data Analytics has to be attributed to the development of certain computing technologies such as Hadoop, HDFS, MapReduce, Google's Bigtables, NoSQL, IoT, etc. These technologies have enabled the managers to convert the intuition to data-backed decisions. The Service Industry has seen an increase in expectation of customers regarding the service. This has coupled with faster transmission of data and ability to service the client from virtual locations making the service delivery model very different. In case of Big Data; the analysis of the data is a crucial component. Recent developments in hardware need to address not simply the storage of large datasets but also it's retrieval and querying. Current research in DBMS [Database Management Systems] has found out the difference between the computing powers needed for storage and that of analysis. Jacobs [11] used PostGre SQL to compare computing times for data storage and data queries. His research indicates that as data volume increases, the time required to perform a query increases. Our research indicates that new technologies will address this computing problem and lead design of integrated decision support systems leading to faster delivery cycles which will help Service Industry.

In this section, few graphs and tables have been presented to reflect future trends. Table 1 and Figure derived from IDC estimates and Wikibon Data[18] and Table 1 and Figure derived from Web Traffic: Cisco Market Forecast by Gartner [11], show some of the global estimates for future.

4 Case Study #1 Cell Service Provider Big Data Analytics

Big Data analytics will be used to take decisions to improve service levels. The customer calls with various issues from billing, coverage, and technical issues. The Tech Support engineer provides a case-by-case solution over the phone. The Cell Service Provider was having a high customer service cost and losing time and opportunity, up sell revenues as the data from CRM and internal systems were not being viewed during problem analysis phase. As the company gets a large number of support calls, it wishes to use Big Data to identify systematic problem areas and analyze call-patterns. Enterprises and organizations are having significant accumulation of data from different sources to use this technique.

For example, if callers from certain areas are having issues then maybe it is a systemic problem rather than the individual customer (Table 2).

Based on our analysis of every data of 2000 customers, we can expect 25 leads for prospective customers. Most of these leads can generate additional revenue activates for the Service Provider. For example, a customer might be interested in an Internet data after 8 PM at a cheaper rate for personal use. This we feel is the right approach to deliver a better customer service (Fig. 1).

Table 1 Wikibon/IDC estimates cisco/gartner estimates [12]

	Global	India	
	US$ billion	US$ million	
2017	4740	5000	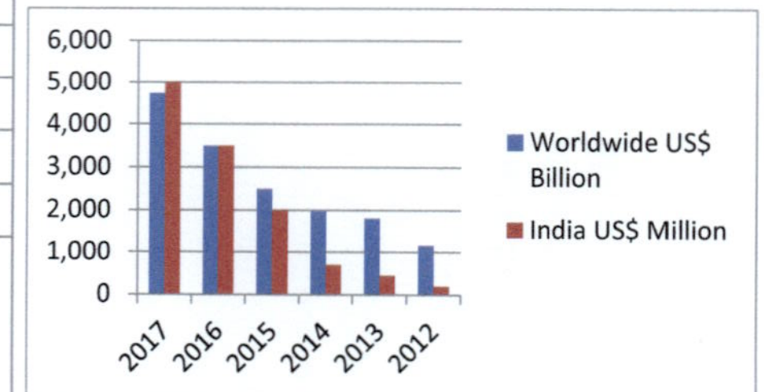
2016	3500	3500	
2015	2500	2000	
2014	2000	700	
2013	1810	450	
2012	1159	200	
Devices/data growth			
Year	# Devices	Traffic	
	Billion	Exabytes	
2020	50	1029	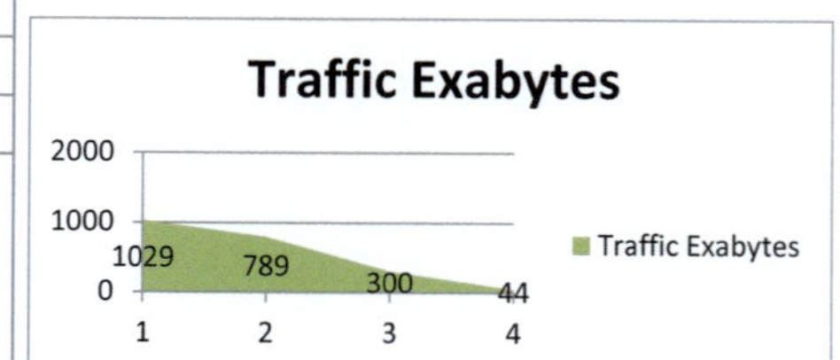
2018	36	789	
2016	28	300	
2014	20	44	

Table 2 Cell-phone call analytics collection data template

Data collection attribute	Details
Name	First name
Phone number	10 digit number
Gender	Male/female
Location	Area/city/tower number
Data usage	2G/3G/4G
Calling time	Early morning/morning/noon/evening/night/late night
Calling duration	Duration of call
Type of call	Personal/professional

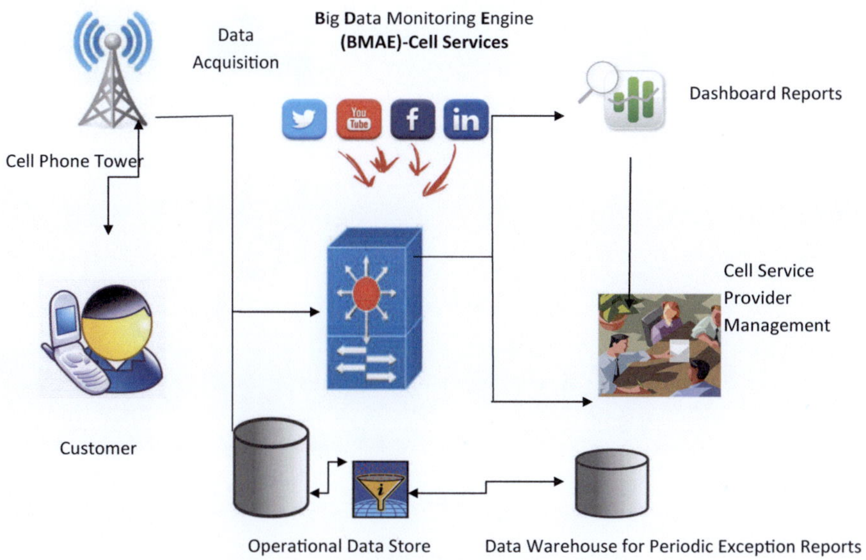

Fig. 1 Cell phone monitoring: big data illustration

5 Case Study #2 E-Commerce Site Analytics

A major Business to Customer (B2C) E-Commerce site to analyze the website statistics to determine the Marketing/Promotion strategy and offer products to a customer based on the prior website visit statistics (Table 3).

A major Business to Customer (B2C) e-commerce site wants to analyze the visitor statistics to determine the promotion strategy and target the interested customer and maintain a wish list of potential purchases and have a mechanism to send him/her promotional pricing as and when it becomes available

Table 3 E-commerce site analytics data template

Name	Phone no.	Address	Demographic data	Married status	Purchased item	Wish list	Bill amt	Purchasing month

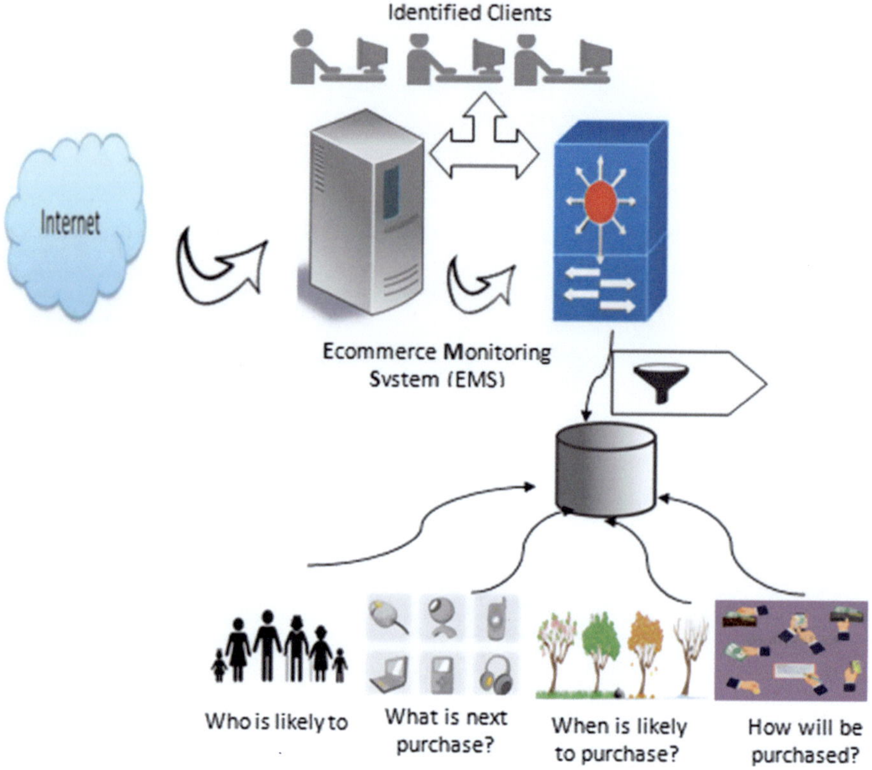

Fig. 2 E-commerce site analytics: big data illustration

We keep the track of the web-visitor statistics and using the EMS we can analyze the data and have the following:

- To keep track of the products which have been clicked by the visitor
- To reach out to visitor when an event related to that product has happened.

For example, if a visitor has been on leather shoes for long and not purchased it, then he is a potential customer for leather shoes. If he has an account with the site then he should be communicated of any special promotion till he buys the product (Fig. 2).

6 Case Study 3 Online Insurance Selling

An insurance company wants to track its new sales to determine if the source of their new sales has been initiated from their own online advertisement and if so what is the website from where it originates. They have a large number of online advertisement which is put on various sites.

The insurance seller has to keep track of its marketing costs and spend money where there is the possibility of a positive outcome as that is the profitable outcome for them.

Problem Analysis: An insurance company wishes to determine its marketing strategy based on the web-based advertisements and best promotion mix of websites based on the positive outcome of advertisement.

- Track its new sales leads and determine the lead generation point from the various online advertisements.
- They want to also analyze the leads from time to progression and closure results.
- Determine the optimal Advertisement mix across the various online portals.

Outline of Solution:

To track the new sales lead can be done based on online advertisement which was clicked. If there is click that has lead to this then they would like to know that source as well.

- The progression of lead from initial click to closure interactions with the customer.
- A positive outcome determination.The determination of advertising mix and budget can be done based on past history usage (Fig. 3; Table 4).

7 Big Data for Service Industry

Big Data will have a huge impact and will redefine the way data can be used for the improvement of the Service Industry.Here are the some of the interesting facts on how the Big Data can be leveraged in Service Industry:

(a) Service Provider Management Team tasked with data analysis, aggregated data from various sources including voter list, social media posts, fundraisers etc.
(b) Multi-variant tests were conducted to understand client's decisions making and designing effective policies to persuade them.
(c) The data analysis included mining customer data, profiling them and sending targeted campaign emails to influence their decision. The analysis also provided crucial insights about the others who are most likely to switch sides and the required triggering points for the switch.

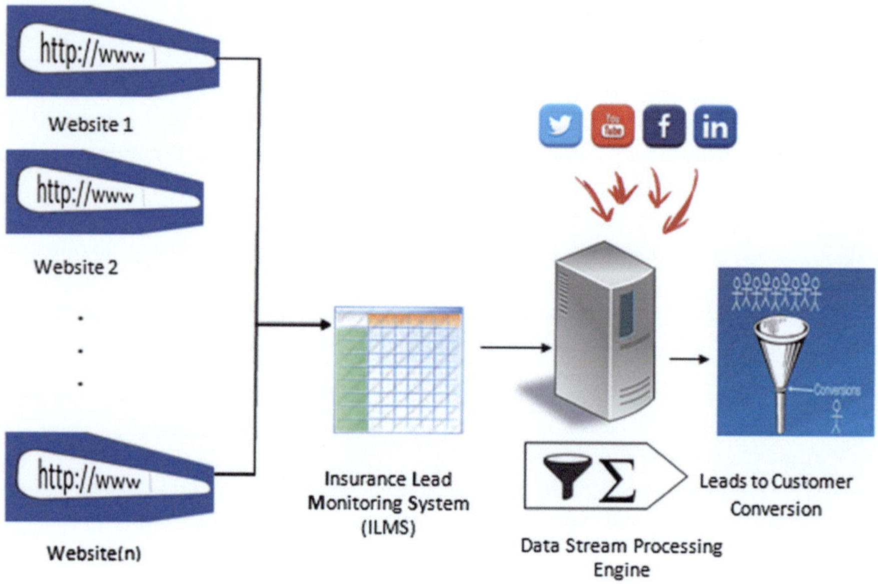

Fig. 3 Insurance cross selling: big data illustration

Table 4 Data collection online insurance selling

Name	Phone no.	Address city	Demographic data	Marital status	Source website

(d) The team built persuasion model with predictive analytics to find out the probability of persuasion among population various geographies.
(e) Analyzing the Big Data was the key differentiator in swinging a good percentage of clients and predicting the results with a greater confidence.

8 Conclusion and Future Research

Majority of data that contribute to Big Data comes from nternet sources or are Internet of Things. We understand that the business is not interested in single data but desires to look at the trend and patterns in the data which might boost the business tremendously, and Internet of things would be creating streams of data needed for this purpose. The objective is to understand the information needed by various industries across verticals to improve the policy to boost the business and the major sources that contribute to this information. Our research indicates that majority of the Big Data systems can be scalable build over various decisions making data systems and information collection systems and will make the workflow more optimal. Big Data can be sourced from the Internet and internal data systems and using simple data collection techniques which can be used to build more complex decision systems. The service industry will be immensely benefited as it can use these to give a better service level into areas as diverse as healthcare and environmental sciences. As per the negative impression, Big Data is seen of Big Brother or invisible intruder, with intrusions in of privacy and attacking civil liberties. Big Data is a more relevant technology to larger corporations and tends to squeeze the small to mid-size corporation due to economies of scale and the sheer volume of data. Whatever way we think of it we feel Big Data will be a potent force as more and more devices connect thru the Internet.

References

1. http://strata.oreilly.com/2010/01/roger-magoulas-on-big-data
2. Ackoff, R.L.: Management misinformation systems. Manag. Sci. **14**(4), 147–156
3. Alavi, M., Carlson, P.: A review of MIS research. J. Manag. Information Systems, 8(4), 45–62 (1992)
4. Dearden, J.: MIS is a mirage. Harvard Business Review, **50**(1), 90–99 (1972)
5. Gorry, G.A., Scott Morton, M.S.: Sloan Manag. Rev. **13**(1), 1–22 (1971)
6. Anthony, R.N.: Planning and Control Systems: A Framework for Analysis (Harvard) (1965)
7. Simon, H.A.: The new science of management decision, rev edn. Prentice-Hall, Englewood Cliffs, NJ (1977)
8. Simon, H.A. A behavioral model of rational choice. Q. J. Econ. **69**(1) (1955)
9. Moorthy, J., Lahiri, R., Biswas, N., Sanyal, D., Ranjan, J., Nanath, K. and Ghosh, P. Big data: Prospects and challenges
10. Math, R., Sharma, N. Big data analytics: In service industry. ISSN 2249–6149
11. Gartner.: Forecast: The internet of things, Worldwide. Retrieved from https://www.gartner.com/doc/2625419/forecast-internet-things-worldwide (2013, December 12)
12. http://wikibon.org/wiki/v/4_Excellent_Big_Data_Case_Studies
13. Jacobs, A.: The pathologies of Big Data. Databases ACM Queue 7(6) (2009)
14. Keen, P.G.W.: DSS: An Organizational Perspective. (1978)
15. http://www.bis.gov.uk/assets/biscore/science/docs/i/11-p123-international-comparative-performance-uk-research-base-
16. Mapping the future big data by patrick tucker the futurist July-August-2013 http://•www.wfs.org
17. http://www.bis.gov.uk/assets/biscore/science/docs/i/11-p123-international-comparative-performance-uk-research-base-2011.pdf

An Analysis of Resource-Aware Adaptive Scheduling for HPC Clusters with Hadoop

S. Rashmi and Anirban Basu

Abstract High-Performance Computing (HPC) is one of the upcoming technologies that represent data-intensive and compute-intensive applications. HPC–on–Cloud is an added advantage to enhance the efficiency of massively parallel applications. Hadoop-MapReduce is a programming paradigm designed to process parallel data on cloud. The key to improve performance of Hadoop-MapReduce lies with Efficient Resource allocation and Scheduling. In this paper, we analyze the behaviour of resource-aware adaptive scheduling which aims to improve resource utilization in MapReduce clusters.

Keywords HPC · Hadoop-MapReduce · Resource allocation · Scheduling · Performance

1 Introduction

HPC [1–3] is an emergent technology that emphasizes parallelism for scientific computing. It solves large problems, which deal with massive data and compute power. Its applications are wider in the areas of Internet search, weather forecasting, traffic control, decision-making systems, and so on. Such applications require the data to be processed in parallel to gain speed up and efficiency.

Cloud computing [4] enables on-demand access to a shared pool of computing resources, such as storage, servers, networking, applications and services. The key characteristics of cloud computing are on-demand self-service, resource pooling,

S. Rashmi (✉) · A. Basu
Department of Computer Science and Engineering,
East Point College of Engineering and Technology, Bangalore, India
e-mail: rashmineha.s@gmail.com

A. Basu
e-mail: abasu@pqrsoftware.com

V.B. Aggarwal et al. (eds.), *Big Data Analytics*, Advances in Intelligent Systems and Computing 654, https://doi.org/10.1007/978-981-10-6620-7_22

rapid elasticity, broad network access, and measured service. It offers easy access to both the user and service provider. With HPC–on–Cloud [5, 6], the challenges of data-intensive computations like handling dynamic data, storage requirements and lack of locality in computations can be assured. Cloud technologies [1, 2] such as MapReduce [7, 8], Hadoop [9, 10] and HDFS [10, 11] prefer moving computations to data for processing.

Hadoop-MapReduce is one the predominant technologies proposed for large-scale data-intensive cloud computing platforms. MapReduce runs multiple map and reduce tasks and parallelize the computations. However, the overall performance of the system essentially depends on efficient resource allocation and scheduling. Scheduling is an approach to allocate the resources of the system such as CPU time, Bandwidth, Memory etc., to improve resource utilization and balance the load across the system. Hadoop comes with three primary schedulers like FIFO, Fair Scheduler [12], and Capacity Scheduler [13], but they have their own limitations. Resource-aware adaptive scheduling (RAS) [14] technique is an efficient resource management framework. In this work, we analyze the behaviour of RAS in multi-job workloads and compare it with the FIFO.

The paper is organized as follows: Sect. 2 gives an overview of Hadoop, MapReduce, fundamental issues influencing the MapReduce performance, scheduling challenges, and the three primary schedulers. Section 3 describes the RAS method, Sect. 4 talks about the working of RAS, Sect. 5 and 6 discuss the evaluation and related work. And finally, we conclude in Sect. 7.

2 Background Knowledge

2.1 Hadoop-MapReduce

Hadoop [9, 10] is a Java open-source implementation of MapReduce. Large IT companies like Google, Yahoo, and Facebook are clients of Hadoop for large-scale data processing. Hadoop uses a distributed file system HDFS and a MapReduce programming paradigm. HDFS can support very large files of size TB or GB. It has a master/slave architecture, a single name node being the master and multiple data nodes serving as slaves. HDFS exhibits characteristics like data replication, data locality, fault tolerance, scalability, and reliability. Figure 1 shows the core components of Hadoop [15].

MapReduce is a parallel programming model for large-scale data sets. It consists of two functions: map and reduce functions. Map accepts as input (key1, value1) pairs. It computes a set of intermediary key-value pairs (key2, value 2).Using key equality, they are grouped as [key2, list (value2)]. Any job executing may go through a set of phases like map, merge, shuffle, sort, and reduce [16].

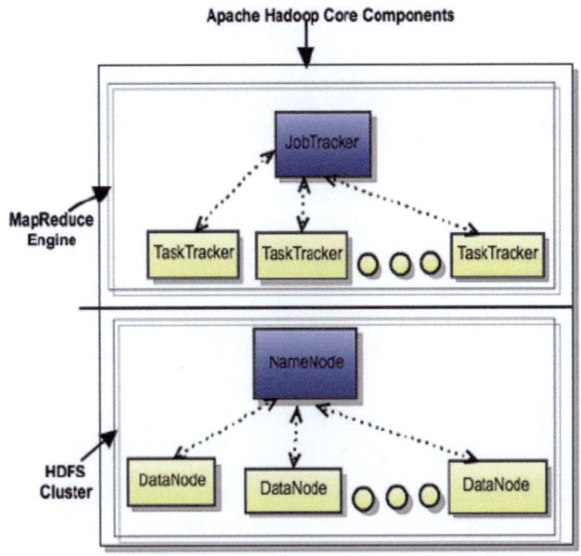

Fig. 1 Core components of Hadoop

2.2 *Fundamental Issues that Influence MapReduce Performance*

Wottrich and Bressoud [17] have identified a set of fundamental issues that influence the performance of MapReduce. At any instance of time, a block read is performed from the datanode that has comparatively least data among the three datanodes that contain the block. This data is again partitioned between the map tasks.

The intermediate phases of MapReduce like merge, shuffle, and sort deals with intermediate data. Finally, the reduce tasks generate the output data. This operational method impacts the MapReduce performance. They can be categorized as

- Quantity of the input data which is partitioned among the map tasks
- Varying amount of intermediate data emitted by the Map tasks at the conclusion of the MapReduce phase of a job which must be shuffled and sorted
- Quantity of the output data emitted at the end of the Reduce phase which gives the job run time
- Varying number of Map tasks generated during the Map phase
- Varying number of Reduce tasks generated during the Reduce phase.

2.3 Scheduling Challenges

A scheduling policy needs to decide the sequence of execution of jobs and then its tasks. Moreover, the jobs would have different complexity, characteristics, and requirements. The tasks also would be of different type and have different data locations. The available node would differ in their speed, capacity, and other hardware characteristics. The scheduling needs to consider all these. An appropriate scheduler must be aware of all these information and also about the currently executing and waiting tasks. An inappropriate scheduling algorithm may result in underutilization of resources; degrade the throughput and performance of the system. It would also fail to exploit the true potential of the system. The complexity of a scheduling problem is said to be NP-Complete [18].

Scheduling algorithms in parallel systems can be broadly classified in different ways [18] based on

(a) Time at which scheduling decisions are taken—Static/Dynamic
(b) Search space —Optimal/Suboptimal or Approximate/ Heuristic
(c) Responsibility of making decisions lie at one single point or distributed—Centralized/ Distributed
(d) Processing capabilities of resources and tasks—Adaptive/Nonadaptive
(e) Goal of improving performance of application or resource—Application centric/Resource centric
(f) Infrastructure of system—Homogeneous/Heterogeneous.

2.4 Primary Hadoop Schedulers

MapReduce in Hadoop comes with a choice of schedulers. The default is FIFO.

1. *FIFO Scheduler*: The default FIFO [12] is a queue-based scheduler. In FIFO scheduling, a jobtracker schedules the oldest job first from the queue. The FIFO scheduling approach does not take into account job priority or job size while choosing a job from the job queue. The algorithm is simple to implement.
2. *Fair Scheduler: The* idea behind Fair scheduler [12] is to evenly allocate the resources among the multiple jobs. Each user has a job pool and each pool has a guaranteed capacity. Tasks are scheduled based on the priority of the job within the pool, cluster capacity, and usage of the pool. Excess capacity in any pool, at any instant of time, is again evenly divided among other users. The fair scheduler was developed by Facebook.
3. *Capacity Scheduler:* The capacity scheduler [13] has several queues instead of job pools as in fair scheduling. Each queue has a guaranteed capacity with a configurable number of map and reduce slots. Each queue can give the portion

of unused slots to other queues. As far as a single queue is concerned, scheduling is done, based on FIFO with priority. The capacity scheduler was developed by Yahoo.

3 Resource-Aware Adaptive Scheduling (RAS)

Hadoop uses slot-based resource allocation. A slot is a computation unit in a node. MapReduce has a fixed size map/reduce slots. But this type of allocation is static and is less suitable for a multi-user, multi-job cluster environment (Fig. 2).

In RAS [14], MapReduce uses Job Profiling technique to obtain information related to utilization of resources of each job. The job profile is created by executing the job in a testing environment resembling the on-site environment. The job is executed a number of times with varying configurations on different nodes. Eg. Once with one map task per node, then two map task per node, etc. The best configuration is used to create a job profile. Figure 3 shows the architecture of RAS [14].

As proposed by Polo et al. [14] in, RAS has five different components: job utility calculator, placement algorithm, job status updater, task scheduler, job completion time estimator. The major role is played by the jobtracker. Jobs are first submitted with their completion Time goal and job profile, which contains information about a number of maps, number of reduces, resource requirements etc., At any instant, the jobtracker maintains two lists: list of executing jobs and their present status and list of tasktracker. Whenever a task completed, the tasktracker sends a notification to the job status updater. Job status updater revises the average task length of the corresponding job. The job completion time estimator determines the number of map tasks required to meet the goal set during job estimation. Placement algorithm and job utility calculator constitute the placement control loop. It creates a placement matrix. The placement algorithm keeps track of tasks of tasktracker, their

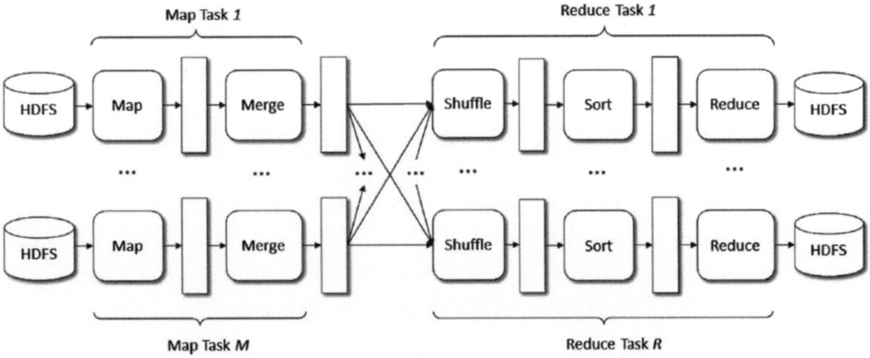

Fig. 2 Phases involved in the execution of a typical MapReduce Job [16]

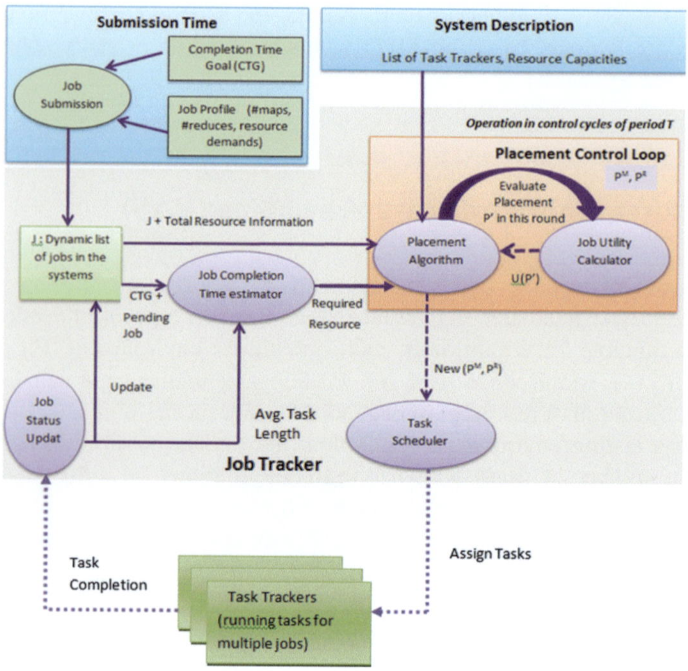

Fig. 3 Architecture of RAS

resource utilization, placement matrix and arrives at the final placement to be used. Job utility calculator finds a utility value which helps placement algorithm to choose the best placement. Task scheduler abides by the placement decision and decides on the new task to be placed. Figures 4 and 5 shows the place reducer and place mapper of the placement algorithm.

4 Working of RAS Scheduler

4.1 Job Initialization

Initialization involves setting up an entity that denotes a job with its tasks and log information to keep track of the tasks' status and progress. When a Job () is submitted by the jobtracker, it inserts it in the queue. Job scheduler then initializes them and creates a number of map tasks based on the number of splits. Reduce tasks are created using the configuration files. As execution progress, the count of map tasks decreases and the count of reduce tasks increases.

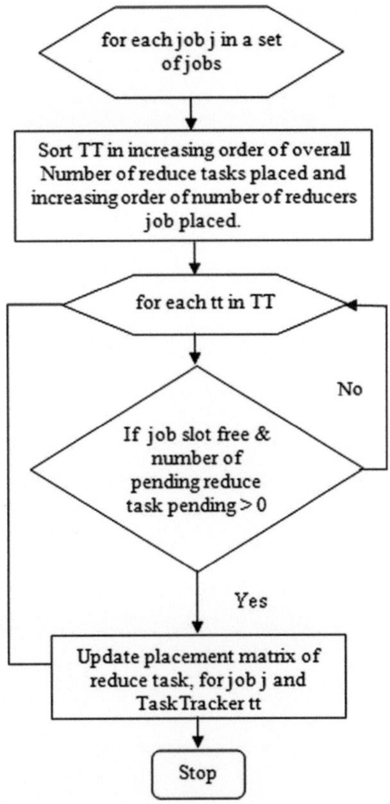

Fig. 4 Place redures of placement algorithm

4.2 *Task Assignment*

A heartbeat signal contains the number of maps and reduce tasks remaining in that particular node. A tasktracker dynamically sends heartbeats signal to the jobtracker to notify that it is alive. It also informs jobtracker whether it is ready for a new task. Upon reception of a new task, it sends a return value. Scheduling comes into the picture at this point when a new task has to assigned. Based on the placement decisions taken by the RAS, a new task will be allotted

4.3 *Task Execution*

After assignment of the task, it has to be executed. The JAR file along with other files is narrowed down to tasktracker. It unloads the JAR file to a local working directory and runs the task. In this way, the tasktracker updates the jobtracker regarding its status every few time units.

Fig. 5 Place mappers of placement algorithm

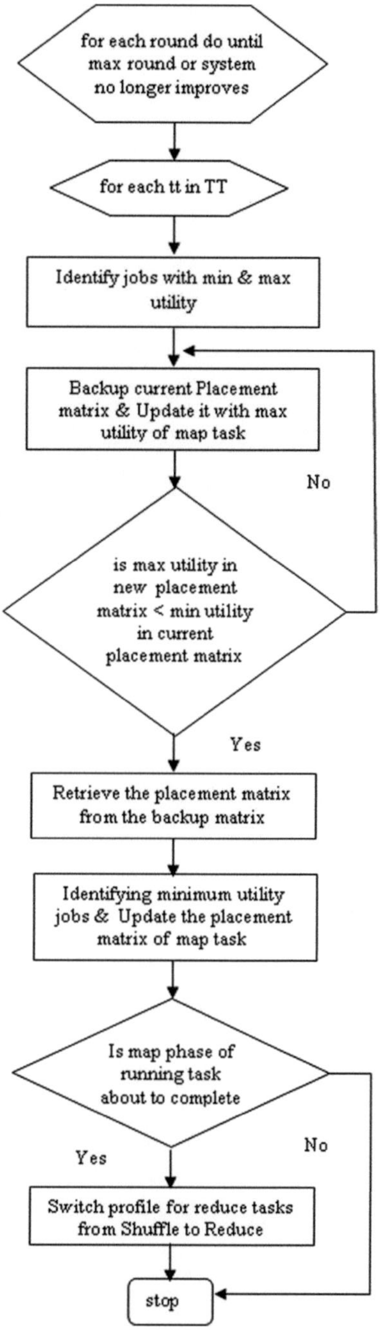

4.4 Progress and Status Updates

Jobs and its tasks have a status such as running, successfully completed etc., when a task executes, its progress must be tracked. If it is a map task, the fraction of the input processing. For a reduce task, the fraction depends on progress of the intermediate phases like shuffle, sort, and reduce

4.5 Job Completion

When the last task of the job finishes, the job status changes to success. The jobtracker and the tasktracker clears the intermediate results and changes its state.

Figure 6 shows the working of RAS in MapReduce

5 Evaluation

To assess the behaviour of RAS [19], a five-node cluster with a capacity of 4 GB of RAM each and with a storage capacity of 250 GB hard disk and the processor speed of 2.2 GHz.

Two jobs, J1 and J2 were submitted in the same order to the default FIFO scheduler. The jobs were of varying sizes, J2 was a smaller job compared to J1.

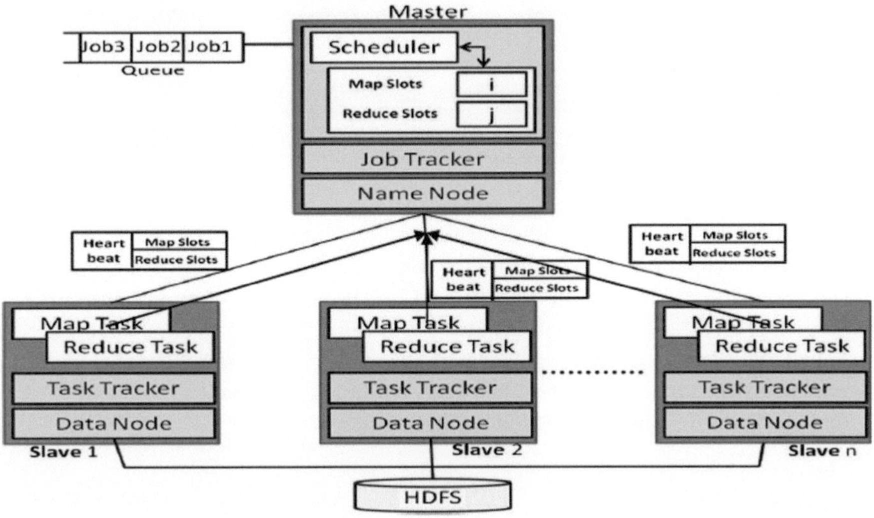

Fig. 6 Working of RAS in MapReduce

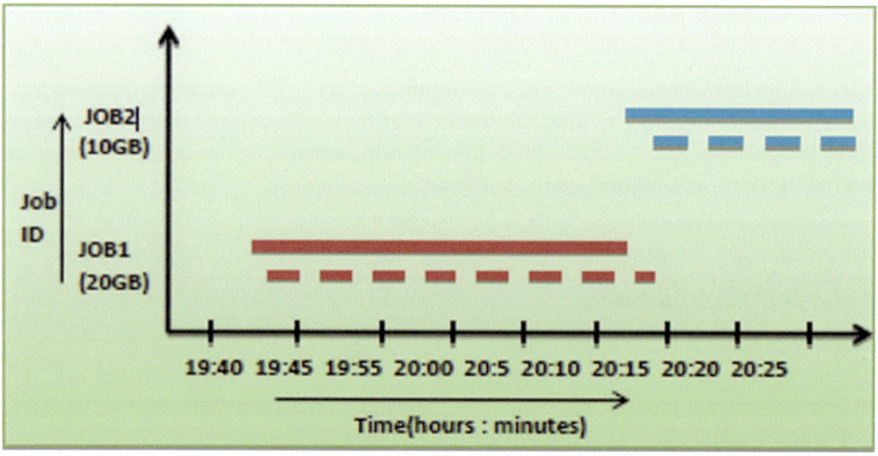

Fig. 7 Behaviour of default scheduler

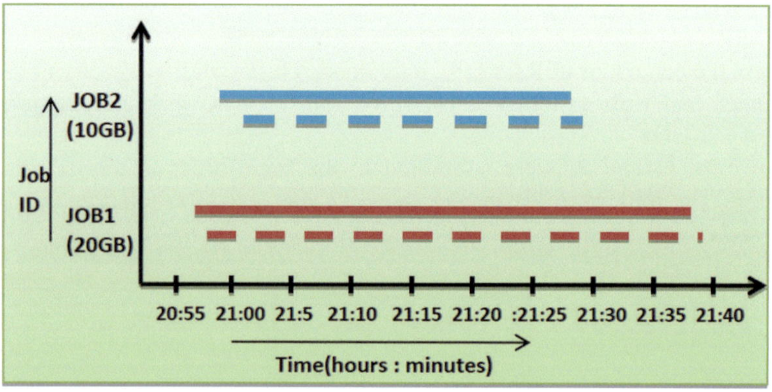

Fig. 8 Behaviour of RAS

It was observed that even though resources were available, they were not utilized for the execution of J2 until J1 completes. Figure 7 shows the graph for Default scheduler. The resource utilization is low and the job completion time is high.

When the same scenario was created using RAS, J1, and J2 were executed simultaneously improving the resource utilization comparatively and Job Completion time. Figure 8 explains the behaviour of RAS.

Table 1 Comparison of schedulers

Algorithm	Dynamic	Adaptive	Data locality	Heterogeneity
FIFO	No	No	No	No
Fair	No	No	No	No
Capacity	No	No	Yes	No
RAS	Yes	Yes	Yes	No

6 Comparison of Schedulers

RAS is a scheduler defined to allocate resources and scheduling jobs for Hadoop-MapReduce. The primary schedulers have many limitations. FIFO has low resource utilization rates and offers no support for multi-user execution environments. FIFO and Fair scheduling neglect heterogeneity, locality and supports static job allocation. This leads to poor performance. Capacity Scheduler can dynamically adjust resource allocation. It also supports parallel execution of multi-users. But it is not suitable for heterogeneous environment. According to the scheduling challenges discussed in Sect. 2, a comparison of the schedulers is shown in Table 1.

7 Conclusion

In this paper, we have shown the behaviour of RAS to prove that it enhances resource utilization and improves job completion time. A comparison of RAS with the default scheduler is made. A set of scheduling challenges have been discussed and an inference is made as to whether these challenges have been met by the primary schedulers and RAS.

References

1. Ekanayake, J., Qiu, X., Gunarathne, T., Beason, S., Fox, G.: High Performance Parallel Computing with Cloud and Cloud Technologies, vol. 34, pp. 20–38 (2010)
2. Ekanayake, J., Fox, G.: High Performance parallel computing with clouds and cloud technologies. 1st international conference on cloud computing, 19–21 Oct 2009
3. Wikipedia. High-performance computing. https://en.wikipedia.org/wiki/Supercomputer
4. NIST Definition of Cloud Computing v15. csrc.nist.gov/groups/SNS/cloud-computing/cloud-def-v15.doc
5. http://www.computer.org/web/computingnow/archive/september2012
6. Ye, X., Lv, A., Zhao, L.: Research of High Performance Computing With Clouds, pp. 289–293 (2010)
7. Dean, J., Ghemawat: MapReduce: Simplified Data Processing On Large Clusters. Google Inc. (2004)
8. Wang, G.: Evaluating MapReduce System Performance:A Simulation Approach (2012)

9. Apache. Hadoop. http://hadoop.apache.org
10. Hadoop: The Definitive Guide, Second Edition, by Tom White, O'Reilly Media, Inc., 1005 Gravenstein Highway North, Sebastopol, CA 95472
11. Hadoop Distributed File System. http://hadoop.apache.org/hdfs
12. Hadoop's Fair Scheduler. https://hadoop.apache.org/docs/r1.2.1/fair_scheduler
13. Hadoop's Capacity Scheduler. http://hadoop.apache.org/core/docs/current/capacity_scheduler.html
14. Polo, J., Castillo, C., Carrera, D., Becerra, Y., Whalley, I., Steinder, M., Torres, J., Ayguadé, E.: Resource-aware adaptive scheduling for MapReduce clusters. In Proceedings of the 12th ACM/IFIP/USENIX international conference on Middleware, in (2011)
15. http://docs.hortonworks.com/HDPDocuments/HDP1/HDP-1.3.0/bk_getting-started-guide/content/ch_hdp1_getting_started_chp2_1.html
16. Zhang, Q., Zhani, M.F., Yang, Y., Boutaba, R., Wong, B.: PRISM: Fine-grained resource-aware scheduling for mapreduce. (2015)
17. Wottrich, K., Bressoud, T.: The Performance Characteristics of MapReduceApplications on Scalable Clusters. MCURCSM (2011)
18. Dong, F., Akl, S.G.: Scheduling algorithms for grid computing: state of art and open problems. Queens University Technicalreport (2006)
19. Shivakumar, N., Rashmi, S., Basu, A.: Hadoop map reduce multi-job workloads using resource aware scheduler. IJARCS (2014)

Analytical and Perspective Approach of Big Data in Cloud Computing

Rekha Pal, Tanvi Anand and Sanjay Kumar Dubey

Abstract Cloud computing is a term which involves delivering services over the Internet at a cheaper cost. Big data is a massive collection of data sets having huge and complicated structures which are difficult to store, analyze and visualize. Cloud computing is the commonly used technology over which big data are managed and stored. The research in this domain has increased over past few years. In order to investigate the usage, issues and challenges by combining the big data in cloud computing, a systematic literature review is conducted. The review included various publications from 2004 to 2014 as a primary study. With the use of search techniques considered, 96 research papers were recognized out of which 23 were identified as relevant papers. The paper presents the various research progresses related to big data in cloud computing. It will also help the researchers to figure out the current and future scenario of research in big data using cloud computing technology.

Keywords Big data · Cloud computing · Hadoop · Data analytics · Distributed data base

1 Introduction

Cloud computing is emerged to be a new paradigm that relies on sharing of computer resources instead of locally handling by personal devices. It is a term which involves delivering services over the internet at a cheaper cost. Cloud

R. Pal · T. Anand (✉) · S.K. Dubey
Computer Science and Engineering Department, Amity University, Sector-125, Expressway, Noida, Uttar Pradesh, India
e-mail: tanvi29anand@gmail.com

R. Pal
e-mail: palrekha106@gmail.com

S.K. Dubey
e-mail: skdubey1@amity.edu

V.B. Aggarwal et al. (eds.), *Big Data Analytics*, Advances in Intelligent Systems and Computing 654, https://doi.org/10.1007/978-981-10-6620-7_23

computing is not about relying on the hard drive for accessing all sort of data but it provides everything that is not physically close to you but can be easily available on the local network. With the development in today's business environment cloud computing serves us many benefits some are like scalability, collaboration efficiency, access to automatic updates, cost efficiency, easy to use and much more. Today suppliers, including AWS, working hard so as to boost public cloud adoption, while IT enterprise is working over hybrid and private cloud architectures so as to manage and control.

Big data is a term that outlines about the bulk amount of organized, semi-organized and unorganized data which mined from the web based application. Big data analytics is linked with cloud computing so as to the analyze the large data sets in real-time which is possible on a platform like Hadoop for storing large volume and variety of data among different distributed cluster and Map Reduce organize, collaborate and compute data from multiple sources. The reason for combine big data with cloud computing is to get the benefit from both the technology, which provides an advantage to an organization to think about how to operate necessary analysis that responds to their actual business requisite rather than still involve in finding ways to accumulate large data. While combining these two technologies user will get benefit with usability, cost-saving, accessibility and disaster management etc. The importance of this review paper is to focus on various issues and challenges that came across while merging these two technologies.

2 Literature Review

This section includes the research done related to big data in cloud computing and what new technologies and issues and challenges that are faced by the researcher during their work within 2004–14. A technique of micro array is used for measuring and reading the mRNA level which accesses a large number of DNA sequences which is done by using cluster and classification [1]. Also by focusing on various techniques of data mining and its future trends, we can have a simplified representation of useful information which will be very effective for coming future which will improve the usability [2]. Various data mining algorithms like k-mean algorithm can be used, which is a Gaussian mixture model for clustering and divide the customer or given set of data into categories which help in the formulation of market strategic planning and guidelines for future [3]. With the help of data mining algorithms, the stored data can be secured without transferring the complete data by using metadata, data segregation, and storage methodology that provide a way to access segregated data [4]. Gene based clustering which is very useful mechanism to extract useful information from noisy and redundant data, unsupervised gene selection can also apply for future selection [5, 6]. According to Satoshi Tsuchiya various technologies for big data processing in cloud computing environment by using key value store technology which distributes our data and offers high performance and high resistance to failure so by combining various functions together that run in cloud will improve complex problems [7]. There are also various data mining privacy and threats on cloud, so to avoid them distributed architecture came which prevent data mining based attacks on cloud [8]. Big data is the term for data sets so large and complicated that it becomes difficult to process using traditional data management tools or processing applications [9]. Big data itself is a large data and varying as well as complex which leads to difficulty while analyzing and storing along with visualizing data for using it to form result [10]. Big data analytics which means analyzing of a large amount of data to select required information, unfold the hidden patterns [11, 12]. Big data analyses service generated big data, the relationship between service logs and also studied big data as a service and discusses its business aspects. We can use tape based service model and combine a large scale tape infrastructure with the cloud [13, 14]. There are various big data applications along with its usefulness in the developing world and its increasing work in the various sector of the organization, there is an increasing need of Hadoop for storing data, but various challenges faced are also there while adapting big data technology in the Hadoop tool [15]. By using integrity verified mechanism will continue to progress then it can meet security challenges faced in the cloud. ICT technology provides improved services of data being received from the cloud [16, 17]. A cloud computing framework can be used which helps in scheduling various distributed application of data mining so as to reduce overall execution time and improve the quality of data provided. With this complexity of cloud is hidden from cloud end users [18–20]. So with the enhancement in cloud computing, the internet or web technologies the data is also increasing and their efficient utilization of that vast data is a big concern [21]. RDBMS is not much capable of handling a large amount of data that's why HDFS comes in the picture because it is fast, secure, consistent and scalable to manage a large amount of unstructured data [22]. Cloud computing is becoming an increasingly popular enterprise model in which computing resources are made available on-demand to the user as needed. The unique value proposition of cloud computing creates new opportunities to align IT and business goals [23].

3 Review Methodology

Present review methodology is related to the literature review that targets various research questions to identify, evaluate, select and incorporate all the high-quality research evidence necessary for the research. Its aim is to present a fair evaluation of research topic by using a trust worthy, rigorous and auditable methodology. Among the available methodologies, paper chooses the journals and research paper methodologies. In the planning the review stage, the need for the review is identified, the research questions are specified, and the review protocol is defined. Finally, in the reporting the review stage, the dissemination mechanisms are specified, and the review report is presented. Papers before 2004 are not considered due to not much work was there in this area.

3.1 Research Questions

The goal of our review is to find the issues and challenges faced while storing a large amount of data in the cloud. During the study following research questions are framed:

RQ1. As per the future aspect how big data is dependent on cloud?

RQ2. How often is the Hadoop technology implemented as a tool?

These review questions allow identifying research gaps in a related area.

3.2 Identification of Primary Studies and Data Inclusion and Analysis Criteria

The main authors were chosen for studies are from IEEE Explore, Springer digital libraries and reputed conferences. We have limited our research with the papers that available online. After completing the search of papers from the year 2004–2014 in the first stage, we made notes (doc file) where we kept the records of all the important keywords that we extracted during the study. In analysis around 100 paper are fetched for study, from this 50 are evaluated and 24 are basically related to analysis.

4 Analysis

4.1 Significance of Review

Present review paper discusses various research progress, issues and challenges related to big data in cloud computing. Security and privacy are one of the main issues found in big data in cloud computing. Various technologies can be used for big data processing in cloud computing environment by using key value store technology which distributes data and offers high performance and high resistance to failure. So by combining various functions together that run in cloud will improve the complex problems

5 Overall Evaluation

The main goal of this paper is to analyze the importance of combine big data in cloud computing as well as research papers in this area. This section produces overall evaluation about the frame research question.

RQ1. As per the future aspect how big data is dependent on the cloud?

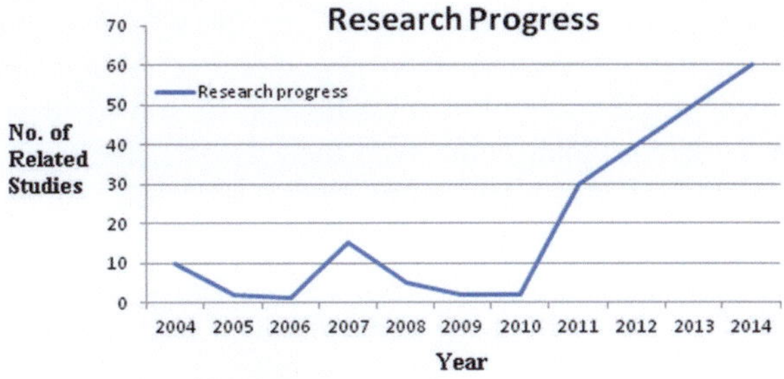

Fig. 1 Research progress (2004–14) for big data in cloud

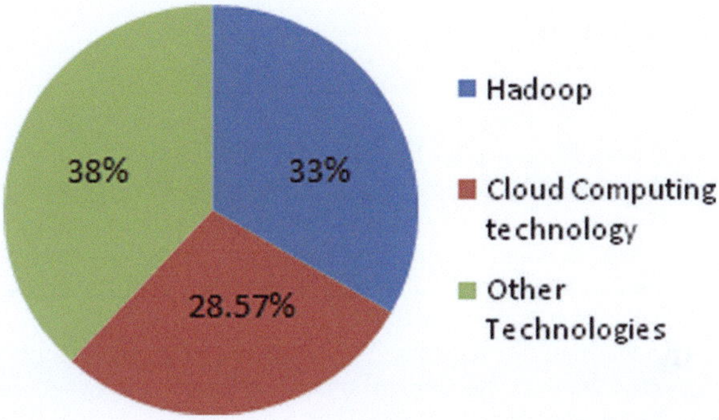

Fig. 2 Mathematical representation of HADOOP

After undergoing much research it is observed that for big data and cloud computing are more productive for building an application with faster and better understanding without worrying about underlying infrastructure. From the study, it is noticed that there is a quite variation in researches in this area as shown in Fig. 1. The graph indicates the growing research in the related area in past 10 years.

RQ2. How often the Hadoop technology is implemented as a tool?

While studying many researches during these 10 years it is observed that there is a quite high increase in the implementation and study of Hadoop technology. From the study conducted it is observed that 1/3rd of researchers used Hadoop as their tool.

From Fig. 2 it is observed 7 papers out of 21 papers reviewed uses specific Hadoop technology, 6 other Cloud Computing technologies and remaining other techniques

6 Conclusion

In this paper, different cloud based big data techniques, approaches are discussed and their usability in the organization is also taken into account. For this purpose, an analytical review is done and also frames research questions in this regard. Selection of primary study and data inclusion/ analysis criteria is also identified.

The present paper also tries to find the solution of framed research questions. By combining various functions together that run in a cloud environment by improving technologies, complex problems can be solved. It is still a big issue in providing security in cloud data. Even there is data, tools are available but there are other issues are also required to improve for efficient usage. Some improvement is required in HADOOP tool so that in future big data using technology will be highly skilled. The correlated technology of big data that are present today is not ideal to deal with challenges so require more examining and analysis.

References

1. Jiang, D., Tang, C., Zhang, A.: Cluster analysis for gene expression data: A survey. IEEE Trans. Knowl. Data Eng. **16**(11), 1370–1386 (2004)
2. Kriegel, H.P., Borgwardt, K., Kroger, P., Pryakhin, A., Schubert, M., Zimek, A.: Future Trends in Data Mining. Springer Science+Business Media, LLC (2007)
3. Chen, X., Gao, L., Zhejiang, Wang, X., Zhang, Z., Wei, Z., Liao Z.: The research on the data mining technology in the active demand management. In: 2011 international conference on internet computing and information services (2011)
4. Subashini, S., Kavihta, V.: A meta data based storage model for securing data in cloud environment. In: International conference on cyber enabled distributed computing and knowledge discovery (2011)
5. Chandrasekhar, T., Thangavel, K., Elayaraja, E.: Gene expression data clustering using unsupervised methods. IEEE, pp. 146–150 (2011)
6. Agrawal, D., Das, S., Abbadi, A.E.: Big data and cloud computing: current state and future opportunities. ACM (2011)
7. Tsuchiya, S., Yoshinori, Tsuchimoto, Y., lee, V.: Big Data processing in cloud environments. Fujitsu Sci. Technol. **48**, 159–168
8. Dev, H., Sen, T., Basak, M., Ali, M.E.: An approach to protect the privacy of cloud from data mining based attacks, sc companion: High performance computing, networking storage and analysis (2012)
9. Li, B., Jain, R.: Survey of recent research progress and issues in big data, pp. 1–13. (2013). Available at: http://www.cse.wustl.edu/~jain/cse570-13/index.html
10. Sagiroglu, S., Sinanc, D.: Big data; a review, pp. 42–47. IEEE (2013)
11. Shilpa, Kaur, M.: Big data and methodology. Intern. J. Adv. Res. Comput. Sci. Softw. Eng. **3** (10), 991–995 (2013)
12. Demchenko, Y., Grosso, P., Laat, L., Membrey, P.: Addressing big data issues in scientific data infrastructure. IEEE pp. 48–55 (2013)
13. Zheng, Z., Zhu, J., Lyu, M.R.: Service generated big data and big data as a service. In: IEEE conference on big data, pp. 403–410 (2013)
14. Prakash, V.S., Wen, Y., Weidong, S.: Tape cloud: Scalable and cost efficient big data infrastructure for cloud computing. In: IEEE sixth conference on cloud computing, pp. 541–548 (2013)
15. Katal, A., Wazid, M., Goudar, R.H.: Big data: Issues, challenges, tools and good practices. IEEE pp. 404–409 (2013)
16. Liu, C., Ranjan, R., Zhang, X., Yang, C., Georgakopoulos, D., Chen, J.: Public auditing for big data storage in cloud computing—A survey 2013. IEEE, pp. 463–468 (2013)
17. Lu, C.-W., Hsieh, C.-M., Chang, C.-H., Yang, C.-T.: An improvement to data services in cloud computing with content sensitive transaction analysis and adaption. In: IEEE 37th annual computer software and application conference workshops, pp. 463–468 (2013)

18. Ismail, L., Masud, M.M., Khan, L.: FSBD: A framework for scheduling of big data mining in cloud computing. In: IEEE international congress on big data , pp. 514–521 (2014)
19. Kadu, P.S., Deshmukh, H.R., Angaitkar, P.G., Karale, S.A.: A review on big data management and its security. Int. J. Pure Appl. Res. Eng. Technol. **2**(9), 1011–1017 (2014)
20. Wang, Y., Zhao, Y.: Transplantation of data mining algorithms to cloud computing platform when dealing big data. In: International conference on cyber-enabled distributed computing and knowledge discovery, pp. 175–178 (2014)
21. Mu, L., Lei, Z.: Big data processing technology research and application prospects. In: Fourth international conference on instrumentation and measurement, computer, communication and control, pp. 269–273 (2014)
22. Dwivedi, K., Dubey, S.K.: Analytical review on Hadoop distributed file system. IEEEXplore, In proceeding of 5th international conference—The next generation information technology summit, confluence-2014, pp. 174–181. Noida, India, 25–26 Sept 2014
23. Insfran, E., Fernandez, A.: A systematic review of usability evaluation in web development. In: Proceedings of 2nd international workshop on web usability and accessibility (IWWUA'08), New Zealand, LNCS, vol. 5176, pp. 81–91. Springer, Berlin (2008)

Implementation of CouchDBViews

Subita Kumari and Pankaj Gupta

Abstract Flexible data model and horizontal scalability are the need of contemporary era to handle huge heterogeneous data. This has lead to the popularity of NoSQL Databases. CouchDB is an admired and easy to use choice among NoSQL Document-Oriented databases. CouchDB is developed in Erlang language. CouchDB's RESTful (Representational State Transfer) APIs (Application Programming Interface) make it special because they allow database access through http (Hyper Text Transfer Protocol) requests. This access in the form of HTTP requests is achieved with the help of command line utility Curl. The Futon, web-based utility of CouchDB, is also used to manage documents, databases, and replication in CouchDB. CouchDB uses a special type of system for querying data than traditional RDBMS (Relational Database Management Systems) i.e. views. This paper explains various unique features of CouchDB which distinguish it from RDBMS. It also includes implementation of temporary and permanent views using MapReduce.

Keywords CouchDB · MapReduce · Views · Futon · Curl

1 Introduction

The database technologies have been evolving at a very fast pace. Database systems are moving from SQL to NoSQL systems to handle datasets of diverse categories. Most NoSQL systems have been developed with the general goal of offering simple operations on flexible data structures. Indeed, they are focused to provide massive throughput and high scalability [1]. NoSQL databases support large data volumes,

S. Kumari (✉)
Computer Science and Engineering, UIET, MDU, Rohtak, India
e-mail: subita.hooda@gmail.com

P. Gupta
Computer Science and Engineering, VCE, Rohtak, India
e-mail: pankajgupta.vce@gmail.com

V.B. Aggarwal et al. (eds.), *Big Data Analytics*, Advances in Intelligent
Systems and Computing 654, https://doi.org/10.1007/978-981-10-6620-7_24

simple and easy copy, eventual consistency and simple API. NoSQL databases are becoming the core phenomena for big data applications. NoSQL databases are broadly classified into three categories: document stores databases, key-value stores databases and column-oriented databases [2]. Today most used document-oriented databases are MongoDB and CouchDB. This paper explores CouchDB documents, databases and views in detail and compares with traditional RDBMS basic architecture. Document-oriented databases provide the alternative of a *'row'* of traditional RDBMS in the form of a more flexible *'document'*. They permit access to data values of database via its content. Documents are hierarchical structures that can be in BSON, JSON, or other formats like XML and therefore consist of more composite elements such as collections, maps or scalar values [3]. There is no need to define schema beforehand means there is a flexibility of defining the size/type of key/value fields of documents on the runtime. This makes it easier to perform operations like insertion and deletion of fields whenever required. Each document is collection of set of fields and is associated with a unique identifier, for indexing and querying purpose.

2 CouchDB Experimental Setup

Developed and maintained by the Apache Software Foundation, CouchDB is an admired and easy to use choice among NoSQL Document-Oriented databases. CouchDB is developed in Erlang language. CouchDB's RESTful APIs make it special because they allow database access through HTTP requests [4]. The software required for the CouchDB setup is:

- CouchDB Version 1.6.1
- Web-Based Interface Futon
- Command Line Utility Curl.

CouchDB makes use of APIs by using the command-line utility *curl*. A very interesting fact is that users are provided insights of the database and great control on HTTP requests by *curl*. Suppose CouchDB is running and the following request is sent to database via curl

```
curl http://127.0.0.1:5984[5]
```

The above curl command will seek an http GET from CouchDB and will return the detailed JSON object as follows:

{"couchdb":"Welcome","uuid":"6c200d933f15fda6543e960e874796a8","version": "1.6.1","vendor":{"version":"1.6.1","name":"The Apache Software Foundation"}}

CouchDB is giving a welcome message with the running version number. Another way to interact with CouchDB is using Futon. It provides default web interface for administration of CouchDB. A full access to features of CouchDB is provided more conveniently by Futon. It provides us the facility to create and remove databases; create, delete, view and modify documents; replicate databases; and compose and run MapReduce views. To load Futon the following link is used in the browser application.

`http://127.0.0.1:5984/_utils/ [5].`

The remaining sections explain the other distinctive features of CouchDB experimentally under above set up.

3 CouchDB Features

3.1 Data Model

CouchDB is composed of databases. Databases are a further collection of variable-schema documents. As opposed to this, RDBMSs are a collection of fixed schema relations which are composed of rows. CouchDB stores JSON (Java Script Object Notation) documents in a binary format. The documents stored fields in the form of key-value pairs. Every document is identified by a unique field "_id". This "_id" may be automatically generated by CouchDB or manually provided by the user. There is no maximum limit for key-value pairs and size of documents. The file extension of database files is .couch. The data model is shown in Fig. 1 [4].

3.2 RESTful API

One of the very outstanding features of CouchDB is its RESTful API. REST architecture explains how to provide services for interaction among machines. REST facilitates the use of HTTP requests for carrying out basic Create, Read,

Fig. 1 CouchDB data model

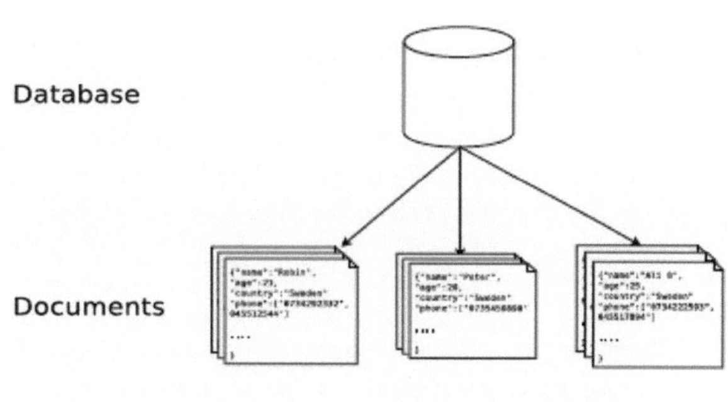

Update and Delete operations (CRUD) on documents [4]. Following HTTP methods are used for performing basic CRUD operations-

- PUT—Create databases/documents/attachments
- POST—Update databases/documents/attachments
- GET—Read databases/documents/attachments
- DELETE—Delete databases/documents/attachments

RESTful architecture gives unique identifiers to databases/documents/attachments etc. in the form of URIs. Suppose a database named "university" is being created on a local CouchDB setup. Using the command-line utility curl following statement will do the needful:

```
curl -X PUT http://127.0.0.1:5984/university
```

The success of the above statement in curl will be replied back by CouchDB in the form of a JSON document, e.g. the creation of database named "university" is notified by:

```
{"ok": true}
```

All other basic operations on documents (CRUD) can be performed with similar curl statements.

3.3 *Documents*

Documents are the fundamental data structure of CouchDB. It is just like a physical document—such as an invoice, an address card, or an invitation card [6]. Documents use the dynamic schema as opposed to relations of RDBMS which use fixed schema. The document contains unique _id and _rev field showing id and revision number of document. Documents are stored by CouchDB using the JSON format in the form of key-value pair. The example below shows one such document of PhD student of the "university" database. "_id" field uniquely identifies the document in the "university" database and "_rev" field shows the version number of the document. Every time a document is updated a new version of the document is created and older versions also remain on the disk. The example below shows the 7th version of the document shown.

```
{
    "_id": "ae288eecf814e1e177e94263870031e7",
    "_rev": "7-de540398f44262de6a80b0d67d72df9d",
    "name": "Reet",
```

```
        "age": 25,
        "doj": "15/06/2015",
        "branch": "Electronics",
        "topic": "Wireless Communication",
        "supervisor": "Deepak",
        "course": "Phd",
        "Marks": {
              "Digital": 88,
              "MicroProcessor": 79,
              "Analog": 62
        }
}
```

The example database "university" contains some other documents containing details of UG, PG and PhD students having different schemas as well as a design document "phd_course" implementing permanent views. A design document is identified by word "_design". Figure 2 shows the snapshot of documents of "university" database from Futon.

3.4 Revisions

CouchDB supports well-built versioning system. It means that when some changes are carried out by user in a document, the next version is created by the CouchDB and it does not overwrite the existing document. CouchDB keeps all versions so that user can later on track earlier amendments. This feature makes it highly available database because this feature is inherent to CouchDB as opposed to RDBMS which does not offer this feature so conveniently [4].

Key ▲	Value
"_design/phd_course" ID: _design/phd_course	{rev: "1-c21a6e878dce4fbb8545161837ff1bf7"}
"ae288eecf814e1e177e9426387000eb7" ID: ae288eecf814e1e177e9426387000eb7	{rev: "1-3b376efbfde851a984622aaa521a8bbc"}
"ae288eecf814e1e177e9426387001689" ID: ae288eecf814e1e177e9426387001689	{rev: "1-8dc6c6f6118a126946904495f3d3dfdf"}
"ae288eecf814e1e177e942638700253d" ID: ae288eecf814e1e177e942638700253d	{rev: "1-1822fc42fc7154e8f011a16c5b091874"}
"ae288eecf814e1e177e94263870029c2" ID: ae288eecf814e1e177e94263870029c2	{rev: "1-058a4a173d9f999d20a8df5e8fbbc1e6"}
"ae288eecf814e1e177e9426387002f6d" ID: ae288eecf814e1e177e9426387002f6d	{rev: "2-085e1a82c21e903f0d88f73b85e203db"}
"ae288eecf814e1e177e94263870031e7" ID: ae288eecf814e1e177e94263870031e7	{rev: "5-c55698601aafc381ae59c00b8e723a8e"}

Fig. 2 Preview of documents of "university" database

3.5 Scaling and Replication

Replicating databases in CouchDB allows easy replication of databases. The databases can be kept in synchronization very easily by the following HTTP request for database replication:

```
POST/replicateHTTP/1.1{"source":"old_database","tar-
get":"http://www.new/database.com/db"}
```

Replication can be performed from the Futon even more easily. Scaling out means splitting the databases across multiple servers of a cluster. CouchDB does not support scaling inherently; instead, CouchDB Lounge9 application serves the purpose of scaling [4].

3.6 Attachments

Like e-mails support attachments, CouchDB also supports binary attachments to documents. Any kind of file can be attached to a document [4]. The example below shows the command to attach an image file to a document:

```
http://www.local-
host:5984/cars/6e4485ed6c37255e54dg12357f18c8af/car_im-
age.jpg
```

3.7 Querying

RDBMS normally use fixed schema means static data and dynamic queries [7]. On the other hand, CouchDB does the opposite. It uses the dynamic schema in the form of JSON documents. Views are used to query data in CouchDB. Views created are of two kinds: temporary and permanent Views. The outcome of MapReduce operations is demonstrated using Views [5]. Map operation carries out parallelism in CouchDB which is its inherent feature as opposed to RDBMS which carries out operations on data in serial order [7]. The user writes statements for Map operations. Each document is traversed by Map function parallel such that the documents with matching criteria only are emitted using emit () function in the form of the key-value pair [4]. Section 3 explains this concept in more detail.

3.8 Indexing

Indexing is required for faster retrieval and better performance of a database. CouchDB inherently provides auto index updating feature. Map functions traverse through all the documents when running for the first time on a data set [7]. The results are then used by CouchDB to make a B-Tree. This is the most suitable and performance oriented data structure for operations like retrieval, insertion, and deletion. On each modification, deletion of a document; CouchDB updates index B-tree automatically [4].

4 CouchDB Views

Views are an old concept which is being used in traditional RDBMSs for long times. There a view behaves like a window based on the original SQL table. It retrieves rows and columns on the basis of criteria and shows the results out of a real table. In CouchDB view are used to query the database and demonstrate the results of MapReduce functions. These functions offer enormous flexibility, being capable of fine tuning to alterations in the structure of document and indexes being automatically and parallel computed. Each document is traversed and passed as an argument to the Map functions. Documents with matching criteria are emitted as key/value pairs. Because of this flexibility, Views in CouchDB are created parallel and incrementally. Some functions carried out by Views are:

- Filter the documents in the database
- Retrieve data from the documents and show it in a particular order
- Build indexes to find documents by any structure that resides in documents
- Carry out all sorts of calculations on the data in the documents.

CouchDB uses two kinds of views for querying the database i.e. temporary view or adhoc view and permanent view or static view.

4.1 Temporary Views

Temporary views are also called adhoc views because their MapReduce functions are changed from Futon in the code section. In "view" drop down box select "Temporary View" to see this view. Emit () function in map function code is used to emit key-value pair. Emit function always takes two arguments i.e. key and value. A default temporary view emits null in key value and document structure in value field. Value field of default view show details of all items of document including _id and _rev field. Figure 3 shows the values of default temporary view of our example database, i.e. "university" database. The value field shows the attributes of all documents. It is clear that various documents have different schema, i.e. different key-value attribute pair. For example, Fig. 3 shows one document having field (name, doj, course, branch, age, marks) and another one having fields (name, doj, course, age, branch, topic, supervisor). These two documents have different schema and have been easily incorporated in same database without need of any kind of joins. This is how CouchDB is different from RDBMS as schema of documents may change on need.

We can change the code of map function to get results according to user query. Suppose from our example database, we want the names of students having age less than 22, and then code of map function would look like the one shown below.

```
function(doc) {
     if(doc.age&&doc.age < 22 && doc.name)
           emit(doc.name , doc.age); }
```

After we run this code, the result would look like as shown in Fig. 4.

Permanent Views

Temporary views are not appropriate for use in production, as they are actually slow for any database with more than a few dozen documents. They can be used to experiment with view functions, but we must switch to a permanent view if it has to be used in an application. Permanent views are also called static views. Permanent views are created with the help of special type of documents called *design* document. Design documents specify these views in the map function. A single design document can have multiple views. We have created a json file named "design2.

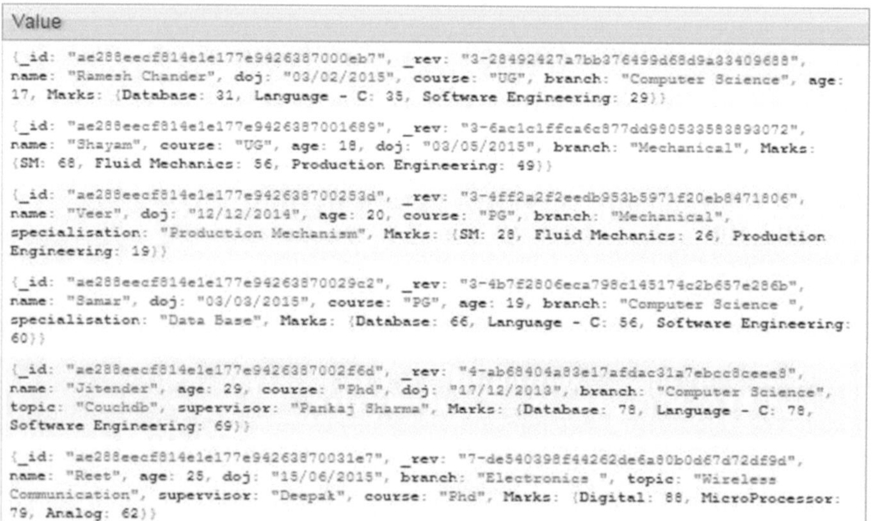

Fig. 3 Default temporary view of "university" database

Fig. 4 Temporary view of name-age pair of "university" database

json" which contains id of the design document "phd_course" and the code of map functions of two view namely "supervisor_detail" and "marks_detail". The file is shown below in Fig. 5.

The below curl command shows how we created our design document "phd_course" with the help of our file "design2.json". `curl-X PUT http://127.0.0.1:5984/university/_design/phd_course-d@desktop/design2.json`

Curl replies with the following JSON document means our design document "phd_course" has been successfully created.

{"ok":true, "id":"_design/phd_course", "rev":"1-ddde17668d269f5cfeb2aa3259e26b1"}

Futon shows our design document containing two views as shown in Fig. 6.

Now to see the result of our view, we select view name "marks_detail" from views drop down box. This view shows the marks of every student in each subject individually and rows sorted by the name of the students as shown in Fig. 7.

CouchDB has given excellent powers to the user in the form of MapReduce functions to design views according to user queries. CouchDB, definitely has some unique features like this incremental MapReduce and indexing which makes it a better fit than traditional RDBMSs for dealing with large datasets.

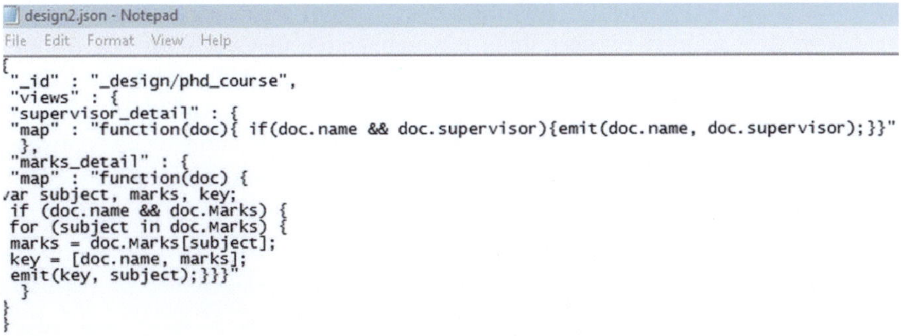

```
{
"_id" : "_design/phd_course",
"views" : {
"supervisor_detail" : {
"map" : "function(doc){ if(doc.name && doc.supervisor){emit(doc.name, doc.supervisor);}}"
 },
"marks_detail" : {
"map" : "function(doc) {
var subject, marks, key;
if (doc.name && doc.Marks) {
for (subject in doc.Marks) {
marks = doc.Marks[subject];
key = [doc.name, marks];
emit(key, subject);}}}"
 }
}
}
```

Fig. 5 Code of design document "phd_course" in "design2.json"

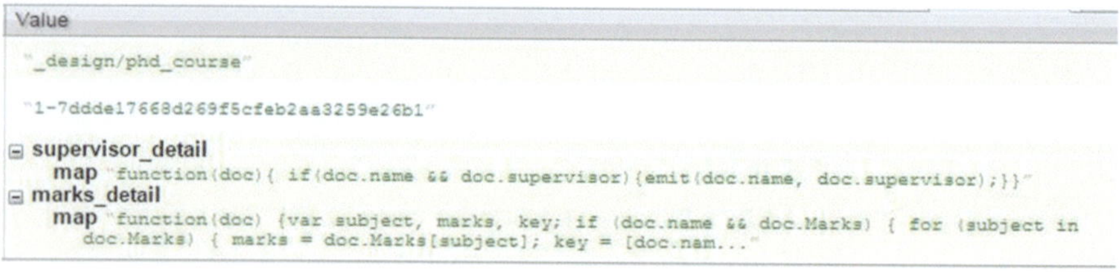

Fig. 6 Design document "phd_course"

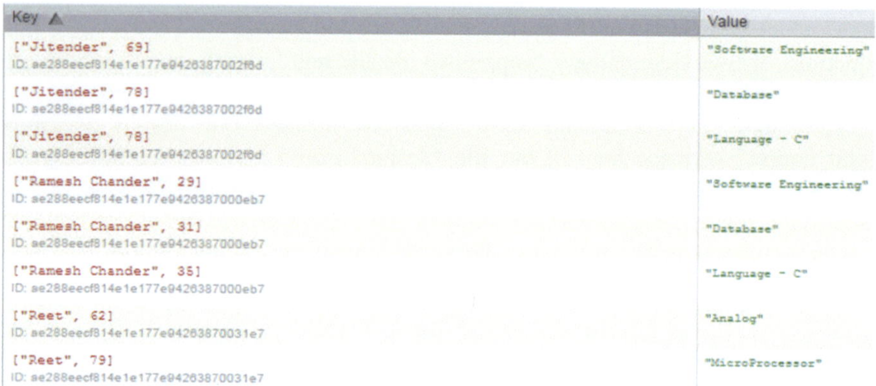

Key	Value
["Jitender", 69] ID: ae288eecf814e1e177e9426387002f6d	"Software Engineering"
["Jitender", 78] ID: ae288eecf814e1e177e9426387002f6d	"Database"
["Jitender", 78] ID: ae288eecf814e1e177e9426387002f6d	"Language - C"
["Ramesh Chander", 29] ID: ae288eecf814e1e177e9426387000eb7	"Software Engineering"
["Ramesh Chander", 31] ID: ae288eecf814e1e177e9426387000eb7	"Database"
["Ramesh Chander", 35] ID: ae288eecf814e1e177e9426387000eb7	"Language - C"
["Reet", 62] ID: ae288eecf814e1e177e94263870031e7	"Analog"
["Reet", 79] ID: ae288eecf814e1e177e94263870031e7	"MicroProcessor"

Fig. 7 Result of permanentview "marks_detail"

5 Conclusion and Future Scope

CouchDB features such as dynamic schema, versioning system, and MapReduce view queries have been explained and compared in-line with traditional RDBMS in this paper. Command line utility Curl and web based utility Futon of CouchDB have been used to implement MapReduce operations of permanent views. Focus on present work is majorly on describing the architecture of CouchDB, key features and implementation of views using futon/curl and inline architectural comparison with RDBMS. The future scope includes using the parallelism of MapReduce on multiple servers and on large and diverse datasets with comparison statistics, graphs, and reports with RDBMS.

References

1. Chen, M., Mao, S., Liu, Y.: Big data: a survey. Springer, Mobile NetwApplFeb (2014)
2. Chaiken, R., Jenkins, B., Larson, P.: Scope: Easy and efficient parallel processing of massive data sets. VLDB, 24–30 August, Auckland, New Zealand (2008)

3. Kumari, S., Gupta, P.: Document store NoSQL Databases. Int. J. Artif. Intell. Knowl. Discov. **5**(3) (2015)
4. Henricsson, R., Gustafsson, G.: A comparison of performance in MongoDB and CouchDB using a Python interface. Technical report, Blekinge Institute of Technology (2011)
5. Anderson, J.C., Lehnardt, J., Slater, N.: CouchDB: the definitive guide. O'Reilly Media Inc (2010)
6. Concept of Views in SQL. http://www.tutorialspoint.com/sql/sql-using-views
7. Khanam, Z., Agarwal, S.: Map-reduce implementations: survey and performance comparison. Int. J. Comput. Sci. Inf. Technol. (IJCSIT) **7**(4) (2015)
8. Dean, J., Ghemawat, S.: Mapreduce: Simplified data processing on large clusters. Commun. ACM **51**(1), 107–113 (2004)
9. Gates, A., Natkovich, O., Chopra, S.: Building a high-level dataflow system on top of map-reduce: the pig experience. VLDB, 24–28 August, Lyon, France (2009)
10. Wei, Z., Pierre, G., Chi, C.: Scalable Join Queries in Cloud Data Stores. In: 12th IEEE/ACM IS On CCG Computing (2012)
11. Sharma, V., Dave, M.: SQL and NoSQL databases. Int. J. Adv. Res. Comput. Sci. Softw. Eng. **2**(8), 2027 (2012)
12. Kanwar, R., Trivedi, P. Singh, K.: NoSQL, a Solution for distributed database management system. Int. J. Comput. Appl. (0975–8887) **67**(2), 6–9 (2013)
13. Dharmasiri, H., Goonetillake, M.: A federated approach on heterogeneous NoSQL data stores. In: International Conference on Advances in ICT for Emerging Region, 234–239 (2013)
14. Changlin, H.: Survey on NoSQL database technology. JASEI **2**(2) (2015)
15. Apache: Apache CouchDB documentation and CouchDB latest Version. https://couchdb.apache.org/
16. Why NoSQL, Couchbase white paper. http://www.couchbase.com

Evolution of FOAF and SIOC in Semantic Web: A Survey

Gagandeep Singh Narula, Usha Yadav, Neelam Duhan and Vishal Jain

Abstract The era of social web has been growing tremendously over the web. Users are getting allured towards new paradigms tools and services of social web. The amount of information available on social web is produced by sharing of beliefs, reviews and knowledge by various online communities. Interoperability and portability of social data are one of the major bottlenecks of social network applications like Facebook, Twitter, Flicker and many more. In order to represent and integrate social information explicitly and efficiently, it is mandatory to enrich social information with the power of semantics. The paper is categorized into following sections. Section 2 describes various studies conducted in context of social semantic web. Section 3 makes readers aware of concept of social web and various issues associated with it. Section 4 describes use of ontologies in achieving interoperability between social and semantic web. Section 5 concludes the giver paper.

Keywords Semantic web (SW) · Social web · Ontology · RDF · FOAF · XFN and SIOC

G.S. Narula (✉)
C-DAC, Noida, India
e-mail: gagan.narula87@gmail.com

U. Yadav · N. Duhan
Department of Computer Engineering, YMCA University of Science and Technology, Faridabad, India
e-mail: usha.yadav.912@gmail.com

N. Duhan
e-mail: neelam_duhan@rediffmail.com

V. Jain
Bharati Vidyapeeth's Institute of Computer Applications (BVICAM), New Delhi, India
e-mail: vishaljain83@ymail.com

V.B. Aggarwal et al. (eds.), *Big Data Analytics*, Advances in Intelligent Systems and Computing 654, https://doi.org/10.1007/978-981-10-6620-7_25

1 Introduction

Combining social and semantic web is a very challenging task. Various studies have been conducted in describing structure of information and maintaining relationship among plethora of web documents. Most of social networking sites are walled websites that means they only provides limited means for users to publish and access social data rather than integration of social data [1]. The era of social websites has gained tremendous height during the past 3–4 years. They have become the medium of marketing and promotions in an innovative way [2].

As the number of social websites increases, the need to achieve secure social data also increases [3]. It has led to an idea of aggregating social data with the help of semantic web technologies. Semantic web consists of various vocabularies/ontologies to deal with social datasets available on different sites in order to allow interoperability through machines rather than XML-based approaches [4]. The paper deal with various constraints associated with social web and describes the capabilities of semantic web technologies which results in evolution of social semantic web. It also examines how semantic web technologies can be used in achieving interoperability among social web applications.

2 State of Art

Halpin and Tuffield [5] presented various issues regarding interoperability of data on social and semantic web, in their paper tilled social network and data portability using semantic web technologies. They also used FOAF and SIOC ontologies to identify persons and deduce their relationship respectively. SIOC is used to represent data for multiple users from different social sites. John G. Bresley et al. briefly described privacy issues, role of semantic web and social web in their article titled “Social Semantic Web”. They presented various suggestions for reducing gap between social web and semantic web. The article also includes survey of semantic web applications like semantic wiki that can be used to analyze social data. Specia and Motta [6] performed study on extracting ontologies from collaborative-tagged systems. Xu et al. [7] led to development of ontology as a unified model of social network and semantics.

3 Social Web

Social web is a collection of social data published and shared by millions of users, which is being spread over various publishing media, networking media, discussion media and sharing media. The term social web was given by Howard Rheingold in 1996 [8]. The use of latest ICT has changed the social web by introducing various second-generation web applications like Wikipedia, blogs, social networking sites (Facebook, twitter), content sharing sites and community sites. The social networking sites are used for maintaining social relations among people all over the world.

User accounts are created by maintaining user profiles based on different preferences. Similarly, community driver websites include quora digest, accdemia.edu that connects group of people to share their common interests and answers via query session either by entering comments or live chat assistance. Content sharing sites enables user to post their informative content on social web. The content may be images text, videos etc. It has led to knowledge sharing through social web (Figs. 1 and 2).

3.1 Issues in Social Web

(a) Indexing: Indexing means generation of metadata. It is known that folksonomies/collaborative tagging is the main source of creation of metadata on social web. But due to its ambiguities and inconsistency, it has not expanded much. With the use of semantic web, it is possible to convert folksonomies to ontologies and generate metadata in Resource Description Framework (RDF) having triples- subject, property and object (Fig. 3).
Example: Ram likes Fosters. In this statement, Ram is object, likes is property and Fosters is resource.
(b) Difficulty in extending and reusing data due to non standards: Social networks focuses on publishing contents of website like songs, images via read only interface rather than using dynamic APIS and interfaces. It has led to portability issues and lack of knowledge representation. To overcome this, there must be usage of semantic applications and browsers to publish content in RDF which eventually leads to interconnection of social networks with multiple data sources.

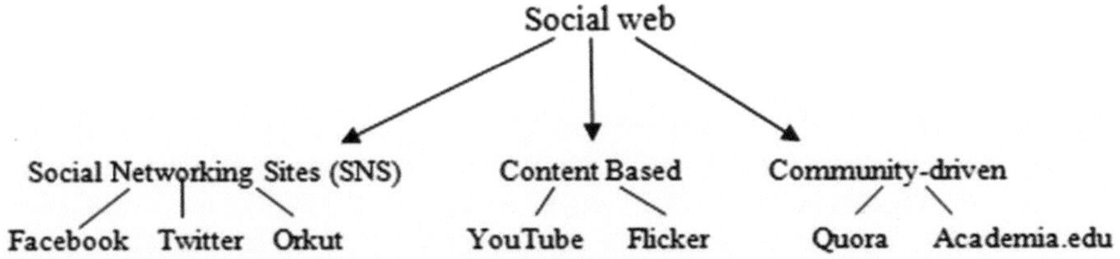

Fig. 1 Ontology on social web [Ontology is abbreviated as FESC (Formal, Explicit, Shared, and Conceptualization) [17]. Formal means that ontology must be understandable by machines. Explicit defines type of constraints associated with it. Shared means that ontology must be visible to group rather than individual. Conceptualization means it should represent some structured from that holds relevant concepts of given domain]

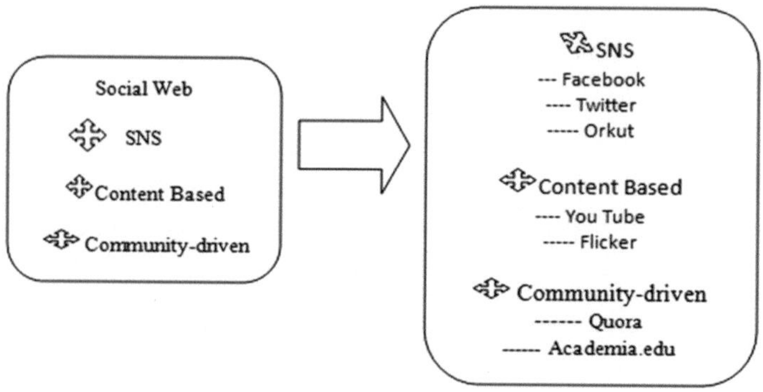

Fig. 2 Defining classes and attributes of social web

Fig. 3 RDF model

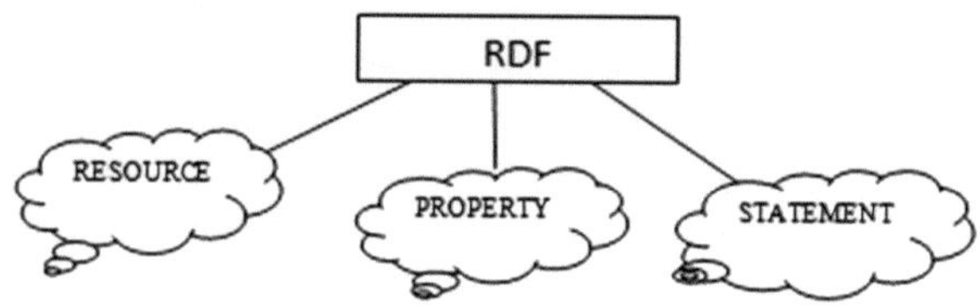

(c) Fake Identity Management: Users make use of different names, aliases and nicknames to create their profiles in different groups. Each group has its terms and conditions that constitutes public privacy as well as closed profiles.
(d) Transformation of social knowledge and facts: It is a cumbersome task to mange and transforms facts associated with social entities into semantic web databases. It might be possible that social and semantic interfaces differ in processing capabilities. Although there are well-defined ontologies related to social networks but there are no mechanisms and heuristics defined for integration and utilization of social results into RDF/OWL format.

3.2 Semantic Web

The idea of semantic web as envisioned by Lee [9] focuses on making data machine understandable as much as it is friendly to humans. Semantic Web aims to abridge knowledge gap between humans and machines. It is characterized by open source, flexible commercial modelling technologies and tools that are being used on various community projects to link public data sets from World Wide Web [10]. Semantic web has an initiative to work on knowledge representation and reasoning of given information [11]. The information may be either in structured, semi-structured and unstructured form. It consists of semantic web documents (SWDS) that are encoded in semantic web languages like OWL (Ontology Web language), RDF, DAML + OIL and many more. Some of the technologies are listed in Table 1.

4 Achieving Interoperability in Social Web Applications

Semantic web consists of various social ontologies to maintain interoperability and portability across various applications. Ontologies/Vocabularies include FOAF (Friend of a Friend), SIOC (Semantically Interlinked Online Communities) and XFN (Friends Network). The brief description of these ontologies is discussed in following subsections.

4.1 FOAF

FOAF is a simple RDF ontology that helps in identifying "who is who" and links them with other persons by using XML/RDF format [12]. It includes mainly three components—ontological definition, ontological properties and empirical properties [13]. One of the most common classes in FOAF ontology is foaf: person. It holds various properties like foaf: name, foaf: email, foaf: gender, foaf: knows and many more (Fig. 4; Table 2).

FOAF profile of above ontology can be created using FOAF-a-Matic application [14]. The result is being generated in RDF (Fig. 5).

4.2 XFN

It is an acronym for friend network. It is one of the social ontologies that describe category wise social relationships among different persons [15]. The category may

Table 1 Semantic web technologies

Technology	Description
1. XML 1.1. XMLs (XML schema)	It is an extensible language that helps users in creating tags to their documents. It provides well-defined syntax for writing content of document It is language for defining XML documents
2. RDF 2.1. RDFs	It is an acronym for Resource Description Framework that is used to express data models consisting of objects, property and relationship It is an acronym for RDF schema. It is a description language for defining vocabularies and represents relationship among objects

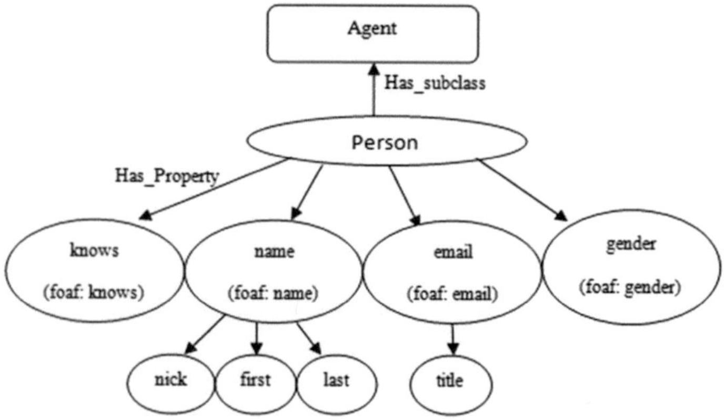

Fig. 4 FOAF ontology with class foaf: person

Table 2 Components of foaf: person class in FOAF ontology

Ontological definition	Ontological properties	Empirical properties (instances)
Agent	foaf: knows foaf: name foaf: email foaf: gender	foaf: nick foaf: first foaf: last foaf: title

include friend, co-worker, neighbour, family, etc. This ontology holds commutative and transitive dependencies. If A is a friend of B then B is also friend of A.

$$A \rightarrow B \Leftrightarrow B \rightarrow A$$

If A is friend of B and B is neighbour of C, then A is neighbour of C but may/may not be friend of C.

$$A \rightarrow B, \quad B \rightarrow C \Leftrightarrow A \rightarrow C$$

4.3 SIOC

Evolution of SIOC: High usage of social sites has led to birth of various constraints like privacy, lack of interoperability, digital signatures and security threats. It becomes difficult to query and interlink social data. So, there must be some unified models/vocabularies to handle these issues. The best way to do this is to combine semantic web technologies with social paradigms in order to propose a new social semantic prototype system. Semantic web technologies include use of RDF, OWL, queries to encode social data into machine understandable format. For combining social and semantic paradigms, there is need to provide some framework for

```
<rdf:RDF
xmlns:rdf="http://www.w3.org/1999/02/22-rdf-syntax-ns#"
xmlns:rdfs="http://www.w3.org/2000/01/rdf-schema#"
xmlns:foaf="http://xmlns.com/foaf/0.1/"
xmlns:admin="http://webns.net/mvcb/">
<foaf:PersonalProfileDocument rdf:about="">
<foaf:maker rdf:resource="#me"/>
<foaf:primaryTopic rdf:resource="#me"/>
<admin:generatorAgent rdf:resource="http://www.ldodds.com/foaf/foaf-a-matic"/>
<admin:errorReportsTo rdf:resource="mailto:leigh@ldodds.com"/>
</foaf:PersonalProfileDocument>
<foaf:Person rdf:ID="me">
<foaf:name>Gagandeep Singh Narula</foaf:name>
<foaf:title>Mr</foaf:title>
<foaf:givenname>Gagandeep Singh</foaf:givenname>
<foaf:family_name>Narula</foaf:family_name>
<foaf:nick>Smily</foaf:nick>
<foaf:mbox_sha1sum>30b2f5faee64d084a0780f724390bff8c0486bf6</foaf:mbox_sha1sum>
<foaf:knows>
<foaf:Person>
<foaf:name>VishalJain</foaf:name>
<foaf:mbox_sha1sum>295863d5ad5b5ea880bde725f16cb21e2d1848fe</foaf:mbox_sha1sum></foa
f:Person></foaf:knows>
<foaf:knows>
<foaf:Person>
<foaf:name>UshaYadav</foaf:name>
<foaf:mbox_sha1sum>b97f8105b2c7820ac793cda0b1865ab2d45a9c0c</foaf:mbox_sha1sum></fo
af:Person></foaf:knows></foaf:Person>
</rdf:RDF>
```

Fig. 5 RDF code snippet

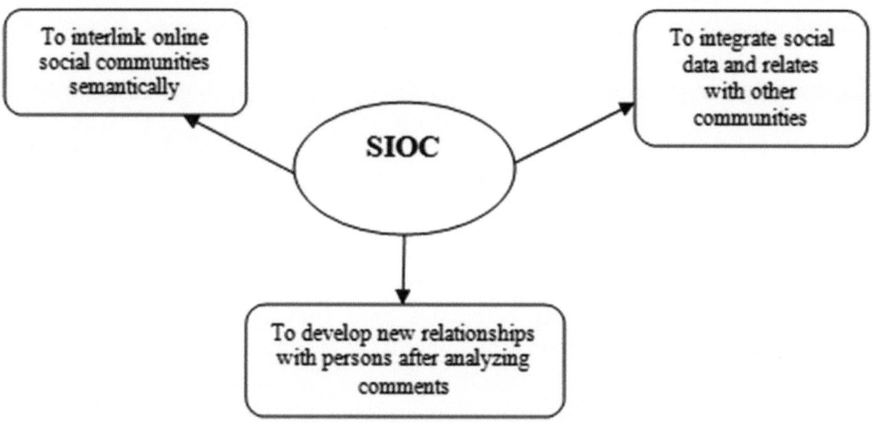

Fig. 6 Functions of SIOC

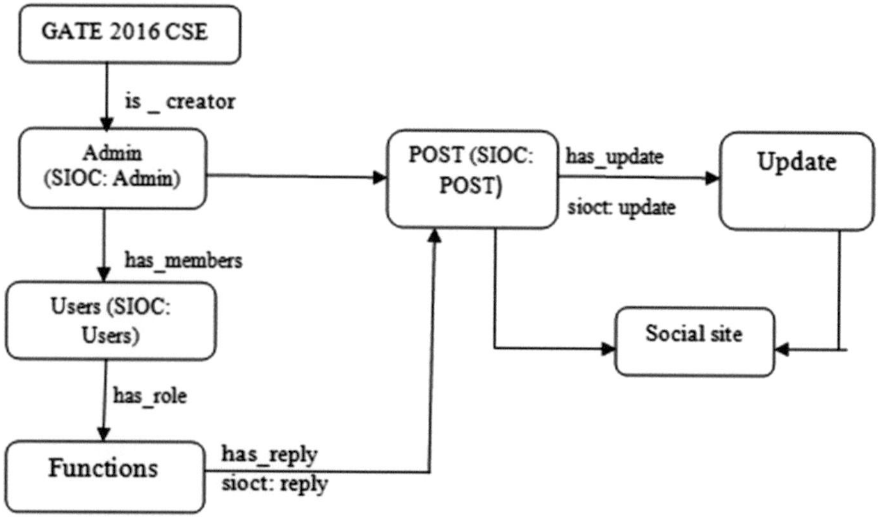

Fig. 7 SIOC ontology model on group "GATE 2016 CSE"

modelling activities and integration of online community information. This framework can be achieved by using SIOC [16].

The functions of SIOC are given in Figs. 6 and 7.

SIOC ontology model deals with various classes and their properties related to user groups created on websites. Consider there is group created by a user named as "GATE 2016 CSE". The creator of this group is marked as Admin and other users are termed as group members. A single ontology class is represented as: SIOC: name of class.

Inverse additional properties like reply, update are represented using sioct: reply and sioct: update respectively. Sioct is an acronym for SIOC types of module.

4.4 FOAF + SIOC

Both ontologies can be used in collaboration to enable a model for interoperability and portability of social data onto semantics. Different user profiles of same person on multiple sites can be combined in single RDF group data.

In Fig. 8, Gagan is a person whose friends are Vishal and Usha. It is represented by foaf: knows property. Gagan has different profile account on sites like Facebook and LinkedIn with different names. Assume NarulaG is admin of group GATE 2016 CSE and Gaggs is one of the members in this group. But both belong to same person Gagan. So these accounts must be merged in single RDF data instead of having multiple accounts.

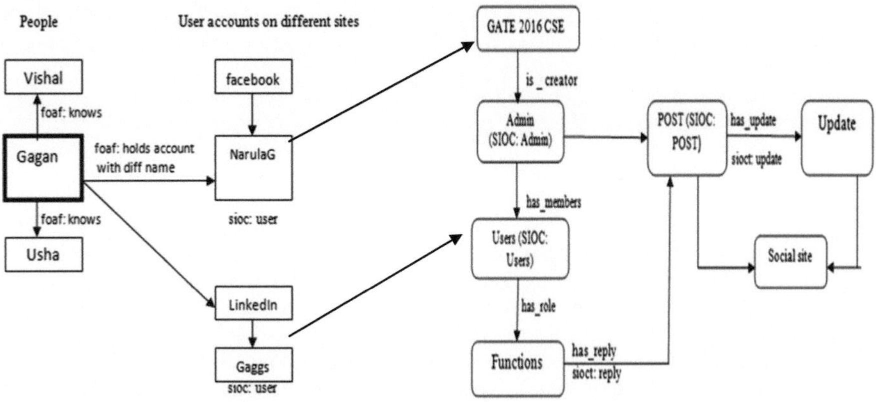

Fig. 8 FOAF + SIOC

5 Conclusion and Future Scope

Although online services of social sites for publishing and accessing data has facilitated the process of information sharing among different groups but it has faced same challenges like predefined API's for each application, lack of knowledge management, fake identity management and many more. So, the paper discusses the need to achieve interoperability in social web applications, access relevant social data and satisfying users to a great extent. Semantic web aims to abridge knowledge gap between humans and machines. Various issues of social sites have been addressed in the following paper. It also provides solutions to cope with these issues by connecting with social ontologies (FOAF, XFN) and interlinking data with online communities (SIOC).

The work can be extended to develop generic interface that is compatible with semantic web technologies and standards. The interface can be used to publish and access data in RDF format which eventually leads to interconnection of social network with different data sources.

References

1. Bojars, U., Breslin, J.G., Peristeras, V. Tummarello, G., Decker, S.: Interlinking the social web with semantics. IEEE Intell. Syst. **23**, 29–40 (2008)
2. Lee, F.: PRISM forum SIG on Semantic web. 12 May 2009
3. Mäkeläinen, S.I.: "Tiedonhallinta Semanttisessa Webissä"-seminar, University of Helsinki (2005)
4. Sloni, D.K.: Safe Semantic web and security aspect implication for social networking. IJCAES, June 2012

5. Halpin, H., Tuffield, M.: A standards-based, open and privacy-aware social web. In: W3C Social Web Incubator Group Report, 6 Dec 2010. W3C Incubator Group Report. Retrieved 6 Aug 2011
6. Specia, L., Motta, E. Integrating Folksonomies with the Semantic web. In: Lect. Notes Comput. Sci. 624–639 (2007)
7. Xu, Z., Fu, Y., Mao, J., Su, D.: Towards the semantic web: collaborative tag suggestions. In: Collaborative Web Tagging Workshop at WWW 2006, Edinburgh, UK (2006)
8. Howard, R.: The virtual community: homesteading on the electronic frontier, p. 334. The MIT Press (2000)
9. Lee, T.B.: The Semantic web. Sci. Am. (2007)
10. Lee, T.B., Hendler, J., Lassila, O.: The Semantic web. Sci. Am. 34–43 (2001)
11. Mika, P.: Social networks and the Semantic web. SIKS Dissertation Series No. 2007-03, 18 Dec 2006
12. Lee, T.B.: The 1st World Wide Web Conference, Geneva, May 1994
13. W3C Semantic web activity. In: World Wide Web Consortium (W3C), 7 Nov 2011. Retrieved 26 Nov 2011
14. http://www.ldodds.com/foaf/foaf-a-matic.html
15. Manola, F., Miller, E.: RDF primer. In: W3C Recommendation, 10 Feb 2004 (2004)
16. Bresley, J.G., Dekkar, S., et al.: SIOC: content exchange and semantic interoperability between social networks. In: W3C Workshop on Social Networking, Barcelona, 15–16 Jan 2009
17. Singh, G., Jain, V.: Information retrieval (IR) through Semantic web (SW): an overview. In: Proceedings of CONFLUENCE 2012—The Next Generation Information Technology Summit at Amity School of Engineering and Technology, pp. 23–27, Sept 2012
18. Giri, K.: Role of ontology in Semantic web. DESIDOC J. Libr. Inf. Technol. **31**(2), 116–120 (2011)
19. Jeremic, Z., et al.: Personal learning environments on the social semantic web. Semantic web-linked data for science and education. ACM DL **4**(1), 23–51 (2013)
20. Singh, G., et al.: Ontology development using Hozo and Semantic analysis for information retrieval in Semantic web. In: IEEE Second International Conference on Image Information Processing (ICIIP) (2013)

Author Biographies

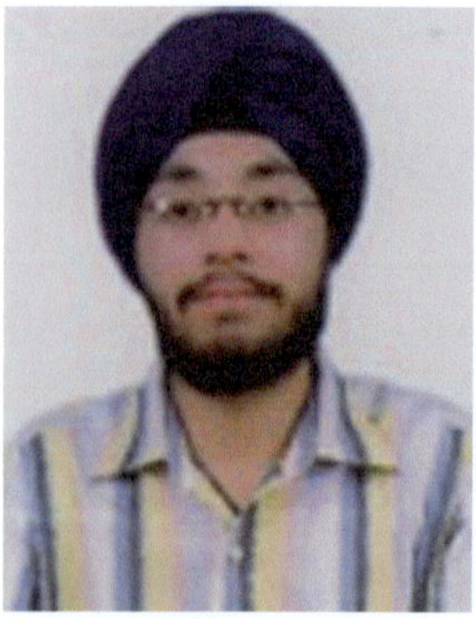

Gagandeep Singh Narula received his B.Tech. in Computer Science and Engineering from Guru Tegh Bahadur Institute of Technology (GTBIT) affiliated to Guru Gobind Singh Indraprastha University (GGSIPU), New Delhi. Now, he is pursuing M.Tech. in Computer Science from CDAC Noida affiliated to GGSIPU. He has published various research papers in various national, international journals and conferences His research areas include Semantic Web, Information Retrieval, Data Mining, Cloud Computing and Knowledge Management. He is also a member of IEEE Spectrum.

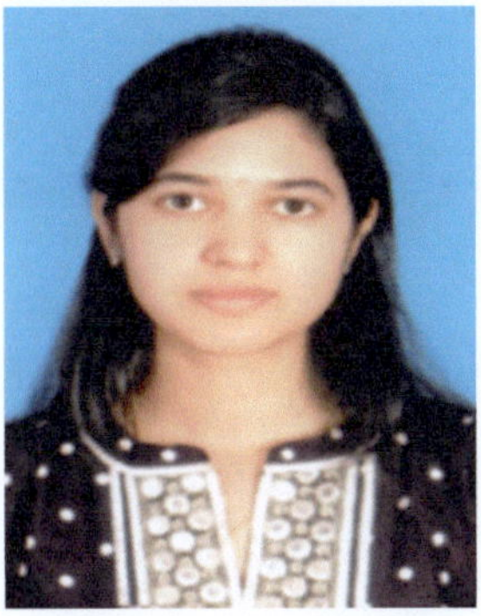

Usha Yadav received her B.E. in Information Technology with Honours from Maharshi Dayanand University, Rohtak in 2009 and M.Tech. with Honours in Computer Engineering from YMCA University of Science and Technology, Faridabad in 2011. She is pursuing her Ph.D. in Computer Engineering from YMCA University of Science and Technology, Faridabad. She is currently working as a Project Engineer in CDAC, Noida and has three years of experience. Her areas of interest are search engines, social web and semantic web.

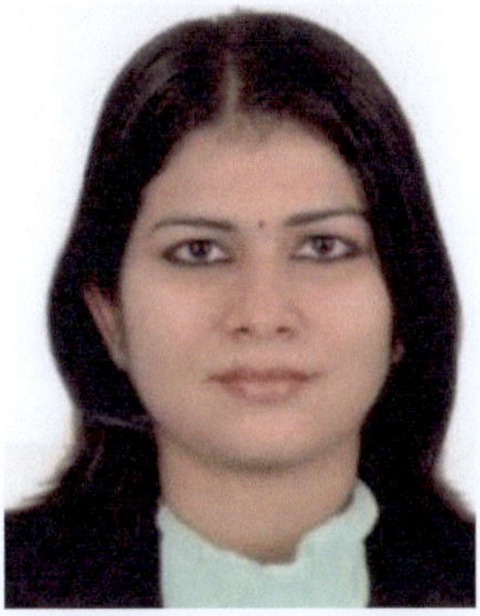

Dr. Neelam Duhan received her B.Tech. in Computer Science and Engineering with Honours from Kurukshetra University, Kurukshetra and M.Tech. with Honours in Computer Engineering from Maharshi Dayanand University, Rohtak in 2002 and 2005, respectively. She completed her Ph.D. in Computer Engineering in 2011 from Maharshi Dayanand University, Rohtak. She is currently working as an Assistant Professor in Computer Engineering Department in YMCA University of Science and Technology, Faridabad and has an experience of about 12 years. She has published over 30 research papers in reputed international Journals and International Conferences. Her areas of interest are databases, search engines and web mining.

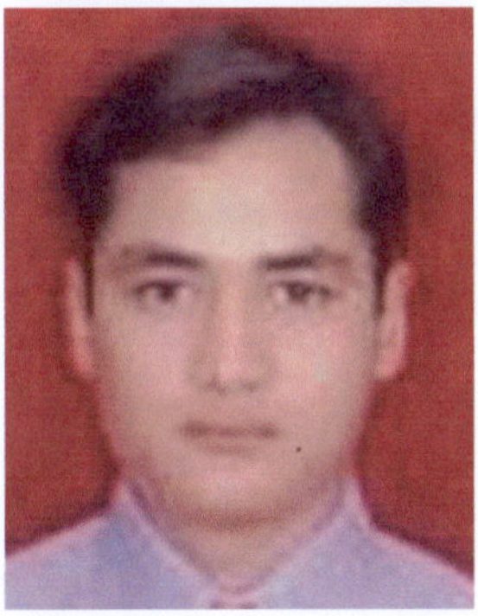

Vishal Jain has completed his M.Tech (CSE) from USIT, Guru Gobind Singh Indraprastha University, Delhi and doing Ph.D. in Computer Science and Engineering Department, Lingaya's University, Faridabad. Presently, He is working as Assistant Professor in Bharati Vidyapeeth's Institute of Computer Applications and Management, (BVICAM), New Delhi. His research area includes Web Technology, Semantic Web and Information Retrieval. He is also associated with CSI, ISTE.

Classification of E-commerce Products Using RepTree and K-means Hybrid Approach

Neha Midha and Vikram Singh

Abstract The paper discusses an algorithm that groups the items on the basis of their attributes and then classifies the clusters. In other words, the proposed algorithms first cluster the items on the basis of property, i.e., attributes available for the dataset. The clustering is performed by K-means clustering. Then this clustered data is classified using the RepTree. In other words, the proposed algorithm is the hybrid algorithm of K-means clustering and the RepTree classification. The proposed algorithm is compared with the RepTree algorithm using the WEKA tool. The comparison is done over clothing dataset downloaded from Internet. The proposed algorithm decreases the mean absolute error as well as the root-mean-square error. The decrease in error results in accurate classification. So the proposed algorithm clusters the items and classifies them on the basis of their attributes more accurately.

Keywords Data mining · Clustering · RepTree · K-means

1 Introduction

The advancement in the technology leads to the digitalization in all the sectors like business, engineering, manufacturing, etc. This leads to the generation of huge amount of data to be processed. This generates the requirement for the automated tools of data mining for knowledge discovery. In the present scenario, the enterprise focuses on automated tools for the data modeling as well as for the data processing.

The data mining is the process to extract the unknown facts or other useful information from existing massive data. But the extract is just a first step for turning

N. Midha (✉)
Chaudhary Devi Lal University, Sirsa, Haryana, India
e-mail: midhaneha.nic@gmail.com

V. Singh
Department of Computer Science & Applications,
Chaudhary Devi Lal University, Sirsa, Haryana, India
e-mail: vikramsinghkuk@yahoo.com

V.B. Aggarwal et al. (eds.), *Big Data Analytics*, Advances in Intelligent Systems and Computing 654, https://doi.org/10.1007/978-981-10-6620-7_26

the data into knowledge and knowledge into action. A variety of data mining techniques exist for the extraction of information and patterns from the database [1, 2]:

- The data consisting of the usage statistics is not considered as data mining techniques. But the evaluation starts from collecting the data. This process used the web-based programs to collect the data and then track features for specific details.
- The classification technique is used to classify the elements based on their class labels. The prediction techniques are used to predict the continuous values. The numeric value results of the prediction lead to the regression.
- Clustering technique is used to group the similar data items and to separate the dissimilar data items. In the clustering, no class is present. Basically, the clustering is unsupervised process. Basic example is pattern recognition.
- The association is used to find the relationship between the different attributes of the dataset. It is used to analyze the pairs that occur in the data frequently.
- Time series analysis checks the deviation in the pattern as well as in rules with the change in time. The analysis must be uninterrupted.

The success of the data mining techniques completely depends upon understanding the various levels of abstraction of the knowledge. Typical example is interactions and learning activities.

The advancement in the e-commerce leads to the automated delivery of products. It generates an automatic system from order to delivery and provides 24 × 7 service to the customers. The customer can customize their purchases, and the increase in the business can be analyzed due to enhancement in the services [3]. It leads to the collection of data electronically. The data of e-commerce is used to analyze the taste of the customer of a particular area by taking care of viewed and the purchased products. This needs the processing of huge amount of the data. The processing of such data is cost-effective as it leads to enhanced business [3].

2 Data Mining Techniques

2.1 RepTree

The RepTree is a decision tree formed on the basis of information gain. The information gain relates to the reduction in variance. The RepTree performs all the basic functioning of the C4.5 and also performs the pruning by sorting the numerical attributes [4]. This algorithm [5] works on the principle of information gain with entropy which results in reduced variance [6]. It reduces the decision tree methods' complexity [5].

Decision tree builds the tree by supervised learning and the tree formed on the basis of divide and rule approach. It repeats the test function recursively until it finds the leaf nodes [6, 7]. The decision tree is used for classification purposes due to good accuracy and easy processing [5–7] Suppose A and B are two distinct variables with values $\{a_1, \ldots, a_n\}$ and $\{b_1, \ldots, b_n\}$. The entropy and conditional entropy of B are shown in Eqs. (1) and (2). After that information gain of A is calculated as shown in Eq. (3):

$$H(B) = -\sum_{i=1}^{k} P(B = b_i) \log P(B = b_i) \tag{1}$$

$$H(B|A) = -\sum_{i=1}^{l} P(A = a_i) H(B|A = a_i) \tag{2}$$

$$IG(B; A) = H(B) - H(B|A). \tag{3}$$

The pruning can be done in two ways, i.e., pre-pruning and post-pruning. In the pre-pruning, the expansion of the tree gets stopped when the information gain due to division is not recognized, while in the post-pruning the process continues until all pure leaf nodes are found [7]. The results of the post-pruning are found to be better than the pre-pruning [8].

2.2 K-means Clustering

The K-means clustering technique is the process to group the elements of a dataset in k-means clusters. The process of clustering is done by calculating the Euclidean distance between the elements and centroid, where centroid is the element with uniform density. The main feature of this algorithm is the simplicity and usability with different data types. But the algorithm results may vary depending upon the position of centroid [9]. The centroid is selected randomly in the initial phase. It is updated in next phases to the optimal value based on distance. However, the testing of large clusters for the different initial sets is not practical [10]. Different methods for the same are given by [11]. The complexity of the k-means algorithm is high [9].

Here k-means clustering divides the datasets into clusters by analyzing the attributes of the elements. The distance is calculated on the basis of the attributes of the elements. The process of clustering continues until centroid converges or maximum iterations achieved [12].

3 A Hybrid Classification Approach

In this work, an algorithm is proposed that groups the items on the basis of their attributes and then classifies the clusters. In other words, the proposed algorithms first cluster the items on the basis of property, i.e., attributes available for the dataset. The clustering is performed by the K-means clustering. Then this clustered data is classified using the RepTree which is already explained in Sect. 3. It means the proposed algorithm is the hybrid algorithm of K-means clustering and the RepTree classification. It can be explained by the following algorithm:

3.1 Proposed Algorithm

1. Define K, i.e., number of clusters.
2. Select K data elements as centroid randomly.
3. For each element in dataset
4. For k=1:K
5. Calculate the distance with k centroid say d(i,k).
6. End for
7. End for
8. Create the clusters on the basis of minimum distance, i.e., Min(d(i,:)).
9. Calculate the mean and select element as new centroid in each group
10. If new centroid != existing centroid
11. Go to step 3
12. End if
13. For j=1:K
14. Calculate the information gain with entropy in the cluster j:

    $H(Y) = -\sum_{i=1}^{k} P(y = y_i) \log P(Y = y_i) \quad (1)$

    $H(Y|X) = -\sum_{i=1}^{l} P(X = x_i) H(Y|X = x_i) \quad (2)$

    $IG(Y;X) = H(Y) - H(Y|X) \quad (3)$
15. If variance of element is not less than the training variance
16. Divide the elements of cluster
17. Go to step 13
18. End if
19. End for

This algorithm can also be explained by the flowchart shown in Fig. 1.

Fig. 1 Proposed algorithm using flowchart

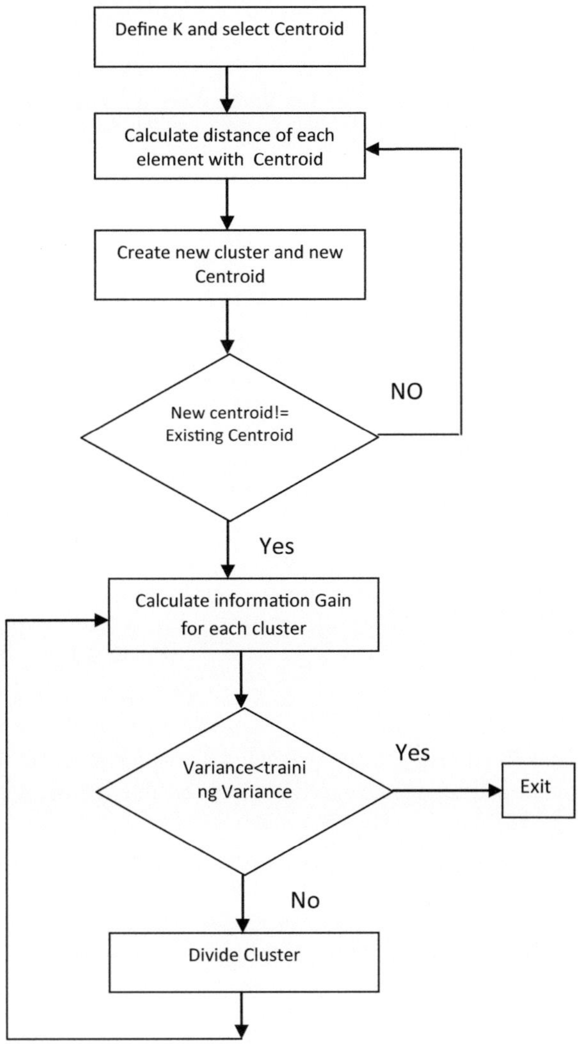

4 Results

The dataset used to analyze the proposed algorithm over WEKA is the clothing dataset. This dataset is downloaded from the "https://github.com/vincentarelbundock/Rdatasets/blob/master/csv/Ecdat/Clothing.csv". The dataset is in CSV, i.e., comma-separated value format. This dataset contains 400 instances each having 14 attributes. The attributes are as srno, tsales, sales, margin, nown, nfull, npart, naux, hoursw, hourspw, inv1, inv2, ssize, and start. These attributes within the dataset explain the size and the sale with a corresponding profit of the t-shirt sale. This is basically dataset that identifies the sales of a product along with other characteristics.

v. Performance evaluation parameters are **root-mean-square**

The root-mean-square is used to estimate the difference between the estimated value and the actual value. It represents the standard deviation and used to analyze the error:

$$\mathrm{RMSE} = \sqrt{\frac{\left(\sum_{i=1}^{n}(\mathrm{actual}_i - \mathrm{estimated}_i)^2\right)}{n}}.$$

Relative Absolute Error

The **relative absolute error** is the similar to RSE except the differences are squared. It is basically the normalized absolute error, where the absolute error is the difference between the observed and the actual value. Mathematically, the **relative absolute error** ERR_i can be given by the following equation:

$$\mathrm{ERR}_i = \frac{\sum_{j=1}^{n}\left|\mathrm{Predicted}_{(ij)} - \mathrm{True}_j\right|}{\sum_{j=1}^{n}\left|T_{\mathrm{rue}j} - \overline{\mathrm{True}}\right|},$$

here $\mathrm{Predicted}_{(ij)}$ is the predicted value for program i of case j; True_j is the target class; and aggregated true is given by the aggregation of true value of each case.

Relative Square Error

It is the normalized version of the squared error, predicted by taking square of the difference of the true and observed value. The normalized value leads to the mean of the total calculated errors. It can be given as

$$\mathrm{Error}_i = \frac{\sum_{j=1}^{n}\left|\mathrm{Pred}_{(ij)} - \mathrm{True}_j\right|}{\sum_{j=1}^{n}\left|\mathrm{True}_j - \overline{\mathrm{True}}\right|},$$

where $\mathrm{Pred}_{(ij)}$ is the predicted value for program i of case j; True_j is the target class; and aggregated true is given by the aggregation of true value of each case.

Mean Absolute Error

The MAE is used to analyze the accuracy of the predication, i.e., how far is the observed value from the actual value. It can be given as

$$\mathrm{MAE} = \frac{1}{n}\sum_{i=1}^{n}|f_i - y_i| = \frac{1}{n}\sum_{i=1}^{n}|e_i|.$$

It is the average of the absolute error and here *f* represents the predicted value and y represents the true value.

Correlation Coefficient

The correlation coefficient between two entities is the division of their covariance by multiplication of their standard deviations. It measures the linear relationship between two entities. It can be given as

$$r_{xy} = \frac{S_{xy}}{S_x S_y},$$

where s_x and s_y are the standard deviations, and s_{xy} is the covariance between x and y entities. The value of correlation near to 1 shows that the entities are linearly related and 0 value shows the weak relation.

The proposed and RepTree algorithms are simulated over the WEKA tool using the clothing dataset. Their performance analysis is shown in the following graphs.

Figure 2 shows that the proposed algorithm decreases the mean absolute error as well as the root-mean-square error. The relative absolute error and the root relative absolute error are also decreased as shown in Fig. 3. The decrease in error results in accurate classification. So the proposed algorithm clusters the items and classifies them on the basis of their attributes more accurately. The relation between the items is derived from the attributes present in the dataset. This relation is used to cluster and classify the items. So the proposed algorithm fully depends on the attributes present in the dataset.

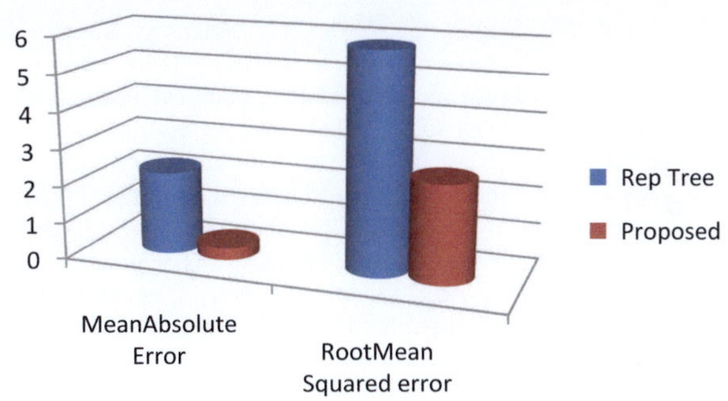

Fig. 2 Comparisons of MAE and RMSE

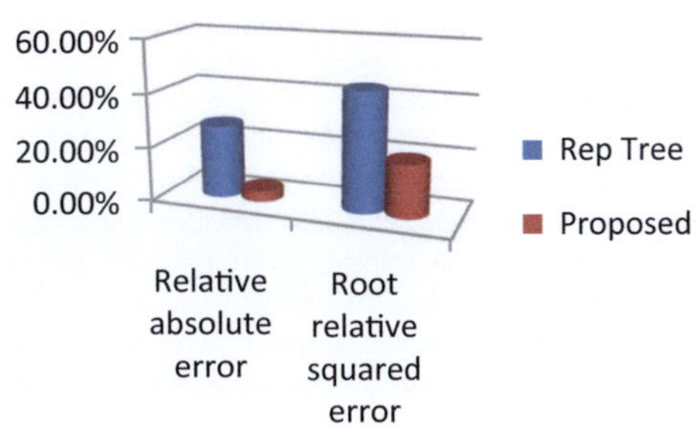

Fig. 3 Comparisons of RAE and RRSE

5 Conclusion

The proposed algorithm is compared with the RepTree algorithm using the WEKA tool. The comparison is done over clothing dataset downloaded from Internet. The proposed algorithm decreases the mean absolute error as well as the root-mean-square error. The relative absolute error and the root relative absolute error are also decreased. The decrease in error results in accurate classification. So the proposed algorithm clusters the items and classifies them on the basis of their attributes more accurately. In future, the algorithm can also be analyzed over other e-commerce datasets. The algorithm can be modified to be applicable for other fields like medicine. The neural network can also be added to the proposed algorithm to enhance the performance.

References

1. Agrawal, R., Srikant, R. Mining sequential patterns. In: Proceedings of the Eleventh International Conference on Data Engineering, 1995, pp. 3–14. IEEE (1995)
2. Cooley, R., Tan, P.N., Srivastava, J.: Discovery of interesting usage patterns from web data. In: Web Usage Analysis and User Profiling, pp. 163–182. Springer, Berlin, Heidelberg (2000)
3. Sanchati, R., Patidar, P.C., Kulkarni, G. Path breaking case studies in E-commerce using data mining. Int. J. Comput. Technol. Electron. Eng. **1** (2011)
4. Mohamed, W., Salleh, M.N.M., Omar, A.H.: A comparative study of reduced error pruning method in decision tree algorithms. In: 2012 IEEE International Conference on Control System, Computing and Engineering (ICCSCE), pp. 392–397. IEEE, Nov 2012
5. Zontul, M., Dogan, G., Aydin, F., Sener, S., Kaynar, O.: Wind speed forecasting using Reptree and bagging methods in Kirklareli-Turkey. J. Theor. Appl. Inf. Technol. **56**(1) (2013)
6. Witten, I.H., Frank. E.: Data mining: practical machine learning tools and techniques. 2nd ed. The United States of America, Morgan Kaufmann Series in Data Management Systems (2005)
7. Alpaydın, E.: Introduction to Machine Learning. The MIT Press, Printed and Bound in the United States of America. ISBN: 0-262-01211-1 (2004)
8. Agrawal, R., Mannila, H., Srikant, R., Toivonen, H., Verkamo, A.I.: Fast discovery of association rules. Adv. Knowl. Discovery Data Min. **12**(1), 307–328 (1996)
9. Sharma (Sachdeva), R.: K-means clustering in spatial data mining using WEKA interface. In: International Conference on Advances in Communication and Computing Technologies (ICACACT) 2012 Proceedings. International Journal of Computer Applications® (IJCA) (2014)
10. Ismail, M., Kamel, M.: Multidimensional data clustering utilization hybrid search strategies. Pattern Recogn. **22**(1), 75–89 (1989)
11. Pena, J.M., Lozano, J.A., Larranaga, P.: An empirical comparison of four initialization methods for the k-means algorithm. Pattern Recogn. Lett. **20**(10), 1027–1040 (1999)
12. Jain, S.: K-means clustering using WEKA interface. In: Proceedings of the 4th National Conference; INDIACom-2010 Computing for Nation Development, 25–26 Feb 2010
13. Pahl, C.: Data mining technology for the evaluation of learning content interaction. Int. J. E-Learn. **3**(4), 47 (2004)
14. Sharma, N., Bajpai, A., Litoriya, R. Comparison the various clustering algorithms of WEKA tools. Int. J. Emerg. Technol. Adv. Eng. **2**(5) (2012)

15. Shrivastava, V., Narayan Arya, P. A study of various clustering algorithms on retail sales data. Int. J. Comput. Commun. Netw. **1**(2) (2012)
16. Quinlan, J.R.: Simplifying decision trees. Int. J. Man Mach. Stud. **27**(3), 221–234 (1987)
17. Bhan, N.: Comparative study of EM and K-means clustering techniques in WEKA inter-face. Int. J. Adv. Technol. Eng. Res. IJATER **3**(4) (2013)

A Study of Factors Affecting MapReduce Scheduling

Manisha Gaur, Bhawna Minocha and Sunil Kumar Muttoo

Abstract MapReduce is a programming model for parallel distributed processing of large-scale data. Hadoop framework is an implementation of MapReduce. Since MapReduce processes data parallel on clusters of nodes, there is a need to have a good scheduling technique to optimize performance. Performance of MapReduce scheduling depends upon various points like execution time, resource utilization across the cluster, data locality, compute capacity, energy efficiency, heterogeneity, scaling, etc. Researchers have developed various algorithms to resolve some or the other problem and reach a near-optimal solution. This paper summarizes most of the research work done in this regard.

Keywords MapReduce · Scheduling algorithms · Hadoop

1 Introduction

The MapReduce [1] model introduced in 2004 is a programing model for parallel distributed processing of large-scale data. MapReduce process comprises two main functions—Map and Reduce [1]. In this system, there are multiple points to be considered to get a robust system and gain good performance. Resource utilization, energy efficiency, heterogeneity, scalability, data locality, and speculative tasks execution are some of them that we include ahead.

Further, the paper is organized as follows. Section 2 highlights the factors affecting scheduling performance followed by the review of the various researches

M. Gaur (✉) · B. Minocha
AIIT, Amity University, Noida, UP, India
e-mail: gaur.manisha2012@gmail.com

B. Minocha
e-mail: bminocha@amity.edu

S.K. Muttoo
University of Delhi, New Delhi, India
e-mail: skmuttoo@cs.du.ac.in

V.B. Aggarwal et al. (eds.), *Big Data Analytics*, Advances in Intelligent Systems and Computing 654, https://doi.org/10.1007/978-981-10-6620-7_27

done on the factors discussed. Finally, we conclude the paper in Sect. 3 with a perspective of future work.

2 Factors Affecting Performance of MapReduce Scheduling

Below we summarize the factors identified to affect MapReduce scheduling.

Data Locality: It refers to the constraint that a task should be executed on a node where the data resides in order to avoid network traffic overhead [2].

Resource Utilization: Three types of resources are used in the system—CPU, Disk input/output, Network input/output. The system can be viewed as a cluster of nodes where each may have multiple slots where data can be executed. Scheduling algorithms need to be defined with an objective to utilize the maximum number of slots of all the nodes with minimum data transfer overhead on the network [3].

Budget and Deadline Constraints: Deadline is a user-defined input indicating the time by which or an interval within which the job must be completed. Budget constraints are however related to the monetary value associated with the pay-as-you-go model of cloud-based services [4].

Other Factors—Network Traffic, Speculative Task Execution, Energy Efficiency, Shared Scan, Heterogeneity, Real-time Scheduling: Network traffic refers to the traffic caused when either the data is being moved toward computation or some speculative tasks have been sent out for fault tolerance [5]. Speculative tasks are those that are run periodically to check for any failed node or failed task execution. Tracking when to run speculative tasks can avoid unnecessary tasks and improve the overall execution time [6]. Energy is consumed on each node and the network. Many researches are being done to maximize the energy efficiency [7]. Many times when the number of jobs is far more than the number of distinct datasets, multiple concurrent jobs end up scanning the same dataset individually. Shared scan is a concept introduced to cooperatively share the read [8]. When the data is too large and scattered in multiple clusters or nodes, there exists data heterogeneity. Also, when multiple clusters come together to form one virtual cluster, there also exists node and cluster heterogeneity in the system [9]. There are a number of factors that affect scheduling in a real-time situation like a number of concurrent users, data placement overhead, etc. These factors have been studied and some amendments have been proposed by researchers for real-time scheduling [10].

Let us see one by one how various researchers have worked upon these factors.

2.1 Data Locality

Hammoud et al. [2] analyzed the advantages and disadvantages of setting early shuffle on to and came out with the Sweet Spot. The proposed Locality-Aware Reduce Task Scheduling algorithm (LARTS), when tested against native Hadoop, appreciatively maximizes the node level and rack level traffic, and minimizes the off-track traffic on a set system size. Luo et al. [11] have presented a hierarchical framework to make multiple clusters work as if it is one big cluster with three functions—Map, Reduce, and GlobalReduce. Two algorithms have been proposed —compute capacity-aware scheduling aiming at optimizing data-intensive jobs and data locality-aware scheduling that runs a job on the cluster where data resides.

Ibrahim et al. [12] presented a two-wave algorithm called Maestro to handle nonlocal network traffic that causes an excessive number of unnecessary speculative execution and an unbalanced map tasks execution across different machines. Tan et al. [13] have worked on the joint optimization of map and reduce tasks and proposed coupling scheduler utilizing random peeking scheduling for map tasks and wait scheduling for reduce tasks. Experimentally, they have proved it more efficient over fair scheduler in terms of improving data locality, mitigating starvation, and improving performance with no harm to single jobs.

Bu et al. [14] worked upon virtual MapReduce clusters and noticed the additional opportunity of data locality for co-hosted virtual machines. They proposed interference and locality-aware task scheduling algorithm that proves better over four other schedulers being used in MapReduce.

2.2 Resource Utilization

Guo et al. [3] presented an opportunistic approach to steal the otherwise-wasted resources for aggressive utilization of the available resources. They proposed benefit aware speculative execution algorithm that predicted the benefit of running any speculative task and thus could avoid a lot of traffic due to unnecessary speculative tasks. Wolf et al. [15] got inspired from the default Hadoop Fair scheduler and designed a flexible scheduling scheme that optimizes a variety of standard theory matrices while maintaining a minimum job slot guarantee for each job. There are two different kinds of scheduling mentioned—Moldable and Malleable schedulings. The proposed FLEX algorithm is said to outperform the Hadoop's default Fair scheduler for a small number of jobs.

Sharma et al. [16] have worked on the problem of dynamic resource allocation and resource contention and proposed MROrchestrator framework that dynamically identifies bottlenecks and resolves them through a fine-grained, on-demand allocation scheme. Experimental results show that this framework reduces the job completion time and increases resource utilization by quite a good percent.

Yao et al. [17] have proposed a scheduler HaSTe for Hadoop YARN ecosystem that leverages the requested resources, resource capacity, and task dependency based on the fitness and urgency of the tasks. Experimentally, the HasTe scheduler proves better than the default Hadoop schedulers—Fair and FIFO on a predefined system configuration. Zhang et al. [18] have focused on the varying requirement of resources throughout the lifetime of a task and divided the entire execution into phases. They have proposed a scheduling algorithm called PRISM, which when compared with Hadoop YARN running capacity and fair scheduler, the benefits of phase-level scheduling and fairness are very evident.

2.3 Budget and Deadline Constraints

Sandholm et al. [4] have examined various schedulers for shared clusters and proposed Dynamic Priority scheduler (DP) extending the capability of fair and FIFO. DP works on the simple principle of bid and buy and can be used by budget and cost corresponding agents as it prioritizes both users and jobs and also allows scaling back when the demand is high and the resources are expensive. However, the admin must monitor the prices to maintain a stable economy.

Chen et al. [19] have utilized bipartite graph modeling and proposed BGMRS scheduler that solves the Minimum Weighted Bipartite Matching problem (MWBM). Experimentally, tested in a simulation environment, this strategy is said to reduce the job elapsed time and the deadline over job ratio by a good number compared to other existing fair and FIFO schedulers.

Wang et al. [20] developed two greedy algorithms—Global Greedy Budget (GGB) and Gradual Refinement (GR). Evaluated on a java-built Budget Distribution Solver (BDS), the algorithms put a step forward for cost-effective infrastructure even though it does not consider the other complex components of Hadoop like speculative tasks execution, dynamic pricing, fault tolerance, etc.

Tang et al. [21] first presented a new distribution model for distributing data as per node's compute capacity and then proposed a two-stage scheduling algorithm MTSD for map and reduce tasks individually. Experimentally, this proves to improve data locality and deadline constraints compared to the default Hadoop schedulers.

Liu et al. [22] focused on the deadline constraint problem of MapReduce and proposed a preemptive approach for job scheduling based on an execution cost model and the current status of the system.

Kc et al. [23] extended the real-time scheduling approach and developed a deadline constraint scheduler that scheduled jobs only if the user-specified deadlines met, not only just meeting the deadlines, but the scheduler also focused on reducing the total completion time of all the jobs. Lai et al. [24] have focused on workload balancing and deadline constraint in MapReduce and proposed a polynomial time algorithm for scheduler design. Evaluated in a simulated environment with a self-proposed resource manager, called CRManager, this algorithm effectively balances the server load, response time, and the deadline satisfaction ratio compared to the traditional approaches used in Hadoop.

2.4 Other Factors—Network Traffic, Speculative Task Execution, Energy Efficiency, Shared Scan, Load Balancing and Heterogeneity, Real-Time Scheduling

Song et al. [5] focused on resource utilization and divided the multilevel scheduling problem into two games—job scheduling game and task scheduling game—and solved each of them using game theory methodologies. The proposed algorithm outperforms the default FIFO strategy.

Zaharia et al. [9] proposed Longest Approximate Time to End (LATE) algorithm which when evaluated in comparison to default Hadoop scheduler and the case when no speculative tasks run, LATE outperforms both. Sun [25] worked upon the same problem of heterogeneity as LATE and SAMR, and proposed enhanced SAMR overcoming the shortcomings of LATE and SAMR. Experimentally, ESAMR is said to outperform LATE and SAMR.

Yigitbasi et al. [7] investigated energy-aware scheduling heuristics including both low-power and high-performance nodes. Mashayekhy et al. [26] proposed Energy-aware MapReduce Scheduling Algorithm (EMRSA) for same modeling of the scheduling problem as an integer program.

Wolf et al. [8] focused on the case where the datasets are reasonably less than the number of jobs and proposed an extended version of the FLEX [13] scheduler that further contributes to making shared scan of datasets possible without much latency. Ahmad et al. [6] contributed toward load balancing in both map and reduce phase in a heterogeneous environment and proposed Tarazu for the same [6]. Experimentally, Tarazu outperforms LATE and default Hadoop schedulers.

In a real-time environment, there are a lot of factors that affect scheduling like concurrent users, data placement, and master scheduling overhead. Phan et al. [10] presented a model and formulated the problem as a constraint satisfaction problem. Dong et al. [27] presented a two-level MapReduce scheduler for mixed real-time and non-real-time scheduling requirement.

3 Conclusion and Future Work

This paper reviews most of the approaches developed to enhance various components of MapReduce scheduling to improve performance in both homogeneous and heterogeneous environments. We discussed the approaches taken but could not compare all of them to a certain standard to realize which is better. As part of future work, we aim to integrate and implement the proposed techniques and come up with a comparison metric to see which algorithm can be preferred in which scenario.

References

1. MapReduce Tutorial. http://hadoop.apache.org/docs/
2. Hammoud, M., Sakr, F.M.: Locality-aware reduce task scheduling for MapReduce. In: Proceeding CLOUDCOM IEEE 3rd International Conference on Cloud Computing Technology and Science, pp. 570–576 (2011)
3. Guo, Z., Fox, G.: Improving MapReduce performance in heterogeneous network environments and resource utilization. In: 12th IEEE/ACM International Symposium on Cluster, Cloud and Grid Computing, pp. 714–716 (2012)
4. Sandholm, T., Lai, K.: Dynamic proportional share scheduling in Hadoop. Job Sched. Strat. Parallel Process. Lect. Notes **V6253**, 110–131 (2010)
5. Song, G., Yu, L., Meng, Z., Lin, X.: A game theory based MapReduce scheduling algorithm. Emerg. Technol. Inf. Syst. Comput. Manage. Lect. Notes Electr. Eng. **236**, 287–296 (2013)
6. Ahmad, F., Chakradhar, S., Raghunathan, A., Vijaykumar, T.N.: Tarazu: optimizing MapReduce on heterogeneous clusters. In: ASPLOS XVII International Conference on Architectural Support for Programming Languages and Operating Systems, pp. 61–74 (2012)
7. Yigitbasi, N., Datta, K., Jain, N., Willke, T.: Energy efficient scheduling of MapReduce workloads on heterogeneous clusters. In: GCM 2nd International Workshop, pp. 1–6 (2011)
8. Wolf, J., Balmin, A., Rajan, D., Hildrum, K., Khandekar, R., Parekh, S., Wu, K.-L., Vernica, R.: On the optimization of schedules for MapReduce workloads in the presence of shared scans. VLDB J. **21**(5), 589–609 (2012)
9. Zaharia, M., Konwinski, A., Joseph, D.A., Katz, H.R., Stoica, I.: Improving MapReduce performance in heterogeneous environments. In: Proceeding OSDI 8th USENIX Conference on Operating Systems Design and Implementation, pp. 29–42 (2008)
10. Phan, T.X.L., Zhang, Z., Loo, T.B., Lee, I.: Real-time MapReduce scheduling. Technical Report, University of Pennsylvania Department of Computer and Information Science
11. Luo, Y., Plale, B.: Hierarchical MapReduce programming model and scheduling algorithms. In:12th IEEE International Symposium on Cluster, Cloud and Grid Computing (2012)
12. Ibrahim, S., Jin, H., Lu, L., He, B., Antoniu, G., Wu, S.: Maestro: replica-aware map scheduling for MapReduce, In: Proceeding CCGRID 12th IEEE/ACM International Symposium on Cluster, Cloud and Grid Computing, pp. 435–442 (2012)
13. Tan, J., Meng, X., Zhang, L.: Coupling task progress for MapReduce resource-aware scheduling. In: INFOCOM pp. 1618–1626 (2013)
14. Bu, X., Rao, J., Xu, C.-Z.,: Interference and locality-aware task scheduling for MapReduce applications in virtual clusters. In: Proceeding HPDC 22nd International Symposium on High-Performance Parallel and Distributed Computing, pp. 227–238 (2013)
15. Wolf, J., Rajan, D., Hildrum, K., Khandekar, R., Kumar, V., Parekh, S., Wu, K.-L., Balmin, A.: FLEX: a slot allocation scheduling optimizer for MapReduce workloads. In: Middleware ACM/IFIP/USENIX 11th International Conference on Middleware Archive, pp. 1–20 (2010)
16. Sharma, B., Prabhakar, R., Lim, S.-H., Kandemir, T.M., Das, R.C.: MROrchestrator: a fine-grained resource orchestration framework for MapReduce clusters. In: IEEE Fifth International Conference on Cloud Computing, pp. 1–8 (2012)
17. Yao, Y., Wang, J., Sheng, B., Lin, J., Mi, N.: HaSTE: Hadoop YARN scheduling based on task-dependency and resource-demand. In: IEEE International Conference on Cloud Computing, pp. 184–191 (2014)

18. Zhang, Q., Zhani, F.M., Yang, Y., Boutaba, R., Wong, B.: PRISM: fine-grained resource-aware scheduling for MapReduce. IEEE Trans. Cloud Comput. **3**(2), 182–194 (2015)
19. Chen, C.-H., Lin, J.-W., Kuo, S.-Y.: Deadline-constrained MapReduce scheduling based on graph modelling. In: IEEE 7th International Conference, pp. 416–423 (2014)
20. Wang, Y., Shi, W. Budget-driven scheduling algorithms for batches of MapReduce jobs in heterogeneous clouds. IEEE Trans. Cloud Comput. 306–319 (2014)
21. Tang, Z., Zhou, J., Li, K., Li, R.: MTSD: a task scheduling algorithm for MapReduce base on deadline constraints. In: 8th International Conference on Semantics, Knowledge and Grids, pp. 2012–2018 (2012)
22. Liu, L., Zhou, Y., Liu, M., Xu, G., Chen, X., Fan, D., Wang, Q.: Preemptive Hadoop jobs scheduling under a deadline. In: 8th International Conference on Semantics, Knowledge, Grids, pp. 72–79 (2012)
23. Kc, K., Anyanwu, K.: Scheduling Hadoop jobs to meet deadlines. In: IEEE Second International Conference on Cloud Computing Technology and Science, pp. 388–392 (2010)
24. Lai, Z.-R., Chang, C.-W., Liu, X., Kuo, T.-W., Hsiu, P.-C.: Deadline-aware load balancing for MapReduce. In: IEEE 20th International Conference on Embedded and Real-Time Computing Systems and Applications (RTCSA), 20–22 Aug 2014, pp. 1–10 (2014)
25. Sun, X.: Thesis on—an enhanced self adaptive MapReduce scheduling algorithm. In: The Graduate College at the University of Nebraska (2012)
26. Mashayekhy, L., Nejad, M.M., Grosu, D., Lu, D., Shi, W.: Energy-aware scheduling of MapReduce jobs. In: IEEE International Congress on Big Data, pp. 32–39 (2014)
27. Dong, X., Wang, Y., Liao, H.: Scheduling mixed real-time and non-real-time applications in MapReduce environment. In: IEEE 17th International Conference on Parallel and Distributed Systems, pp. 9–16 (2011)

Outlier Detection in Agriculture Domain: Application and Techniques

Sonal Sharma and Rajni Jain

Abstract Outliers are those values that do not comply with the general behavior of the existing data. Outliers vary quantitatively from rest of the data, according to any outlier-selection algorithm. Normal data values or objects follow a common generating mechanism, whereas the abnormal objects deviated from that mechanism and it seems that they have been generated from some different mechanisms. These abnormal data objects are referred as "Outliers". In this paper, authors have tried to explore various applications and techniques of outlier detection. Further, an algorithm for detecting the outliers in agriculture domain has been proposed and its implementation through hand-coded ETL tool, AGRETL, has been discussed. The results show the significant improvement, when the algorithm was validated on the real-time dataset.

Keywords Outlier detection · Agriculture · ETL process

1 Introduction

Outliers are those values that do not comply with the general behavior of the existing data. It is quite different to what one understands for anomaly. As anomaly is a data value observed, which deviates qualitatively from what is considered as normal, according to the area experts, "An outlier is an observation, which deviates so much from the other observations as to arouse suspicions that it was generated

S. Sharma (✉)
Uttarakhand Technical University, Dehradun, India
e-mail: sonal_horizon@rediffmail.com

S. Sharma
Computer Application Department, Faculty of Management and Business Studies, Uttaranchal University, Dehradun, India

R. Jain
NIAP, New Delhi, India
e-mail: rajnijain67@gmail.com

V.B. Aggarwal et al. (eds.), *Big Data Analytics*, Advances in Intelligent Systems and Computing 654, https://doi.org/10.1007/978-981-10-6620-7_28

by a different mechanism". Outliers vary quantitatively from rest of the data, according to any outlier-selection algorithm. Normal data values or objects follow a common generating mechanism, whereas the abnormal objects deviated from that mechanism and it seems that they have been generated from some different mechanisms. These abnormal data objects are referred as outliers. They are different from or inconsistent with the remaining set of the data. It may be caused by measurement or execution error. For example, the age of the person being mentioned in the dataset as −99, this is actually not possible. Same ways, the salary of an executive officer could seem to be an outlier, as all the junior staff members must be withdrawing less salary than him. While one is detecting these types of values from the dataset, the result may be just eliminating/deleting them. This results in the loss of information, as one's noise could be others' signal. Other may be interested in knowing those patterns and correlating them for some sort of analysis. Outliers are different from noise. Noise is a random error or variance in any measured variable and it should be removed before outlier detection. The various application areas where outlier detection plays a significant role are insurance fraud detection, finding the probability of non-reimbursement or non-payment of loan amount, telecom fraud, customer segmentation, and many more. Outlier detection methods have been suggested for numerous applications, such as clinical trials, credit card fraud detection, data cleansing, voting irregularity analysis, network intrusion, geographic information systems, severe weather prediction, and other data mining tasks. Outlier detection is one of the important activities that have to performed while modeling the ETL process for ensuring good quality of data in the data warehouse. Though various conceptual and logical models for ETL process have been proposed in the literature, none of them has been accepted as a standard. Here, an algorithm is proposed and implemented through a tool, called AGRETL, to handle outliers in the agricultural dataset. Section 2 explains literature review on the conceptual and logical models proposed by various researchers as well as it explores the application of outlier detection in different domains. Section 3 provides a classification of outliers in various categories. Sections 4 and 5 focus on the challenges and techniques of outlier detection, respectively. In Sect. 6, the proposed algorithm is elaborated, whereas Sect. 7 represents the implementation of the algorithm through hand-coded ETL tool called AGRETL. Section 8 presents performance analysis of the algorithm on the real-time dataset. The entire work has been concluded in Sect. 9.

2 Literature Review

Extraction–Transformation–Loading (ETL) tools are responsible for the extraction of data from multiple sources, their pre-processing, insertion, and customization into a data warehouse [1, 2]. There are three different conceptual approaches to model ETL process, which are witnessed in literature [3–12]. These approaches are

- Modeling based on mapping expressions and guidelines.
- Modeling based on conceptual constructs.
- Modeling based on UML environment.

Muller and Rahm [13] presented conceptual modeling based on UML for ETL process using various UML-based mechanisms to execute the ETL operations like filtering, join, merge, wrapper, aggregation, and conversion but these methods in turn inherit all the pros and cons of UML modeling techniques.

Kimball [14] provided an informal documentation layout for the entire process of ETL where the methodology grouped as tips and guidelines have been included.

Cappiello et al. [15] have suggested that the quality of data is often explained as "fitness for use", i.e., its ability lies in the data collection to meet user requirements. The evaluation of data quality parameters must realize the intensity, at which data satisfy user's requirement.

But none of the conceptual modeling techniques as proposed by various researchers from time-to-time has been accepted as a standard. Hence, there lies lots of scope for the improvement in the methodology.

The literature review on logical modeling process has been presented, keeping user interfaces, functionality, interoperability with ETL tools, and internal representation of the data in main focus. As laid by the research community, there exist two different approaches to perform logical modeling of the ETL process.

Orchid: Dessloch et al. [16] proposed an ETL tool, named Orchid, which is modeled to integrate ETL processes and the schema mappings which is a three-layer architecture. Basic operators, which are available in Orchid Hub Model, are Filter, Join, Format, Aggregate, Union, and Copy. Orchid is a commercial tool by IBM and is not available for the research community.

Arktos: Vassiliadis et al. [17] proposed another model for logical modeling of the ETL process. Arktos II, which is a three-layer architecture to describe the semantics of the processes, is a graphical representation of the ETL activities designed with the help of the template containing name, expression, mapping, and parameter list for each activity. Table 1 summarizes the ETL operators available with these tools.

None of the logical models implements the procedure to detect the outliers existing in the data. The review firmly suggests that if the dataset contains such type of data element, then surely the interpretation based on them would lead to the incorrect analysis. The outlier detection focuses on finding hidden patterns, which do not comply with the expected behavior. It has multiple applications in various domains ranging from defense surveillance to detecting fraud in credit card or insurance sector. The importance of outlier detection lies in the mere fact that it can

Table 1 Summarized operator implementation in detail

Approach	Operator						
	Filter	Join	Format	Aggregate	Union	Sort	Copy
Orchid	•	•	•	•	•	–	•
Arktos II	•	•	•	•	•	•	–

deduce the actionable information from the given data. A large amount of sudden traffic in the computer network could mean that a hacked system is transmitting bulk information to the unauthorized/unreliable system. An outlier in the credit card entries may reflect the theft of the card and thus help to identify theft or some abnormal observation in the aircraft sensors may indicate component failure [18].

1. **Fraud Detection** Fraud is defined as any criminal activity, which occurs in some commercial ventures. They may be some banks, insurance companies, mobile phone companies, stock market, or any other setup wherever some monetary matters are involved. Falsified user enacts like a customer of the organization. The purpose of this type of detection is to identify such persons and catch hold of them. A very simple approach that could be used in such cases is to maintain user profiles and regularly monitoring their performance and transactions performed in the system. Any deviation from the normal activity could be the alarm of fraud. Credit card fraudulent usage could be depicted by maintaining the data records over various dimensions like user id, the amount of time spent in accessing, high rate of purchase, purchasing goods, which are never ever purchased before are some of the parameters, which could be used in fraud detection. Purchasing behavior from the credit card usually changes when the card is stolen. Abnormal buying patterns can characterize credit card abuse.
2. **Medicine** The type of data, which exist in the patient record system, is of various categories like blood group, weight, age, etc. This data may be temporal as well as spatial such as data gathered due to abnormal patient condition or recording failures caused due to instrumentation errors. The approach used to identify outlier in such data is semi-supervised as the data labels are for the healthy person too. Unusual symptoms or test results may indicate potential health problems of a patient. Whether a particular test result is abnormal may depend on other characteristics of the patients (e.g., gender, age). The occurrence of a particular disease, e.g., tetanus, scattered across various hospitals of a city to indicate problems with the corresponding vaccination program in that city. Whether an occurrence is abnormal depends on different aspects like frequency, spatial correlation, etc. Outlier detection in this domain is very crucial as it has to be precise and it is quite expensive too.
3. **Sports Statistics** In many sports, various parameters are recorded for players in order to evaluate the players' performances. Outstanding (in a positive as well as a negative sense) players may be identified as having abnormal parameter values. Sometimes, players show abnormal values only on a subset or a special combination of the recorded parameters.
4. **Detecting Measurement Errors** The data gathered from the sensor fault detection application or from intrusion detection events are very interesting for analysis. Any single sensor may be collecting information comprising different types and formats like binary, continuous, audio, discrete set, and video. As a consequence, this entire project is to ample amount of challenges for the analysts. Abnormal values could provide an indication of a measurement error. Removing such errors can be important in other data mining and data analysis

tasks. "One person's noise could be another person's signal". On the basis of various types of quantitative deviations, outliers can be broadly classified into various categories.

Hence, it becomes essential to implement the model which could effectively detect the outlier values from the given dataset but could also handle them. The next section discusses outlier classification based on the quantity/value of stored data element.

3 Outlier Classification

Depending upon the type of attribute and the dataset, in which the attribute exists and the co-relation of that instance with rest of the data, outliers can be classified into three categories as follows [18–20]:

- **Global Outliers (point anomaly)**: When an object O_c deviates significantly from rest of the data like population of any densely populated area as 1 or 0, now this single object attains anomalous behavior from rest of the data as a result, and this is referred as the point outlier. In real example, the credit card fraud detection and transaction, in which large amount is spent as compared to the normal range of expenses, would be considered as a point outlier.
- **Contextual Outlier (conditional outlier)**: If the object O_c deviates significantly based on a selected context, it is referred as contextual outlier. For example,, the temperature of Dehradun in scorching summer cannot be 4 °C but the same could be recorded in winter. So what seems, an outlier at a particular period of time may be a valid data value at some other time period of year. Here, the notion of data object is influenced by the value of other instances. This is the reason that it is also referred as conditional outlier. The attribute, which influences, is called as the contextual attribute and the other one is stated as the behavioral attribute. The value of behavioral attribute within specific context determines the anomalous behavior. For example, in credit card, fraud detection time can be considered as a contextual attribute and the amount spent as behavioral. Let us assume a card owner normally go for the purchase of rupees 30,000 per month. But a purchase in the month of Diwali, let us say of rupees, 1 lakhs is normal though it deviates from the regular value. Now if the same amount of purchasing is being done in the month of June, it would be referred as contextual outlier. The contextual outlier detection technique helps to establish such correlations in the data and depicts these outliers. This approach seems easy to be implemented but it is not that simple.
- **Collective Outlier**: A subset of data objects, which collectively deviates significantly from the whole dataset, even if the individual data objects may not be outliers, is categorized as collective outliers. For example, during the drought period, the range of rainfall may be same for some period in that particular

region. Here looking at collection of data values, no data object would be an outlier in the sample but when compared at large scale or may be across a decade, the same sample itself becomes an outlier.

The next section elaborates various challenges, which are faced while performing outlier detection technique on any dataset.

4 Challenges of Outlier Detection

- Application-specific outlier detection: The object elements that could be the outliers deeply depend on the type of application one is analyzing.
- Modeling normal objects and outliers properly.
- Handling noise in outlier detection.
- Understandability.
- Voluminous datasets.

5 Techniques for Outlier Detection

As such there are various techniques for detecting outlier from the given dataset [18, 19]. The basic idea behind them being that, out of n data objects or data points, k is the expected outliers. In order to find top k such elements, the methodology could be based on exception, dissimilarity, and inconsistency. These techniques can be easily handled by addressing them in two phases: first, data could be considered as the outliers and second, a method to mine outliers so defined.

There are three different traditional techniques for outlier detection: Distance based, clustering based, and approach based (on local outlier factor). Clustering algorithms are optimized to find clusters rather than outliers. Accuracy of outlier detection depends on how good the clustering algorithm captures the structure of clusters. A set of many abnormal data objects that are similar to each other would be recognized as a cluster rather than as noise/outlier. Sometimes, it has been observed that what seems as an outlier is actually a real-time information existing in the dataset due to some or the other reasons, for example, in the agriculture domain, there is a sudden decrease in the population of Uttar Pradesh, Andhra Pradesh, Madhya Pradesh, and Bihar. The reasons being were not due to any calamity but purely on the fact that these states were geographical divided into subparts. Therefore, if any outlier detection algorithm is fired on that dataset, it may find the new values with sudden decrease as an outlier. Actually, the data is accurate. The another example is that the sudden increase in production of a crop in a state may occur in the dataset because of the introduction of good high variety of seeds, usage of good quality of fertilizer, and better irrigation facilities, but the same may be treated as an outlier when compared with the past information.

This now becomes a crucial state to identify a real outlier to the actual information, as witnessed through the literature review that neither of the conceptual or logical models for modeling ETL process has any technique for handling outlier. Here, authors have presented a partial work of AGRETL tool for modeling ETL process while ensuring good quality of data in agricultural domain. This tool handles various quality issues in agricultural domain, outlier detection being one of them. AGRETL provides this facility to the user to take the appropriate action depending upon the dataset and his own wisdom to choose the action and technique to handle the detected outlier elements. The action taken could be to just ignore the element as they are the part of acceptable trend or delete such information. If required a metadata facility is also available with AGRETL to save the information for other references as and when required.

6 Proposed Algorithm for Outlier Detection

There are various algorithms for outlier detection which has been discussed in the literature. Around hundreds of outlier tests have been designed depending upon the distribution of data, knowledge about the distribution parameters like mean and variance, the total number of expected outliers that may exist in the data, and the upper and lower limit of the outlier, i.e., the expected outliers. Due to these dependencies, there exist some serious problems like that of single attribute outliers; as a result they cannot be used for the multidimensional dataset and the data values are distribution based. The easiest of all to detect the outlier within the given dataset would be to provide the range of expected value for the attribute.

The AGRETL facilitates to identify the outlier on the selected attribute by various techniques:

(1) **Range Specification**: Specifying the valid range as provided by the user, which means all those values which do not lie in the specified range in the data set would be retrieved as the outliers. Now the user may take in the appropriate action depending on his discretion based on his understanding and domain knowledge.
(2) **Ignoring**: The other approach for handling the outlier could be just ignoring that tuple set.

Algorithm:
AGRETL_Outlier__Procedure
Input: Data Source
STEPS

1. Select the data source
2. Mark the attribute for which outlier detection has to be performed
3. Get Upper_limit for the attribute
4. Get Lower_limit for the attribute
5. I ←0
6. For I !=EOF
   If $attrib>lower_limit | | $attrib<upper_limit
   Select the tuple for output
   Display and the result
   Ask the user for the action to be taken
   If Action←ignore
   Leave the data set as it is
   else if Action←delete
   delete those tuples from the output
   Increment I by 1
   Loop
7. Display and save the result after outlier detection.

7 Implementation and Results

The algorithm proposed has been implemented with the help of the ETL tool, AGRETL, developed in C#. This tool performs modeling of ETL process to improve the quality of data in agricultural data warehouse. It contains various modules to accomplish the desired task of ETL modeling, one of the very important being presented in through this research paper. Authors have been working on rest of the modules which are likely to be completed very soon. Figure 1 represents the screenshot of AGRETL model to handle outliers. As depicted in figure the user has to select the source, and thereafter mention the attribute to be checked for outlier as well as he also has to choose whether the process is statewise or districtwise.

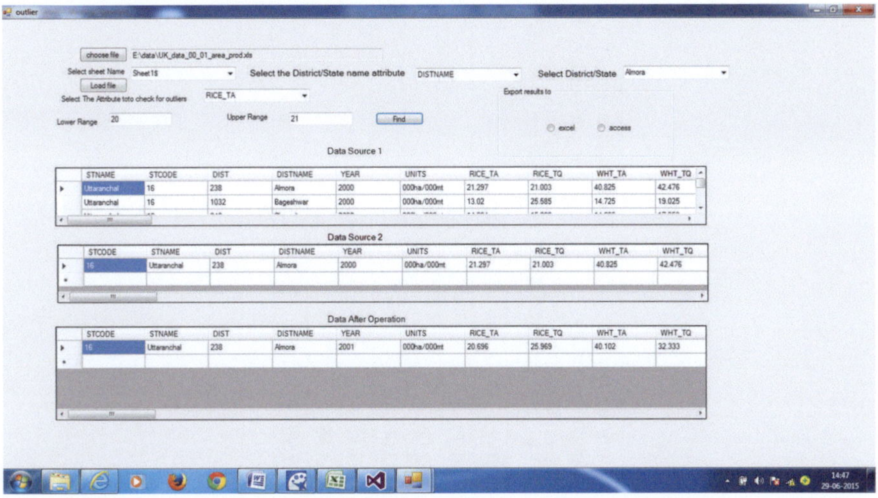

Fig. 1 AGRETL screenshot to handle outliers

Along with the value ranges for the selected attribute, once all the required information is provided by the user, the data is processed into two data grids. One grid containing outlier record set and the other consisting of processed information. As one's noise could be others' signal, both the data record sets can easily be saved into separate files in the required formats. The sample outcome of the dataset is presented in Tables 3 and 4 as enclosed in the Appendix.

8 Performance Analysis

This research work was carried, with the aim of implementing data modeling for ETL process, which is a key factor for successful dimensional data analysis through data warehouse project. A model, AGRETL, for fulfilling this aim was designed and implemented. The work presented here focuses on the outlier detection. The proposed outlier detection algorithm has been analyzed, using average function. As discussed earlier, outlier detection and its handling are very important. Otherwise, the computed results and the decision based on them would not be precise and acceptable. In order to analyze the performance of AGRETL tool, for outlier detection, a dataset was selected from the agriculture domain containing the details of crop production of all the districts of state, as shown in Table 3. This is the original dataset, which does not contain any outlier. The attribute referred was CERL_TA. First of all, the average production of CERL_TA, through this dataset,

Table 2 Performance comparison of outlier detection algorithm on using average function

No. of outliers in the data set	Attribute	Average based on the data set containing outlier	Average based on data set not containing outlier	Average based on actual value	Error in data set containing outlier $= \left(\frac{\lvert(V-III)\rvert}{V}\right) \times 100$	Error in data set containing no outiler $= \left(\frac{\lvert(V-IV)\rvert}{V}\right) \times 100$
I	II	III	IV	V	VI	VII
1	CERL_TA	75.64	75.1	75.06	0.77	0.05
2	CERL_TA	84.77	75.56	75.06	12.94	0.67
3	CERL_TA	84.07	75.83	75.06	12.00	1.03
4	CERL_TA	82.66	75.27	75.06	10.13	0.28
5	CERL_TA	72.3	73.25	75.06	3.68	2.41
Average error (%)					7.90	0.89
Error reduced (%) = (7.90−0.89) = 7.01%						

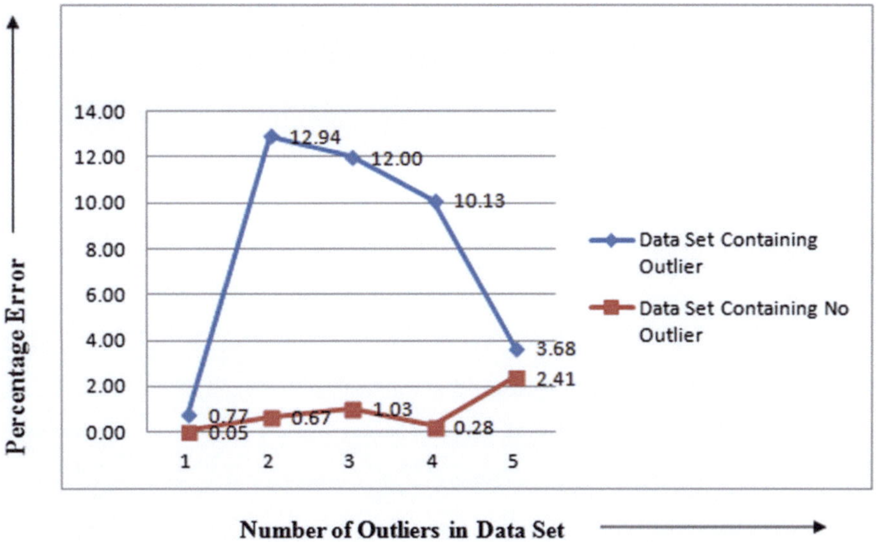

Fig. 2 Performance comparison of outlier detection algorithm on using average function

for Uttarakhand state was computed. It was found to be 75.06. Then, deliberately an outlier was introduced. The production data for Pithoragarh in the year 2001 was raised to 117.50. Now, the new average was computed, which was 75.64. On this dataset, when outlier detection algorithm of AGRETL tool was applied, the average production was recorded to be 75.01. Likewise, every time the number of outliers was introduced in the dataset and then the AGRETL tool was applied. The averages for both the instances were recorded. Further, the error percentage in dataset containing outliers and error percentage in imputed value were computed, as shown in Table 2. The result thus obtained was plotted against a number of outliers introduced and the percentage error, as shown in Fig. 2. When the AGRETL tool was used to handle the outliers in the dataset, it was seen that the error was reduced; the results were much closer to the original dataset results. Overall error is reduced by 7.01%:

9 Conclusion

In this paper, authors have discussed various reasons for outlier existences, its techniques to detect the outliers from the data. Also an algorithm is being proposed to handle the outliers effectively so as to improve the data quality. It is very important for ETL activities. The proposed approach is the part of a module in a hand-coded ETL tool called AGRETL, which cleanses the data source and thus enhances data quality and henceforth the decision-making capability of the organization. The results proved that the average error percentage was reduced significantly from 7.90 to 0.89%, i.e., overall the performance of the system was improved by 7.01%.

Appendix

See Tables 3 and 4.

Table 3 Original data source for sugarcane crop with outliers

Stcode	Stname	Dist_code	Dist_name	Year	Sugarcane
16	Uttaranchal	238	Dehradun	2002	373.73
16	Uttaranchal	1032	Haridwar	2002	3762.86
16	Uttaranchal	240	Nainital	2002	402.44
16	Uttaranchal	1035	Udhamsingh nagar	2002	2292.42
16	Uttaranchal	244	Dehradun	2005	339.57
16	Uttaranchal	243	Haridwar	2005	3941.96
16	Uttaranchal	527	Nainital	2005	392.83
16	Uttaranchal	237	Udhamsingh nagar	2005	2284.60
16	Uttaranchal	239	Dehradun	2006	316.01
16	Uttaranchal	1043	Haridwar	2006	4665.59
16	Uttaranchal	242	Nainital	2006	352.90
16	Uttaranchal	1030	Tehri garhwal	2006	0.30
16	Uttaranchal	241	Udhamsingh nagar	2006	2351.10
16	Uttaranchal	238	Champavat	2007	0.37
16	Uttaranchal	1032	Dehradun	2007	316.19
16	Uttaranchal	240	Haridwar	2007	3452.58
16	Uttaranchal	1035	Nainital	2007	237.89
16	Uttaranchal	244	Udhamsingh nagar	2007	10.10
16	Uttaranchal	243	Champavat	2008	0.37
16	Uttaranchal	527	Dehradun	2008	326.87
16	Uttaranchal	237	Haridwar	2008	3394.98
16	Uttaranchal	239	Nainital	2008	209.59
16	Uttaranchal	1043	Udhamsingh nagar	2008	1129.92
16	Uttaranchal	242	Dehradun	2009	2333.00
16	Uttaranchal	1030	Tehri garhwal	2009	0.30
16	Uttaranchal	241	Udhamsingh nagar	2009	2351.10

Table 4 Data source after performing outlier procedure

Stcode	Stname	Dist_code	Dist_name	Year	Sugarcane
16	Uttaranchal	238	Dehradun	2002	373.73
16	Uttaranchal	1032	Haridwar	2002	3762.86
16	Uttaranchal	240	Nainital	2002	402.44
16	Uttaranchal	1035	Udhamsingh nagar	2002	2292.42
16	Uttaranchal	244	Dehradun	2005	339.57
16	Uttaranchal	243	Haridwar	2005	3941.96
16	Uttaranchal	527	Nainital	2005	392.83
16	Uttaranchal	237	Udhamsingh nagar	2005	2284.60
16	Uttaranchal	239	Dehradun	2006	316.01
16	Uttaranchal	1043	Haridwar	2006	4665.59
16	Uttaranchal	242	Nainital	2006	352.90
16	Uttaranchal	1030	Tehri garhwal	2006	0.30
16	Uttaranchal	241	Udhamsingh nagar	2006	2351.10
16	Uttaranchal	238	Champavat	2007	0.37
16	Uttaranchal	1032	Dehradun	2007	316.19
16	Uttaranchal	240	Haridwar	2007	3452.58
16	Uttaranchal	1035	Nainital	2007	237.89
16	Uttaranchal	243	Champavat	2008	0.37
16	Uttaranchal	527	Dehradun	2008	326.87
16	Uttaranchal	237	Haridwar	2008	3394.98
16	Uttaranchal	239	Nainital	2008	209.59
16	Uttaranchal	1043	Udhamsingh nagar	2008	1129.92
16	Uttaranchal	1030	Tehri garhwal	2009	0.30
16	Uttaranchal	241	Udhamsingh nagar	2009	2351.10

References

1. Simitsis, A., Vassiliadis, P.: A method for the mapping of conceptual design to logical blueprint for ETL processes. Decis. Support. Syst. Data Warehouse. OLAP **45**(1), 22–40 (2008)
2. Simitis, A.: Modeling and managing ETL process. Available at http://ftp.informatik.rwtaachen.de/Publications/CEUR-WS/Vol-76/simitsis.pdf
3. Inmon, W.H.: Data warehousing and data mining. Commun. ACM **39**(11) (1996)
4. Luzan-Mora, T.J., Song, L.-Y.: Multidimensional modeling with UML package diagrams. In: Spaccapietra, S., March, S.T., Kambayashi, Y. (eds) ER 2002, LNCS, vol. 2503, pp. 199–213. Springer (2002)
5. Dobre, A., Hakimpour, F., Dittrich, K.R.: Operators and classifications for data mapping in semantic integration. Conceptual Modeling—ER 2003, LNCS, vol. 2813, pp. 534–547. Springer (2003)
6. Jarke, M., Lenzerini, M., Vassiliou, Y., Vassiliadis, P.: Fundamentals of data warehouses, 2nd ed. Springer, Berlin, Heidelberg (2003). ISBN 3-540-42089-4

7. Jovanovic, P., Romero, O., Simitis, A., Abello, A.: Requirement-driven creation and deployment of multidimensional and ETL designs. In: ER Workshops 2012, LNCS, vol. 7518, pp. 391–395 (2012)
8. Sapia, C., Blaschkka, M., Hofting, G., Dinter, B.: Extending the E/R model for multidimensional paradigm. LNCS, vol. 1552, pp. 105–116. Springer (1998)
9. Sharma, S.D., Singh, R., Rai, A.: Integrated national agriculture resources information system. http://www.inaris.gen.in
10. Sharma, S., Kumar, H.: Data warehouse design issues in forestry: eucalyptus tereticornis. IJCIR **7**(1), 109–114 (2011)
11. Sharma, S., Jain, R.: Comparison between various architectural approaches in data warehousing: a discriminatory analysis. In: Proceedings of 9th National Conference on Smarter Approaches in Computing Technologies & Applications (SACTA-2014), India (2014)
12. Sharma, S., Jain, R.: Modeling ETL process in data warehouse: an exploratory study. In: Proceedings of 4th International Conference on Advanced Computing & Communication Technologies (ACCT2014), India (2014). Available at IEEE eXplore
13. Muller, R., Rahm, E.: An integrative and uniform model for metadata management in data warehousing environments. In: Proceedings of the International Workshop on Design and Management of Data Warehouses (DMDW'99), Germany (1999)
14. Kimball, R.: The Data Warehouse Toolkit: Practical Technique for Building Dimensional Data Warehouses. Wiley, New York (2004)
15. Cappiello, C., Francalanci, C., Pernici, B.: Data quality assessment from the user's perspective. In: Proceedings of IQIS'04, pp. 68–73, ACM, USA (2004)
16. Dessloch, S., Hernández, M.A., Wisnesky, R., Radwan, A., Zhou, J.: Orchid: integrating schema mapping and ETL. In: Proceedings of the 24th international conference on data engineering (ICDE), pp. 1307–1316, Mexico (2008)
17. Vassiliadis, P., Vagena, Z., Skiaopoulos, S., Karayannidis, N., Sellis, T.: Arktos: towards the modeling, design, control and execution of ETL Processes. Inf. Syst. **26**, 537–561 (2001)
18. Singh, K., Upadhyaya, S.: Outlier detection: applications and techniques. IJCSI Int. J. Comput. Sci. **9**(3) (2012)
19. Mohammad, Z.P., Umesh, N.: A comparative study on outlier detection techniques. Int. J. Comput. Appl. **66**(24) (2013). ISBN: 0975-8887
20. Upadhyaya, S., Singh, K.: Classification based outlier detection techniques. Int. J. Comput. Trends Technol. **3**(2), 294 (2012). ISSN: 2231-2803
21. Javed, B., Shadab, H.: Data quality—a problem and an approach. White Paper available at http://www.utopianic.com
22. Demarest: The Politics of Data Warehouses. Available at http://dssresources.com/papers/features/demarest/demarest07232004.html
23. Han, J., Kamber, M.: Data Mining: Concepts and Techniques. 2nd ed. Elsevier (2007)
24. Rai, A.: Data Warehouse and its Applications in Agriculture. Available at http://www.inaris.gen.in
25. Vassiliadis, P., Bouzeghoub, M., Quix, C.: Towards Quality-Oriented Data Warehouse Usage and Evolution. Inf Syst **25**(2), 89–115 (2000)
26. Irad, B.-G.: Outlier detection. In: Data Mining and Knowledge Discovery Handbook: A Complete Guide for Practitioners and Researchers, Kluwer Academic Publishers (2005). ISBN: 0-387-24435-2

A Framework for Twitter Data Analysis

Imran Khan, S.K. Naqvi, Mansaf Alam and S.N.A. Rizvi

Abstract As the number of users increases on the Internet, the data is also increasing with the exponential rate. A number of websites are available where terabytes of data is generated daily. As the e-commerce sites are gaining popularity, the data from the various customers, reviews, transactions logs, web search logs, etc. is being generated on daily basis. Other than e-commerce sites some other very important sources of data on the internet are social network sites and web search engines. Social networking sites like Facebook and Twitter have billions of users which generate petabytes of data with a high rate that emerges a new era in the field of data science and that is "Big Data". In this paper, we have proposed a framework that could analyze Twitter data which is one of the major sources of big data. In our study, we have focused on the political domain and proposed a framework that extracts the tweets from any location and classifies them as political or not. After classification out system also extracts the sentiments from those tweets in order to understand the emotions regarding various political issues at a particular place.

Keywords Twitter data · Tweet Classification · Big Data · Hadoop

I. Khan (✉)
BVICAM, New Delhi, India
e-mail: imrankhan.ee2531@gmail.com

S.K. Naqvi
CIT, JMI, New Delhi, India
e-mail: sknaqvi@jmi.ac.in

M. Alam
Department of Computer Science, JMI, New Delhi, India
e-mail: malam2@jmi.ac.in

S.N.A. Rizvi
JMI, New Delhi, India
e-mail: dr.snarizvi@gmail.com

V.B. Aggarwal et al. (eds.), *Big Data Analytics*, Advances in Intelligent Systems and Computing 654, https://doi.org/10.1007/978-981-10-6620-7_29

1 Introduction

The Internet is growing with a constant rate as more and more users and businesses are connecting to it which increases the data on the internet at an exponential rate. According to the figures given by eMarketer, the number of Internet user has exceeded from 3 billion (2015) and are increasing 6.2% next year so that it becomes 42.4% of the entire world's population [1]. eMarketer also estimates that by the year 2018, the users will exceed 3.6 billion which will be 50% of the total world's population.

As the number of users increases on the internet, the data is also increasing with the exponential rate. A number of websites are available where terabytes of data is generated daily. As the e-commerce sites are gaining popularity, the data from the various customers, reviews, transactions logs, web search logs, etc. is being generated on daily basis. Other than e-commerce sites, some other very important sources of data on the internet are social network sites and web search engines. Social networking sites like Facebook and Twitter have billions of users which generate petabytes of data with a high rate that emerges a new era in the field of data science and that is "Big Data".

The emergence of big data has changed the way of managing and analyzing data as big data deals with the very high amount of data and in order to manage it special systems are needed as it is not possible to manage that data using traditional database system. Big data is often characterized by its "3Vs" and they are volume, velocity, and variety. Traditional systems focused on structured data management and cannot meet the changing behavior of big data. The analysis of big data is gaining momentum as academic and industrial world focuses to leverage big data. Big organizations like Facebook and Twitter produce massive data that could be used to analyze the behavior or their customers and to increase their profit. For example, when it comes to analyze social media big data, one can get valuable insights about the behavioral aspects of people.

Social media technologies are an integral part of almost everyone's life. Social media sites like Facebook allow to share the views of any user in the form of posts, messages, images, videos, etc., and analysis of big data from these sites plays an important role in many applications, for example, we can predict the sentiments of people on any of the events that happened in the world. A number of researches identified that interaction of people on social media can be analyzed to predict the psychological information about attitudes and behaviors. Twitter is another source of big data where users share a short message to express their feelings. Twitter is a rich source of information for the researches nowadays because the data of Twitter can be analyzed for a number of researches. Some of the other sources of big data are LinkedIn, yahoo, Google, and many more. Although a number of sources are available from where we can get a huge amount of data, we are still lacking in having a unified framework that could analyze this data. One of the common reasons behind this is the amount of unstructured data which is difficult to process. In this paper, we have proposed a framework that could analyze Twitter data which is one of the major sources of big data. In our study, we have focused on the political domain and proposed a framework that extracts the tweets from any location and classifies them as political or not. After classification out system also extracts the sentiments from those tweets in order to understand the emotions regarding various political issues at a particular place.

2 Related Work

Big data is buzz word in current scenario and a number of systems are there that are the prime generator of big data. In order to manage that high-velocity high variety and high-velocity data, a number of frameworks and systems have been proposed. As in [2], a data model is proposed that classifies the variety of data and provides a unified schema for big data. Although a number of organizations are there in the market that are the major sources of big data, social media is one of the important sources that provide a vast amount of data and that can be used to find the insight from the data and Twitter is one of such sources. A lot of work is going on to find the valuable information contained in the 140 character tweet from Twitter. Researchers are working to find the political preference or sentiment from the tweet [3, 4]. A tweet can be used to predict the election results or sentiments using the words contained in it [5–10]. In [5], LIWC software is used to find the sentiments of the tweet based on 12 parameters using unsupervised learning technique. In order to process real-time data processing, an infrastructural and sentiment model is proposed in [6] that process real-time data and extract sentiments. Some supervised learned model has also been developed as in [7]; the model is trained using manually labeled tweets. A semi-manual two-phase approach is being used in [7], where the model is trained with the SVM on unigram features of the tweet. Twitter has also been used as source form word-to-mouth marketing as done in [11].

In this work, we have proposed a framework for analyzing Twitter data of any location and we have focused on the political domain. We have used Twitter streaming API to collect streaming data and perform our classification algorithm to classify whether the tweet is political on that data. Once the data is classified, we have applied sentiment analysis on the classified data in order to understand the sentiments of any particular subject extract from the politically classified tweets.

3 Proposed Framework

There are four phases in our framework:

1. Data collection phase
2. Data Loading Phase
3. Tweet classification and Storage
4. Sentiment Analysis (Fig. 1)

1. **Data Collection Phase** (Fig. 2)

The Twitter Application Programming Interface (API) provides three types of APIs: Streaming API, REST API, and Search API [12, 13]. Twitter Streaming API provides nearly real-time tweets, replies, etc., and it required a persistent connection to http server. The API uses basic HTTP authentication and requires a valid Twitter account while data can be retrieved in XML/JSON format. Once the user is authenticated, public tweets are retrieved which we can store in any text or csv file.

2. **Data Loading Phase** (Fig. 3)

When the sufficient data is stored, it is being transferred to the hadoop ecosystem for analyzing the tweets and finding the tweeter trend for that timestamp. Hadoop is an open-source software platform by the Apache Foundation for building clusters of servers for use in distributed computing. Server clustering is really nothing new or revolutionary but Hadoop is designed specifically for mass-scale computing, which involves thousands of servers. Based on a paper originally written by Google about their MapReduce system, Hadoop leverages concepts from functional programming to solve large computing problems. Hadoop is an ideal solution for working with large volumes of data in a variety of applications.

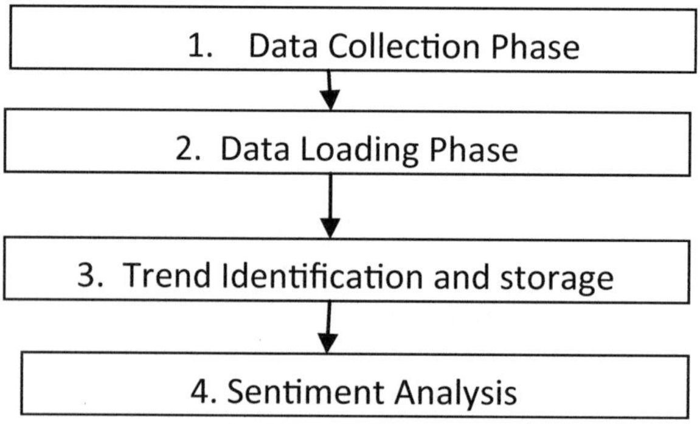

Fig. 1

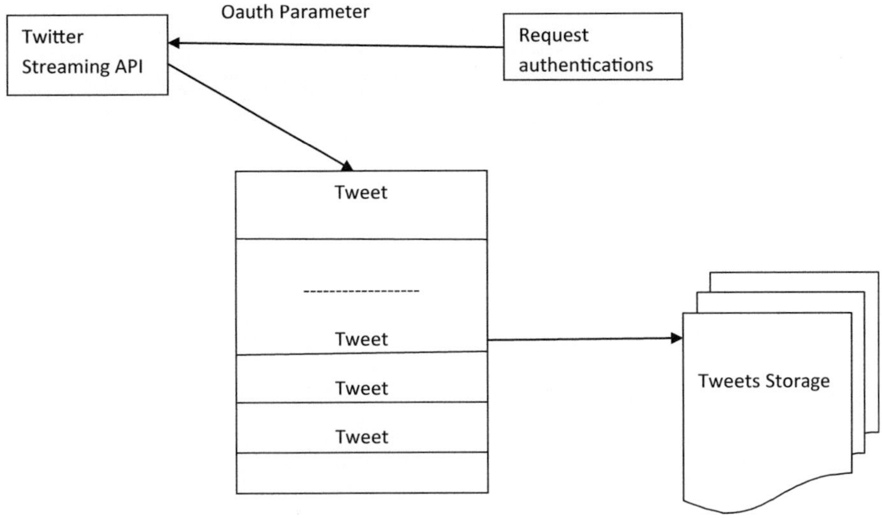

Fig. 2

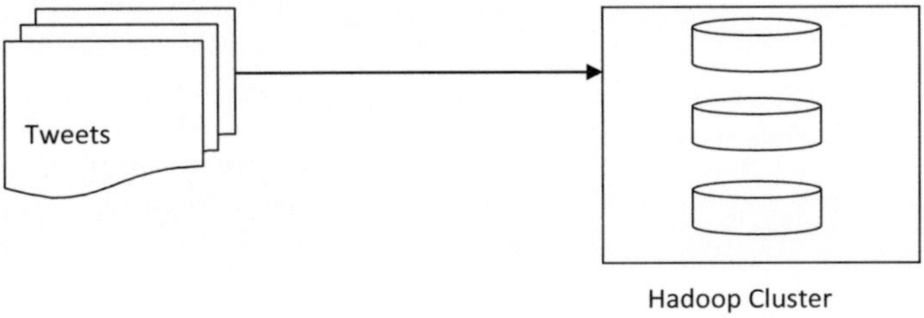

Fig. 3

3. **Tweet Classification and Storage** (Fig. 4)

The tweets are loaded and being parsed to analyze using JSON parser. We are using Python as the programming language for this analysis. The parsed tweet streams will be structured in such a way that we can extract each word separately. Once the tweets got framed, we can use Rapid Miner for counting the frequency of trending words and that word count could be used as a way to find the current trend of the tweeter.

4. **Sentiment Analysis** (Fig. 5)

Once all the tweets are classified as political or non-political, we will perform sentiment analysis on the political tweets. In order to find out the sentiment of a particular tweet, we have a list of positive and negative words. From each of the tweets collected as political, we first find out the frequency of positive and negative words from the tweet. Then we will find the ratio of positive and negative words.

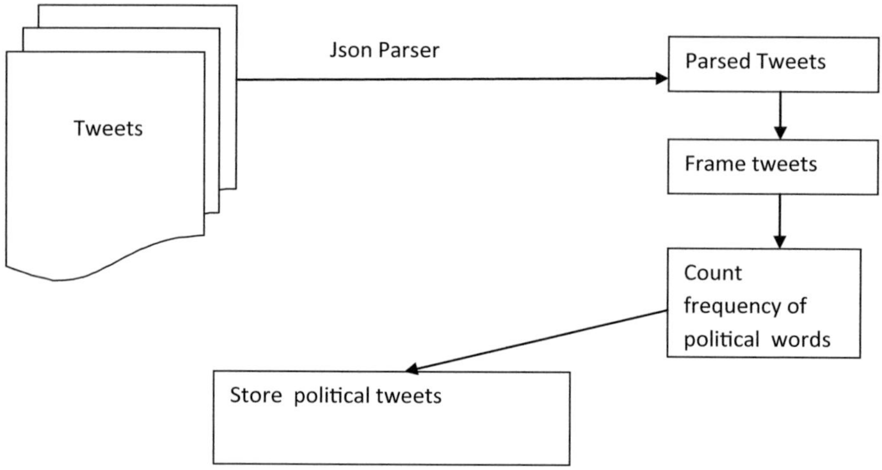

Fig. 4

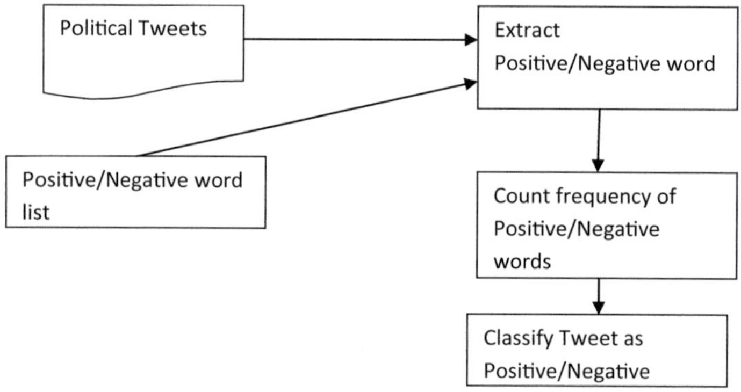

Fig. 5

We classify a tweet as positive if the ratio of positive to negative words is greater than or equal to 1 and negative if the ratio is less than 1 and is neutral if it is zero.

4 Results and Conclusion

Twitter is a large source of information used nowadays. By analyzing the short messages that are known as tweets, a number of results can be evaluated. A number of researchers are working on a number of domains and they are taking data from the Twitter. In this paper, we have presented a method for analyzing Twitter data. In our study, we have proposed a way to classify the tweets and also perform sentiments analyses on them. The results can be used to produce a number of applications.

References

1. http://www.emarketer.com/Article/Internet-Hit-3-Billion-Users-2015/1011602
2. Khan, I., Naqvi, S.K., Mansaf, A., Rizvi, S.N.A: Data model for Big Data in cloud environment. In: 2nd International Conference on Computing for Sustainable Global Development (INDIACom), 2015, pp. 582–585, 11–13 Mar 2015
3. Makazhanov, A., Rafiei, D., Waqar, M.: Predicting political preference of Twitter users. Soc. Netw. Anal. Min. **4**(1), 1–15 (2014)
4. Agarwal, A., et al.: Sentiment analysis of Twitter data. In: Proceedings of the Workshop on Languages in Social Media. Association for Computational Linguistics (2011)
5. Tumasjan, A., Sprenger, T.O., Sandner, P.G., Welpe, I.M.: Predicting elections with Twitter: What 140 characters reveal about political sentiment. ICWSM **10**(1), 178–185 (2010)
6. Wang, H., Can, D., Kazemzadeh, A., Bar, F., Narayanan, S.:A system for real-time Twitter sentiment analysis of 2012 U.S. presidential election cycle. In: ACL (System Demonstrations), pp. 115–120 (2012)
7. Conover, M., Goncalves, B., Ratkiewicz, J., Flammini, A., Menczer, F.: Predicting the political alignment of Twitter users, In: Social-Com/PASSAT, pp. 192–199 (2011)
8. Conover, M., Ratkiewicz, J., Francisco, M., Goncalves, B., Menczer, F., Flammini, A.: Political polarization on Twitter. In: ICWSM (2011)
9. Marchetti-Bowick, M., Chambers, N.: Learning for micro blogs with distant supervision: Political forecasting with Twitter. In: EACL, pp. 603–612 (2012)
10. Choy, M., Cheong, M.L.F., Laik, M.N., Shung, K.P.: A sentiment analysis of Singapore presidential election 2011 using Twitter data with census correction. CoRR, vol. abs/1108.5520 (2011)
11. Jansen, B., Zhang, M., Sobel, K., Chowdury, A.: Twitter power: Tweets as electronic word of mouth. J. Am. Soc. Inform. Sci. Technol. **60**(11), 2169–2188 (2009)
12. Green, A.: Twitter API programming tips, tutorials, source code libraries and consulting. http://140dev.com/twitter-api-programming-tutorials/twitterapi-database-cache/ Accessed May 2011
13. Twitter API programming tips, tutorials, source code libraries and consulting. http://140dev.com/free-twitter-api-source-code-library/twitter-databaseserver/code-architecture/ Accessed May 2011
14. Myslı´n, M., et al.: Using Twitter to examine smoking behavior and perceptions of emerging tobacco products. J. Med. Internet Res. **15**(8), e174 (2013)
15. Young, S., et al.: Extrapolating psychological insights from Facebook profiles: a study of religion and relationship status. Cyberpsychol. Behav. **12**, 347–350 (2009)

Web Structure Mining Algorithms: A Survey

Neha Tyagi and Santosh Kumar Gupta

Abstract World Wide Web (WWW) is a massive collection of information and due to its rapid growing size, information retrieval becomes more challenging task to the user. Web mining techniques such as web content mining, web usage mining, and web structure mining are used to make the information retrieval more efficient. In this paper, study is focused on the web structure mining and different link analysis algorithms. Further, a comparative review of these algorithms is given.

Keywords Web mining · Information retrieval · Web usage mining · Web content mining · Link analysis · Web structure mining

1 Introduction

In today's era, everyone is dependent on the WWW to get information about any query. As Internet is the huge source of information and the amount of information in WWW is increasing dynamically day by day, user faces information overload problem while finding appropriate information in response to the query [5]. As the user interacts with the web to retrieve information about the posed query, the following problems are encountered [1] :

(i) In finding relevant information on the web, users use the search service. Lists of webpages are produced in response to the user query but the searching tools face the low precision and low recall problems because of inapplicable search results and inadequacy to tabulate all the information, respectively [3].

N. Tyagi (✉) · S.K. Gupta
Department of Computer Science and Engineering,
Krishna Institute of Engineering and Technology, Ghaziabad, India
e-mail: nehaktyagi@gmail.com

S.K. Gupta
e-mail: santoshg25@gmail.com

V.B. Aggarwal et al. (eds.), *Big Data Analytics*, Advances in Intelligent Systems and Computing 654, https://doi.org/10.1007/978-981-10-6620-7_30

(ii) Extraction of helpful information from the web documents raised the problem of new knowledge creation from accessible information.
(iii) Information personalization problem occurred as user faces different types and representation of the web content.
(iv) User perception involves the problem of learning about consumers or individual as various users pose distinct query for the same result.

The collection of web data is increasing day by day thereby leading to the information overload situation. And to solve this problem, web mining techniques can be used as a direct or indirect approach. In the direct approach, web mining techniques are used as the main method to extract information from the web data. On the other hand, in indirect approach, web mining techniques are used with other methods.

This paper is arranged as follows: Sect. 2 is an overview of web mining and its classification. Section 3 consists of existing link analysis algorithms for web structure mining. Section 4 shows comparative review of the link analysis algorithms. Section 5 contains the related work, and Sect. 6 is the conclusion.

2 Web Mining

The task of discovering and extraction of information using data mining techniques from web documents is known as web mining [2]. Web mining has two different approaches namely process-centric view and data-centric view, according to first approach data mining is set of tasks in sequence [2], and according to later approach data mining is based on the type of data to be mined [4]. Web mining process disintegrated in subtasks as resources finding to retrieve pledged web documents, selection and preprocessing of information, generalization to discover general patterns, and analysis to certify and/or explicate the mined patterns [1, 2].

2.1 Web Mining Categories

On the basis of type of data, web mining is classified into three parts: web content, web usage, and web structure mining [6, 7] which have been shown in Fig. 1, and are described in next subsections.

2.1.1 Web Content Mining

In Web Content Mining (WCM), web document is used as the source data for extracting useful information [8]. The data contained in the web documents may be structured, semi-structured, or unstructured. WCM is further categorized into two:

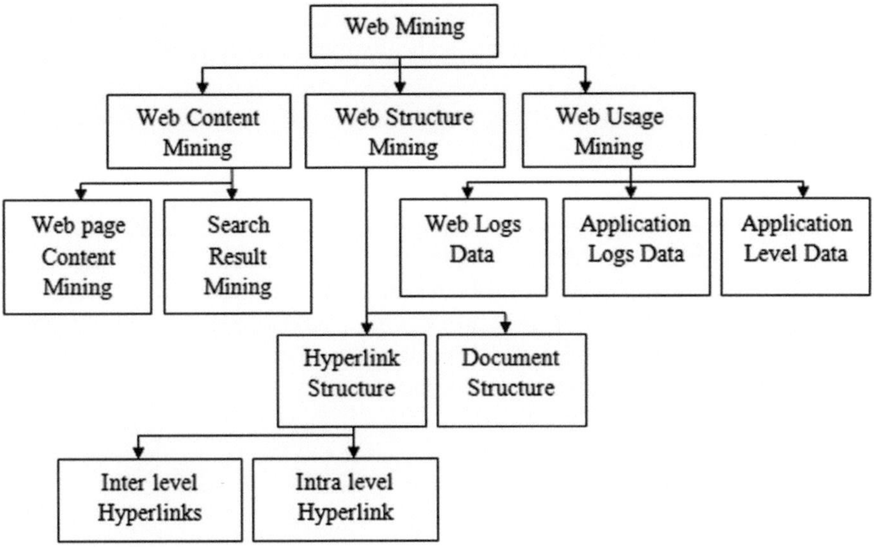

Fig. 1 Web mining categories [6, 7]

Webpage content mining and search result mining. First is a conventional approach which used web data (html, xml, text, and multimedia) to extract useful information, and second used previous search results in order to search new webpages [25].

2.1.2 Web Usage Mining

In Web Usage Mining (WUM), useful information is extracted from the derived interesting navigational pattern (usage data [11]) on the basis of user interaction during web surfing. The data sources for WUM are Web Servers, Web Clients, and Proxy Servers [1, 12].

2.1.3 Web Structure Mining

Web Structure Mining (WSM) concerned with the structure of web the structure may be intra-document (within the web document) or inter-document (within the web itself) [1]. Website structure information helps to improve index quality of search engines and extraction and mining of structured data. The link structure of web contains important information that helps to rank the pages as per their popularity. Structure mining is further categorized into two classes: hyperlink structure and document structure [18]. A hyperlink is used to connect the locations of intra-documents or inter-documents [18]. Inter-level hyperlink connects two different webpages with a hyperlink; on the other hand, intra-level hyperlink connects two different locations to the page itself. According to various HTML and XML tags, web content can also be arranged in tree-structure format [18], and Document Object Model (DOM) structure is automatically extracting from web document.

3 Link Analysis Algorithms

On the basis of link analysis of the webpages, there are several algorithms such as Page Rank (PR) algorithm, Weighted Page Rank (WPR) algorithm, Hypertext-Induced Topic Search (HITS) algorithm, etc. Some variations of PR algorithm and HITS algorithm are shown in Fig. 2. Several link analysis algorithms exist in the literature but PR and HITS algorithms are mostly being used. Link analysis algorithms are explained next in detail.

3.1 Page Rank

Page Rank (PR) algorithm [23] measured the relative significance of webpage and is important while searching on the web. There are two classes of page rankers: Connectivity-based rankers and content-based rankers. Content-based rankers focused on the matches of the terms, number of counts of terms, etc.; on the other

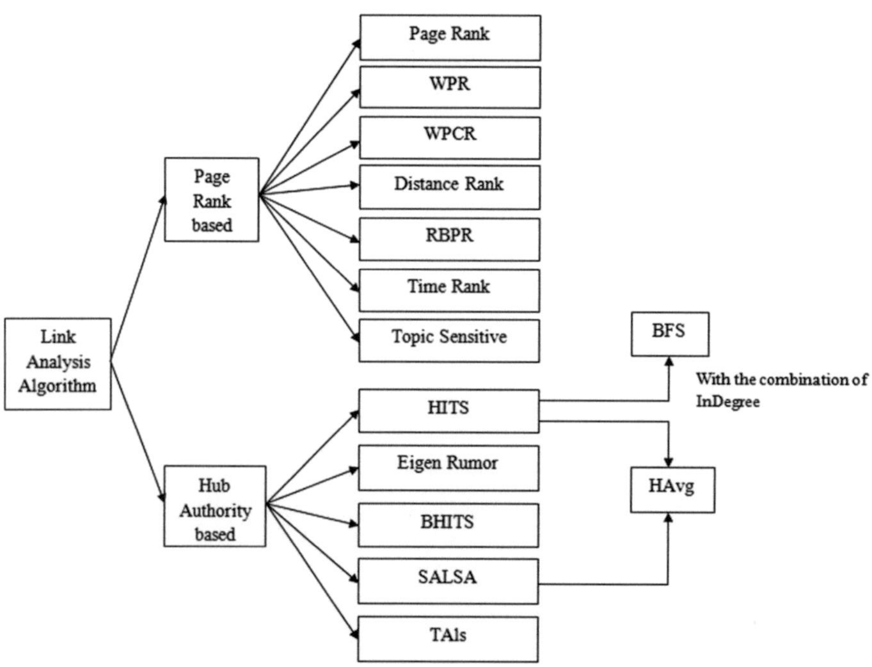

Fig. 2 Link analysis algorithms

hand, connectivity-based rankers focused on the analysis of the links through which the webpages are connected. Page rank of a webpage is calculated as Eq. (1). In Eq. 1, d_f is the damping factor (probability to request a random page when the user getting bored with the current page) set as $0 < d_f < 1$, and $(1 - d_f)$ is used to avoid the webpages those do not have the out-links, P_{rank} (N_i) is the page rank of N_i, that points to another webpage, and O_{link} (N_i) is the number of out-links of N_i:

$$P_{\text{rank}}(M) = (1 - d_f) + d_f \left(\frac{P_{\text{rank}}(N_1)}{O_{\text{link}}(N_1)} + \cdots + \frac{P_{\text{rank}}(N_n)}{O_{\text{link}}(N_n)} \right). \quad (1)$$

3.2 Weighted Page Rank

Weighted Page Rank (WPR) algorithm [10] assigns more linkage to the popular webpage and less linkage to the less popular webpages. In the WPR algorithm, two terms are introduced in-links popularity IN_{Wt} (a, b), and out-links popularity OUT_{Wt} (a, b). IN_{Wt} (a, b) is defined as the weight of the link (a, b) of in-links of page b and the number of in-links of all reference pages of page a, OUT_{Wt} (a, b) is defined as the weight of the link (a, b) of out-links of page b, and the number of out-links of all reference pages of page a. These in-links and out-links weights are used in modified PR algorithm formula, and then the WPR formula to find the rank of the webpages is defined as in Eq. (2):

$$\text{Wt}_{\text{PR}}(b) = (1 - d_f) + d_f \sum_{a \in \text{B}(b)} P_{\text{rank}}\,(a)\,\text{IN}_{\text{Wt}}\,(a,\,b)\,\text{OUT}_{\text{Wt}}\,(a,\,b) \quad (2)$$

3.3 Weighted Page Content Rank

Weighted Page Content Rank (WPCR) algorithm is used to give a sorted order numerical values for webpages in response to the user query. There are two steps in WPCR algorithm: first step is relevance calculation and the second one is rank calculation [17]. In relevance calculation step, there are two factors to be focused content weight and probability weight. Content Weight (CW) is the webpage's weight of content with respect to the query terms. Probability weight is the ratio of query terms to the total query terms. In rank calculation step, the values of CW and PW used to calculate the rank of webpage "b" as Eq. (3):

$$\text{WPCR}(b) = (1 - d_f) + d_f \sum_{a \in \text{B}(b)} P_{\text{rank}}\,(a)\,\text{IN}_{\text{Wt}}\,(a,\,b)\,\text{OUT}_{\text{Wt}}\,(a,\,b) * (\text{CW} + \text{PW}) \quad (3)$$

3.4 Distance Rank

Distance rank algorithm [28] is used to calculate the rank of page on the basis of distance between webpages, where a number of average clicks are the distance. Initially, this algorithm started with basic definition to simplified idea as the weight of link (*a*, *b*) is equal to $\log_{10}O(a)$, where $O(a)$ is the forward links of "*a*". The distance rank of page "*b*" is calculated as in Eq. (4), where "*a*" belongs to the pages that point to "*b*", $O_{\text{degree}}(a)$ is the out degree of "*a*", η is the user's learning rate, and t is the time:

$$D_{\text{rank}_t}(b) = (1-\eta) * D_{\text{rank}_{t-1}}(b) + \eta * \min_i\left(\log\left(O_{\text{degree}}(a) + d_{\text{rank}_{t-1}}(a)\right)\right). \quad (4)$$

3.5 Relation-Based Page Rank

Relation-Based Page Rank (RBPR) [29] algorithm is used to enlarge the information retrieval correctness by utilizing the relations of semantic web resources. The algorithm depends on the information that could be extracted from the user queries and expounded resources.

3.6 Time Rank

Time rank [9] algorithm is used to visit time to calculate the rank of pages and improves the rank score by assuming that the user may stay on a page if he/she interested in the page's content; otherwise, the user looks forward to the next page. Working of time rank algorithm proceeds in three steps: in the first step, the topic-sensitive page rank is computed for each page according to the [19], and the second step is the computation of similarity between keywords and topics using Bayesian theory. The last one is time accumulation step in which visited time vector for each page is obtained through the user's visiting order. The time rank is computed by Eq. (5):

$$\text{Time}_{\text{rank}}x(m) = \text{TSPR}x(m) * t(x). \quad (5)$$

3.7 Topic Sensitive

Topic-Sensitive Page Rank (TSPR) [19] algorithm uses the concept of computing a set of PR vectors unlike the original PR algorithm which computes a single vector using the link structure of the web for the pages satisfying the query. The TSPR for page 'v' is calculated as Eq. (6), where Jm(x) represents the jump of user from one page to another:

$$\text{TSPR}x(v) = \alpha * \sum_{x \epsilon \text{B}} \frac{\text{TSPR}(x)}{|E_x|} + (1 - \alpha) * \text{Jm}(x) \tag{6}$$

3.8 *HITS (Hypertext-Induced Topic Search)*

HITS [16] method proposed two distinct forms of webpages namely hubs and authorities, where authorities are defined as the web pages that contained the important information and hubs are that guiding user to the authorities. HITS algorithm consists of two steps: sampling and iterative; first, high authority pages are retrieved as a subgraph S from G. Next, using Eqs. (7) and (8), hubs and authorities are found. Here, H_{j} is the page's hub score, A_{j} is the page's authority score, I_{j} is page J's reference pages set, and B_{j} is page J's referrer pages set:

$$\text{HUB } (H_{\text{J}}) = \sum_{k \in I_{\text{J}}} A_{\text{J}} \tag{7}$$

$$\text{AUTHORITY } (A_{\text{J}}) = \sum_{k \in B_{\text{J}}} H_{\text{J}}. \tag{8}$$

3.9 *Eigen Rumor*

Eigen rumor [22] algorithm uses agents and objects for blogger and blog entries, respectively, and then the rank is calculated using information evaluation (hub score) and information provisioning (authority scores). Although PR and HITS are abetting blogs to obtain the rank values, some issues arise with the implementation of these algorithms in this particular area.

3.10 *BHITS*

An incremental connectivity analysis approach BHITS [20] is used to address the problem of topic distillation (the process of finding query's quality documents). The upshot of this method is to extend the algorithm based on previous connectivity analysis which has three problems such as mutually reinforcing relationship between hosts, automatically generated links, and nonrelevant documents, to overcome them.

3.11 SALSA

SALSA (Stochastic Approach for Link Structure Analysis) [21] algorithm is used to find authoritative webpages. In salsa algorithm, consider G (bipartite graph) with two parts as hubs and authorities, a link between hub "*h*" and authority "*a*" shows the informative link from *h* to *a*. By examining random walks, highly visible sites are identified more periodically than others.

3.12 Hub Averaging

Hub Averaging (HAvg) [25] algorithm is a combination of HITS and SALSA algorithms. The "*O*" operations are performed as the HITS algorithm to update the authority weights and "*I*" operations are performed as SALSA algorithm to update the hub weights. HAvg algorithm is used to overcome the problem with HITS algorithm that a large number of authorities pointed by a hub even those authorities do not have a good quality.

3.13 Threshold Algorithms

Hub threshold, authority threshold, and full threshold come into the category of Threshold Algorithms (TAls) [25]. Hub threshold algorithm considers only those hubs whose weights are greater than or equal to the average hub weight of all the webpages that point to a particular page. Authority threshold algorithm considers the top "*k*" authorities only. Full threshold algorithm is the combination of both hub threshold and authority threshold algorithms.

3.14 Breadth-First Search

Breadth-First Search (BFS) [25] combines the idea of both the in-degree and the HITS algorithms. Algorithm considers a node as starting point and then visit its acquainted in breadth-first sequence, consecutive between rearward and onward steps. Algorithm starts with node weight modification according to the link which is moved further from the starting node and stops either all the links have been traversed or the destination nodes are weary.

Table 1 Comparison of link analysis algorithms

Criteria algo	Mining method used	Description	I/P parameter	QoR	Cxty	Rlvncy	Limitations
PR	WSM	Score is computed at indexing time and results are based on page's importance	Backlinks	Medium	O(log n)	Less	Query independent, dangling pages
WPR	WSM	Important pages assigned with the large values and rank value of a page is not evenly divided among its out-link pages	Backlinks, forward links	Higher than PR	O(log n)	Less	Ignore the relevancy
WPCR	WSM and WCM	Generates sorted order of webpages with numerical value to response user query	Backlinks and content	Medium	O(log n)	More	Numerical value based webpages order
Distance rank	WSM	Based on reinforcement learning with consideration of webpages logarithmic distance	Inbound links	High	O(log n)	Average	Insertion of new pages involve large calculations
RBPR	WSM	Input is keywords and return the pages considering keywords and associated concept	Keywords	High	O(log n)	High	Annotated webpages with some ontology
Time rank	WUM	Consider visiting time to compute the score of the page	PR and server logs	Average	O(log n)	High	Idle time of pages provides incorrect input
TSPR	WSM and WCM	Computes the scores of webpages according to the importance of content	Backlinks, forward links and content	High	O(log n)	More	Mines text data
HITS	WSM and WCM	Scores of highly relevant pages are computed	Backlinks, forward links and content	Less than PR	O(log n)	More	Topic drift and efficiency problem
Eigen rumor	WSM	Adjacency matrix that is obtained from agent to object link is used	Agent/ objects	Higher than PR and HITS	O(log n)	High	Used only for blogs mining

(continued)

Table 1 (continued)

Criteria algo	Mining method used	Description	I/P parameter	QoR	Cxty	Rlvncy	Limitations
BHITS	WSM and WCM	Find quality document using incremented analysis algorithm	Backlinks, forward links and content	Higher than HITS	O(log n)	More	Limited to the topics
SALSA	WSM and WCM	Perform a random walk alternating between hubs and authorities	Backlinks, forward links and content	Less than PR	O(VE)	Average	Query dependent
HAvg	WSM and WCM	Update the authority weights as HITS algorithm and hub weights as SALSA algorithm	Backlinks, forward links and content	Medium	O(log n)	More	Identical hubs point equal no. of equally good authorities
TAls	WSM and WCM	Hub weight of a node is set to the sum of largest authority weights of the authorities pointed to by that node	Backlinks, forward links and content	Medium	O(log n)	Average	Irrelevant pages may have the higher rank
BFS	WSM	Rank the nodes according to their reach ability	Backlinks, forward links	High	O (V + E)	High	Best for small search space

Algo Algorithm, *QoR* Quality of Results, *Cxty* Complexity, *Rlvncy* Relavancy

4 Comparative Review

In Sect. 3, different link analysis algorithms are discussed and on the basis of some parameters, link analysis algorithms are compared and the result is shown in Table 1.

5 Related Work

Internet is a huge collection of web documents and webpages. Through page ranking algorithms, webpage's popularity can be calculated, though there are several page ranking algorithms, but HITS and Google page ranks are widely used. An algorithm [24] is suggested that used the user interaction time to compute average response time and then the webpage's rank is predicted on the basis of it. Web documents require a distinct and structural framework which provides an ease of navigation; for this, WSM is used which is based on the link-oriented similarity measures [13]. To increase WSM precision, navigation system mining [14] is used, in which Navigation Structure Graphs (NSGs) are examined rather than the whole web graph. This deep examination provides an information architecture that is much closer to the human viewpoint and identifies site boundaries and content hierarchies. A topical web crawling algorithm [15] based on WCM and WSM with the collaboration of neural network's characteristics is used to discover the relevance between webpages and topics which provide an improvement in the accuracy and efficiency of collected information. In e-commerce industry to satisfy the customer's need, the website should be well designed and well organized because for the customer websites are the faces of their respective companies. A newly improved mining [26] is suggested to restructure the website and helps to implement intelligent web mining.

6 Conclusion

Three categories of web mining namely web content mining, web usage mining, and web structure mining have been discussed. In the web structure mining, methods are based on the link analysis algorithm. This study focuses on the exploration of link analysis algorithms and their comparison. According to the comparative review from all the link analysis algorithms, breadth-first search is the best one but for small search space, though all the algorithms having some limitations, PR and HITS algorithms are mostly used for the web mining.

References

1. Kosla, R., Blockeel, H.: Web mining research: a survey. SIGKDD Explor. **2**, 1–15 (2000)
2. Etzioni, O.: The world wide web: quagmire or goldmine. Commun. ACM **39**(11), 65–68 (1996)
3. Chakrabarti, S.: Data mining for hypertext: a tutorial survey. ACM SIGKDD Explor. **1**(2), 1–11 (2000)
4. Cooley, R., Mobasher, B., Srivastava, J.: Web mining: information and pattern discovery on the world wide web. In: Proceeding Ninth Int'l Conference Tools with Artificial Intelligence '97, pp. 558–567 (1997)
5. Maes, P.: Agents that reduce work and information overload. Commun. ACM **37**(7), 30–40 (1994)
6. Borges, J., Levene, M.: Data mining of user navigation patterns. In: Proceedings of the WEBKDD'99 Workshop on Web Usage Analysis and User Profiling, pp. 31–36 (1999)
7. Madria, S.K., Bhowmick, S.S., Ng, W.K., Lim, E.-P.: Research issues in web data mining. In Proceedings of Data Warehousing and Knowledge Discovery, First International Conference, DaWaK'99, pp. 303–312 (1999)
8. Liu, B., Chang, K.: Editorial: special issue on web content mining. SIGKDD Explor. **6**(2), 1–4 (2004)
9. Jiang, H., Ge, Y.X., Zuo, D., Han, B.: TIME RANK: a method of improving rank scores by visited time. In: Proceedings of the Seventh International Conference on Machine Learning and Cybernetics, Kunming, pp. 1654–1657, 12–15 July (2008)
10. Xing, W., Ali, G.: Weighted PageRank algorithm. In: Proceedings of the Second Annual Conference on Communication Networks and Services Research (CNSR'04), IEEE, pp. 305–314 (2004)
11. Eirinaki, M., Vazirgiannis, M.: Web mining for web personalization. ACM Trans. Internet Technol. (TOIT) **3**(1), 1–27 (2003)
12. Facca, F.M., Lanzi, P.L.: Mining interesting knowledge from weblogs: a survey. Data Knowl. Eng. **53**(3), 225–241 (2005)
13. Lee, W.: Hierarchical web structure mining. In: Proceedings of Data Engineering Workshop (DEWS) (2006)
14. Keller, M., Nussbaumer, M.: Beyond the web graph: mining the information architecture of the www with navigation structure graphs. In: Proceedings of International Conference on Emerging Intelligent Data and Web Technologies, Tirana, Albania, pp. 99–106 (2011)
15. Qian, R., Zhang, K., Zhao, G.: A topic-specific web crawler based on content and structure mining. In: 3rd International Conference on Computer Science and Network Technology (ICCSNT), pp. 458–461 (2013)
16. Kleinberg, J.M.: Authoritative sources in a hyperlinked environment. In: Proceedings of the Ninth Annual ACM-SIAM Symposium on Discrete Algorithms, pp. 668–677, 25–27 January (1998)
17. Sharma, P., Bhadana, P., Tyagi, D.: Weighted page content rank for ordering web search result. Inter. J. Eng. Sci. Technol. **2**(12), 7301–7310 (2010)
18. Srivastava, J., Desikan, P., Kumar, V.: Web mining—concepts, applications and research directions. In: NGDM. MIT/AAAI Press (2004)
19. Haveliwala, T.H.: Topic-sensitive pagerank: a context-sensitive ranking algorithm for web search. IEEE Trans. Knowl. Data Eng. **15**(4), 784–796 (2003)
20. Bharat, K., Henzinger, M. R.: Improved algorithms for topic distillation in a hyperlinked environment. In Proceedings of the 21st Annual International ACM SIGIR Conference on Research and Development in Information Retrieval, pp. 104–111 (1998)
21. Lempel, R., Moran, S.: SALSA: the stochastic approach for link-structure analysis. ACM Trans. Inf. Syst. (TOIS) **19**(2), 131–160 (2001)
22. Fujimura, K., Inoue, T., Sugisaki, M.: The EigenRumor algorithm for ranking blogs. In: WWW 2005 2nd Annual Workshop on the Weblogging Ecosystem (2005)

23. Page, L., Brin, S., Motwani, R., Winograd, T.: The pagerank citation ranking: bringing order to the Web. In: Technical Report, Stanford Digital Libraries SIDL-WP 1999-0120 (1999)
24. Jain, N., Dwivedi, U.: Ranking web pages based on user interaction time. In: International Conference on Advances in Computer Engineering and Application (ICACEA), pp. 35–41 (2015)
25. Segall, R.S., Zhang, Q.: Teaching web mining in the classroom: with an overview of web usage mining. In: Proceedings of the Thirty-Ninth Annual Conference of the Southwest Decision Science Institute, vol. 39 (2008)
26. Verma, N., Singh, J.: Improved web mining for e-commerce website restructuring. In: IEEE Computational Intelligence & Communicational Technology (ICICT), pp. 155–160 (2015)
27. Borodin, A., Roberts, G.O., Rosenthal, J.S., Tsaparas, P.: Finding authorities and hubs from link structures on the World Wide Web. In: Proceedings of the 10th International Conference on World Wide Web, pp. 415–429, 01–05 May (2001)
28. Bidoki, A.M.Z., Yazdani, N.: DistanceRank: an intelligent ranking algorithm for web pages. Inf. Process. Manag. **44**(2), 877–892 (2008)
29. Lamberti, F., Sanna, A., Demartini, C.: A relation-based page rank algorithm for semantic web search engines. IEEE Trans. KDE **21**(1), 123–136 (2009)

Big Data Analytics via IoT with Cloud Service

Saritha Dittakavi, Goutham Bhamidipati and V. Siva Krishna Neelam

Abstract This publish conceptualizes the origin of data accumulated with the help of Internet of Things and analysis, storage, providing security to data, measures taken to meet the demands of market with the help of cloud services. Big data emphasizes the organization for marketing effectively by reaching to communally noteworthy issues. Big data is centralized on developing variable and highly attained computing, analytics as well as governance in a model such that organization can be related with variety of fields like health care.

Keywords Cloud · Big data · Analytics · Internet of things · Data analytics as a service · Analytics as a service · Data access · Data storage · Data privacy

1 Introduction

Big Data (BD) usually refers to voluminous data irrespective of the medium like digital, traditional, machine sources around us in which data has been gathered or generated. The data can be either structured, multi-structured or unstructured [3].

S. Dittakavi (✉)
Computer Science and Engineering Department,
GVP College for Degree and PG Courses,
Visakhapatnam, Andhra Pradesh, India
e-mail: sarithad@gvptc.edu.in

G. Bhamidipati
Hyderabad, Telangana, India
e-mail: gouthambhamidipati@hotmail.com

V.S.K. Neelam
Physics Department, GVP College for Degree and PG Courses,
Visakhapatnam, Andhra Pradesh, India
e-mail: vsk.neelam@gvptc.edu.in

V.B. Aggarwal et al. (eds.), *Big Data Analytics*, Advances in Intelligent Systems and Computing 654, https://doi.org/10.1007/978-981-10-6620-7_31

Big Data Analytics explains a computational and systematic analysis of data, providing an insight of future, processing the data in clinical way by attaining an inner view on data generated, and procuring insight in the future. This helps in being organized for covering the crests and troughs in future.

Internet of Things (IoT) let us get into concept by diverging the name itself. "Internet" basically a known normal term to every individual who is using smart ways to perform their work, learn any concept, get updated with latest information. Internet has many purposes which can't be listed as few. "Things" usually are tangible objects which we can come into contact with. So, how these things are related to Internet to form "Internet of Things"? IoT can be defined as a scenario or nonetheless as a growing movement where things are implanted with a smart chip and accessed from remote location via Internet.

For example, consider an automobile with built-in sensor which helps in transmitting the data about the machine condition or level of fuel in the tank or now a day's seat belt reminder. The best example for IoT is "Smart Watch" from well-known mobile manufacturing companies which help us to monitor our heart beat, pulse rate, etc.

2 Big Data with IoT

Nowadays, big data has been collected and maintained by very few organizations due to its form factors for maintenance [10].

- **V's of Big Data**

  Basically, V's of big data represent

- **Volume** of the data collected from any machine source usually be in smaller volume like chunk, bytes of data. But when we put together all the collected data, it forms considerably larger amount of size. Based on an analysis in recent years, which is done by collaboration of EMC Corporation and International Data Corporation IDC, data collected in all the means consumes 4.4 Zettabytes (1 Zettabyte $\approx$ 1 trillion gigabytes). It is also expected to reach 40 Zettabyte by 2020.
- **Velocity** of the data i.e., speed at which the data is collected from the devices and generated by the devices plays a prominent role in the big data. The speed at which the data gets changed and also the speed at which data has to be analyzed matter a lot in the real-time world.
- **Variety** of the data can be in various forms based on the source from which it has been collected. Data can be digital, analog data, and either continuous or discrete. All types of data have to be processed and should be handled (Fig. 1).

These three V's define the big data. As the adoption of big data has been grown rapidly, users are defining some more V's for big data (Fig. 2).

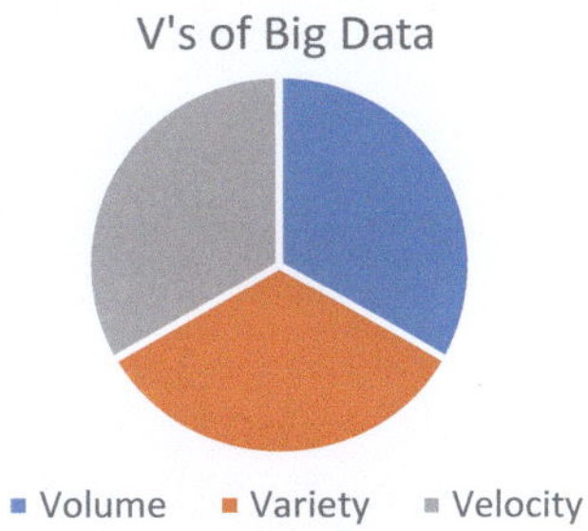

Fig. 1 Explains the V's of big data [8]

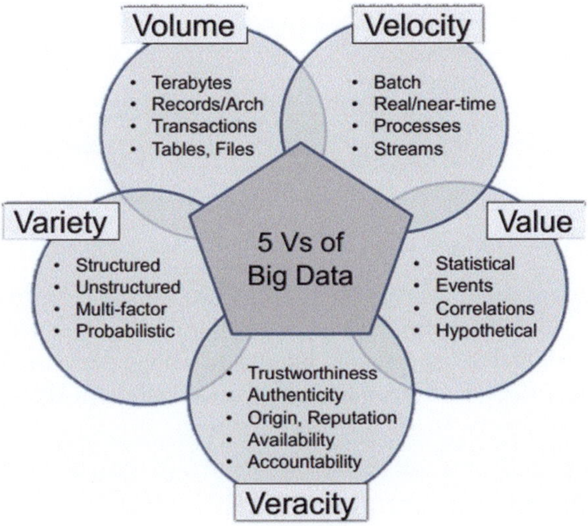

Fig. 2 5 V's of big data [8]

- **Things in IoT**

  Imagine hand-held devices, human beings, machines, almost all connectable devices as things for a short period. Basically, IoT hasn't been recognized until a decade and a half or so years, but the concept has been there since 1980s. The first device which has been connected and accessed over the network was a "Coke Machine" at a University located in USA. That was the first "Internet Appliance" in this concept. Now, based on recent researches and surveys, the appliances that connected over the network reached to 14.8 billion, and the expected figure by 2020 is at around 50 billion appliances.

When IoT will be adopted to a higher extent, then enormous data collected from the things connected over the network obviously triggers the phenomenon for the need of big data. This evolution results in an open chance for more devices to be connected causing a huge change from Internet of Things (IoT) to Internet of Everything (IoE).

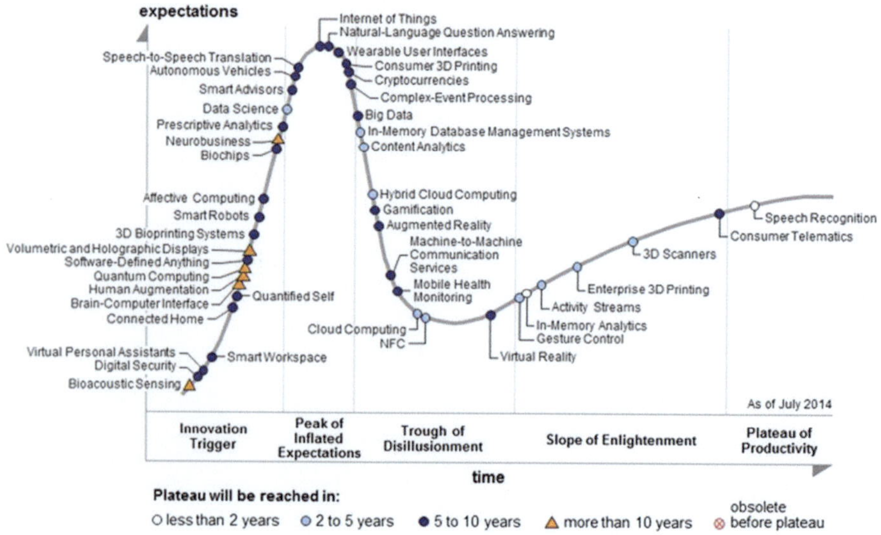

Fig. 3 Gartner's hype circle explaining about emerging technologies [5]

Based on this Hype Circle provided by Gartner in 2014, we can come to an insight that big data and Internet of Things are considered as achievable targets in a foreseeable future. Check Fig. 3 for Gartner's Hype Circle.

3 Big Data Analytics Over Cloud

Nowadays, as the evolution from traditional data collecting and computing techniques, consumers who are adopting big data techniques are increasing rapidly. Upon the needs of the consumer, data is stored at either single or multiple physical locations. But as the heap keeps on voluminously increasing, cloud storage is opted to store data. If BD and IoT handshake together, hinging on the above calculations, we might find they will be leveraging on cloud-based platforms not only to store but also secure and handle data more than both individual technologies rather than concepts are now.

On the grounds of growing data intake, cloud service providers are being sought out to provide infrastructure for both storing and also analyzing data virtually through cloud. The reason for this need was the time taken to process the data collected into individual data sets, analyze, generate data request to get what is needed by business analysts, and store this excess data on their personal systems for faster access resulting in risking compliance and privacy.

The solution available in the market for sustaining above discussed demands and hassles is "**Data Analytics as a Service**" (**DAaaS or AaaS**). In AaaS, the service offered is bit part of all cloud services offered currently in market. With this service as an option, consumers or organizations are beneficiary by providing the data to cloud securely along with business context for analyzed reports. By this leap, process reduces the effort put in differentiating data and dealing with it [1].

AaaS also obliterates the delays in knowledge transfer from organizational staff like business analysts and consumers face and, on the other hand, enables data analysts to exchange data sets reciprocated and elicit more insights swiftly (Table 1).

Data sources that are being connected together and with cloud for storing data are at rapid growth in the form of machine to machine communication, social media, etc. Therefore, AaaS can provide a flexible and productive services with proper intake of information if given.

Data access or data sharing/storing into the cloud plays a vital role in AaaS. As the data intake is bulk, the data collected will accommodate user information, machine information, surveyed information i.e., used for analyses along with unwanted garbage data accordingly. With the data in hands, sharing might be strenuous as the data contains user private data and data actually needed for analysis [2].

Figure 4 explains the data intake from various public social media. Every minute of the day helps us to calculate the volume of user private data in cloud that has to be analyzed and predict the interests of a particular user [11].

4 Security Challenges for Big Data in Cloud

Upon the point made by Fig. 4, accessing any form of data illegally in big data could lead to a catastrophic situation. There is a flair chance for exploitation of data in illicit manner. In the way to nullify such activities, service providers and consumers have to face few challenges that are discussed below,

- **Data Access**
  - **Data Analytics Systems** could be considered as a major challenge that big data is fronting in current market. Systems in which data is analyzed are to be developed robust and capable of handling voluminous data without any outage or delay. It should be able to store digital signatures of the data like the storage and creating date-time for the future use.
  - **Data Validity or Normalization** has to be checked thoroughly to avoid miscalculations or spiteful manipulations. As the data is collected from various system devices in different formats, in general, for data storage and

Table 1 Deriving analytics as a service from existing services

Services	Service offered medium
Infrastructure as a service (IaaS)	Storage capacity for big data collected
Platform as a service (PaaS)	Software platform for accessing analytic tools
Software as a service (SaaS)	Developing and deploying analytic tools

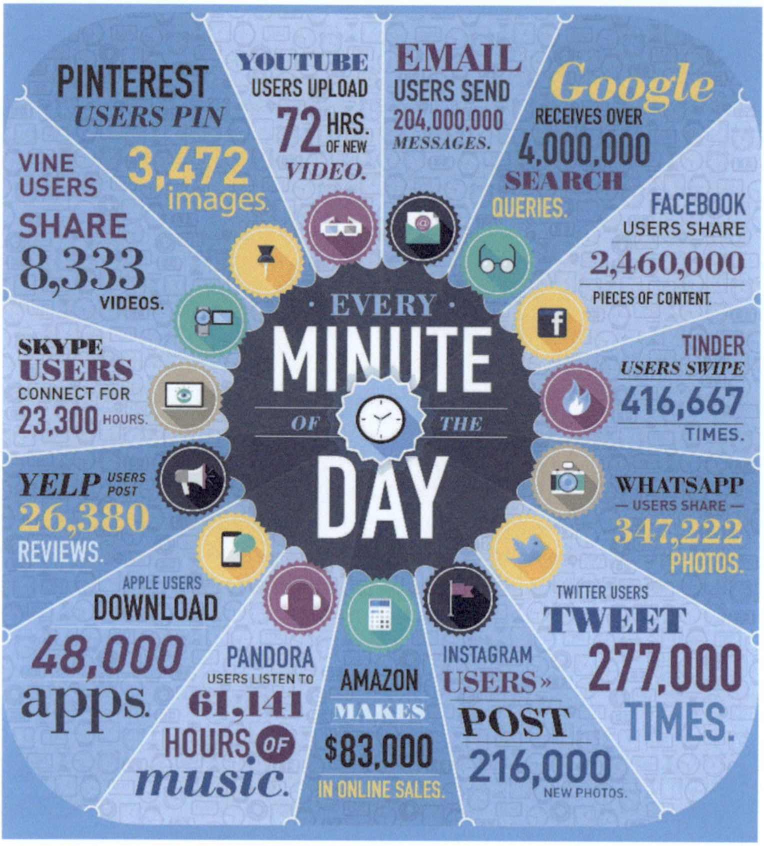

Fig. 4 Data accessed/stored every minute [7]

access in cloud, a distributed architecture is used. Data analysts perform same set of analytic algorithm on different subsets of a particular data set. Therefore, one-self cannot certify that particular data set is trustworthy.

- **Input Validation** is one of the crucial facets in AaaS. While data is collected, the device itself has to inspect whether the data is appropriate with the help of algorithms or sensors-driven mechanisms. If the validation doesn't pass the baseline, it might lead to malicious data sent for analysis.
- **Monitoring** helps us to foresee the alarms and provide real-time security. But, as the data could be inconsistent which results in generating false alarms, it requires human power to address. This situation would put IT Department to monitor the whole data activities in real time which is unendurable. The security can be increased, if and only if audits on the data collected are managed from granular level at regular time spans.

- **Data Storage**
  - **Multi-tiered Storage** could be considered as one of the major challenges in storing big data. As the data is accumulated from various sources and in various data forms, storing them in a traditional data storage models use multi-tiered storage architecture. Data upon the value it prevails is ranked from lower level to higher level. Lower level ranked data is stored in farther location on different media. But voluminous big data prevails the value until unless it is matched to find inconsistent patterns. Therefore, multi-tiered storage isn't pragmatic solution. To suffice this problem, automated storage tiering (AST) is developed which automatically manages the data according to the process. It also maintains a metadata regarding the locations where the data is stored.
  - **Non-relational Databases (NRDB)** came into existence as a part of large framework where middleware technologies are secured. With big data in the play, 90% of the data is collected as unstructured data sets. Data security is never intended in NRDB but this is the best solution to process the obtained data sets. As there is voluminous growth in data generated or collected, securing the data is very highly prioritized.
- **Data Privacy**
  - **Privacy Risk** of the data is at stake with the integration of BD and Cloud. Data collected and stored in different can be accessed, analyzed to identification for further association with one's personal information. Private cloud is also available but due to the variance of the data, privacy might be compromised with different ways of accessing. To avoid this impediment, cryptographically administered access control along with invulnerable communication is implemented to ensure the private data is allowed to access with valid authorizations. But private data stored without any encryption in BD due to privacy policies.
  - **Controlled Access** is ensured with authentication protocols and also by providing granular level access which in turns helps to share the required data precisely. Data has to be shared, stored, and accessed through private cloud with the help of controlled secure keys. Data provenance results in more complication with voluminous, variant data. The metadata in such cases helps data analytic experts to investigate and predict the accuracy of the data source. Access should be allowed and controlled at very granular level.

5 Literature Survey [6]

Big data had a true potential to lead an organization to real business value by real-time decisions based on facts. Let us consider recent crisis in both IT and financial sectors which resulted them to consider thousands of old data as a single entity leading to failure of assessing risk. With the help of BD, we can prevent such cases by assessing the risk and mitigating at very lower rather than individual level.

In big data, there is rule that states "analysis would be more accurate if the data sample is larger." BD analyzes the samples to enhance the end results. But organizations are restricted to use subsets of their data for basic and simple analysis. The data which is collected hugely will go in vain if it's not processed. This scenario left the organization to choose between the choices below,

- **Usage of Voluminous Data in Analytics** leaves the organization puzzled about the necessity of the usage. But if it results in better analytics, we can achieve accurate results. Now and then voluminous data cannot be analyzed with traditional approaches and need to use analytics like In-Database/Memory Analytics for better and fast computations and risk assessment from ware house.
- **Data Relevance determination** has to be done before using the data for analytics. The relevant data shall be used for analytics, and the non-relevant data will be hoarded for future references using cloud services.

Either of options distinct organization from all the hassles resulting their independency over analysis of the data subsets available.

6 Case Study [4]

To speak up for big data analytics via IoT with cloud services, let us consider a case study which has recently implemented in health management system.

Traditional health management system does all the monitoring and processing manually which could be prone to human error or inaccuracy. Data related to equipment, patient, and surgery, test reports were manually handled and analyzed by a hierarchy of personnel. Monitoring of patients used to happen by several calls over regular intervals which results in poor visibility to patient flow. This system also costs in high utilization of revenues, patient satisfaction, etc. To avoid such problems, Tagnos provided a de facto standard solution (Fig. 5).

Real-Time Location Solution monitors patient flow, ward and room readiness/utilization, alert's staff, provides analytics and insights regarding patient treatment with the help of their test reports, health condition, and last but not least it also updates the family members and patients about their location in the hospital if any changes are done. RTLS is combination of real-time location tracking along with both data analytics and workflow of a health management system.

RTLS monitoring is done as follows:

- Assign a specific ID tags which can be monitored to staff, equipment, and patients as they enter into environment. These tags help the hospital-monitoring staff to monitor the patients wait time, notifies staff if wait time is too long based on the hospital metrics.

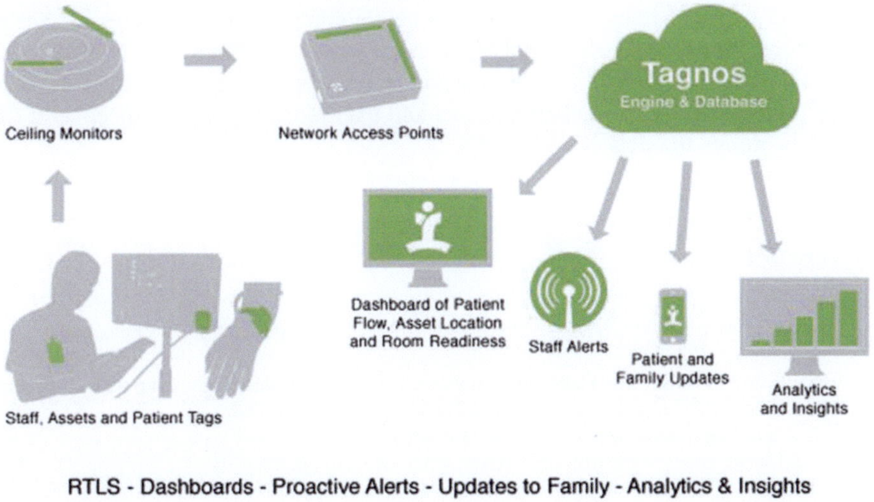

Fig. 5 Real-time location system for health management system [9]

- Once patient is attended and moved to ward or room, required equipment is automatically located and gathered to patient's room for diagnose.
- If there are any changes in patient's location, RTLS notifies the patient and his/her family member about the new location so that they can feel less tense and stay comfortable.
- Apart from these operations, RTLS also monitors, interpret patient's data regarding diagnoses held and health conditions, and notifies the pertinent staff which helps them to be in sync with all the required equipment, processes ready.

With RTLS, we can achieve improved patient satisfaction, high monitoring efficiency, equipment management. It helps in reducing the operational costs, regulated staffing, and also to gain patient's confidence and satisfaction.

RTLS was implemented by Tagnos in White Memorial Medical Center. WMMC is benefitted with improved patient satisfaction from 45 to 90% and saved around thousands of dollars for the management.

7 Conclusion

Big data analytics via IoT over cloud yield flexible data communication between consumers and service providers for faster analysis. With Big Data analytics adoption, few of the consumers are benefitted with befitted prediction analysis. As there is an ascend in volume, variety and velocity of the data over network Data analytics as a service has been introduced for sustainability of process and systems regardless of the sources of the data.

DAaaS or AaaS reduces the IT department's complexities and generates faster predictions compared to traditional big data analytics algorithms and processes. But service providers along with the consumers who opted AaaS in cloud have to ensure that ever security challenge is met and data security prior irrespective of the device or things the data is collected.

References

1. Analytics as a Service (AaaS): http://www.techopedia.com/definition/29893/analytics-as-a-service-aaas
2. AaaS aims to solve Big Data's big problems: http://searchcloudcomputing.techtarget.com/feature/Analytics-as-a-Service-aims-to-solve-big-datas-big-problems
3. Big Data: http://www.webopedia.com/TERM/B/big_data.html
4. Case Study: https://www.youtube.com/watch?v=HeA4bYjd2FI
5. Gartner's Hype Circle: http://www.gartner.com/newsroom/id/2819918
6. Literature Survey: www.sas.com/content/…/big-data-meets-big-data-analytics-105777.pdf
7. Managing Big Data: http://www.smartdatacollective.com/gunjantripathi/332791/managing-big-data-make-sure-you-know-challenges
8. Modelling Cloud Service for Big Data: http://www.researchjournals.in/QIMRJ/2015/4.3/4319.pdf
9. Real—time location system for health management system: http://www.nhfca.org/psf/Materials3/feb15/tagnos_slide_deck_for_hasc-hqi_event[1].pdf
10. The Internet of the Things and Big Data unlocking the Power: http://www.zdnet.com/article/the-internet-of-things-and-big-data-unlocking-the-power
11. The Road to AaaS: http://www.forbes.com/sites/oracle/2014/09/26/the-road-to-analytics-as-a-service

A Proposed Contextual Model for Big Data Analysis Using Advanced Analytics

Manjula Ramannavar and Nandini S. Sidnal

Abstract Big Data has numerous issues related to its primary defining characteristics of the three V's: Variety, Volume and Velocity. A greater segment of Big Data is attributed to semi-structured or unstructured text that emanates from social interactions on the web, emails, tweets, blogs, etc. Conventional approaches are overwhelmed by the data deluge and fall short to perform. These challenges consequently create scope for research in developing models to analyze data and extract actionable insights to realize the fourth V, i.e., Value. The purpose of this paper is to propose a contextual model for Resume Analytics that utilizes Semantic technologies and Analytic (Descriptive, Predictive and Prescriptive) procedures to find a befitting match between a job and candidate(s). The related work, issues and challenges and design requirements are presented along with a discussion of the analytical framework for the opted use case.

Keywords Big data · Descriptive analytics · Predictive analytics · Prescriptive analytics · Semantic technologies

1 Introduction

The Internet, web, social media, smartphones and other online work based-tools generate humongous digital data affecting our daily lives. Big Data refers to massive datasets, ranging beyond terabytes, which are heterogeneous and generated at an ever-increasing rate. Unstructured text contributes to around eighty per cent [13] of the total digital data generated by companies due to machine generated logs, call detail records, e-commerce, emails, etc. The conventional tools and technologies are beleaguered by the distinctive dimensions of Big Data [16]. Hence efficient

M. Ramannavar (✉) · N.S. Sidnal
KLS Gogte Institute of Technology, Belagavi, India

V.B. Aggarwal et al. (eds.), *Big Data Analytics*, Advances in Intelligent Systems and Computing 654, https://doi.org/10.1007/978-981-10-6620-7_32

algorithms, methods and tools need to be devised to capture, process and analyze this data in an intelligent automated fashion to draw inferences. Advanced Analytics [15] entails application of a multitude of analytic processes to address the diversity of Big Data to yield responsive information in the form of descriptions, predictions and prescriptions. The inferences drawn may guide strategic decision-making to enable an organization to gain a competitive edge. Big Data and Advanced Analytics thus come together to become critical enablers of the modern economy.

1.1 The Resume Analytics Problem

Human Resources (HR) [25] are an important asset to any organization. The strength of an organization lies in its right HR workforce. A Resume or Curriculum Vitae represents the functional aspects of a job aspirant and consists of several sections, namely qualification, experience, skills, personal details, etc. It is used to screen applicants; the ones that get through are selected for subsequent round, generally, an interview. In the context of automated Resume Analytics, the following two stakeholders are identified:

Job Provider: This role is represented by an individual, a group or an organization. A Job Provider is often faced with the problem of finding the talent pool, i.e., the most befitting candidate to fill up a vacancy. A job description indicates the requirements, i.e., qualification, skill set and experience needed for a job. In the event of a vacancy, job provider calls for posts online by floating job descriptions.

Job Seeker: This role is represented by an individual who is a job aspirant. A prospective candidate prepares a resume to reflect his personality in an appealing manner and uploads it, anticipating a call for the recruitment process.

The Resume Analytics problem is to find the most appropriate fit between a job description and prospective candidate(s), given a pool of resumes and a job description. Commercial tools such as ALEX [1], Daxtra [9], RChilli [20], Sovren [24], Textkernel_hr_suite [27] are available for job and resume parsing and mapping a job to resume. However, open-source contributions to the specified problem are solicited for the benefit of the masses. This proposition is an attempt towards developing a suite of components to deal with the Resume Analytics problem.

The rest of the paper is organized as follows: Sect. 2 reviews related work. Section 3 identifies issues and challenges based on literature survey. The design requirements for the model are enumerated in Sect. 4. Section 5 utilizes the Big Data Value Chain or the Big Data Analysis Pipeline to suggest the intended model, and Sect. 6 concludes the paper with directions for future work.

2 Related Work

This section reviews the literature to summarize the contributions made by various researchers towards resume parsing and allied fields.

The authors in [2] have worked on ontology-based ranking of documents using Graph Databases. Attribute values are extracted from resumes and mapped onto RDF. Resumes are ranked based on cosine similarity measures. Experiments for retrieval time for three cases are compared: Single RDF, Four RDFs and Three RDFs.

Latent Semantic Analysis (LSA) and ontological concepts are used to support e-recruitment in the teaching domain in [4]. Ontology is built, and vector is generated by applying LSA. Semantic similarity is found between job posting and CV.

Ontology based Resume Parser (ORP) system is proposed in [7] for Kariyer.net company that has more than 6,000,000 unstructured and freestyle résumés as MS Word. The architecture, working mechanism, similarity of concept, matching techniques and inference mechanism are introduced, and a case study for a Turkish resume is presented. The proposed ORP system in [7] is implemented in [6] which transforms an input résumé into structured format by splitting it into explicit segments, parsing it, normalizing it and finally applying classification and clustering task. [8] extends work done in [6] by incorporating Semantic Web Rule Language (SWRL) inference mechanism.

Machine learning-based CV Parser system is used in [10] to extract information from Hungarian, English and German CVs for a Career Portal. The system converts CVs into text files and extracts relevant data using maximum-entropy Markov model (MEMM).

Deductive model and an Ontology-Based Hybrid Approach are used to match job seeker and a posting in [11]. Similarity-based approach is used to rank applicants.

Most of the methods extract information from resume while in [17], a resume is selected from a group of resumes by extracting Special Skills type and Special Skill Values thereby improving performance.

Linked Data allows resources to be openly published and well connected to other resources thereby enabling discovery of highly relevant information. The authors in [18] publish Resume data in RDF into Web of Data using the Linked Data approach. Information may be consumed by machines using RDF and by humans using HTML. Issues of heterogeneity, interoperability and data reusing between multiple data sources are addressed using Linked Data.

A Semantic Web enabled System for Résumé Composition and Publication is implemented in [19]. The system assists a user to write a resume using domain ontologies and also annotate with reference to a common ontological vocabulary. It also enables a user to create his own tag-bag which would better expose the candidate on the web for crawlers.

A Framework is proposed in [21] for semantic annotation of Urdu web documents based on domain ontology. It deals with Urdu web documents that are free format, imprecise and in unintelligible formats.

In [22], a system for Candidate-Task matching in the E-Recruitment field is detailed. The system uses a web-based interface that allows one to enter required skills and desired skills and retrieve candidate(s) accordingly.

A system for information extraction from a resume based on Named Entity Clustering algorithm is presented in [23]. A resume is segmented. Chunkers recognize named entities which are then clustered and normalized.

Large Scale Skill Matching through Knowledge Compilation is the core theme in [28]. Knowledge Compilation approach is used where the knowledge base in Description Logics is converted into relational database. SQL queries are then executed over the database for skill matching. Job request is semantically matched against the candidates. Strict requirements and preferences may be specified.

It can be seen that most of the works utilize domain ontology to characterize background knowledge for information extraction and semantic representation. The focus is more on transforming an unstructured resume into a structured semantic format to facilitate information exchange and expert finding on the web. The authors in [13] discuss a host of machine learning techniques and methods used for automated categorization of text documents. According to editorial [14], Linked Data and Big Data together constitute the 4th paradigm in computing. Linked Data is a part of the Big Data Landscape and an ideal test bed for research on Big Data issues. There is a necessity to adopt the Big Data approach to solve the use case.

3 Issues and Challenges

A Big Data initiative needs to have a well-planned strategy and the right set of tools to cope with heterogeneity, speed and scalability concerns. A study of related work in Sect. 2 indicates the following research issues and challenges for the Resume Analytics problem:

- Resumes are uploaded in different formats at various sites. Collection and aggregation of these resumes is a challenge.
- A resume is free text and hence is of semi-structured or unstructured nature. It typifies the Variety dimension of Big Data. Suitable methods need to be devised to efficiently store, analyze and extract knowledge.
- The concepts of a resume and underlying relationships between them need to be clearly understood. This issue may be handled by capturing domain knowledge through ontologies.
- The information extracted from a resume has to be stored to facilitate querying and retrieval. Resource Description Framework (RDF) and Linked Data technologies can be used to enable data from different sources to be connected and queried.

- Resumes and job descriptions are continually uploaded by the two stakeholders all over the world. The Volume and Velocity aspects call for solutions to deal with the issues of scale and speed. Scalable-distributed computing frameworks have to be exploited to address these issues.
- Finding the most appropriate fit between job description and resume(s) necessitates innovative ways of applying techniques of Advanced Analytics in order to perform computational analyses in an optimal and effective manner.

4 Design Requirements

In the light of the above-stated issues, existing studies in allied disciplines have raised the need for a model [26] to aid the stakeholders in the recruitment process. Considering these domain-driven motivational needs, the following design (functional and non-functional) requirements ought to be met:

4.1 Functional Requirements

To articulate formalized repository of domain knowledge: A job description and a resume embed domain knowledge of distinctive aspects such as objective/summary, skill set, experience, education. Distributed architectures and domain-based ontology need to be exploited to allow optimal storage and retrieval.
To identify relevant concepts/entities related to the recruitment process: To extract different sections and build a concept map. Synonyms, for example qualification and education and same terms expressed in different forms have to be identified as the same concept.
To perform Resume Analytics: To discover correlations (explicit and hidden) between extracted concepts based on the concept map. For example, Hierarchical relationship: Skill → Programming Languages → C. Ranks need to be assigned on the basis of qualitative evaluation of resumes using techniques of Advanced Analytics. Job description also needs to be ranked. Resumes are to be clustered according to the ranks.
To present the extracted knowledge: To present the results in the form of resumes satisfying the job requirements along with implications. Also seek the most appropriate fit between a job and candidate(s).

4.2 Non-functional Requirements

Scalability, Reliability and Availability: It is needed to develop solution(s) that operate in parallel and distributed architectures offering fault-tolerance and replication.
Resilience and Speed: The solution(s) should provide quick responses and provide an acceptable level of service in the event of faults.

5 Proposed Model for Big Data Analysis

The proposed model in Fig. 1 meets the aforementioned functional requirements while the architecture in Fig. 2 satisfies the non-functional requirements of the above-stated design requirements. The Big Data Value Chain or the Big Data Analysis Pipeline [3] serves as the blueprint for the proposed model for Big Data Analytics. It consists of multiple distinct phases: Acquisition/Recording,

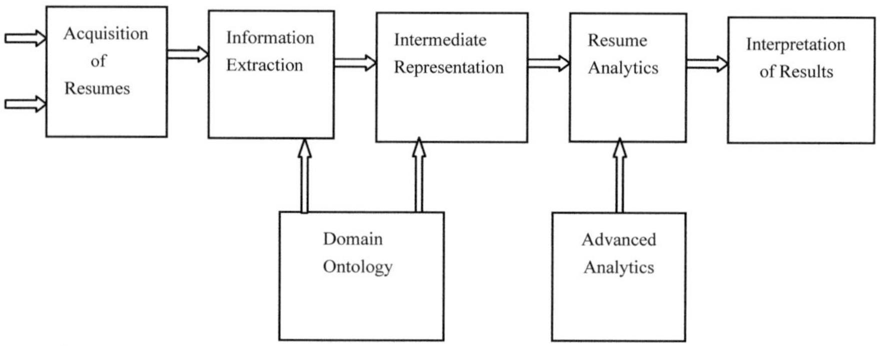

Fig. 1 Proposed model for Big Data Analysis

Fig. 2 Architecture of the proposed model

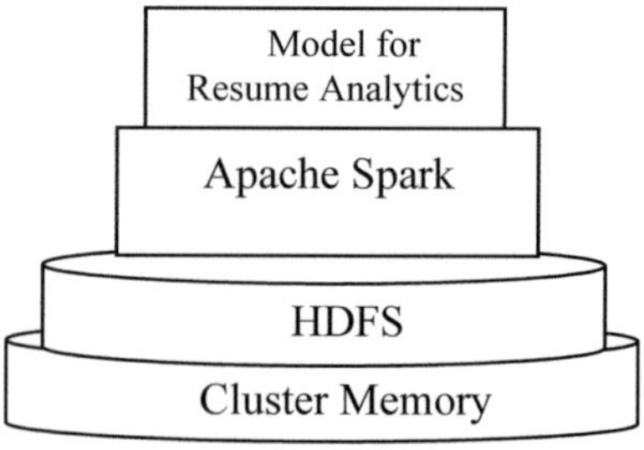

Information Extraction and Cleaning, Data Integration, Aggregation, and Representation, Query Processing, Data modelling, and Analysis and Interpretation. Figure 1 gives a picture of the proposed model for the Resume Analytics problem.

5.1 *Phases of the Model*

Acquisition: Resumes are collected from various sources such as emails, job portals, LinkedIn and recorded for the subsequent phases.
Information Extraction: Relevant concepts pertaining to skills, experience, qualification etc. are extracted from the resumes to build a concept map. Background knowledge in the form of domain ontology assists in semantic extraction of information.
Intermediate Representation: The extracted information is stored in an intermediate representation suitable for subsequent analysis. The representation should be chosen to enable quick and easy access. RDF and Linked Data technologies may be used for optimal semantic storage and retrieval.
Resume Analytics: Every resume in the intermediate representation is analyzed using the techniques of Advanced Analytics based on the various criteria against the job requirement and assigned a rank.
Interpretation of Results: The resumes satisfying the job requirements are visualized as results along with decision enabling indicators. The most appropriate fit between the job description and the candidate(s) also serve as the analytic results.

5.2 *Analytics*

There are three types of analytics: Descriptive analytics is a set of processes and technologies that summarize data to infer what is happening now or what has happened in the past. Predictive analytics is a set of processes that look into the past to predict the future. Prescriptive analytics not only enables to look into the future but also suggests actions to benefit from the predictions and shows the decision maker the implications of each decision option. While descriptive analytics look into the past, Advanced Analytics in the form of predictive and prescriptive analytics provide a forward-looking perspective and make use of techniques encompassing a wide range of disciplines including statistics, machine learning, optimization, simulation. The proposed work intends to integrate Advanced Analytics models to map a job to resume(s).

Figure 2 depicts the architecture to be used for the Resume Analytics Model.

Apache Spark [5] is an open-source scalable cluster computing platform that is much faster than Hadoop [16] due to in-memory computing primitives. It allows data to be directly loaded into cluster memory. Spark is also well suited to machine learning algorithms and can interface with a variety of distributed storage including Cassandra, Hadoop Distributed File System (HDFS), and Amazon S3. HDFS [12] is a highly available, highly fault-tolerant distributed file system designed to operate on commodity hardware. The proposed model shown in Fig. 1 would be implemented on top of Spark.

6 Experimental Results

In this section, the results of preliminary work are presented. To evaluate the performance, the work was applied on real data set of resumes, containing around 200 resumes of postgraduate and undergraduate students. Experiment is based on resume information where a dataset containing description of resume information is generated, and then, search queries are used to find the required information from the resume. This dataset is assumed as a part of the Web of Data and is used for experimental purpose. A CV dataset contains information about business and academic information, skill, company, title, etc.

Resume processing like building concepts and analyzing phase is done in Hadoop. To build concepts of resumes, multiple resumes are processed through MapReduce jobs. The qualitative measure 'coverage' can be taken as value denoting how many sections and subsections are covered in a resume. The next job was then to see how many concepts from a class are covered in a resume. This required extraction of concepts and performing matching. If all the concepts are covered in the resume, as per resume grammar, then that particular resume is considered as complete resume or else incomplete. To compute comprehensibility, each line in resume is fed to mapper which gives comprehensibility of that line. Reduce sums up all the results and gives comprehensibility of each resume as output. Figure 3 shows the selected resumes that match a job description.

Once MapReduce jobs are done, it gives summary of each resume called as Comprehensive Quality. It gives summary on missing information of header and data. After summing up the comprehensibility, each resume is ranked according to the coverage and comprehensibility. Finally, for a given job description, it lists all the resumes along with the ranks as shown in Fig. 4.

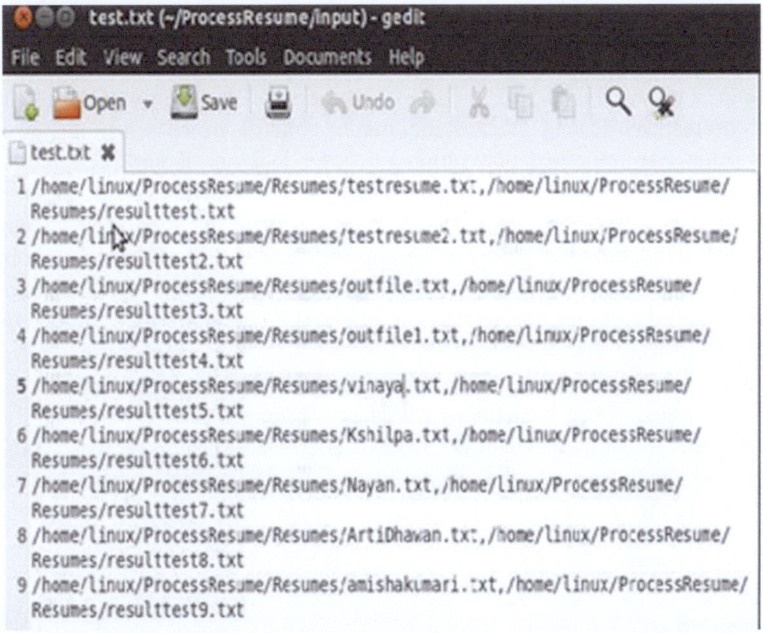

Fig. 3 Selected resumes that match job description

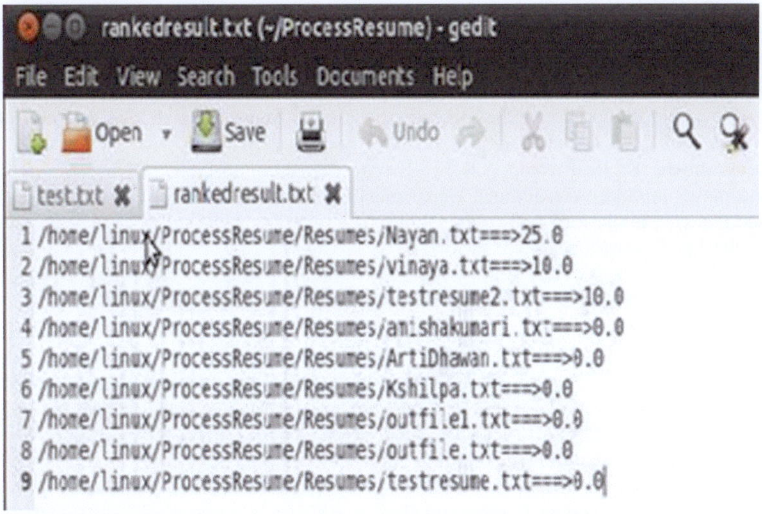

Fig. 4 Ranked resumes

7 Conclusion and Future Work

Big Data and Analytics are the front runners of innovation and technology advancements. While Big Data is inevitable, analytic processes probe through it (which otherwise remained unexplored) to infer insights of unprecedented worth. Semi-structured or unstructured data contributes to a major chunk of Big Data. Managing it is a huge challenge that implores several avenues for research. This paper considered the case study of Resume Analytics and reviewed various contributions in its realm. A research proposition has been formulated stating the objectives and design requirements. The planned architecture and model to realize the objectives were also discussed.

Future work would focus on a deeper study of the constituent elements of the model. Attempts would be made towards developing a prototype for the various modules incorporated in the model from implementation perspective. The model would also have to be evaluated taking into account associated metrics followed by rigorous validations.

References

1. ALEX Resume Parser: http://www.hireability.com/ALEX
2. Abirami, A.M., Askarunisa, A., Sangeetha, R.: Ontology based ranking of documents using graph databases: a big data approach, smarter planet and big data analytics workshop. In: Co-located with International Conference on Distributed Computing and Networking, 4 Jan 2014, Amrita University, Coimbatore
3. Agrawal, D., et. al.: Challenges and opportunities with big data. A community white paper developed by leading researchers across the United States through Collaborative Writing between Nov 2011 to Feb 2012
4. Al-lasassmeh, K.Q., Kayed, A.K.A.: Latent Semantic analysis (LSA) and ontological concepts to support e-recruitment. Department of Computer Science, Faculty of Information Technology, Middle East University, June 2013
5. Apache Spark: https://spark.apache.org/
6. Çelikelik, D., Elçi, A.: An ontology-based information extraction approach for Résumés. In: ICPCA-SWS 2012, LNCS 7719, pp. 165–179 (2013). Springer, Berlin
7. Çelikelik, D.: Towards a semantic based information extraction system for matching résumés to job openings. Computer Engineering Department, Istanbul Aydin University, Turkey
8. Çelikelik, D., et. al.: Towards an information extraction system based on ontology to match Résumés and jobs. In: 2013 IEEE 37th annual computer software and applications conference workshops, Kyoto, Japan, 22–26 July 2013. doi:10.1109/COMPSACW.2013.60
9. Daxtra Intelligent Recruitment Solutions: http://www.daxtra.com
10. Farkas, R., Dobó, A., Kurai, Z., Miklós, I., Nagy, A., Vincze, V., Zsibrita, J.: Information extraction from Hungarian, English and German CVs for a career portal. In: Prasath, R., et al. (eds.) MIKE 2014, LNAI 8891, pp. 333–341 (2014). Springer International Publishing, Switzerland
11. Fazel-Zarandi, M., Fox, M.S.: Semantic matchmaking for job recruitment: an ontology-based hybrid approach. In: 8th International Semantic Web Conference (2009)
12. Hadoop Distributed File System (HDFS): https://hadoop.apache.org/docs/r1.2.1/hdfs_design.html

13. Halper, F., Kaufman, M., Kirsh, D.: Text analytics: the Hurwitz victory index report. Technical Report (2013). http://www.sas.com/news/analysts/Hurwitz_Victory_Index-TextAnalytics_SAS.PDF
14. Hitzler, P., Janowicz, K.: Linked data, big data, and the 4th Paradigm. Editorial. Semantic Web Journal by IOS Press. Feb 2013. http://www.semantic-webjournal.net/system/files/swj488.pdf
15. Kaisler, S.H., Espinosa, J.A., Armour, F., Money, W.H.: Advanced analytics—issues and challenges in the global environment. In: 47th Hawaii international conference on system science, Hilton Waikoloa, Big Island, pp. 729–738, 6–9 Jan 2014. doi:10.1109/HICSS.2014.98
16. Katal, A.,Wazid, M., Goudar, R.H.: Big data: issues, challenges, tools and good practices. In: Sixth International IEEE Conference on Contemporary Computing (IC3), Noida, India, pp. 349–353, 8–10 Aug 2013
17. Maheshwari, S., Sainani, A., Krishna Reddy, P.: An approach to extract special skills to improve the performance of resume selection. In: 6th International Workshop on Databases in Networked Information Systems (DNIS2010), Centre for Data Engineering, International Institute of Information Technology, Hyderabad, India, Mar 2010
18. Marjit, U., Sharma, K., Biswas, U.: Discovering resume information using linked data. Int. J. Web Semant. Technol. (IJWesT) **3**(2) (2012)
19. Mirizzi, R., Noia, T.D., Sciascio, E.D., Michelantonio, T.: A Semantic Web enabled System for Résumé Composition and Publication. In: 3rd IEEE International Conference on Semantic Computing (ICSC 2009), Berkeley, CA, USA, 14–16 Sept 2009. doi:10.1109/ICSC.2009.40. http://www.researchgate.net/publication/221406004_A_Semantic_Web_Enabled_System_for_Rsum_Composition_and_Publication
20. Overview of RChilli Resume Parser Copyright © 2014 RChilli Inc.: http://rchilli.com/wp-content/uploads/2014/12/Overview-of-RChilli-Resume-Parser.pdf
21. Rajput, Q.: Ontology based semantic annotation of Urdu language web documents. In: 18th International Conference on Knowledge-Based and Intelligent Information & Engineering Systems (KES 2014), Gdynia, Poland, 15–17 Sept 2014, pp. 662–670. doi:10.1016/j.2014
22. Saellstrom, P.: A system for candidate-task matching in the e-recruitment field. Umea University, Department of Computing Science, Sweden, July 2013
23. Sonar, S., Bankar, B.: Resume parsing with named entity clustering algorithm. http://www.slideshare.net/swapnilmsonar/resume-parsing-with-named-entity-clustering-algorithm
24. Sovren Resume/CV Parser: http://www.sovren.com
25. Suen, H.: The effect of end user computing competence on human resource job performance: mapping for human resource roles. Afr. J. Bus. Manage. **6**(28), 8287–8295 (2012). doi:10.5897/AJBM11.577. ISSN 1993-8233 © 2012 Academic Journals. http://www.academicjournals.org/AJBM
26. Tao, J., Deokar, A.V., El-Gayar, O.F.: An Ontology-based information extraction (OBIE) framework for analyzing initial public offering (IPO) prospectus, pp. 769–778. In: 47th Hawaii International Conference on System Science, Waikoloa, HI, USA, 6–9 Jan 2014. doi:10.1109/HICSS.2014.103
27. Textkernel_hr_suite. Empowering Recruitment: www.textkernel.com
28. Tinelli, E., Colucci, S., Giannini, S., Sciascio, E.D., Donini, F.M.: Large Scale Skill Matching Through Knowledge Compilation. Foundations of Intelligent Systems, Lecture Notes in Computer Science, vol. 7661, pp. 192–201 (2012). http://link.springer.com/chapter/10.1007%2F978-3-642-34624-8_23

Ranked Search Over Encrypted Cloud Data in Azure Using Secure K-NN

Himaja Cheruku and P. Subhashini

Abstract Commercial cloud service providers are approached to maintain huge data and run the applications on their platforms. But when sensitive data is to be outsourced, the data owners expect privacy for their data from being known to the cloud management. In such cases to incorporate privacy and security, encrypted cloud services are of supreme requirement. Unfortunately, traditional encryption methods are not fair for this purpose. So here we define a method using which the cloud data can be encrypted allowing the best relevant document search. Based on secure kNN computation, this method is made to evaluate similarity measure for the user's search keyword while allowing encryption. The method includes encryption of documents before outsourcing to the cloud environment using a random matrix. For enriched privacy, keyword encryption is made and finally, top-k documents are retrieved. The approach is compared with multiple similarity measures like Euclidean, Manhattan, and Cosine distances, to find the best relevant document for the user's query.

Keywords Cloud computing · Encrypted cloud · Privacy preserving · Ranked search · Security

1 Introduction

Security in the cloud is an emerging concern in network security and cloud data privacy. Today, service providers are turning their groundwork and framework into a bulky cloud computing environment, which enables them to run the applications of the users on their platforms. The moment an organization chooses to host their services as applications on the public cloud, it simply means that, there is not any

H. Cheruku (✉) · P. Subhashini
MVSR Engineering College, Osmania University, Hyderabad, India
e-mail: himacheruku@gmail.com

P. Subhashini
e-mail: subhashini.pallikonda@gmail.com

V.B. Aggarwal et al. (eds.), *Big Data Analytics*, Advances in Intelligent Systems and Computing 654, https://doi.org/10.1007/978-981-10-6620-7_33

access for them to the servers and therefore the data. As a result, probably business required, receptive, confidential, and private data are at risk. According to a recent alliance report, among multiple contingences being faced, insider attacks are the major risk for cloud environment.

In this context, while using the public cloud, exclusive information including both business data and related information, should not be exposed to unlicensed, illegal parties. To protect the data from these attacks, privacy is obligatory on such a service model and data running on the platform.

In this view, encryption of data is aimed. Cloud encryption is the renovation of a cloud service customer's data into ciphertext. Cloud encryption is alike in-house encryption with one significant difference. The customer must have knowledge about the provider's policies, the encryption technique, and the key management. This encryption must also match the sensitivity level of customer's data being hosted. As this results in processor overhead, many cloud providers offer only primary, primitive encryption on key fields like passwords and account numbers. At this point, encrypting data before deploying to the cloud is concentrated.

In the literature, a technique where encrypted data are considered as documents allowing user to search through a single keyword and retrieve documents of interest is known as searchable encryption [1–9]. However, applying these approaches to a large cloud would not be necessarily suitable and secure, as they cannot accommodate requirements like system usability, keyword searching experience, and easy information discovery. Although to support Boolean keyword search [10–18], some techniques have been proposed, they are not enough for relevancy retrieval.

Being aware of this, the prior works of Wang et al. [19, 20] have provided solutions limiting to queries consisting of single keyword. When it comes to multiple search words given by user as a single word (called as multi-keyword), the retrieval is very difficult as it is to be done over encrypted cloud, and hence, we focus on retrieval on multi-keyword ranked search in our work.

Though the cloud providers are able to accommodate multiple services to the users with their cloud environment, security plays a major role. In this paper, we illustrate and work out the issue how the data is being deployed while allowing privacy and security. While using public cloud services, the data owners blindly provide their data to the cloud services, in this context, security breach occurs and unauthorized data access can be expected, hence, we consider the problem of encryption of data before deploying to the cloud. Using k-nearest neighbor (kNN) computation over an encrypted collection, we get the k-top-relevant documents from the cloud. We analyze the encryption process with multiple distance measures for best relevant document retrieval.

The remainder of this paper is standardized as follows: Sect. 2 describes system model and two existing schemes of encryption. Section 3 describes secure encryption and retrieval of documents, and we conclude the paper in Sect. 4. Sections 5 and 6 include future enhancements and results of the work done.

2 Problem Conception

2.1 System Model

Hosting data in the cloud involves three different entities, the data owner, the data user, and the cloud server. Assume the data owner holds documents *D*, which are to be outsourced to the cloud after the encryption, Let *C* be the encrypted documents. The text searching procedure is to be done over the encrypted collection *C*. To search the document collection *C* for the "*t*" given keywords, the user must be authorized with search control mechanisms like broadcast encryption [4]. The cloud server checks the authorization of the user and returns the corresponding encrypted documents set, based on the user requirement, i.e., the query "*Q*." For improving the accuracy of the result, the cloud server must be capable to rank the search result, conferring to some ranking criteria.

Finally, the access control mechanisms are employed for decryption process.

2.2 SkNN and MRSE Schemes

Secure kNN is the base of all methods used to retrieve the encrypted data over the cloud. SkNN in simple is the kNN computation applied on SCONEDB model. This method of data retrieval was introduced due to the results obtained from DRE [21], distance-recoverable encryption. According to Wong et al. [21], considering an encryption function *E*, and a key *K*, let *E*(*f*, *K*) be the encrypted value of a point *f* in DB. *E* is called as distance—recoverable if and only if there exists a computational procedure '*f*' such that

$$\forall p1, p2, K, f(E(p1, K), E(p2, K)) = d(p1, p2)$$

DRE resulted in attacker knowing the distance between the data points before and after encryption. Randomizing ASPE [27] and DRE, SkNN was introduced. SkNN which deals with stronger attacks concentrates on dimension extension and splitting the vector values of documents. Any number of equations can be tried by the attacker to decrypt the data; hence to make the scheme harder to crack, one process is to introduce randomness. To achieve this, considering the database point p, we split the value at each dimension randomly, in simple, we generate two d-dimensional point's p_a, p_b, such that p[i] = p [i] and thus we write $p = p_a + p_b$. As this technique does not secure the data, d-dimension vectors are considered, which can be achieved by adding artificial dimensions. The padding values can be 0 or 1.

MRSE is another scheme with improved security [22]. Here to quantitatively gage the similarity measure "coordinate matching," inner-product similarity [23] is used. Specifically, D_i is the binary vector for document F_i, where each bit,

$D[k]$ belongs to {0, 1}, represents the existence of keyword W_k, in the dictionary. The relevancy score can be stated as the inner product of query vector and data vector. These are the major concepts concentrated by MRSE.

Retrieval of Encrypted Documents by Euclidean Method
According to [21], Euclidean distance operator is used to obtain the perfect documents relevant to the user query.

Distance comparison operator
If F_1 and F_2 are two different documents whose encrypted points are F_1^1, F_2^1, then considering Q as the search word and its encrypted point as Q^1, the most relevant document to Q^1 can be found by $(F_1^1 - F_2^1) \cdot \mathrm{Q}^1 > 0$.

This method clearly compares the distance between the documents and outputs the best most relevant document. If we observe, we can clearly notice that the time complexity of retrieval using Euclidean method is same as a linear scan over unencrypted data.

Both the search and access controls are above the scope of this paper where, the prior illustrates how unauthorized users acquire keys and later explains managing access to outsourced data.

3 Secure Encryption and Retrieval of Documents

Usually, the texts we have are not the one we analyze. We likely want to break up a long text (such as a book-length work) into smaller chunks so we can get a sense of the variability. Search engines today (Google) most probably are avoiding the stemming process, and this trend may perhaps increase in future. Query expansion and wildcard queries can be used to emulate stemming.

"*Regex*" is the regular expression, which is used here for preprocessing the text. Once the text documents are uploaded, the words in the documents are gathered, (i.e.,) after tokenization and stemming processes a *collection* of words is made, which is named as the "*dictionary.*" Based on the terms, and their positions in the dictionary, our feature vectors are generated.

3.1 Feature Vector Generation

A document can be represented as a *vector* having binary values [1, 0]. Every document has its own vector representation, and this is defined as "*Document Vector*" of that particular document. The vector generated for a query is called as "*Query Vector.*" The meaning of the documents is conveyed by the words used, if a document is represented by its vector, it is probable to compare documents with search words to conclude how alike their content is. If a search word is considered to be like a document, a *Similarity Measure* that measures the similarity between the query and the document can be computed. Documents with content similar to the search word as per computation or the vector are considered the most relevant. The position of the term in the document is also given importance.

If a vector space model is considered, then the most similar document is the one pointing the same direction of the query vector. The angle between the document and the query vector represents similarity between them. We generated the document vectors for every document based on the collection of terms called a dictionary. Once the documents are uploaded, preprocessing is done and the terms are collected from the documents. These terms are further sorted into alphabetical order. Every time a new document gets uploaded, new terms are added to the dictionary and duplicates are emulated. Thus, dictionary is maintained.

Consider a document collection with merely two distinct terms, "A1" and "B1." All the vectors contain only two constituents, the first represents occurrences of "A1," and the second represents occurrences of "B1" within that document or query. The simplest means of building, a vector is to place a "1" in the corresponding vector component if the term appears, and a "0" if the term does not appear. Consider a document "D1" that contains two occurrences of term "A1" and 0 occurrence of term "B1." The vector $\langle 1, 0\rangle$ represents that document using a binary representation. This binary representation can be used to produce a similarity coefficient, but it does not consider the frequency of a term within a document.

Distance from the query to the two vectors is the similarity coefficient between query and documents. The document having the least distance from query vector will have the highest rank in the result set.

3.2 Encryption Process

The core objective of the scheme is to secure the data from being known to the cloud management. Documents selected by the data owner are uploaded to the cloud only after the encryption procedure is successfully completed, this is from the owner's point of view. Similarly, if we consider from users view, they typically wish to keep their search words from being wide-open to others like the cloud server, the most important concern is to hide what they are searching, i.e., the keywords. If some background data from the collection is known to server management, it would help them reverse engineer the actual data from the keyword. Hence, encryption is made both to the data set and the search query.

Encryption Requirements

1. **Key**: A key K is required for the encryption and decryption processes. A $d * d$ invertible matrix "*M*," (where d = number of terms in dictionary or size of vector)
2. **Document Encryption**: Consider a Document Vector D, then Encrypted Document is written as $P^1 = M^T * D$

3. **Query Encryption**: Consider a Query Vector Q, and then Encrypted Query is written as $Q^1 = M^{-1} * Q$

Document vectors need to be encrypted using the encryption key. We consider a matrix of size (d * d) as an encryption key, where d = the number of terms in the dictionary or it can also be defined as the size of the document vector or the query vector. The encryption process starts by representing the document vectors as column matrices.

After the column matrices are formed, every document is multiplied with the secret key we take. Depending on the size of the vectors, a random matrix of the same size is considered as the secret key. The encryption process used here is a symmetric key encryption.

Assuming $M = \begin{bmatrix} 1 & 0 & 0 \\ 0 & 1 & 1 \\ 1 & 0 & 1 \end{bmatrix}$ as the encryption key generated randomly and considering 3 terms in the dictionary. The inverse and the transpose of matrix M are written as

$$M^{-1} = \begin{bmatrix} 1 & 0 & 0 \\ 1 & 1 & -1 \\ -1 & 0 & 1 \end{bmatrix} \quad M^T = \begin{bmatrix} 1 & 0 & 1 \\ 0 & 1 & 0 \\ 0 & 1 & 1 \end{bmatrix}$$

These are used for encryption of documents and search terms.

3.3 *Retrieval of Encrypted Documents*

The encoded documents stored in the cloud are retrieved when the user requests a search keyword. Since the retrieval is to be done over the encrypted cloud data, traditional techniques are not sufficient, keeping in view the large number of data users and documents in the cloud, it is very much needed to allow multi-keyword search and return the most relevant documents to the user, hence, among different retrieval methods introduced earlier, *secure kNN* and *MRSE* are referred. As mentioned above, the retrieval of encrypted documents is done using distance comparison operator. Here, we also analyze the most relevant with three other distance measures (i.e.,) Euclidian, Manhattan, and Cosine distances. Figure 2 in results section shows the differences in results retrieved to the given query and documents in the cloud. The distance between the documents and user search word is considered with various similarity measures.

4 Conclusion

We illustrated and given the solution for keyword preserved ranked search over encrypted cloud data and provided a variety of privacy requirements. Among various multi-keyword semantics, we choose the efficient similarity measure of "coordinate matching," i.e., as many matches as possible, for capturing the best relevant documents to the search keywords and use "inner-product similarity" to quantitatively evaluate such similarity measure. We finally evaluate the process with other similarity measures for performance analysis.

5 Future Enhancements

In our future work, we will explore checking the integrity of the rank order in the search result and concentrate on how the access control which managed. If the symmetric key encryption is used, then the key management and transferring of the key while preserving the privacy using different methods can be explored.

6 Results

See Figs. 1, 2 and 3.

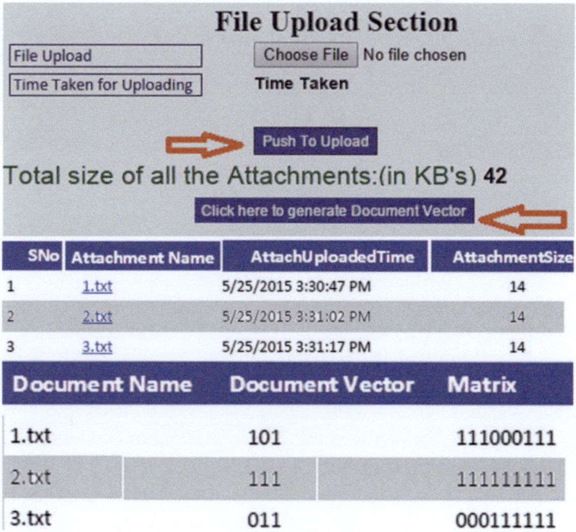

Fig. 1 Data owner view

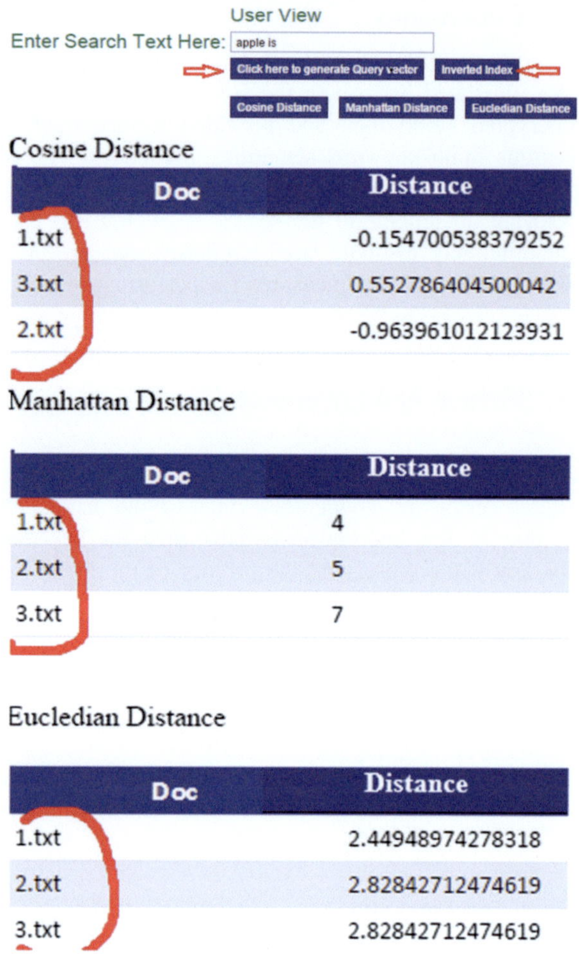

Fig. 2 User view

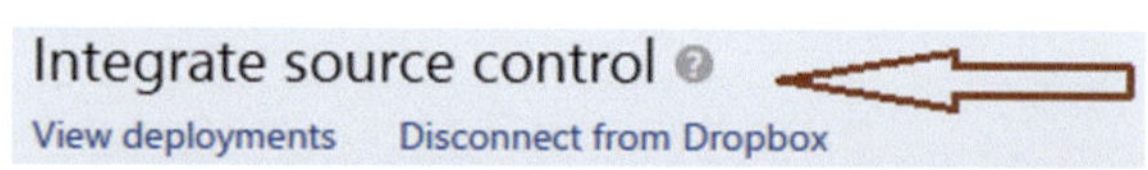

Fig. 3 Option in Azure to deploy the app

References

1. Song, D., Wagner, D., Perrig, A.: Practical techniques for searches on encrypted data. In: Proceedings of IEEE Symposium on Security and Privacy (2000)
2. Goh, E.-J.: Secure indexes. Cryptology ePrint Archive (2003). http://eprint.iacr.org/2003/216
3. Chang, Y.-C. , Mitzenmacher, M.: Privacy preserving keyword searches on remote encrypted data. In: Proceedings of Third International Conference on Applied Cryptography and Network Security (2005)

4. Curtmola, R., Garay, J.A., Kamara, S., Ostrovsky, R.: Searchable symmetric encryption: improved definitions and efficient constructions. In: Proceedings of 13th ACM Conference on Computer and Communications Security (CCS '06) (2006)
5. Boneh, D., Crescenzo, G.D., Ostrovsky, R., Persiano, G.: Public key encryption with keyword search. In: Proceedings of International Conference on Theory and Applications of Cryptographic Techniques (EUROCRYPT) (2004)
6. Bellare, M., Boldyreva, A., ONeill, A.: Deterministic and efficiently searchable encryption. In: Proceedings of 27th Annual International Cryptology Conference on Advances in Cryptology (CRYPTO '07) (2007)
7. Abdalla, M., Bellare, M., Catalano, D., Kiltz, E., Kohno, T., Lange, T., Malone-Lee, J., Neven, G., Paillier, P., Shi, H.: Searchable encryption revisited: consistency properties, relation to anonymous IBE, and extensions. J. Cryptol. **21**(3), 350391 (2008)
8. Li, J., Wang, Q., Wang, C., Cao, N., Ren, C., Lou, W.: Fuzzy keyword search over encrypted data in cloud computing. In: Proceedings of IEEE INFOCOM, Mar 2010
9. Boneh, D., Kushilevitz, E., Ostrovsky, R., Skeith III, W.E.: Public key encryption that allows PIR queries. In: Proceedings of 27th Annual International Cryptology Conference on Advances in Cryptology (CRYPTO '07) (2007)
10. Golle, P., Staddon, J., Waters, B. : Secure conjunctive keyword search over encrypted data. In: Proceedings of Applied Cryptography and Network Security, pp. 31–45 (2004)
11. Ballard, L., Kamara, S., Monrose, F.: Achieving efficient conjunctive keyword searches over encrypted data. In: Proceedings of Seventh International Conference on Information and Communications Security (ICICS '05) (2005)
12. (a) Boneh, D., Waters, B.: Conjunctive, subset, and range queries on encrypted data. In: Proceedings of Fourth Conference on Theory Cryptography (TCC), pp. 535-554, 2007. (b) Brinkman, R.: Searching in encrypted data. PhD thesis, University of Twente (2007)
13. Hwang, Y., Lee, P.: Public key encryption with conjunctive keyword search and its extension to a multi-user system. Pairing **4575**, 2–22 (2007)
14. Katz, J., Sahai, A., Waters, B.: Predicate encryption supporting disjunctions, polynomial equations, and inner products. In: Proceedings of 27th Annual International Conference on Theory and Applications of Cryptographic Techniques (EUROCRYPT) (2008)
15. Lewko, A., Okamoto, T., Sahai, A., Takashima, K., Waters, B.: Fully secure functional encryption: attribute-based encryption and (hierarchical) inner product encryption. In: Proceedings of 29th Annual International Conference on Theory and Applications of Cryptographic Techniques (EUROCRYPT '10) (2010)
16. Shen, E., Shi, E., Waters, B.: Predicate privacy in encryption systems. In: Proceedings of Sixth Theory of Cryptography Conference Theory of Cryptography (TCC) (2009)
17. Vaquero, L.M., Rodero-Merino, L., Caceres, J., Lindner, M.: A break in the clouds: towards a cloud definition. ACM SIGCOMM Comput. Commun. Rev. **39**(1), 50–55 (2009)
18. Cao, N., Yu, S., Yang, Z., Lou, W., Hou, Y.: LT codes-based secure and reliable cloud storage service. In: Proceedings of IEEE INFOCOM, pp. 693–701 (2012)
19. Wang, C., Cao, N., Li, J., Ren, K., Lou, W.: Secure ranked keyword search over encrypted cloud data. In: Proceedings of IEEE 30th International Conference on Distributed Computing Systems (ICDCS '10) (2010)
20. Wang, C., Cao, N., Ren, K., Lou, W.: Enabling secure and efficient ranked keyword search over outsourced cloud data. IEEE Trans Parallel Distrib Syst **23**(8), 14671479 (2012)
21. Wong, W.K., Cheung, D.W., Kao, B., Mamoulis, N.: Secure kNN computation on encrypted databases. In: Proceedings of 35th ACM SIGMOD International Conference on Management of Data (SIGMOD), pp. 139–152 (2009)
22. Cao, N., Wang, C., Li, M., Ren, K., Lou, W.: Privacy-preserving multi-keyword ranked search over encrypted cloud data. In: Proceedings of IEEE INFOCOM, pp 829-837, Apr 2011
23. Witten, I.H., Moffat, A., Bell, T.C.: Managing Gigabytes: Compressing and Indexing Documents and Images. Morgan Kaufmann Publishing, Burlington (1999)
24. Kamara, S., Lauter, K.: Cryptographic cloud storage. In: Proceedings of 14th International Conference on Financial Cryptograpy and Data Security, Jan 2010

25. Singhal, A.: Modern information retrieval: a brief overview. IEEE Data Eng Bull **24**(4), 35–43 (2001)
26. Li, M., Yu, S., Cao, N., Lou, W.: Authorized private keyword search over encrypted data in cloud computing. In: Proceedings of 31st International Conference on Distributed Computing Systems (ICDCS '10), pp. 383–392, June 2011

DCI^3 Model for Privacy Preserving in Big Data

Hemlata and Preeti Gulia

Abstract Big Data is like a hot cake in the market. It is an important discussion topic of different areas, like marketing management, research in science, security areas, etc. Nowadays, everyone is curious about the privacy risks of big and thereof legal issues emerge from the breach of privacy. In this paper, we have tried to cover major privacy and legal issues specific to Big Data. We have summarized different method to tackle the breach of privacy. Also, we have proposed DCI^3 legal model to reduce the legal problems for the security of data and information. Some legal cases from different areas specific to Big Data are also presented in the end.

Keywords Big data · Privacy · Security · Legal implications · DNT · DNC · DCI^3 legal model · IPR

1 Introduction

Big Data provides a big opportunity for the economy of the world in a variety of fields from credit risk analysis to urban planning and from marketing to medical research. But nowadays this positive side of Big Data is blackened by the data privacy and security issues. It is the biggest challenge to reach at equilibrium between privacy and benefits of Big Data [1]. Choices can be made between organization's policies and individual's rights. Different policies can be the law enforcement, efficient use of resources, security, etc., and individual rights can be the right to privacy, equality, speech, etc. The potential for Big Data is huge when it deals with marketing by Big Data Analytics. With the help of it, the marketers specifically target consumers by advertisements and special offers of products and

Hemlata (✉) · P. Gulia
Department of Computer Science and Applications,
M.D. University, Rohtak, India
e-mail: hemlatachahal@gmail.com

P. Gulia
e-mail: preeti.gulia81@gmail.com

V.B. Aggarwal et al. (eds.), *Big Data Analytics*, Advances in Intelligent
Systems and Computing 654, https://doi.org/10.1007/978-981-10-6620-7_34

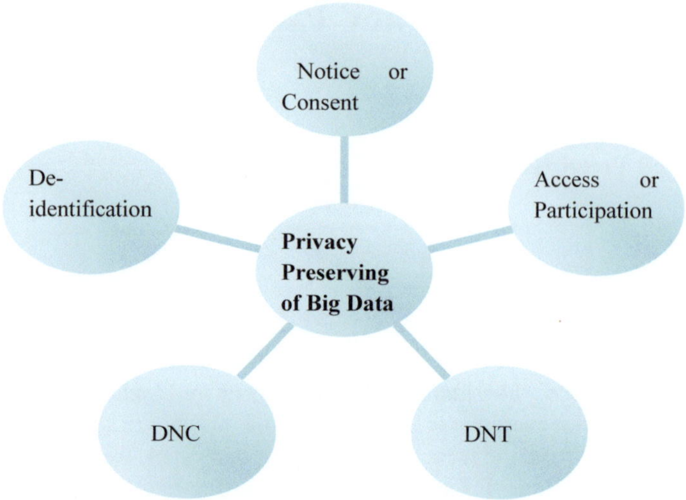

Fig. 1 Privacy preserving methods of Big Data

services. Through mobile's geo-spatial tracking, Big Data provides the individual with information that is highly relevant, delivered at right time and at the right place. Most important legal challenge of utilizing Big Data is privacy. Here, different methods for preserving privacy and providing security to data are presented (Fig. 1).

1.1 Notice or Consent

Data protection and privacy can be achieved through notice or awareness and consent or choice. While applying the rule of notice and awareness, the individual or organization must be disclosed how their personal information will be used, and to whom it will be accessible [2]. The people must understand how their data is being used by the organizations and give their consent to use it. If the data collected is collected by the organization for a particular purpose will be used for an altogether different objective or purpose, the organization should be liable to make the users aware about its use [3]. The notice allows the individual to choose whether his personal information should be collected and used. There are two problems here:

1. The individuals or consumers do not know where their personal information will go. Also, it can be joined with any another existing information which extracts more about the person.
2. The person is unaware about the interpretations and inferences which can be drawn from his personal data using techniques of Big Data mining and Big Data Analytics.

1.2 Access or Participation

Fair Credit Reporting Act (FCRA) [4] gave this principle of access and participation. According to this principle, the individual accesses his own data to be confident that if it is accurate and complete. It also allows them to correct inaccurate information. This access to their personal data is being given by different Credit reporting agencies.

In this Big Data era, it is a big challenge to satisfy the access/participation principle. Mostly, the consumers do not have a direct relationship with the company which is using their data, and also these companies do not receive the data directly from the individuals. Even if a consumer can find the company which has his or her profile, he or she may not take any legal action because of lack of contract conditions.

The Federal Trade Commission (FTC) calls on the representatives of the companies who collect and analyze the data for the purpose of marketing and ask them to design a centralized website to [5]:

1. Represent before the consumers how they use their data.
2. Describe all the access rights which they provide for their customers [5].

1.3 DNT and DNC

Another privacy-affected area is Do Not Track (DNT) [6]. Do Not Track (DNT) means the consumer's data should not be used for targeted advertising. Federal Trade Commission (FDC) states the concept of DNT which prohibits the targeting of individuals and individual's personal information collection (Do Not Collect). While the individual's information collected from multiple sources, the companies are able to identify the identity of users and preferences of users. This collection reveals the sensitive information i.e., health information, financial information, likes, dislikes, and behavior.

Tracking and collecting individual's personal information are a serious breach of privacy. There should be strict laws to stop it. The companies should be allowed only after sharing the information with the person himself or herself that it is using the information for the specified objective. This gives the company the consent of using the personal information.

1.4 De-identification and Re-identification

Another problem with Big Data is de-identification and anonymization. Anonymization refers to the process of preventing the data identity of the data owner from any future re-identification in all conditions [7, 8]. De-identification is the process of preservation of identifying information of the data owner [8]. Strict guidelines have been issued by the Department of Health and Human Services for de-identification of data related to health. The civil rights office has identified two methods for de-identification under HIPAA [9]:

1. expert determination
2. safe harbor

European data protection laws state that anonymized data should not identify the concerned data even by the intermingling of anonymized information [10]. Anonymized data can re-identify individuals if de-identification is not done properly. There are many examples in which re-identification has occurred. One popular example of re-identification is Netflix. In a contest, the customers were asked to make a movie recommendation engine. For this, the company gave an anonymous set of data of 480,000 customers. Some researchers claimed that they have identified some of the customers by retrieving and analyzing already available information publically [11]. Afterwards, the contest led to a lawsuit against Netflix [12]. In another popular example, a researcher claimed that from an anonymous healthcare database, she had re-identified some of the individuals on the basis of their voter records available publicly. She re-identified the information of Massachusetts governor [13].

2 Literature Review

After the emergence of the concept of Big Data Analytics, problems like security and privacy came into existence. This is relatively a new analysis, and hence legal problems emerge out of it. Due to its recent development, there is a limited literature on it. The legal framework is formally not chalked out. In this section, we summarize different methods which can be treated as equivalent to legal framework of the privacy of Big Data.

2.1 Legal Framework in UK [14]

The legal framework for the law enforcement in UK(United Kingdom) and implemented by EU(European Union) is as follows:

- Human Rights—The law enforcement should safeguard the human rights of each and every user whose data is to be saved.
- Purpose Limiting—The compilation of different types of data should be fora specific purpose.

- Further Processing—The stored data should be processed for further mining and extracting useful data from it.
- Public Trust and Confidence—The storage and processing of data should be of such level that it should have the trust of the public that their data will not be misused. If the confidence of public is not with the processing organization, there are chances of legal cases.

2.2 European Legal Framework [14]

Since the inception in 1970s, this framework has faced many developments and alterations due to technological advancements. The two steps according to this framework for the data protection are:

- Directive 95/46/EC and Revision 2012
- Data Retention Directive

2.3 Italian Legal Framework [14]

This framework clearly defines the difference between data protection rights and secrecy rights. Former can be defined as the protection of data and information and its use. The latter can be defined as the right not to publicize the private and family data and knowledge. According to it, the Government has the authority to protect one's personal data, and it cannot be challenged. The privacy is protected by the law, namely, The Italian Privacy Code. The objective of this code is to give protection to data on the principal of harmonization and simplification. It defines different provisions on different categories of data:

- Sensitive Data
- Judiciary Data
- Semi-sensitive Data
- Traffic Data

3 DCI^3 Legal Model

The existing frameworks as depicted in the earlier section are specific to the rules of a particular region like Italy, Europe, etc. So, there are problems while implementing them universally. Also, these frameworks do not include the exact steps for minimizing the legal problems arising out of the data storage, processing and mining new data without losing the privacy of data owner.

Fig. 2 DCI^3 legal model

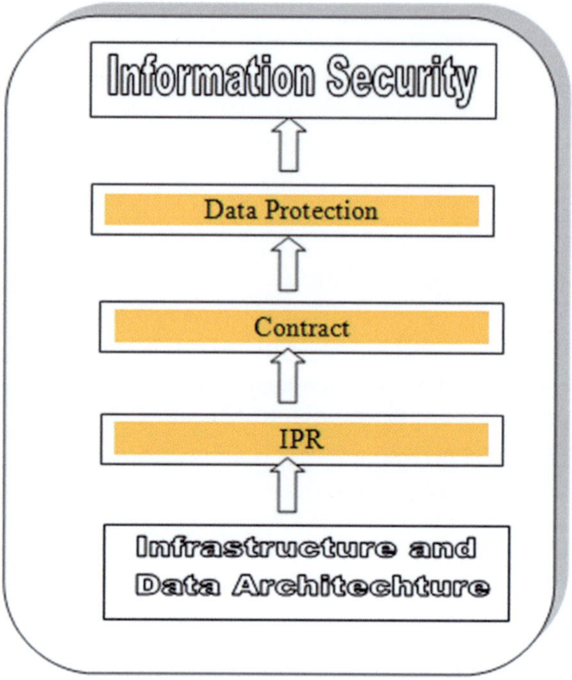

In light of the limitations encountered, we propose a model (Fig. 2) which provides five steps to protect data legally. In this model, we have tried to make a foolproof system of data protection and privacy which can be implemented universally.

In the model, three levels (IPR, Contract, and data protection) are sandwiched between **i**nfrastructure and architecture from the lower and information security from the upper side. This model depicts that as we go up from one level to another our privacy and security of data increases. In the topmost level i.e., information security, not only the data stored, but also information extracted is also secure and free from all legal issues.

3.1 Infrastructure and Data Architecture

Physical infrastructure consists of storage devices, routers, gateways, network servers, and the software of these devices like operating system, data connectivity software, etc. In light of the law, software copyright issues arise. Copyright is a formal remedy of protecting expression. Hence, while creating or inventing any hardware device or creating any software for this hardware everyone should go for **copyright**, in order to avoid any legal complexity.

Data Architecture includes data structure, design, schemas, format, model as a representation of data flows through data entities, attributes, and interrelationships. This is protectable by copyright rules in the EU (Chapter II, Article 3 of the Database Directive) [15]. One should have copyright for the data structures, database design, and schemas to be safe from high-level copying act. This is the safest way to avoid any legal problem.

3.2 IPR (Intellectual Property Right)

"Intellectual Property Rights" means the rights attained to protect ones original creations [16]. These rights can be of two types [16]:

1. Industrial Property Rights—It includes patents, industrial designs, and trademarks.
2. Copyright—It means the right of the creator.

In light of data, IPR includes copyright, database right, confidentiality, patents, right to inventions, and trademarks. Copyright, database right, and confidentiality are directly related to data but patents and trademarks are not directly related to data. Patents apply to software and business process, and trademarks apply to data products.

Copyright [16]: The mechanism which protects the original work from copying without accessible rights is copyright. In true sense of the word, it means the rights attached to the tin. For copyright of the data or software, the documentations such as written statements and technical details should be considered. The related laws and regulations should be initiated so that copyright of data is not infringed.

Database right [16]: Database right was launched on January 1, 1998, by the Database Directive, implementing EU legislation. The owner of database right is the maker, the person who takes the risk of obtaining, verifying, and presenting its contents. The duration of database right is of 15 years [16]. Database right is violated if a user uses the whole or part of data without permission [16]. The individual who wants to build his database rights should claim and assert the rights in relevant systems. He should amend processes and internally and externally available documentation.

Confidentiality: Confidentiality is a set of rules that controls access or puts restrictions on different types of information [17]. In the medical field, confidentiality is the most important duties of medical practice. Health care providers must keep a patient's personal health information secret unless consent is provided by the patient [18]. Confidentiality is right for protection without a contract. In a contract, it is shown that the information is not accessible publicly. There are different rules for different organizations which express their inability to disclose all their data publically—it is an example of confidentiality.

3.3 Contract

Contract is an authorized agreement to enforce responsibilities and grant rights of the data between parties. To grant cogent rights, strict liability is the rule of contract. The UK High Court in 2006 said that the data owner can use the data as a user with or without having the IP rights [19]. Contract rights operate 'in person am' i.e., it can be enforceable only on the concerned parties not anyone else. Contract rights are applicable only to the concerned party of agreement. Some important points while making a contract can be:

License—The agreement should contain all the rules regarding reservation of rights and should be personal to the licensee.

Derived Data—The contracting parties should be well aware of the fact that a party of agreement can use the data for procuring new knowledge from the concerned data. The parties must know which rights are owned by them in the acquired data.

Intermingling—Intermingling data is the data in which the user takes the data as input from one or more source and creates altogether new intermingled data (in the same way as we mix two colors and creates a third and all together new color). The contract should cover exactly what will happen. Confidentiality can provide some help in intermingling.

Data Minimization—The contracting parties should agree on the use of minimum data for specific purpose. They should not use unnecessarily everything for their small objective.

Termination—The most important question is that what will happen after contract termination. Most of the contracts are silent for post-term use. The user or licensee should know if can use it after cessation of the contract.

The contract should cover all data and the confidential information that is relevant. It should include all the present and future rights of the data concerned. One level up now, the rights has strong liabilities, and the licensee is legally more responsible if conditions of contract not followed. So, contract law is much stronger than IPR.

3.4 Data Protection

The greatest barrier to the advancement of Big Data is data protection. Data protection means imposing rights and responsibility of processing personal data. Data regulation states that the data should be processed in a lawful manner i.e., it should be adequate, accurate, and precise.

After Contract, there should be some regulating authorities who can regulate the IPR as well as contract of data. These regulatory authorities should check specific-rule formulations for specific industries. Data protection is not only for any sector-specific industry. The specific industry rules are relevant to the data of the sector concerned. From generations, the main objectives of legal profession are confidentiality and privilege given to clients [16].

3.5 Information Security

The topmost level of legal model is information security. At this level, we are concerned with the security and privacy of information and not of data. In all the four lower layers, data is secured by copyright, IPR, Contract, and regulations imposed by regulatory authorities. The information derived or extracted from the data should also be secure from unauthorized and illegal use. Different standards are set up by different organizations for their information security. Here, the data is processed and translated into information which should be secured. Payment Card Industry (PCI) published and operates DSS (Data Security Standards). ISO (International Standard Organization) has also published 27,000 series of ISMS (Information Security Management Systems). SSAE 16 is the new "attest" standard given by the Auditing Standards Board of the American Institute of Certified Public Accountants [19]. These are some of the standards setup for information security. In the Big Data world, these are not sufficient as data comes in big quantity and big velocity. So these standards should be modified and strict as per present day requirement. Also, there should be more strict and severe fines and punishments for the infringement of these laws.

3.6 Summary of the DCI^3 Model

The model provides a novel approach to deal with the privacy and security of Big Data and thereof its legal implications. The success of the model lies in the fact that how accurate is the compliance of the steps of the model. It is true to say here that it is easy to make rules and regulations, but very difficult to implement them in real life.

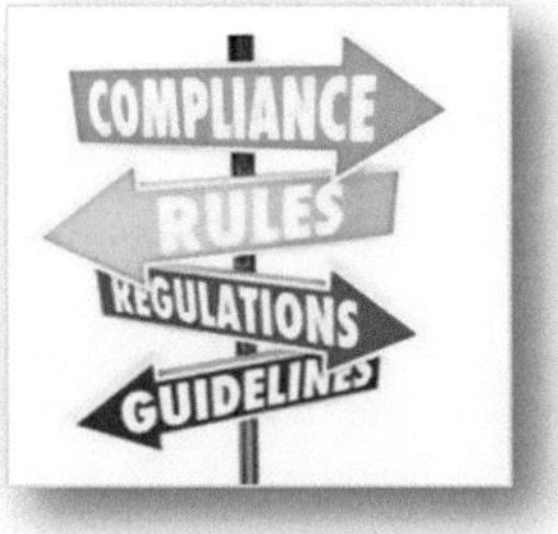

4 Data Protection Legal Cases

Some of the related legal cases are presented along with the decisions of the court for ready reference.

4.1 Copyright Case [16]

In 2003, District Court of Maryland decided a copyright case, Lowry v Legg Mason. Legg Mason was found guilty of willful copyright infringement and breach of contract. Lowry is a publisher, and Legg Mason is a firm of financial services. The firm was guilty of unauthorized copying and distribution of the financial newsletter. Legg mason was awarded $19,725,270 as a fine for damages.

4.2 DNT and DNC Case [20]

A store of Minneapolis tracked the buying habits of customers and sent some coupons to the father of a teenager girl. The coupons were related to pregnancy. After receiving them father lodged a complaint against the store. But after analysis it was found that the predictive model of the store was correct, and the girl was pregnant about which the father was unaware. Subsequently, the man apologized to the store.

4.3 Copying Data Case [16]

In August 2010, UBS was sued in the UK courts for allegedly copying of articles from oil and gas publication, reprinting them, and distributing it to clients.

4.4 Contract Breach Cases [16]

1. In November 2010, a breach of contract was identified between Tullett Prebon and BGC Capital Partners for the reproduction of US Treasury data.
2. In May 1982, US District Court of New York heard a case Standard & Poor's Corp v Commodity Exchange Inc. The Commodity Exchange Inc. misused the equity stocks created by the Standard & Poor's Corp for future contracts and misused its trade name and reputation.

3. In November 2004, The British Horseracing Board ("BHB") versus William Hill case came into light for database right infringement. BHB created a stud list which included fixture lists. European court of Justice(ECJ) decided that Mr. William Hill infringed the database right of BHB by using its data on internet site for its personal benefits.

4.5 Database Copyright Case [16]

Again another important decision for database copyright case was Football Dataco Ltd. vs Brittens Pools Ltd. Football Dataco Ltd. initiated football league matches in Scotland and England. So the company had commercial rights for holding license to sell fixture lists. But Brittens Pools Ltd. is a gambling organization which used the fixtures list without license. Justice J Floyd asserted that the data was protected under Article 3, which involved labor and skill.

4.6 Trademark Case [16]

In 1987, a trade mark case came into the limelight—Golden Nugget Inc vs American Stock Exchange. American Stock Exchange (ASE) issued and used Golden Nugget's stock without its consent. Golden Nugget sued that ASE is involved in unfair means to infringe the Golden Nugget trade mark.

5 Conclusion and Future Work

In the Big Data era, privacy and security are the most important legal issues. Some of the steps to save the privacy of the data are presented in the paper. A new model is proposed in this regard which can be beneficial to some extent. But there is a lot of scope in this field of research. Researchers can develop altogether new paradigm to keep our data/database secure from others. Government can also develop new laws in this regard. Companies or organizations should issue strict orders to the workers for not disclosing the private data to the third party.

References

1. Ira Rubinstein, Big Data: The End of Privacy or a New Beginning? 3 INT'L DATA PRIVACY L. 74, 77–78 (2013)

2. Tene, Omer, Polonetsky, Jules: Big data for all: privacy and user control in the age of analytics, 11 NW. J. Tech. Intell. Prop. **239**, 240–242 (2013)
3. Consent of Customer to Use Personal Data: http://www.ftc.gov/reports/privacy3/
4. Big Data and Data Protection, ICO Informations Commissioner's Office
5. Fair Credit Reporting Act (FCRA), 15 U.S.C. § 1681, et. seq
6. Young, M.: The technical writer's handbook-protecting consumer privacy in an era of rapid change. University Science, Mill Valley, CA (1989)
7. http://www.infolawgroup.com/2012/03/articles/data-privacy-law-or-regulation/ftc-looks-to-link-donottrack-big-data-privacy-concerns-seeks-solutions/
8. Godard, B., et al.: Data storage and DNA banking for biomedical research: Informed consent, confidentiality, quality issues, ownership, return of benefits. A professional perspective. Eur. J. Hum. Genet. (2003)
9. De-identification of Customer Data: http://en.wikipedia.org/wiki/De-identification
10. Annonymised and De-identification of Information: http://www.hhs.gov/ocr/privacy/hipaa/understanding/coveredentities/De-identification/hhs_deid_guidance.pdf
11. European Union Directive 95/46/EC
12. Robust De-annonymization of Large Data Sets: How to break anonymity of the netflix prize data set. http://arxiv.org/PS_cache/cs/pdf/0610/0610105v2.pdf
13. Example of Anonymous Data: http://www.wired.com/images_blogs/threatlevel/2009/12/doe-v-netflix.pdf
14. Akhgar, B., et al.: Application of Big Data for National Security—A Practitioners Guide to Emerging Technologies. Elsevier, Amsterdam (2015)
15. Example of Legal Case: http://www.cs.duke.edu/~ashwin/pubs/BigPrivacyACMXRDS_final.pdf
16. Example of Legal Case: http://eur-lex.europa.eu/LexUriServ/LexUriServ.do?uri=CELEX:31996L0009:EN:HTML
17. Kemp, R., et al.: Legal rights in data (27 CLSR [2], pp. 139–151), or Practical Law at http://uk.practicallaw.com/5-504-1074?q=Big+Data+Kemp
18. Confidentiality of Personal Data: http://en.wikipedia.org/wiki/Confidentiality
19. Confidentiality of Personal Data: https://depts.washington.edu/bioethx/topics/confiden.html
20. DNT and DNC Case: http://isae3402.com/ISAE3402
21. Navetta, D.: Legal implications of big data. ISSA J. (2013)
22. Data Security Standards: http://www.bailii.org/ew/cases/EWHC/Ch/2005/3015.html
23. Nelson, S.D., Simek, J.W.: BIG DATA: big pain or big gain for lawyers? Law Pract. Mag. EBSCO Host Connect. **39**(4)
24. Stanford Law Review Online.: Special issue for the proceeding of the Workshop conducted by Future of Privacy Forum and Center for Internet and Society at Stanford Law School, vol. 66, p. 25 Sept 2013
25. Kemp, R.: Legal aspects of managing Big Data. White papers of IT+, Sept 2014
26. Cloud Security Alliance: Top ten Big Data security and privacy challenges, Nov 2012

Study of Sentiment Analysis Using Hadoop

Dipty Sharma

Abstract In the current world of Internet people express themselves, present their views and feelings about specific topics or entities using various social media application. These posts from users present a huge opportunity for the organizations to increase their market value by analyzing the posts and using information in decision making. These posts can be studied using various machine learning and lexicon-based approaches for extracting its sentiments. With more and more people moving to internet, huge data is being produced every second and challenge is to store this large data and process it efficiently in real time to infer knowledge from this data. This paper presents different approaches for real-time and scalable ways of performing sentiment analysis using Hadoop in a time efficient manner. Hadoop and its component tools like MapReduce, Mahout, and Hive are being surveyed in different scholar articles for this paper.

Keywords Sentiment analysis · Twitter · Hadoop · MapReduce · Hive · Mahout

1 Introduction

As e-commerce is gaining popularity, more and more e-commerce sites are being launched. These sites are constantly in need to keep its customers happy and to identify ways to overcome competition. One way to achieve customer satisfaction is to be able to present and display the products based on customer's interests. With sites like Twitter, Facebook etc., users are provided with a platform to post emotions, views, and likings about various topics, people, product, and services. Opinions expressed in social media can be classified to determine the orientation (negative, positive, and neutral) of the posted text. Sentiment strength and intensity

D. Sharma (✉)
IBM India, Bengaluru, India
e-mail: diptysha@gmail.com

D. Sharma
UIT, Barkatullah University, Bhopal, India

V.B. Aggarwal et al. (eds.), *Big Data Analytics*, Advances in Intelligent Systems and Computing 654, https://doi.org/10.1007/978-981-10-6620-7_35

of the post are determined with the aim to identify opinion and emotion of the user about a specific product or service.

Sentiment of textual posts can be analyzed in three different levels:

- Document Level

Analytical study performed for the whole document, determining the polarity (positivity, negativity or neutrality) of the document on the subject as a whole.

- Sentence Level

Analytical study performed for each statement or sentence where each sentence is expressed as positive, negative or neutral.

- Aspect Level

Analytical study performed at fine-granular level. Each aspect or feature of product is analyzed, and polarity is determined for each feature.

Technically, following are ways to perform sentiment analysis.

1. Machine learning Approach

Sentiment analysis process can be performed using various machine learning algorithms like Naïve Bayes. These learning approaches are based on building classifiers from labeled instances of textual posts. They perform well for the domain on which they are trained.

2. Lexicon-Based Approach

These approaches calculate emotional orientation of a document from the semantic orientation of words or phrases in the document. These dictionary-based approaches consist of dictionary of number of words annotated with their polarity, strength, and semantic orientation.

With increase in access to Internet and more people coming online and using e-commerce. Textual information on internet is increasing every second, and it is a challenge to read and process this vast data set in efficient manner.

Hadoop provides a framework (Fig. 1) commonly used by academic and industry for Big Data analysis. It allows collection, storage, retrieval, management, and distributed processing of huge data sets using cluster of computers and simple programming models. Each machine in Hadoop cluster has local storage and can perform local computation. Hadoop is highly performance intensive, scalable, and flexible development framework for parallel processing. Hadoop framework offers reliable service availability by detecting and handling failures at application layer itself.

Audience of this paper are professionals and practitioners who intend to perform sentiment analysis using Hadoop. Section 2 shows how the steps in sentiment analysis process maps with different components of Hadoop. Section 3 describes scholarly articles on sentiment analysis using Hadoop. Section 4 provides detailed

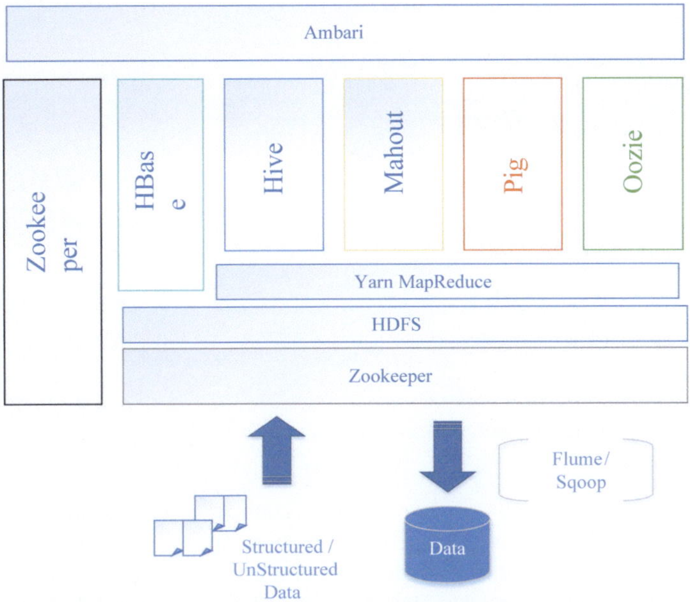

Fig. 1 Hadoop eco system

review on various aspects for performing sentiment analysis in Hadoop. Section 5 concludes on using Hadoop for sentiment analysis.

2 Implementation of Sentiment Analysis in Hadoop

Process of sentiment analysis involves collection of textual data from various sources like blogs, reviews, social sites etc., processing this vast volume of data to remove unwanted, undesirable text, analyzing, extracting sentiment of collected data and integrating with applications to help decision making. A simple process of sentiment analysis is shown in Fig. 2 involves following steps (1) Data Collection (2) Data Preprocessing (3) Analysis.

Following section lists one to one mapping of sentiment analysis process steps in Hadoop Framework Fig. 7.

2.1 Data Collection and Storage

HDFS and Hive provide data storage capabilities in Hadoop. Hadoop Distributed File System (HDFS) provides distributed file system that can store data in different

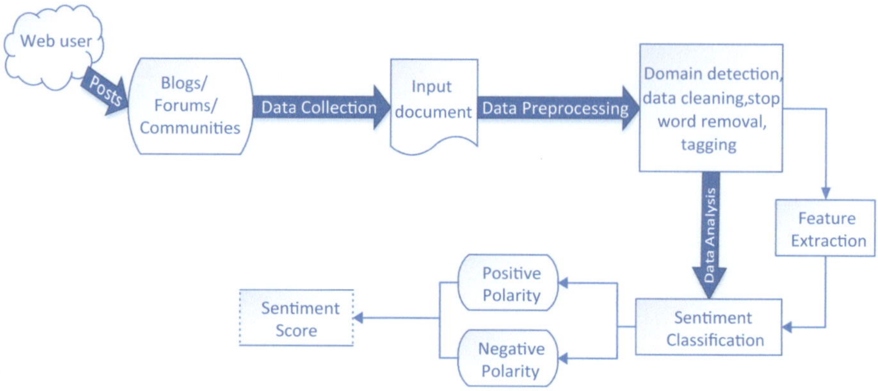

Fig. 2 Process flow of sentiment analysis

formats. It provides high-throughput access to application data. Data present in logs or files can be read using MapReduce programming and stored in HDFS. MapReduce core component of Hadoop. It is a java-based framework for writing easy applications which process vast amounts of data in parallel. A MapReduce *job* splits the input data set into independent chunks which are processed by the *map tasks* in a completely parallel manner Fig. 3. The framework sorts the outputs of the maps, which are then input to the *reduce tasks* Fig. 4. Both the input and the output of the jobs are stored in a HDFS. The framework takes care of scheduling tasks, monitoring them and re-executes the failed tasks.

Real-time data from Twitter can be streamed into HDFS using Flume. Flume [1] has a simple and flexible architecture efficiently collecting, aggregating, and moving large amounts of log data. Data from Twitter in the form of Json can be partitioned based on posted dates and stored in Hive for processing. Hive is a data warehouse infrastructure that provides data summarization and ad hoc querying using SQL like commands. Large data present in relational database can also be loaded into HDFS, Hive using Sqoop. Sqoop [2] imports and exports data from numerous relational databases. Figures 5 and 6 show the process architecture of Flume and Sqoop.

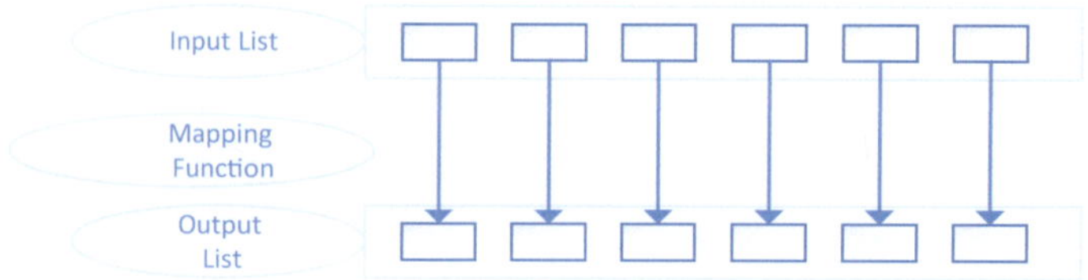

Fig. 3 Mapper function

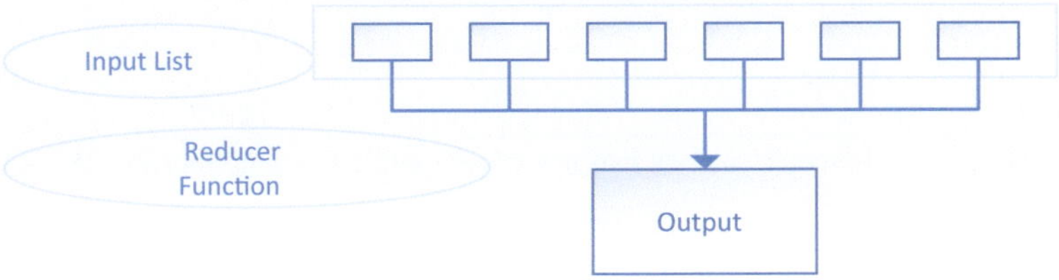

Fig. 4 Reducer function

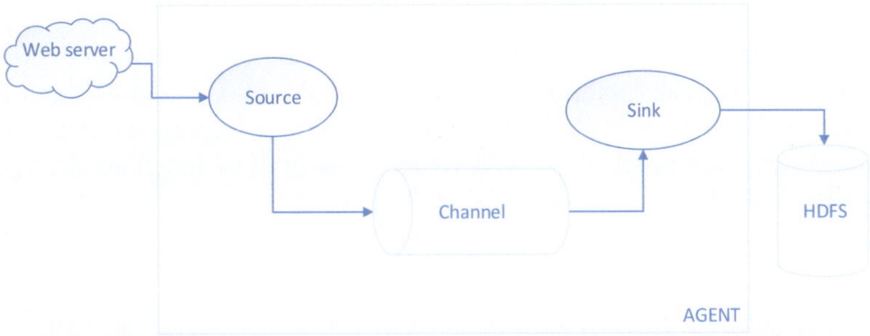

Fig. 5 Flume architecture

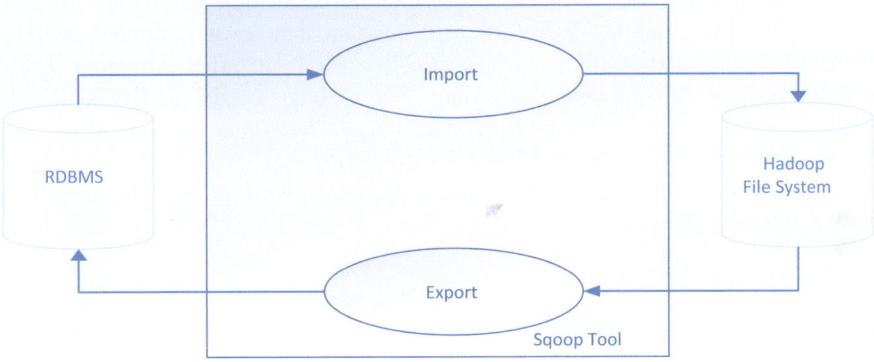

Fig. 6 Sqoop data flow

2.2 *Data Preprocessing*

Data preprocessing is natural language processing steps required to clean the textual data from all the unwanted text from the collection of data. Data preprocessing involves cleaning the data: removal of stop words, spell check, conversion of unstructured data into structured data (e.g., happpyyy → happy), conversion of slangs (e.g., luv → love, OMG → oh my god), conversion of hash tags and

Table 1 Hive pre-post processing functions

Built-in functions	Usage	Output
Sentences	Tokenizes a string into words and sentences, returns an array of words	Array
Explode	Returns one row for each element from the array	Rows
get_json_object	Returns json string of the extracted json object	String
json_tuple	Returns a tuple of values using one function from json string	Tuple

emoticons and extracting important features, removing duplicates, and converting data formats. External Libraries like NLTK python library and OpenNLP java library can be plugged with MapReduce or User Defined Functions (UDFs) in Hive for natural language processing. A Hive provides built-in functions for text pre-processing Table 1.

2.3 *Sentiment Classification*

Sentiment analysis of text data is essentially the classification of text, based on the strength and polarity (positive/negative) of the opinion words that defines the text. Hadoop provides framework for users to develop their own sentiment analysis algorithms using lexicon dictionary, available APIs or external programs. These algorithms can be implemented using MapReduce or Hive UDFs [3] in Hadoop. Hive also provides built-in text analysis functions Table 2. Hive uses N-gram Probabilistic language Model for predicting next word in a sequence of words. Mahout provides machine learning library consisting of different inbuilt classifiers [4–6] (Fig. 7).

Table 2 Hive built-in classifier

Built-in functions	Usage	Output
ngrams	Find important topics using a stop word list, trending topics	k most frequently occurring n grams
Context_ngrams	Extract intelligence around certain keywords, pre compute search look ahead	k most frequently occurring n grams

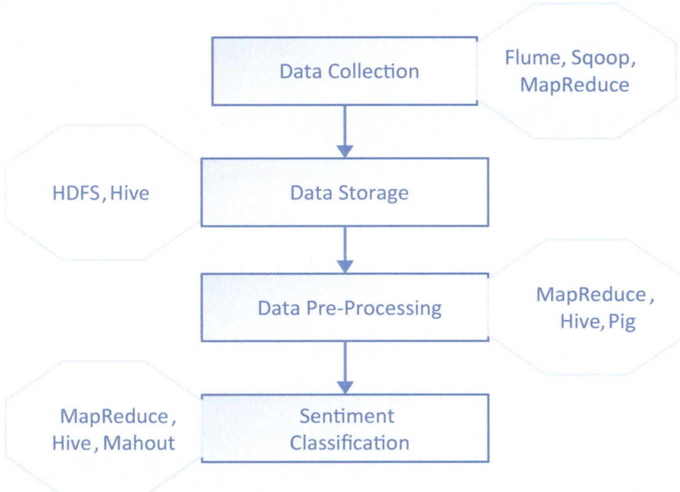

Fig. 7 Step by step mapping on hadoop

3 Literature Survey

A Speedy Data Uploading Approach for Twitter Trend and Sentiment Analysis Using Hadoop

Gaurav et al. [7] in their paper demonstrated how open source framework of Hadoop can help organizations with real time, cost effective and secure social analytics. Their study presents a distributed Hadoop system using HDFS, Pig, Hive and Oozie for Twitter trend analysis. Querying Twitter post in RDBMS is difficult because of multiple retweets of same post. It is important to identify who is prominent. Their proposed work combined open source software and hardware phenomenon. Data download speed is increased with the help of network-based application. Latency and network delays are removed. Reliable connection between source and sink is established using application on Twitter side. Their work shows how data available in HDFS is processed with help of Hive and Pig. To coordinate and schedule the processes, they used Oozie. Zookeeper helped maintain the configuration information providing distributed synchronization. Their work shows how Hadoop can help increase organization profits by reducing cost, time delays, and security issues.

Real Time Sentiment Analysis of Twitter Data Using Hadoop

Mane et al. [8] use MapReduce programming framework lexicon dictionary-based sentiment analysis at sentence level. Data is collected in real time using Twitter streaming API and stored in HDFS. Collected data is preprocessed to remove the stop words, convert unstructured text to structured text and convert emoticons into words using OpenNLP implementation. Lexicon dictionary of sentiment words using SentiWordNet is generated. All possible usage of a word is obtained to determine the overall sentiment of the word and updated in the dictionary. They used numbering approach to assign suitable range for different sentiments. To reduce the search time dictionary is stored local memory. Naïve Bayes algorithm is implemented using chained MapReduce jobs to process each tweet and assign sentiment to each word. PMR-IR algorithm is implemented to determine orientation of phrases. Sentiment of tweet is computed by aggregating the sentiments for each word in tweet. Overall accuracy of 72% is achieved. Time efficiency is achieved for large data set using Hadoop.

The Evaluation of the Public Opinion a Case Study: MERS-CoV Infection Virus in KSA

Zarrad et al. [9] based their study on methods similar to [10]. Their work is to detect sentiments on Arabic Tweets on MERS Virus using multiple Hive UDFs (User defined functions) using Arabic lexicon. Keyword-based search performed on certain words like MERS-CoV virus is done using Twitter Rest API. Tweets are collected and stored into HDFS using Flume. Because of the complexities of Arabic language, a custom text preprocessing module is developed to clean the text. Sentiment analysis module is developed using Hive UDF. Lexicon based on MPQA is manually updated with 1100 negative and 850 positive words. Lexicon is translated into Arabic for this work. Their proposed sentiment detection algorithm can search up to 5 consecutive composite words in polarity lexicon and can detect negation on opinion. Proposed algorithm can identify positive word affected by non-consecutive negative word. To get the satisfaction measure of efforts undertaken by Heath Ministry on controlling MERS-CoV virus, they collected tweets for four months and evaluated public opinion.

Big Data Sentiment Analysis Using Hadoop

Ramesh et al. [11] proposed sentence level sentiment analysis using lexicon dictionary-based approach. The study shows how accuracy of sentiment detection can be achieved while focusing on speedy processing on vast data sets using Hadoop. They created dictionary of sentiment words with strength (strong, weak) and polarity (positive, negative, negation, and blind negation) for each word. Dictionary consists of all forms of words to avoid stemming each word to increase processing time. Negation and blind negation words that reverse the polarity of sentence are included in the dictionary. Sentiment analysis is performed by combining the polarity of the word its strength to compute the sentiment score with score 0 as neutral polarity. Sentence polarity is aggregation of words score. Polarity of sentence is reversed when blind negation word is identified in the sentence. Their study shows how lexicon-based sentiment analysis implemented in Hadoop performs better than machine learning approaches for the real-time data that is not domain specific.

Cloud-Based Predictive Analytics

Kalvdiya et al. [12] studies are based on machine learning based text classification on cloud environment. They suggested category-based text classification of e-mails, to automatically classify incoming news feeds into appropriate categories. The classification results contained the index of the category label and best associated score output.

For classification training data, they collected set of e-mails from Mahout and Hive user list to train Naïve Bayesian algorithm. E-mails were stored in HDFS, and Mahout Command was used to train the classifier model. Data for training is represented in word-vector format using TF-IDF (term frequency–inverse document frequency), which involves counting word frequencies over large corpus of documents. Feature document vector was created with TF-IDF weighting implemented by Mahout to give more weight to specific topic words. Naïve Bayes classifier model was performance tested by running Mahout testnb command.

To use the classifier model for new text files java program was written using Mahout Libraries. Files in directories were converted into sequential format, and TF-IDF sparse vectors were generated and then classified using the model. Model was run on the cloud using Maven to manage dependencies. During their work they identified that Mahout scales well with massive data sets and performs comparable to other machine learning algorithms.

Research on Public Opinion Based on Big Data

Shang et al. [13] demonstrate how Mahout algorithms can be efficiently used for processing large scale and complex Big Data. Mahout text mining algorithms are presented to handle high-dimensional data. Preprocessing of data was done using TF-Gini algorithm, and processing of text is performed using Mahout algorithms. Their research demonstrated clustering algorithms: canopy and k-means algorithms. Canopy algorithm differs from traditional algorithm as it uses two computing distance methods and computes only overlapping data vectors. Mahout's built-in Naïve Bayes algorithm for classification, Apriori and FP-tree algorithms for pattern mining are presented. Mahout used Parallel Frequent Pattern Mining. Firstly identifying one-dimensional frequent items and then dividing original data set into different groups based on frequent items. FP-tree is computed for each group. FP-tree is mining to get frequent items, and result is obtained by merging each FP-tree frequent items. The proposed system using parallel computing function of Hadoop Mahout.

Scalable Sentiment Classification for Big Data Analysis Using Naive Bayes Classifier

Liu et al. [14] present scalable implementation of Naïve Bayes algorithm to analyze sentiment sentences of millions of movie reviews. They build Big Data analyzing system using simple MapReduce analyzing jobs and work flow controller (WFC), user terminal, result collector and data parser.

Movie reviews collected was preprocessed through data parser in desired data format. Unwanted context such as punctuation, special symbols, and numbers was deleted and each review was split into one line in data set tagged with sentiment and document id. Data parser would return the desired number of positive and negative reviews on request to WFC. WFC manages work flow of the whole system and stores data set in HDFS for training. Training job, combining job, and classifier job were executed in sequence. The training job builds a model that computes the polarity of each word based on the frequency of word. The combining job generates an intermediate table by associating the test data with the model, excluding the words that appear in test data but not in the model. Classifier job then classifies reviews into positive or negative and output the results into HDFS. The statistics of true positive, true negative, false positive, and false negative were recorded. Result collector would retrieve the model, intermediate table, classification result, and statistics of test from HDFS. User terminal was used to submit user jobs and results were accessible in user terminal after result collected finished collection. The scalability of the algorithm in Hadoop was tested with accuracy of 82% with changing the data set size from one thousand to one million in each class.

Scaling Archived Social Media Data Analysis Using a Hadoop Cloud

Conejero et al. [15] present COSMOS platform for Twitter data analysis on socially significant events. Cardiff Online Social Media Observatory (COSMOS) platform provides mechanisms to capture, analyze and visualize results of real-time data. They demonstrated how this system can scale using OpenNebula Cloud environment with MapReduce using Hadoop for Big Data. COSMOS ingest and archives the spritzer stream using Twitter Streaming API. Approximately, 3.5 million messages per day can be processed using COSMOS API. Collection of virtual machines makes Hadoop cluster. OpenNebula helps decide size and characteristics of Hadoop cluster. Kernel-based Virtual Machine (KVM) manages virtualization within resources. MapReduce paradigm processes each tweet in parallel using SentiStrength. SentiStrength estimates the strength of word in scale of −1 to −5 for negative opinion and 1–5 for positive opinion. They demonstrated the feasibility of MapReduce using Hadoop for COSMOS and performance benefits achieved by using multiple virtual worker nodes. Greater the number of virtual nodes better the performance.

DOM: A Big Data Analytics Framework for Mining Thai Public Opinions

Prom-on et al. [16] present DOM (Data and Opinion Mining) a mobile data analytics engine for mining Thai public opinions. They present keyword-based sentiment analysis using MapReduce. Messages collected from social networks, blogs, and forums are stored in MongoDB. Twitter data is collected using Search API, and Facebook data is collected using Graph API. Each message is processed using natural processing techniques using MapReduce technique on Hadoop. MapReduce accelerated the analysis speed. Lexicon-based algorithm is developed to measure sentiment of score of each word. They defined five corpora which includes positive, negative, modifiers, conjunction, and point of interest words with sentiment rating ranging from −5 to 5. LexTo tool is used to tokenize words in each sentence. DOM implements MapReduce program to generate jobs that detects words in each sentence in parallel. Non-related sentences were discarded by matching words in point of interests. DOM then computes the sentiment score using positive and negative words in corpora. Sentiment score is inverted when modifier is adjacent to sentiment words. DOM engine can classify messages and perform sentiment analysis with accuracy of over 75% when compared to Human analysis. DOM engine was tested on general public opinion expressed in social network to determine political climate around end of 2013.

Customer Preference Analysis Based on SNS Data

Kim et al. [10] proposed feature based sentiment detection of social network sites using Hadoop. Twitter data is collected using TwitterAPI, Twitter4J stored and analyzed in multi-dimensional fashion to identify factors that affect customer preferences on smart phones. Their approach used Hannanum Java-based morphological analyzer to process the data into sentiments. Morphological analyzer consists of text preprocessing, morphological analysis, and POS tagging. Synonyms and acronyms in Twitter are collected and processed. They performed multi-dimensional analysis to find the sentiment of each attribute of mobile. Each Twitter table has 4-dimensional tables: mobile and its attributes, sentiment words, mobile carrier, brand, and maker. Analysis on each of this dimension table is done using implementation in Hive and R. Three aspects of Big Data volume, variety, and velocity were handled by making real-time feed from Twitter and analyzing in multi-dimensional fashion to address variety and volume in Hadoop.

The Impact of Cluster Characteristics on HiveQL Query Optimization

Joldzic et al. [17] analyzed the impact of cluster characteristics on HiveQL query optimization. Non-relational databases were developed to improve processing of Big Data. In this paper, they discussed the transfer of data from relational databases MySQL to distributed data storage HDFS using Apache Sqoop. MapReduce is used by Sqoop to import and export data using parallel operations in fault-tolerant manner. Sqoop uses database table reading table row by row into HDFS. Transfer process can be customized by specifying delimiters, file formats, row ranges, columns etc. Data is imported into non-relational database Hive for query analysis. They illustrated the comparative analysis of different queries in MySQL and Hive. HiveQL requires runtime optimization in order for jobs to run efficiently and with acceptable execution times.

4 Critical Review on Sentiment Analysis Using Hadoop

Hadoop addresses all the aspects of Big Data analysis for sentiment determination. Hadoop helps collect loads of volume of data. Hadoop provides speedy data download for real-time sentiment analysis. Hadoop framework helps distribute the work among different clustering machines, thus, achieving high performance. Sentiment analysis performance is improved in Hadoop by splitting the data into modules, processing in different machines, reducing response time, and improved fault tolerance by replicating the data. Hadoop helps in collection of variety of unstructured data from multiple sources in multiple formats, across domains and efficiently processing them in multi-dimensional fashion. HiveQL can be optimized at runtime improving the execution time.

Studies show that process of sentiment analysis can be performed without compromising on accuracy and speed. It can scale to bigger data sets with better performance. Machine learning algorithms like Naïve Bayes when implemented using MapReduce gives high accuracy for large volumes of data. Machine learning algorithms provided in Mahout scales well for high-dimensional large volume and complex data and can be used in several different applications. Apache Open Source platform using Hadoop also provides reduced cost application to perform sentiment analysis thus help increasing the profit of organization.

5 Conclusion

Hadoop implemented sentiment analysis has less complex business logic implementation easily extendible and better understandability and high performance at lower cost. Table 3 shows difference between MapReduce and Hive. MapReduce or Hive UDFs help process large volume of data with accuracy and time efficiently. Machine learning algorithms implemented in Hadoop are simpler and modular with

Table 3 Comparitive analysis of MapReduce and hive

Sentiment classification	MapReduce	Hive
Hadoop component	Inner	Tool
Built-in classifiers	N	N
Performance	Better	Poor
Programming model	Java	SQL
Data	Hierarchical/structured/unstructured	Structured
Development time	More	Less
Flexibility	More	Less
Robust	More	Less
Code branching	Easy	Difficult
Complexity	More	Less

few lines of code. Code written in Hadoop can be easily extended. Mahout provides scalable and time efficient build-in classifier.

Hadoop supports effective sentiment analysis process for Big Data. Hadoop with it components addresses three aspects of Big Data velocity, volume, and variety. Hadoop can effectively collect data in real time from social media sites or relational database using Flume and Sqoop tool, respectively. Large data sets can be efficiently stored and retrieved from Hadoop HDFS and Hive. Hadoop supports both machine learning and lexicon-based sentiment analysis of text using MapReduce or Hive. Sentiment analysis implemented in Hadoop framework provides high accuracy with efficient processing time and lower cost.

Acknowledgements The author is grateful to (Dr.) Divakar Singh, HOD, Department of CSE, UIT, Barkatullah University, Bhopal for his valuable suggestions and comments in writing this paper. The author wish to thank Puneet Sharma, for his continuous encouragement, inspiration and guidance with his abode of experience in data mining.

References

1. The Apache Software Foundation, https://flume.apache.org
2. The Apache Software Foundation, https://sqoop.apache.org
3. Dataiku, http://www.dataiku.com/blog/2013/05/01/a-complete-guide-to-writing-hive-udf.html
4. IBM, http://www.ibm.com/developerworks/java/library/j-mahout/
5. IBM, http://www.ibm.com/developerworks/library/j-mahout-scaling/
6. Pillar, http://www.3pillarglobal.com/insights/how-to-tame-the-machine-learning-beast-with-apache-mahout
7. Rajurkar G.D., Goudar R.M.: A speedy data uploading approach for twitter trend and sentiment analysis using HADOOP. In: 2015 International Conference on Computing Communication Control and Automation, pp. 580–584. IEEE, Pune (2015)
8. Mane S.B., Sawnt Y., Kazi S., Shinde V.: Real time sentiment analysis of twitter data using hadoop. In: International Journal of Computer Science and Information Technology, vol. 5(3), pp. 3098–3100, IJCSIT (2014)
9. Zarrad A., Aljialoud J.: The evaluation of the public opinion a case study: MERS-Cov infection virus in KSA. In: 7th International Conference on Utility and Cloud Computing, pp. 664–607. IEEE, London (2014)
10. Kim J.S., Yang M.H., Hwang Y.J., Jeon S.H., Kim K.Y., Jung I.S., Choi C.H., Cho W.S., Na J.H.: Customer preference analysis based on SNS data. In: Second International Conference on Cloud and Green Computing, pp. 609–613. IEEE, Xiangtan (2012)
11. Ramesh R., Divya G., Divya D., Kurian M.K.: Big data sentiment analysis using hadoop. In: International Journal for Innovative Research in Science & Technology, vol. 1. IJIRST (2015)
12. Hammond K., Varde A.S.: Cloud based predictive analytics. In: 13th International Conference on Data Mining Workshops, pp. 607–612. IEEE, Dallas, TX (2013)
13. Shang S., Shi M., Shan W., Hong Z.: Research on public opinion based on big data. In: 14th International Conference on Computer and Information Science, pp. 559–562. IEEE, Las Vegas, NV (2015)
14. Lui B., Blasch E., Chen Y., Shen D., Chen G.: Scalable sentiment classification for big data analysis using naive bayes classifier. In: International Conference on Big Data, pp. 99–104. IEEE, Silicon Valley, CA (2013)

15. Conejero J, Burnap P., Rana O., Morgan J.: Scaling archived social media data analysis using a hadoop cloud. In: Sixth International Conference on Cloud Computing, pp. 685–692. IEEE, Santa Clara, CA (2013)
16. Prom-on S., Ranong S.N., Jenviriyakul P., Wongkaew T., Saetiew N., Achalakul T.: DOM: a big data analytics framework for mining Thai public opinions. In: International Conference on Computer, Control, Informatics and Its Applications, pp. 1–6. IEEE, Bandung (2014)
17. Joldzic O.V., Vukovic D.R.: The impact of cluster characteristics on HiveQL query optimization. In: 21st Telecommunication Forum, pp. 837–840. IEEE, Belgrade (2013)
18. The Apache Software Foundation, https://hadoop.apache.org/

OPTIMA (OPinionated Tweet Implied Mining and Analysis)

An Innovative Tool to Automate Sentiment Analysis

Ram Chatterjee and Monika Goyal

Abstract The prevalent social media usage ramification has recently directed the research into the area of "Sentiment Analysis" producing potpourri of interesting results to analyze and apply in diverse domains. Among its existence in several forms, "Twitter" (an instance of the social media) is the most popular micro-blogging platform. Hence, contextually, "Sentiment analysis" connotes to assortment of user's opinions expressed over the "Twitter," into positive and negative classes. To exemplify and establish the essence, significance, and incidence of Opinion Mining, a corpus of tweets on "Windows 10" has been collected and built, with an objective to provide aid in customer feedback loop during its beta release. This paper focuses on the significance of sentiment analysis in a reasoned manner by epitomizing the working methodology of opinion mining techniques via its automated implementation. To address the purpose, an innovative tool has been developed named OPTIMA (OPinionated Tweet Implied Mining and Analysis) ver. 1.0.0., to automate the process of sentiment analysis and the results have been presented in a graphical form, in an analytical and comprehensive manner.

Keywords Naïve Bayesian · NLP · Opinion mining · Package · Sentiment analysis · SVM · Tweets

1 The Preamble

Idealistically, the feedback of other people about a product, process, or service has always been one of the prominent influencing factors in finalizing ones own decision about the same/similar product, process, or service in terms of buying the

R. Chatterjee (✉) · M. Goyal
Department of Computer Science and Technology,
Manav Rachna University (MRU), Faridabad, India
e-mail: ram@mru.edu.in

M. Goyal
e-mail: monikagoyal27@gmail.com

V.B. Aggarwal et al. (eds.), *Big Data Analytics*, Advances in Intelligent Systems and Computing 654, https://doi.org/10.1007/978-981-10-6620-7_36

product, implementing the process, and/or availing the service. It is here where the tool "OPTIMA" finds its role and significance by serving to fulfill the need of making a better and befitting decision by a customer/user in the context of acquiring the product, process, or service. To further explicate in a lucid manner, we reinstate Sentiment Analysis [1] as the process to automatically determine the sentiments expressed in a piece of plain text using some natural language processing (NLP) techniques. Elucidating further, the opinions expressed on anything, for example, a product, an individual, or a topic, over some prominent micro-blogger such as "Twitter," are utilized in various forms, for instance—users are able to narrow down their options based on the opinions expressed by others. Moreover, it also helps manufacturing companies to improve product quality and influencing its marketing based on customer's feedback. Opinion Mining helps software engineers form decisive judgment on beta releases of the products leading to incorporation of more befitting amendments before its final release to ameliorate the product marketing and acceptance. Policy makers can analyze user reviews and opinions to get instant and comprehensive feedback which may procreate novel ideas to enhance and promote the policy. Hence, Sentiment Analysis is a crucial activity in today's world aiming to present recapitulated pros and cons on features about products, laws, or policies by mining reviews, discussions, forums, etc. [2].

2 Theoretical Underpinnings of Tweet Retrieval and Analysis

In particular, this paper emphasizes on the automation of Sentiment Analysis on "tweets" and for the readers' interest and knowledge, we specify the Twitter relevant fundamentals. Twitter allows only 140 character status updates (popularly known as "tweets") and has various special properties like hash tags, targets, emoticons. Moreover, the Twitter data is available publically for analysis; there are APIs which can pull data from Twitter Web site [3]. There are plethora of techniques available for the tweet retrieval which can be broadly categorized as "programming" and "non-programming" techniques. The programming techniques include "R" programming language which is a statistical language for tweet retrieval and its analysis and works well on Windows, Mac, and UNIX platforms. "R" language can be easily interfaced with java, C, C++ using the various inbuilt packages of "R" [4]. "R" is widely used in variety of applications including data mining and visualizations. Python is another programming language used for similar task. On the other hand, non-programming techniques include various online applications named as "Streamcrab," "Topsy," "Sentiment 140," "Sentiment, viz.," "Trackur" and the likes. They are actually a time saver in order to get what users want. Users only need to provide a keyword for which one wants to extract tweets, and within a minute, hundreds of tweets are displayed on the users screen. However, the suitability of the ease and flexibility of non-programming methods is contradicted by the difficulties faced while exporting tweets into an Excel file and making them available for preprocessing. Owing to this hitch, we have proceeded with the task choosing the programming language "R," as obligatory, to retrieve Tweets.

3 Intricacies of the Machine Learning Algorithms Applied

For consolidation of the underlying concepts, it is essential to mention that the aim of machine learning is to develop an algorithm so as to optimize the performance of the system using example data or past experience. The machine learning provides a solution to the classification problem that involves two steps:

(1) Learning the model from a corpus of training data
(2) Classifying the unseen data based on the trained model.

Artificial intelligence (AI) uses information provided by the NLP and applies various machine learning techniques, viz., Naïve Bayes (NB), Support Vector Machine (SVM), Decision Tree, Random Forest, Maximum Entropy to determine the accuracy of the system of classification [5]. This paper primarily focuses on automation of two such machine learning classifiers, viz., NB and SVM. The Naive Bayes classifier uses Bayes Theorem as stated in Fig. 1 [6], which discovers the probability of an event given the probability of another event that has already occurred. Naive Bayes classifier performs extremely well for problems which are linearly separable.

The prior probabilities are calculated as in Eq. (1):

$$\gamma(\alpha) = \frac{N_c}{N} \tag{1}$$

where

N_c the number of document in class α and
N total number of documents.

Readers may note that the estimation on the probability of occurred event is calculated as in Eq. (2).

Fig. 1 Bayesian formula

$$\gamma(\alpha \mid \beta) = \frac{\gamma(\alpha) * \gamma(\beta \mid \alpha)}{\gamma(\beta)}$$

Where α : Specific class
β : Document wants to classify
$\gamma(\alpha)$ and $\gamma(\beta)$: Prior probabilities
$\gamma(\alpha \mid \beta)$ and $\gamma(\beta \mid \alpha)$: Posterior probabilities

$$\gamma(\omega|\alpha) = \frac{\text{count}(\omega,\alpha) + 1}{\text{count}(\alpha) + |V|} \tag{2}$$

where

count(ω,α) number of occurrences of ω in training documents from class α
count(α) number of words in that class
$|V|$ number of terms in the vocabulary.

In cognizance to the emphasis laid by the experimental study [7], the Support Vector Machines (SVMs) have been shown to be highly effective at traditional text categorization, generally outperforming Naive Bayesian. They are large margin, rather than probabilistic, classifiers, in contrast to Naive Bayesian. The concept of SVM algorithm is based on decision plane that defines decision boundaries. A decision plane separates group of instances having different class memberships.

In general, the performance of sentiment classification is evaluated by using the following indexes. They are precision, recall, and F1-score. The common way for computing these indexes is based on the confusion matrix [7] as shown in Fig. 2. In general, positive = identified and negative = rejected. Therefore:

True positive = correctly identified
False positive = incorrectly identified
True negative = correctly rejected
False negative = incorrectly rejected

Precision is the portion of true positive-predicted instances against all positive-predicted instances. Recall is the portion of true positive-predicted instances against all actual positive instances. F1 is a harmonic average of precision and recall [8]. To consolidate the concept discussed so far, we present below these indexes that can be defined by the following equations:

- $\text{Precision} = \frac{\text{TP}}{\text{TP} + \text{FP}}$
- $\text{Recall} = \frac{\text{TP}}{\text{TP} + \text{FN}}$
- $\text{F1} = \frac{2 \times \text{Precision} \times \text{Recall}}{\text{Precision} + \text{Recall}}$

#	Predicted positives	Predicted negatives
Actual positive instances	Number of True Positive instances (TP)	Number of False Negative instances (FN)
Actual negative instances	Number of False Positive instances (FP)	Number of True Negative instances (TN)

Fig. 2 Confusion matrix

4 Synopsis of the Tool—OPTIMA Version 1.0.0

A. *Prologue on the Tool*

For the reader to decipher the working of the tool analytically, we commence with the brief introduction on the tool. OPTIMA as stated has been developed in "R" programming language and in fact has been portrayed as a Web application that consolidates the various phases of Opinion Mining [9], viz., tweet extraction, text preprocessing, application of machine learning algorithms for classification into single integrated form.

B. *Tool Portrayal*

To leverage the technical intricacies of OPTIMA, an inherent and coherent explanation necessitates it worth mentioning that several "R" packages have been used to query the Twitter search API in order to collect tweets into R for Opinion Mining, mandating establishment of a secured connection between the R console and the Twitter [10].

The tool assimilates an inbuilt function to extract tweets based on the "search keyword" given by the user. Additionally, the tool is characterized with the capability of generating "word cloud" connoting to the most frequent terms in the "corpus" formed from the extracted tweets. To clarify further, the initial tool interface has been shown in Fig. 3 in labeled form for readers' clear

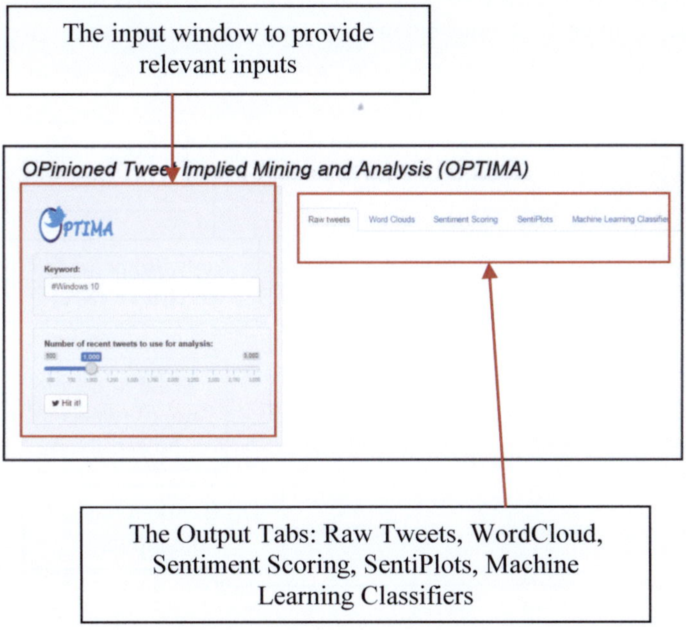

Fig. 3 Tool interface

comprehension. As depicted in the figure, the tool implicates two initial inputs and five output tabs, providing the provision to the user to switch among the tabs in order to view the multifarious outputs produced by the tool in the context of the given "search keyword".

C. *Illustrating the tool input and output*

To augment the discussion on the tool input further, besides the "search keyword" (that has been set as "Windows 10" by default) serving as an input parameter, the "count of tweets" (that is desired to be extracted) serves as a second input parameter, with the flexibility of setting this count value on the given scale as per the requirement, as has been depicted in Fig. 4. Promoting the generalization on the input parameter "search keyword," the end user may enter any desired subject matter as an input for which tweets need to be retrieved from the Twitter Web site. Analogously, the input parameter "number of recent tweets to use for analysis" can also be customized for retrieving the desired number of tweets from the Twitter Web site, as depicted in Fig. 4.

Demarcating the outputs from the inputs, we have been depicting the outputs from Figs. 5 to 10 in self-explanatory manner which are being corroborated with the following detailed discussion.

Figure 5 portrays the first output—the list of retrieved tweets which are the "raw tweets" comprised of stop words, punctuation marks, and hashtags. Being in raw form, these tweets are subjected to text processing [11] where the result of text processing is exported into a word cloud, as illustrated in Fig. 6, which forms the second output. For the ease of understanding of the readers, we state that word clouds are graphical demonstrations of word frequency that give superior

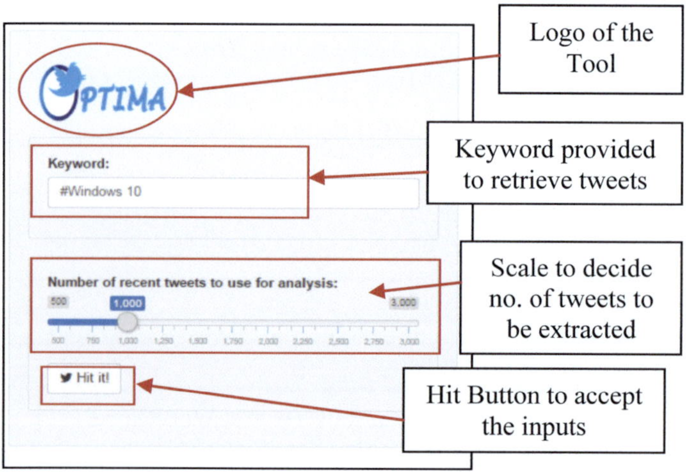

Fig. 4 Input window

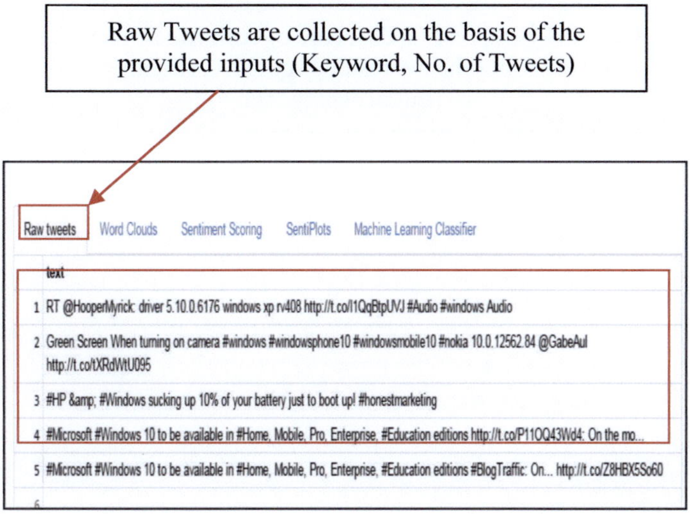

Fig. 5 Output tabs showing raw tweets

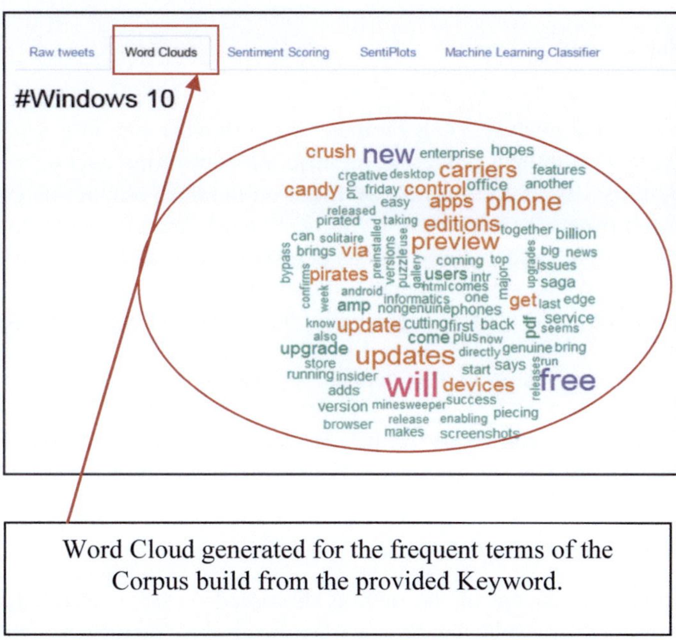

Fig. 6 WordCloud of "Windows 10"

importance to words that appear more recurrently in a source text. The more a word is found to be common in the documents, the bigger is its appearance in the visual form in the word cloud. Visualization of this kind corroborates evaluators with

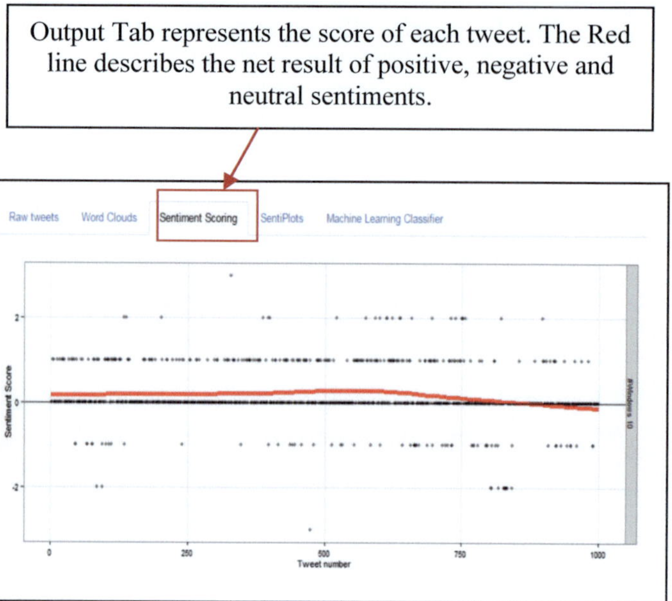

Fig. 7 Scoring of tweets

investigative textual analysis [12]. Further, such visualizations also serve in communicating most prominent point and premise inherent in the tweets.

Proceeding the discussion further, we focus on the third output that connotes to "scoring of the tweets," as depicted in Fig. 7. Readers are advised to comprehend score "1" as positive tweet, score "−1" as negative tweet, and score "0" as neutral tweet, where positive, negative, and neutral terms refer to the underlying sentiment, inherent in the retrieved tweets. Technically, the "score" is calculated as:

$$\text{Score} = (\text{Sum of Pos. words}) - (\text{Sum of Neg. words}).$$

Supplementing the discussion further, readers may note that "SentiPlots" are plotted against "scoring of tweets," "Polarity Classification," and "Emotions Classification".

D. *Detailing Deployment of the Tool*

To consolidate the concept of the outputs discussed so far, it is for the readers' appreciation and crisp understanding, we explicate the "SentiPlots" further. The polarity plot (Fig. 8) categorizes the polarity (e.g., positive or negative) of a set of texts. The polarity describes the absolute log likelihood of the document expressing a positive/negative sentiment [13]. Hence, the plot helps to identify the percentage of positive and negative sentiment.

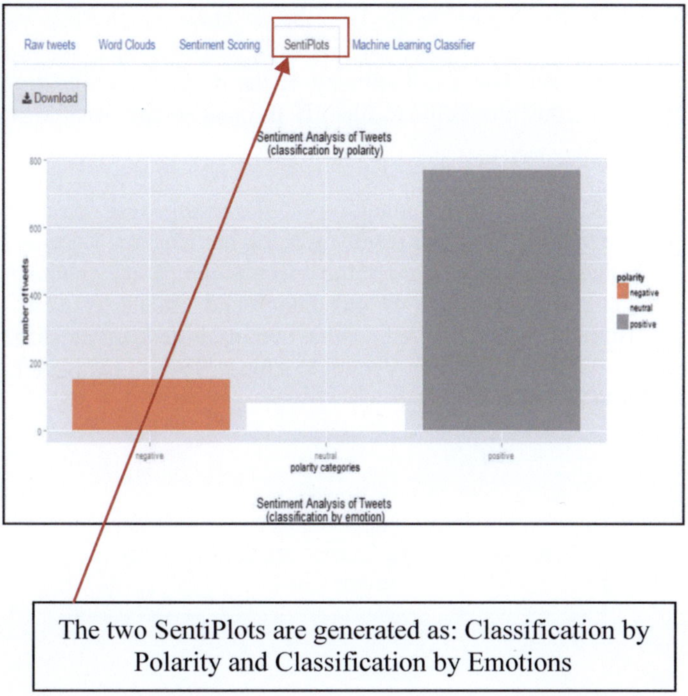

Fig. 8 Plot distribution of polarity

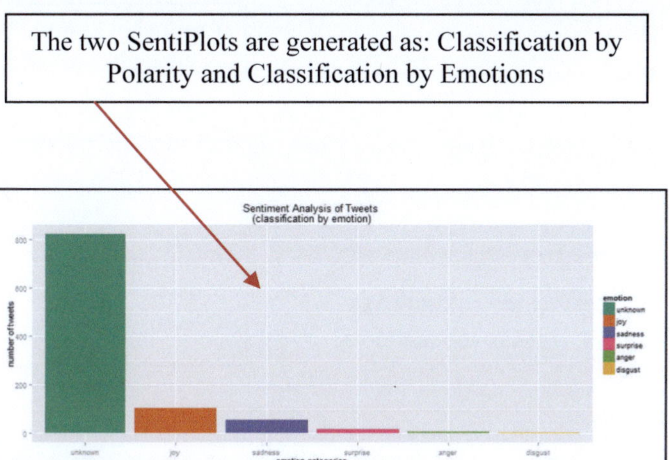

Fig. 9 Plot distribution of emotion

Supplementing the discussion further, the emotion graph (Fig. 9) plots the emotion (e.g., anger, disgust, fear, joy, sadness, surprise) of a set of texts. The emotion depicts the absolute log likelihood of the document expressing that sentiment [13]. Hence, this plot helps to identify the percentage of various emotions.

E. *Outlining the Tool Output*

Technically speaking, the predominant aspect prevailing over sentiment analysis process is to gain confidence of the results by applying machine learning classifiers. In other words, determining the score of the tweets is not enough; authenticating the exactness of the retrieved results is mandatory and crucial as well. Hence, to establish the accuracy of the retrieved results, two machine learning classifiers, viz., Naïve Bayesian (NB) and Support Vector Machine (SVM) [14] have been implicated in the tool OPTIMA.

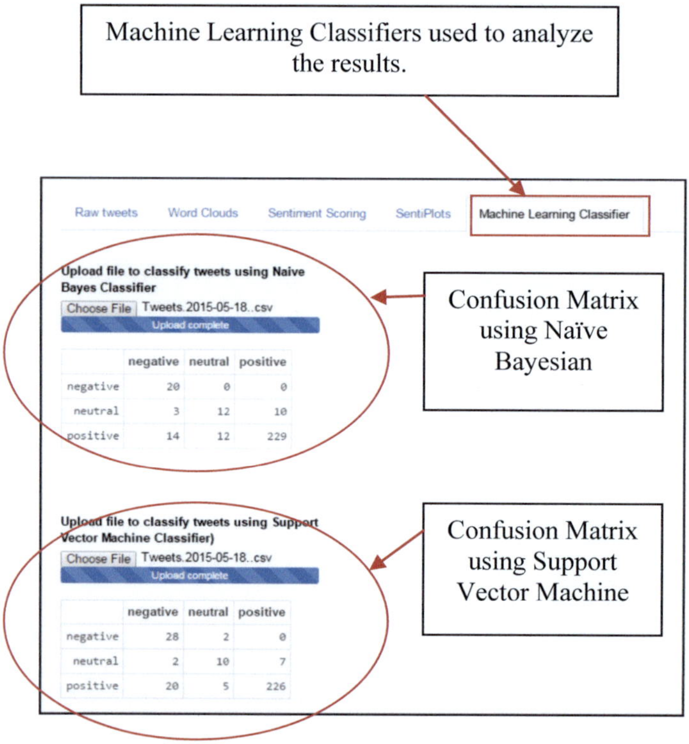

Fig. 10 Confusion matrix

These classifiers generate a "confusion matrix" which serves as the basis for calculating several performance parameters. To consolidate the conversation further, readers may note that the classified tweets (that have been classified as positive, negative, and neutral) which formed the outcome of scoring serve as an input for the machine learning classifier, generating "confusion matrix" as the output (illustrated in Fig. 10). The mentioned figure is labeled properly for the ease of understanding of the readers.

5 Result Analysis

In the context of the "classification model," the crucial aspect lies in the model's ability to correctly predict or separate the classes. The "confusion matrix" serves in delineating the errors made by a classification model under consideration. Our case is distinguishable with having three class problems, viz., negative, neutral, and positive classes. The depiction, illustrated in Fig. 10, connotes to the confusion matrix generated for the search keyword "Windows 10" resulting into extraction of 1000 tweets. Among these 1000 tweets, 70% is classified as training data and the rest constitutes the testing data. In the context of Fig. 10, the rows communicate the known class of the data, i.e., the labels in the data. The columns connote to the predictions made by the model. Consequently, the diagonal elements represent the number of correct classifications made for each class, and the off-diagonal elements depict the errors made. The precision and recall values are computed for each classifier as depicted in Tables 1 and 2, respectively. It is noteworthy to mention for the scholars' interest and knowledge that in the context of the given search keyword "Windows 10," for each class, Support Vector Machine outperforms the Naive Bayesian classifier as evident in Tables 1 and 2. However, these computed results may likely vary with the inputs provided, viz., the search keyword and the scale factor determining the count of the tweets intended to be retrieved.

Table 1 Precision value

Classifier	Classes		
	Positive (%)	Negative (%)	Neutral (%)
NB	95	54	50
SVM	96	56	58

Table 2 Recall value

Classifier	Classes		
	Positive (%)	Negative (%)	Neutral (%)
NB	89	100	48
SVM	90	93	52

6 Conclusion and Future Work

The paper strives to demonstrate the significance and role of sentiment Analysis in corroborating the Twitter data. To facilitate the analysis of the retrieved tweets, the opinion mining techniques, viz., preconstructed opinion lexicons and machine learning classifiers, have been discussed, primarily emphasizing elaboration on Naïve Bayesian and Support Vector Machine classifiers. Relevant to the context of discussion on the above-mentioned opinion mining techniques, the need to automate them and detail of the working procedure of the automated tool OPTIMA (OPinionated Tweet Implied Mining and Analysis) ver. 1.0.0. have been explained and illustrated in a lucid manner. The paper culminates presenting discussion on the automated tool's facility to plot graphs, highlighting the classification on the basis of polarity and emotions. This helps the user to form an idea about the classified tweets as positive, negative, and neutral sentiments as prevailing over the Twitter.

The future work entails remodeling the tool with better and improved opinion mining techniques like working with emoticons such as ☺ ☹ 😐 during preprocessing of tweets, in order to yield more accurate results of sentiment analysis, congenial to the query submitted by the user. Our emphasis is to compare and contrast the results of the underlying search techniques in the prospective remodeled tool on the basis of their corresponding precision and recall values.

References

1. Buche, A., Chandak, M.B., Zadgaonkar, A.: Opinion mining and analysis: a survey. Proc. Int. J. Nat Lang. Comput. **2**(3), 39–48 (2013)
2. Sidorov, G. et al.: Empirical study of machine learning based approach for opinion mining in tweets. MICAI (2), Vol. 7629 of the series Lecture Notes in Computer Science, pp. 1–14 (2014)
3. Pak, A., Paroubek, P.: Twitter as a corpus for sentiment analysis and opinion mining. Proc. Int. Conf. Lang. Resour. Eval. **1**, 433–441 (2010)
4. Zhao, Y.: R and Data Mining: Examples and Case Studies. Academic Press, Elsevier (2012)
5. Vinodhini, G., Chandrasekaran, R.M.: Sentiment analysis and opinion mining: a survey. Proc. Int. J. Adv. Res. Comput. Sci. Softw. Eng. **2**(6), 282–292 (2012)
6. Dhande, L.L., Patnaik, G.K.: Analyzing sentiment of movie review data using Naive Bayes neural classifier. Int. J. Emerg. Trends Technol. Comput. Sci. **3**(4), 313–320 (2014)
7. Khairnar, J., Kinikar, M.: Machine learning algorithms for opinion mining and sentiment classification. Int. J. Sci. Res Publ. **3**(6), 1–6 (2013)
8. Singh, P.K., Husain, M.S.: Analytical study of feature extraction techniques in opinion mining. CS & IT-CSCP **57**(13), 85–94 (2013)
9. Liu, B.: Sentiment Analysis and Opinion Mining. Morgan & Claypool Publishers, California (2012)
10. Jeff Gentry.: Twitter client for R [Online]. Available: https://sense.io/api/v1/projects/ryanswanstrom/twitter-text-analysis-project/files/R/twitteR/doc/twitteR.pdf 24 Mar 2014
11. Feinerer, I.: Introduction to the tm package text mining in R [Online]. Available: https://cran.r-project.org/web/packages/tm/vignettes/tm.pdf 3 July 2015

12. Williams, G.: Hands-on data science with R text mining [Online]. Available: http://handsondatascience.com/TextMiningO.pdf 5 Nov 2014
13. Jurka, T.P.: Package-Sentiment [Online]. Available: https://cran.r-project.org/src/contrib/Archive/sentiment/ (2012)
14. Meyer, D.: Support vector machines _the interface to libsvm in package e1071[Online]. Available: https://cran.r-project.org/web/packages/e1071/vignettes/svmdoc.pdf 5 Aug 2015

Mobile Agent Based MapReduce Framework for Big Data Processing

Umesh Kumar and Sapna Gambhir

Abstract This chapter gives the information regarding Big Data, MapReduce Framework, and Stragglers in MapReduce Network, their current situation, their impact, and scope in today's reality. Paper proceeds with information about MapReduce strategy for Big Data handling and the vicinity of stragglers in MapReduce Network. Further, the significance of mitigating straggler is talked about, alongside their effects. This paper also introduces the mobile agent technology for processing Big Data utilizing MapReduce system and its implementation results.

Keywords Big data · MapReduce · Mantri · Mapper · Reducer · Mobile agent · Straggler · JADE

1 Introduction

It is observed that there are lots of systems proposed for the recognition of stragglers in parallel processing information systems; however, none of them utilized mobile agents. Advancement of the Internet invokes the requirement for Web applications across heterogeneous systems. From the investigation of existing solutions for straggler handling, LATE and Mantri [1] offer a productive calculation for straggler mitigation using the speculative cap for the number of speculative copies of a single task can run at the same time, however, the execution can further

11th International Conference on Wirtschaftsinformatik, 27th February–01st March 2013, Leipzig, Germany.

U. Kumar (✉) · S. Gambhir
Computer Science Department, YMCA University of Science and Technology, Faridabad, India
e-mail: umesh554@gmail.com

S. Gambhir
e-mail: sapnagambhir@gmail.com

V.B. Aggarwal et al. (eds.), *Big Data Analytics*, Advances in Intelligent Systems and Computing 654, https://doi.org/10.1007/978-981-10-6620-7_37

be enhanced using mobile agents. Mobile agents have not been examined for parallel computation problems. Due to stragglers, a part of resources gets wasted because we have multiple speculative copies of a single task running at the same time but we need only one for one final execution. So if we can limit the number of speculative execution to a single copy at any time, we can have a hundred percent resource utilization for the users because we run only one instance for any file at a time. In the next section, we will discuss big data processing and related issues.

2 Big Data Processing

Big Data [2] is considered to be a data collection that has grown so large it cannot be effectively or affordably managed (or exploited) using conventional data management tools: e.g., classic relational database management systems (RDBMS) [3] or conventional search engines [4], depending on the task at hand. The 3 Vs that define Big Data are Variety, Velocity, and Volume.

(a) *Variety:* Data can be stored in multiple formats. For example, database, excel, csv, access, or for the matter of the fact, it can be stored in a simple text file. Sometimes the data can be in the form of video, SMS, pdf, or something we might have not thought about like SMS and profile of users. This variety of the data represents *Big Data*.
(b) *Velocity:* Today, most of the users rely on social media for information retrievals like Facebook and Twitter. The information updating is almost real time and the update window is updated at fraction of seconds. This high-velocity data represent *Big Data*.
(c) *Volume:* Terabytes and petabytes of the storage system are very common these days. This big volume of data represents *Big Data*.

MapReduce Paradigm

MapReduce is a programming framework popularized by Google [5]. This is a methodology, which is used to handle extensive scale Web applications. This methodology is used for creating machine learning, data mining, and search applications in data centers. The point of interest is that it permits programmers to restrain from the issues of booking, parallelization, parceling, replication, and concentrates on creating their application.

MapReduce Execution Framework

The *Map* invocations are distributed across multiple machines by automatically partitioning the input data into a set of M *splits*. The input splits can be processed in parallel by different machines. *Reduce* invocations are distributed by partitioning the intermediate key space into R pieces using a partitioning function (e.g., hash (key) mod R). The number of partitions (R) and the partitioning function are

Fig. 1

specified by the user. Figure 1 shows the overall flow of a MapReduce operation in our implementation [6]. The developer submits the job to the node of the cluster and execution environment takes care of further processing [7].

Mappers and Reducers

In MapReduce, the developer creates a mapper and a reducer as shown below [8]:

$$\text{map: } (k_1, v_1) \rightarrow [(k_2, v_2)]$$
$$\text{reduce: } (k_2, [v_2]) \rightarrow [(k_3, v_3)] \quad [\ldots] \text{ denotes a list here.}$$

3 Related Work

There are a number of straggler mitigation and detection algorithms currently available like Hadoop native scheduler, MonTool, Mantri, Dolly, and LATE. Hadoop native scheduler [9] works on the basis of advancement score between 0 and 1. The execution of tasks is basically separated into three phases: Duplicate phase, Sort phase, and Decrease phase.

In every phase, score is the function of processed data. Hadoop computes the average score for each process to assign a limit for speculative execution. If the score of task advancement is 0.2 less than normal of its class, it is identified as a straggler.

LATE [10] uses a different idea that approximates the time for task completion to predict potential stragglers. Calculation of progress rate is done as advancement score/T where the value of T is task-running time. Estimation of time to finish is done by (1-progress score)/progress rate. Tasks, which have the advancement rate less than 25‰, are identified as stragglers.

Mantri [11] relies on the basis of real time reports. So identification of straggler is done by Mantri somewhat early as compared to other techniques. Mantri identifies spots at which tasks are not able to make progress at a normal rate. Mantri identifies the straggler with the help of cause awareness and resource perception.

MonTool [12] uses the mechanism of tracing system calls and doing analysis on that. With the help of this analysis, MonTool tries to find straggler and its reasons.

Dolly [13] uses an interesting mechanism like by launching clones of a task and using the result of a clone, which completes first.

4 Problem Identification

As we have seen, there are some techniques available for straggler detection and mitigation. Each of the technique finds the straggler in a different way using different approaches but then reschedules them to other location in the nearly similar way. They speculatively execute them on other comparatively faster machines available in the vicinity of the staggering machine. Initially, one may assume that straggler detection will be an easy task, simultaneously speculating tasks that are sufficiently slower. Several issues, which were identified, are as follows:

(a) Firstly, speculative assignments will require other resources for execution, for example, a system with other running tasks.
(b) Secondly, how to select the node to run speculative task is as significant as selecting the task.
(c) Thirdly, how to recognize nodes that are marginally slower than the mean and stragglers.

At last, Stragglers ought to be expected on time. So our main concern is how we can overcome these issues. The agents [14] are software entities having the certain kind of intelligence associated with them. The basic dictionary definition of agent is one who acts and responds [15]. Agents also communicate with other agents and give result back to the user.

5 Proposed Work

Agent-based Web applications make the full capabilities of the existing network infrastructures and information available in the network. A new straggler detection and mitigation approach using mobile agents is proposed in this section.

5.1 Mobile Agent Based MapReduce (ABMR) for BigData Processing

Assumptions: Some of the important assumptions that have been made to clearly specify the applicability of technique are as follows:

- Each of the machines should have JADE [16]; the agent execution environment preinstalled, which provides efficient mobile agent development and execution environment for parallel data processing. In the execution environment, an agent can hide its code and data integrity and also its owner identification.
- The Big Data file should be splitted evenly so that each agent gets an equal share of the load, and hence the score computed is even in all.
- Each agent gets only a single split of the file, i.e., the number of agents is equal to the number of the splits in the network.
- An intermediate location is already set to store the intermediate data from the various map agents.
- The big data file is located at the main host itself.

Methodology: During the literature survey, it was found that the methods were using some kind of heuristics for straggler detection and then were speculatively executing them at two different locations at the same time in order to mitigate their effect. The core of our proposed solution for processing big data is the scheduler agent, which supports mobile agent creation and rescheduling if they are not performing near the average performance of all the agents.

5.2 Algorithm

The proposed ABMR algorithm uses one mobile agent for each split, it gets from the user and then that mobile agent moves from one location to another based on how the scheduler schedules it based on the performance score the agent has sent to the scheduler as shown in Fig. 2. The scheduler maintains two arrays one for slower machines and one for faster machines. The scheduler reschedules the agents running on slower machines to the faster machines one at a time. The scheduler finally recollects all the results after each agent has done its work and then presents it to the original user of the application. Pseudocode for the same has been shown in Fig. 3.

(a) *Algorithm for Scheduler*

1. All hosts in the network which want to take part in big data processing register themselves with their IP Addresses.
2. These IP addresses are used to create agent containers in the main program.
3. A Scheduler agent is created in by the main application, which takes a file name as an argument and finds all the agent containers running on the home platform.

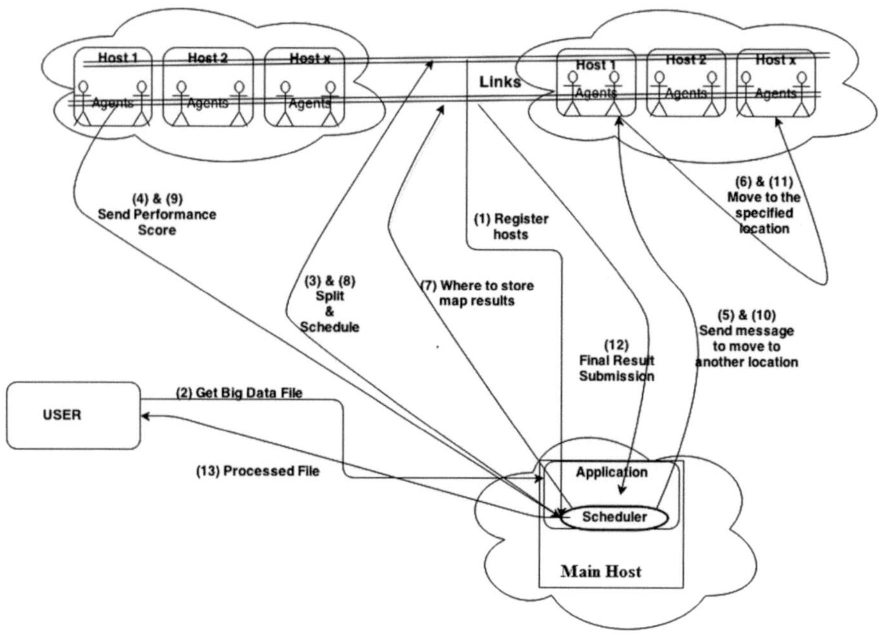

Fig. 2 ABMR working

4. Scheduler agent creates the mobile agents after splitting the file and assigns a file split to each of them.
5. Each agent sends its performance score to the scheduler after every Ts seconds. **score_agent[i] = Total executed/Total to be executed * Ts**
6. Meanwhile, when the agent moves from one location to another, it saves its current state so that they can start from the very same place where they stopped the execution.
7. After performing all the operations, the agent submits the result back to the scheduler.
8. The scheduler forwards the result to the user after the accumulation of results from all the reducers.

(b) *Agent Life Cycle Functions*

setup(File_Split, Location)
Agent is created using this function. Agent is loaded with a file and a location where it initially has been placed. This file_split and the location are provided by the scheduler while creating an agent.

map_execution(split): The agent in this phase executes the map operation, here defined as a word count algorithm, the map function counts the number of time a word appears in the split assigned to this agent.

```
  MainScheduler(file[],containers[])
        ratio=file.length/container.length
        for j=1 to container.length
            for i=1 to ratio
            container[j].createAgent(file[i],container[j]
        )
      for j=1 to file.length
            score[j] =(receive (msg[j]);
            avg+=score/file.length;
         for i=1 to no of agents
            if score[i]<0.5 * avg
            slowContainers[k++]=container[i];
            else if score[i]>= avg
            fastContainers[k++]=container[i];
         for i=1 to no of slowContainers
            agent[i].move(fastContainer[i])
         if allMessageFinished
return
```

Fig. 3 Pseudocode

TickerBehavior (time): This behavior is used for sending the score messages to the scheduler. As the name implies this executes its code after a particular time specified by its time parameter.

action(split, type): This method specifies the type of action(map/reduce) to be executed on the specific split and then the particular execution method is called.

reduce_execution(split): This method defines the reduce function for a particular split assigned by the scheduler. The scheduler based on the hashing function calculates which split is to be assigned to which reducer and then assign that particular split to that reducer by calling this method.

move (location): The agent class contains this method, which helps in its movement from one location to the other. The scheduler sends the location parameter to the agent, which in turn calls this method on itself with the location parameter.

destroy()

The agent class contains this method, which helps in freeing all the resources, which the agent had earlier used.

Working Steps

1. **Registration Phase**: Each of the nodes who want to be the part of the computing grid first of all registers itself with the main node where the application has been running. This registration process is carried out for a fixed-time period. Each node sends its IP Address to the main application so that it can further communicate with these nodes. These IP addresses are stored in the array and a corresponding agent container is launched in the jade runtime environment for each of the agents. This agent container controls all the operations to be performed on a particular agent. Each node registering itself admits that it is meeting all the conditions it is required to fulfill and is readily offering its services to the parallel processing network.
2. **File Fetching and Scheduler Agent Creation**: In this step, the address of the big data file to be processed it is fetched, and then the scheduler agent is created along with the file address and the array of the agent containers created earlier. The scheduler then contacts all the agent containers and they are then used for the creation of agents. The scheduler in the meantime splits the file among multiple pieces based on the size of the split, which it takes from the user.
3. **Agent Score Calculation**: Each agent calculates the score based on the number of words it has processed in unit time out of the total number of words it had to process using the formula.

   - Score = (Number of words processed/Total number of words to be processed) * (unit time) where the Number of words processed is counted by a variable,
   - the Number of words to be processed is found by the string library in JAVA,
   - unit time is a constant set to 100 ms.

4. **Agent Score Submission**: Each agent then submits its partially calculated score and then sends it back to the scheduler; the agent uses the message format from the agent class in JADE execution environment to send the score of the current execution. The application has an array for the slowest and fastest running agents to store the exact values.
5. **Agent Relocation**: The arrays stored for slowest and fastest machines are used to send the location where the slow agents have to move where they can complete the original activity of the agent. The location is sent to the agent in a message particularly to the agent, which the scheduler declares the straggler.
6. **Agent Result Submission**: The agent then submits the result to the application, which then merges all the results into the main result and then directs the final result to the user. The final result is in the form of the file, which contains the overall result.
7. **Final Result Submission**: The application then sends the result back to the users who have requested the task.

5.3 *Result and Analysis*

The proposed algorithm is tested on both scenarios for split sizes as well as for various setting up of stragglers. This section describes the results collected by the experiments and provides the comparison of the results with results of other technique proposed for solving the problem of straggler detection and mitigation. At the end of the section, further optimization is also proposed, which will make the execution of the algorithm faster.

Testing

The implementation of the proposed algorithm is tested on an Intel i5 laptop with 6 GB RAM is used for the execution of the program for both scenarios with a 450 MB text file. The map and reduce operations are defined for word count procedures. JADE is used for creating agents on the various machines. The algorithm is run with the parameter values as shown in Table 1. The values of these parameters can be fine-tuned according to the network properties as they vary with large amounts. This gives the algorithm the flexibility to be applied to various types of networks. By varying these parameters, one can get different execution times. If one provides values which are below or beyond those constrains, the results will not be same. The algorithm is tested to provide good results with these values of the parameters within constraints.

Comparison with HADOOP Native Scheduler based on Straggler Percentage

The proposed algorithm is compared with the HADOOP Native Scheduler and Table 2 clearly shows that the proposed technique outperforms this technique in execution time for randomly generated graphs. Not only it outperforms the Hadoop Native Scheduler in its execution time but also it does so without any DFS. It simply saves the extra time Hadoop takes to create the DFS and then resumes them from the place where they have left earlier.

The proposed algorithm is compared with the HADOOP Native Scheduler for its straggler detection and mitigation technique's wide implementation. The following Fig. 4 clearly shows that the proposed technique outperforms this technique in execution time for randomly generated graphs for various split sizes. Our algorithm provided better results than the algorithms used for comparison. Not only it outperforms HADOOP Native Scheduler in its execution time but also it does so without any DFS. Split sizes, however, can increase our problems because we used

Table 1 Parameter values

Parameter	Value
Size of Big Data file	450 MB
Agent containers per main container	2–3
Agents per agent container	3–10
Mapping technique	Word count

Table 2 Execution overview on straggler %

Straggler (%)	HADOOP native scheduler time (ms)	Mobile agent based MapReduce time (ms)
10	48,587	51,237
20	58,548	54,893
40	87,373	74,120
50	120,252	99,365

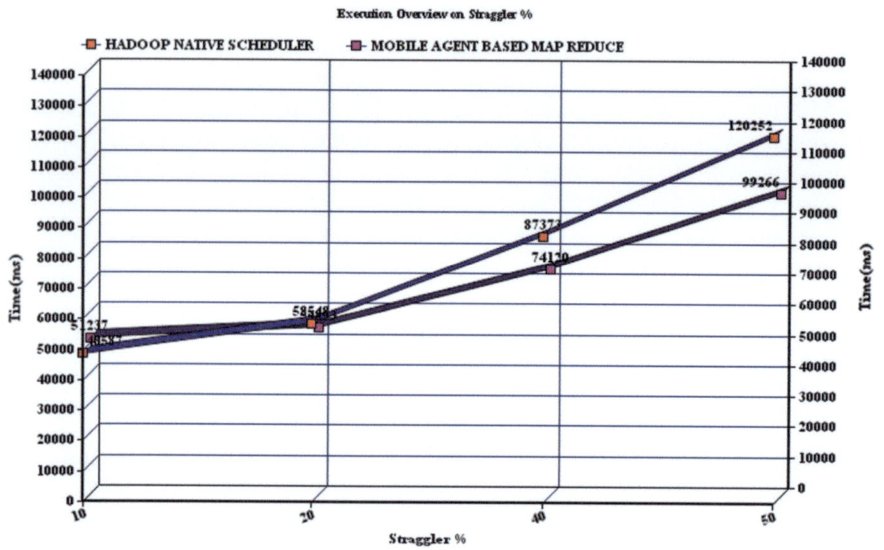

Fig. 4 Graph showing performance comparison with HADOOP based on split sizes

the network to transfer information from one machine to the other. While the information or splits are being transmitted the network speed comes into picture, which can increase the overall execution time.

From the previous section, it is evident that the MBMR Algorithm performs well on a single machine as well as for a network of machines. The algorithm improves theexecution time for a single machine and can serve the same purpose for if we have enough bandwidth. Table 3 shows execution overview on the basis of various split sizes.

The significant insights from the result of the implementation of MBMR are as follows: (i) Outliers or stragglers are detected and are then rescheduled to other machine without wasting a single machine cycle because it reschedules them in an efficient manner. (ii) Rescheduling process is delayed so that if a node has stuck in some other useful work it is not marked straggler and can continue its work. This delay does not cost us much because we are using mobile agents, which are known

Table 3 Execution overview on the basis of various split sizes

Setup scenario size * container * agents/container	HADOOP native scheduler time (s)	Mobile agent based MapReduce time (ms)
50 * 3 * 3	45	48
45 * 2 * 5	47	48
30 * 3 * 5	50	49
15 * 3 * 10	55	55

for their ability to start from the very place, they left their execution. (iii) There is a significant improvement in the execution time as compared to existing algorithms, i.e., about 10–12% and that as well without using any DFS.

6 Conclusion

Straggler detection and mitigation approaches have attracted a lot of attention of researchers in recent years and there is a considerable increase in the number of algorithms published for solving the issue as it has applications in various domains like big data processing and parallel computation. The main goal was to come up with a technique, which is better than the current state of art solutions. The proposed technique performs well as compared to the classical algorithms and the current state of art algorithms.

References

1. Kumar, U., Kumar, J.: A comprehensive review of straggler handling algorithms for MapReduce framework. Int. J. Grid Distrib. Comput. **7**(4), 139–148 (2014). ISSN: 2005-4262
2. Wilber, L., Mills, S., Perlowitz, B.: Demystifying Big Data. Notices of TA Foundation (2009)
3. Olofson, C.W., Perry, R.: IDC analyze the future. White Paper **104**, 36–41 (2011)
4. Guimerà, R., Sales-Pardo, M., Amaral, L.A.N.: Search engine architectures from conventional to P2P. Phys. Rev. E **70**, 025101 (2012)
5. Dean, J., Ghemawat, Sanjay: MapReduce: simplified data processing on large clusters. Commun. ACM **51**, 107–113 (2004)
6. Farkas, I., Abel, D., Palla, G., Vicsek, T.: Map reduce execution framework. New J. Phys. **9** (6), 180 (2010)
7. Kumpula, J.M., Kivela, M.: Sequential algorithm for fast straggler detection. Phys. Rev. E **78** (2), 026109, (2007)
8. Freeman, L.C.: Finding stragglers in parallel computation. ACM **1**, 215–239 (2009)
9. http://hadoop.apache.org/
10. Zaharia, M., Konwinski, A., Joseph, A.D., Katz, R., Stoica, I.: Improving MapReduce performance in heterogeneous environment. In: OSDI'08 Proceedings of the 8th USENIX Conference on Operating Systems Design and Implementation, pp. 29–42 (2008)

11. Ananthanarayan, G., Ghodsi, A., Shenker, S., Stoica, I.: Effective straggler mitigation: attack of the clones. In: Proceedings of the 10th USENIX Conference on Networked Systems Design and Implementation, pp. 185–198 (2013)
12. Gandhi, R., Sabne, A.: Finding stragglers in Hadoop. In: European Conference on Computer Systems (2012)
13. Ananthanarayanan, G., Kandula, S., Berg, A.G., Stoica, I., Harris, E., Shaha, B.: Reining in the outliers in MapReduce clusters using Mantri. In: 9th USENIX Symposium on Networked Systems Design and Implementation (2010)
14. Wu, Z., Lin, Y., Wan, H., Tian, S.: A fast and reasonable method for straggler detection and mitigation. In: ISKE Conference, 376–379 (2010)
15. Franklin, S., Graesser, A.: Is it an agent, or just a program?: A taxonomy for autonomous agents, vol. 1193. Springer, Berlin, Heidelberg, pp. 21–35 (1997)
16. Stonebraker, M., Abadi, D., DeWitt, D.J., Madden, S., Paulson, E., Pavlo, A., Rasin, A.: MapReduce and parallel DBMSs: friends or foes? Commun. ACM **53**(1), 64–71 (2010)

Review of Parallel Apriori Algorithm on MapReduce Framework for Performance Enhancement

Ruchi Agarwal, Sunny Singh and Satvik Vats

Abstract Finding frequent itemsets in the large transactional database is considered as one of the most and significant issues in data mining. Apriori is one of the popular algorithms that widely used as a solution of addressing the same issue. However, it has computing power shortage to deal with large data sets. Various modified Apriori-like algorithms have been proposed to enhance the performance of traditional Apriori algorithm that works on distributed platform. Developing efficient and fast computing algorithm to handle large data sets becomes a challenging task due to load balancing, synchronisation and fault-tolerance issue. In order to overcome these problems, MapReduce model comes into existence, originally introduced by Google. MapReduce model-based parallel Apriori algorithm finds the frequent itemsets from large data sets using a large number of computers in distributed computational environment. In this paper, we mainly focused on parallel Apriori algorithm and its different versions based on approaches used to implement them. We also explored on current major open issues and extensions of MapReduce framework along with future research directions.

Keywords Frequent itemsets · Parallel Apriori · Big data · Hadoop · MapReduce

R. Agarwal (✉) · S. Singh · S. Vats
Department of Computer Science and Engineering, Sharda University, Greater Noida, India
e-mail: ruchi.agarwal@sharda.ac.in

S. Singh
e-mail: aryans1027@gmail.com

S. Vats
e-mail: satvik.vats@gmail.com

V.B. Aggarwal et al. (eds.), *Big Data Analytics*, Advances in Intelligent Systems and Computing 654, https://doi.org/10.1007/978-981-10-6620-7_38

1 Introduction

We are living in Big Data era where data is growing exponentially with time and size of data is moving from terabytes to petabytes [1]. This trend brings out challenges to store this vast amount of data effectively and demands for analytical technology. Analysis of Big Data helps the organizations as well as government in decision-making and setting polices to provide better services to people. Various data mining tools are available from last decades to extract useful information, but they failed to process the large data sets because of time and space complexity. Association rules mining (ARM) technique [2] is used to find out the interesting patterns, sequences or itemsets from large database [3]. Apriori algorithm is used to implement ARM, but effectiveness of this algorithm reduces as the size of the data sets increases to compute, because of its iterative fashion of working which leads to further increment in the value of time complexity. Lots of work has been done to make Apriori algorithm run parallel to reduce the time complexity of traditional Apriori, originally proposed by R. Agarwal. As a result, several parallel Apriori algorithms come into existence such as count distribution (CD), candidate distribution (CaD) and data distribution (DD). These algorithms provide some key features such as dynamic itemset counting [4], data and task parallelism [5]. However, these algorithms come with some major weakness of synchronisation of data, communication issues due to message passing interface (MPI) framework which mainly support for homogeneous environment rather than heterogeneous environment and only work with low-level language like C and FORTRAN [6, 7]. Further, workload balancing [8] and fault-tolerance issue make them incapable to handle Big Data in distributed environments. Above problems lead to the development of MapReduce programming model, introduced by Google [9] for processing large database which enables the programmer to write programming code using map and reduce functions to run parallel applications. Google's MapReduce framework [10] is one of the current approaches which are available to process the Big Data using commodity machines or nodes in distributed computational environment. Hadoop provides platform to run the MapReduce programming model [11, 12] and enables the developers to code analytical applications under the hood of strong fault tolerance where guarantee is offered by Hadoop. Despite of various advantages of MapReduce model, it has also been criticised in terms of its limitation and complexity [13]. This leads to extensive research on MapReduce characteristics, to identify various issues in terms of performance and complexity of the model and current implementations [14–16]. To overcome these difficulties, various extensions are proposed where each one of the extensions fix one or more limitations and drawbacks of MapReduce framework. The scope of this paper is strictly limited to open issues and extensions of MapReduce model to enhance it, not to discuss generalised data-flow systems such as Spark, Dryad and Stratosphere.

This paper is organised as follows. Section 2 presents an overview of Big Data and MapReduce as a programming model under the title background study. Section 3 presents the parallel Apriori algorithm and its implementation on

MapReduce framework. Section 4 presents the open issues as limitations of MapReduce model and various extensions of MapReduce to improve it. We conclude in Sect. 5 with possible future research direction.

2 Background Study

2.1 Big Data and Its Characteristics

Generally, Big Data term is used to describe the data that is very large in size and yet growing exponentially with time. It can be characterised by using following four parameters, commonly known in terms of "4 V" parameters: (i) volume: refers to the size of data, (ii) velocity: refers to the speed of generation of data, (iii) variety: refers to the nature of data whether it is structured or unstructured data and (iv) variability: refers to inconsistency in the data. In current scenario, Big Data and its analysis are at the centre point of current science and business.

2.2 MapReduce as a Programming Model

MapReduce intends to perform flexible information processing in the cloud [9]. Many Programming models have been proposed under the name process models such as generic processing model, graph processing model and stream processing model to solve domain-specific applications. These models are used to improve the performance of NoSQL databases. MapReduce programming model comes under generic processing model that used to address the general application problems. MapReduce programs can be seen in two phases, map phase and reduce phase which consist of map function and reduce function, respectively, and input to each

Table 1 Classification of MapReduce algorithms

Class	Description	Example
First	Algorithms which are fundamentally based on single execution of MapReduce model	Factoring integers
Second	Algorithms which are adapted as a sequential execution of a constant number of MapReduce model	Clustering LARge Application (CLARA) [28]
Third	Algorithms which are iterative in nature and where each iteration requires execution of single MapReduce model only	Partitioning around medoids (PAM) [28]
Fourth	Algorithms which are iterative in nature and content of single iteration is significantly denoted as an execution of multiple MapReduce models	Conjugate gradient (CG) [29]

function are key-value pairs. MapReduce algorithms can be categorised into four classes, as shown in Table 1.

3 Parallel Apriori Algorithm

3.1 *Parallel Apriori Algorithm on MapReduce*

First and foremost, it is required to write parallel Apriori algorithm code in terms of map and reduce functions to run the application on MapReduce model. These two main functions of MapReduce model get the inputs in key-value pairs and generate the output in the key-value form also. The key step in parallel Apriori algorithm is to find out the frequent itemsets. Figure 1 shows the work flow of generation of frequent 1-itemsets.

First, HDFS divides the transactional database into data-chunks (default size of data-chunk is 64 MB) and distributes them among different machines in key-value form where key represents the Transactional ID (TID) and value denotes the list of items. Each mapper running on different machines fed by this key-value pairs and generates the output (key-value) pairs after reading one transaction at a time where key is further refined to represent each item and value is frequency of occurrence of item in the database. These outputs of mapper functions also are known as intermediate values, because these values are fed to combiner before to submit to reducers. Combiner has the task to shuffle and exchange the values using shuffle sort algorithm and consequently prepares a list having values linked with the same key. Here, key represents the item and value represents the support count $\geq$ minimum support of that item.

Reducer function has the main task to aggregate all key-value pairs and generates final output [17]. Here, frequent 1-itemsets are generated at the end into HDFS (storage unit) as output. Frequent k-itemsets are generated by each mapper after reading frequent itemsets from previous iteration and generate candidate itemsets on that basis. This process is done in iterative fashion to get frequent k-itemsets where each iterative step is same as generation of frequent 1-itemsets [7, 18].

3.2 *Various Proposed Implementations of Parallel Apriori Algorithm on MapReduce*

To reduce the time and space complexity of parallel Apriori algorithm, various Apriori-like algorithms have been proposed which execute on MapReduce framework. Broadly, these algorithms can be further classified based on 1-phase of MapReduce and combiner and k-phase of MapReduce approach which is used to

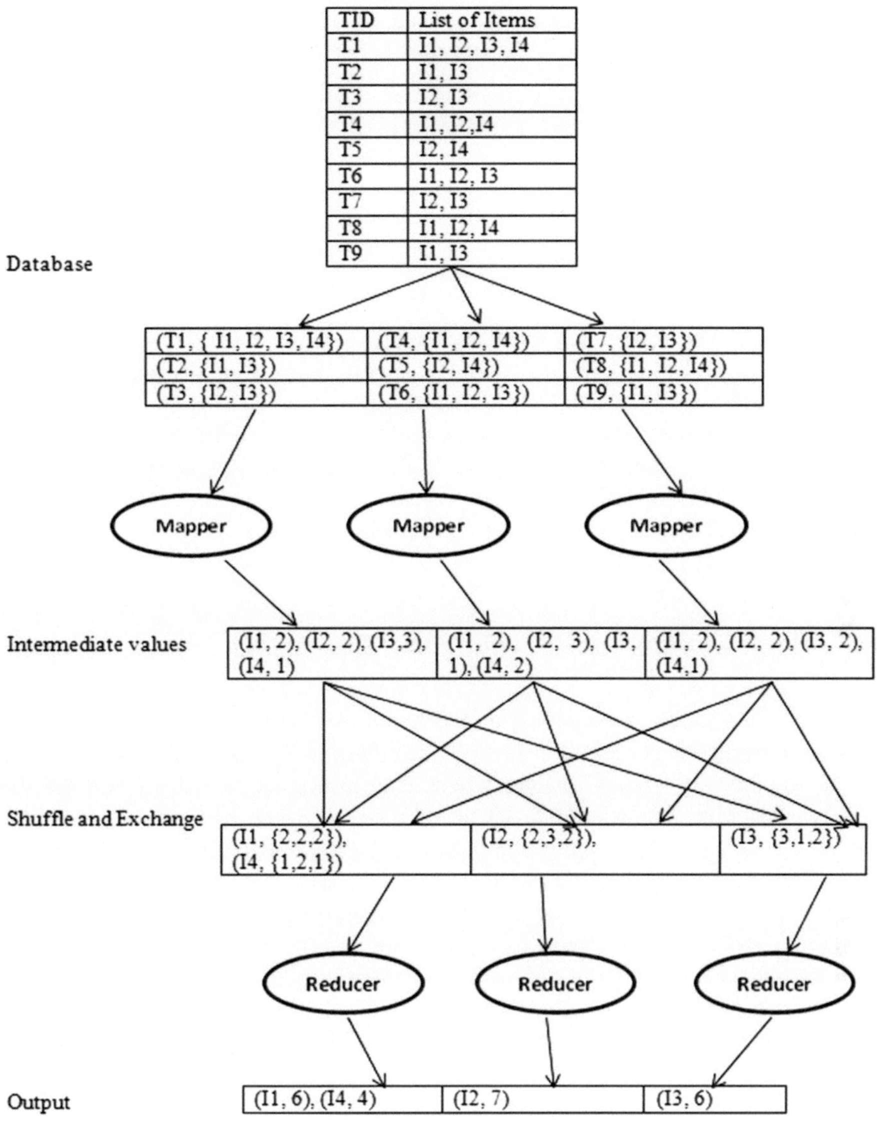

Fig. 1 Finding of frequent 1-itemsets

develop them. Algorithms having 1-phase of MapReduce approach execute single iteration of MapReduce job to extract all frequent itemsets. On the other hand, algorithms having *k*-phase of MapReduce approach execute multiple iterations of MapReduce job [19]. As a result of continuous research, an improved Apriori algorithm [20] comes into existence which further minimises the time complexity of parallel Apriori algorithm from $O(|L_k|^2)$ to $O\ (|V_{key}|^2/q)$ where L_k is the set of large

k-itemsets, V_{key} is the value list of ith key and q is the number of reducers. Further, pruning step of this algorithm is improved that leads to Improved Pruning Apriori (IP-Apriori) [21].

4 MapReduce Open Issues and Extensions

4.1 Performance Issues

MapReduce platform provides some key features such as scalability, fault tolerance to handle the data at large scale, but overall performance of this platform highly depends on the nature of application that is executed in distributed computational environment. To make MapReduce framework more suitable for Big Data handling and to improve the performance, various Hadoop extensions are suggested over the period such as index creation [22], data co-location, reuse the previously computed results and mechanisms dealing with computational skew.

4.2 Programming Model and Query Processing Issues

To code MapReduce applications, understanding of both system architecture and programming skills is required. The programming model of MapReduce has the limitation under its "batch" nature where data is needed to upload into the file system even when the same data set needs to be analysed many times. This programming model is also inappropriate for many classes of algorithm where results of one MapReduce job serving as the input for the next in case of complex queries analysis process. Consequently, a set of domain-specific systems have been emerged to extend the MapReduce programming model where high-level languages such as Java, Ruby, Python and various abstractions have been built to support MapReduce application development environment. Researchers proposed some model to implement iterative algorithms using MapReduce framework such as Hadoop, iHadoop [23], iMapReduce [24], Twister [25] and CloudClustering [26]. Apart from that, users have to spend more time in writing programs in the absence of expressiveness just like SQL. Therefore, it is required to enhance the MapReduce query capabilities [27].

4.3 MapReduce Extensions

To eliminate the limitations of MapReduce framework, researchers try to integrate the key features of parallel database and database to MapReduce programming

Table 2 MapReduce extensions and advantages

MapReduce extensions	Advantages
Hadoop++ [30]	Enhanced performance by injecting joining and indexing capabilities into Hadoop
Manimal [31]	Enables the MapReduce to analyse MapReduce programs automatically
CoHadoop [32]	Supports data storage of linked data at the same compute nodes
SkewReduce [33]	Handles workload by equally dividing input data to mitigate computational skew
SkewTune [34]	Reduces skew using both map and reduce phases at run-time
MapReduce Online [35]	Helps in online aggregation and stream processing to improve resource utilisation
EARL [36]	Allows incremental computations for early results using bootstrapping technique that is used to estimate the error in sampling data [36]
HAIL [37]	Binary PAX representation [38] is used in HAIL to maintain each physical block copy in a different sort order and preserves Hadoop's fault-tolerance properties
MRShare [39]	Provides the optimal grouping of queries to support sharing opportunities
ReStore [40]	Stores and reuses intermediate results of script after completion of tasks or sub-tasks

model which results in MapReduce extensions. Various MapReduce extensions with key advantages are listed in Table 2.

5 Conclusion and Future Research Direction

Based on our survey, both Apriori (traditional Apriori) and parallel Apriori algorithm versions are suffering from the problem of scanning the database multiple times, specially those based on *k*-phase of MapReduce approach which incurs high processing cost and generation of candidate itemsets that needs more memory space. We also focused on MapReduce capabilities, limitations as open issues and various proposed extensions. Open issues lead to various extensions or enhancements, and major enhancements are the result of integration of database with MapReduce, integration of indexing capabilities to MapReduce, integration of MapReduce with data warehouse capabilities and adding skew management in MapReduce.

Future research can be carried out in two dimensions to enhance the performance of parallel Apriori algorithm. One dimension leads to modification in joining and pruning steps of existing algorithm to enable it to support pipelining or use of alternative Apriori-like algorithms which are free from the problem of multiple times scanning of database. Second dimension of research leads to use of advanced

MapReduce framework such as i^2 MapReduce model which supports incremental problem-based algorithm or hybrid algorithms also to enhance the overall throughput of system.

References

1. Assunção, M.D., Calheiros, R.N., Bianchi, S., Netto, M.A., Buyya, R.: Big data computing and clouds: trends and future directions. J. Parallel Distrib. Comput. **79**, 3–15 (2015)
2. Agrawal, R., Ramakrishnan, S.: Fast algorithms for mining association rules. In: Proceedings of the 20th International Conference on Very Large Data Bases, VLDB, vol. 1215, pp. 487–499 (1994)
3. Agrawal, R., Imieliński, T., Swami, A. Mining association rules between sets of items in large databases. ACM SIGMOD Rec. **22**(2), 207–216 (1993)
4. Brin, S., Motwani, R., Ullman, J.D., Tsur, S.: Dynamic itemset counting and implication rules for market basket data. ACM SIGMOD Rec. **26**(2), 255–264 (1997)
5. Dunham, M.H., Xiao, Y. Gruenwald, L., Hossain, Z.: A survey of association rules (2008). Retrieved 5 Jan 2001
6. Oruganti, S., Ding, Q., Tabrizi, N.: Exploring HADOOP as a platform for distributed association rule mining. In: FUTURE COMPUTING 2013, The Fifth International Conference on Future Computational Technologies and Applications, pp. 62–67 (2013)
7. Lin, M.-Y., Lee, P.-Y., Hsueh, S.-C.: Apriori-based frequent itemset mining algorithms on MapReduce. In: Proceedings of the 6th International Conference on Ubiquitous Information Management and Communication, p. 76. ACM (2012)
8. Agrawal, R., Shafer, J.C.: Parallel mining of association rules. IEEE Trans. Knowl. Data Eng. **6**, 962–969 (1996)
9. Dean, J., Ghemawat, S.: MapReduce: simplified data processing on large clusters. In: Proceedings of the Operating Systems Design and Implementation (OSDI), pp 137–150 (2004)
10. Dean, J., Ghemawat, S.: MapReduce: simplified data processing on large clusters. Commun. ACM **51**(1), 107–113 (2008)
11. He, H., Du, Z., Zhang, W., Chen, A.: Optimization strategy of Hadoop small file storage for big data in healthcare. J. Supercomput. 1–12 (2015)
12. Schneider, R.D.: Hadoop for Dummies®. Special edn. Wiley, Canada (2012)
13. Pavlo, A., Paulson, E. Rasin, A., Abadi, D.J., DeWitt, D.J., Madden, S., Stonebraker, M.: A comparison of approaches to large-scale data analysis. In: Proceedings of the 2009 ACM SIGMOD International Conference on Management of Data, pp. 165–178. ACM (2009)
14. Lee, K.-H., Lee, Y.-J., Choi, H. Chung, Y.D., Bongki, M.: Parallel data processing with MapReduce: a survey. ACM SIGMOD Rec. **40**(4), 11–20 (2012)
15. Jiang, D., Ooi, B.C., Shi, L., Wu, S.: The performance of Mapreduce: an in-depth study. Proc. VLDB Endowment **3**(1-2 (2010): 472-483
16. Goyal, A., Dadizadeh, S.: A survey on cloud computing. In: University of British Columbia Technical Report for CS 508, 55–58 (2009)
17. Kovacs, F., Illes, J: Frequent itemset mining on hadoop. In: 2013 IEEE 9th International Conference on Computational Cybernetics (ICCC), pp. 241–245. IEEE (2013)
18. Li, N., Zeng, L., He, Q., Shi, Z.: Parallel implementation of Apriori algorithm based on MapReduce. In: 2012 13th ACIS International Conference on Software Engineering, Artificial Intelligence, Networking and Parallel & Distributed Computing (SNPD), pp. 236–241. IEEE (2012)

19. Li, L., Zhang, M.: The strategy of mining association rule based on cloud computing. In: 2011 International Conference on Business Computing and Global Informatization (BCGIN), pp. 475–478. IEEE (2011)
20. Al-Maolegi, M., Arkok, B. An improved Apriori algorithm for association rules. arXiv preprint arXiv:1403.3948 (2014)
21. Sequeira, J.V., Ansari, Z.: Analysis on improved pruning in Apriori algorithm. Int. J. Adv. Res. Comput. Sci. Softw. Eng. (IJARCSSE) **5**, 894–902 (2015)
22. Kang, W.L., Kim, H.G., Lee, Y.J.: Efficient indexing for OLAP query processing with MapReduce. In: Computer Science and Its Applications, pp. 783–788. Springer, Berlin, Heidelberg (2015)
23. Song, J., Guo, C., Zhang, Y., Zhu, Z., Yu, G.: Research on MapReduce based incremental iterative model and framework. IETE J. Res. **61**(1), 32–40 (2015)
24. Zhang, Y., Gao, Q., Gao, L., Wang, C.: Imapreduce: a distributed computing framework for iterative computation. J. Grid Comput. **10**(1), 47–68 (2012)
25. Ekanayake, J., Li, H., Zhang, B., Gunarathne, T., Bae, S.-H., Qiu, J., Fox, G.: Twister: a runtime for iterative mapreduce. In: Proceedings of the 19th ACM International Symposium on High Performance Distributed Computing, pp. 810–818. ACM (2010)
26. Dave, A., Lu, W., Jackson, J., Barga, R.: CloudClustering: toward an iterative data processing pattern on the cloud. In: 2011 IEEE International Symposium on Parallel and Distributed Processing Workshops and Phd Forum (IPDPSW), pp. 1132–1137. IEEE (2011)
27. Thusoo, A., Sarma, J.S., Jain, N., Shao, Z., Chakka, P., Zhang, N., Antony, S., Liu, H., Murthy, R.: Hive—a petabyte scale data warehouse using Hadoop. In: 2010 IEEE 26th International Conference on Data Engineering (ICDE), pp. 996–1005. IEEE (2010)
28. Kaufman, L., Rousseeuw, P.J.: Finding Groups in Data: An Introduction to Cluster Analysis, vol. 344. Wiley (2009)
29. Shewchuk, J.R.: An introduction to the conjugate gradient method without the agonizing pain (1994)
30. Dittrich, J., Quiané-Ruiz, J.-A., Jindal, A., Kargin, Y., Setty, V., Schad, J.: Hadoop++: making a yellow elephant run like a cheetah (without it even noticing). Proc. VLDB Endowment **3**(1–2), 515–529 (2010)
31. Jahani, E., Cafarella, M.J., Ré, C.: Automatic optimization for MapReduce programs. Proc. VLDB Endowment **4**(6), 385–396 (2011)
32. Eltabakh, M.Y., Tian, Y., Özcan, F., Gemulla, R., Krettek, A., McPherson, J.: CoHadoop: flexible data placement and its exploitation in Hadoop. Proc. VLDB Endowment **4**(9), 575–585 (2011)
33. Kwon, Y.C., Balazinska, M., Howe, B., Rolia, J.: Skew-resistant parallel processing of feature-extracting scientific user-defined functions. In: Proceedings of the 1st ACM Symposium on Cloud Computing, pp. 75–86. ACM (2010)
34. Kwon, Y.C., Ren, K., Balazinska, M., Howe, B., Rolia, J.: Managing skew in Hadoop. IEEE Data Eng. Bull. **36**(1), 24–33 (2013)
35. Condie, T., Conway, N., Alvaro, P., Hellerstein, J.M., Elmeleegy, K., Sears, R.: MapReduce Online. NSDI **10**(4), 20 (2010)
36. Laptev, N., Zeng, K., Zaniolo, C.: Early accurate results for advanced analytics on mapreduce. Proc. VLDB Endowment **5**(10), 1028–1039 (2012)
37. Dittrich, J., Quiané-Ruiz, J.-A., Richter, S., Schuh, S., Jindal, A., Schad, J.: Only aggressive elephants are fast elephants. Proc. VLDB Endowment **5**(11), 1591–1602 (2012)
38. Ailamaki, A., DeWitt, D.J., Hill, M.D., Skounakis, M.: Weaving relations for cache performance. VLDB **1**, 169–180 (2001)
39. Nykiel, T., Potamias, M., Mishra, C., Kollios, G., Koudas, N.: MRShare: sharing across multiple queries in MapReduce. Proc. VLDB Endowment **3**(1–2), 494–505 (2010)
40. Elghandour, I., Aboulnaga, A.: ReStore: reusing results of MapReduce jobs. Proc. VLDB Endowment **5**(6), 586–597 (2012)

A Novel Approach to Realize Internet of Intelligent Things

Vishal Mehta

Abstract In this era of emerging technologies, Internet of Things is one which is ready to change the world on how it works. Today, a new breed of generation of human beings has evolved which love to be always "connected" to the other part of world, publish their opinions on social networks, and tweet about their sentiments on Twitter. Human beings are surrounded with physical objects. Is there a way so that these surrounding objects become part of the human community and the answer is YES: Internet of Things, where everything is connected to everything else. But connecting the "Things" is not just the answer we are looking to. In this paper, we are trying to propose a framework which does not tell that the things are mere an abstraction but also they are "intelligent" enough like human beings, they have the intelligence to take decision on their own, and they can also post their sentiments on social networks like human beings. In this paper, we are trying to implement a system which can automatically contact the manufacturer, block a calendar for the maintenance, and drop an e-mail to the owner to make a credit card payment to get the maintenance done before it breaks.

Keywords IOT internet of things · RPi · Agent · Prosumer

1 Introduction

A "Thing" is an entity or a system composed of subsystems where every subsystem becomes the integral component of the system and makes a thing as "Thing". If we break the thing abstraction, we can find that every subsystem has a behavior. Now the question is how we can understand a thing in isolation. To understand the behavior of "Thing," we need to understand what are the basic subcomponents of

V. Mehta (✉)
Mphasis Limited, Cybercity Tower IV, Magarpatta City, Hadapsar,
Pune, Maharashtra, India
e-mail: sirius.mehta@gmail.com

V.B. Aggarwal et al. (eds.), *Big Data Analytics*, Advances in Intelligent
Systems and Computing 654, https://doi.org/10.1007/978-981-10-6620-7_39

the system (thing) and then we need to understand the behavior of these subsystems to understand the behavior of the thing as a whole.

To understand these subcomponents, these subcomponents are deployed with sensors or better said agents, and these agents are not just electronic sensors but also they are equipped with the capability to learn the behavior of the subcomponent and log the behavior data of that subcomponent for that "Thing" which has a unique ID onto the cloud so that this sensed data for the thing can be further analyzed to extract "Thing Dynamics" a coin termed similar to Human Dynamics.

2 Working of "Thing"

2.1 Architecture of Thing

As we can see in Fig. 1, we have a conceptual diagram of Thing including its sub component. The subcomponents are deployed with learning agent (sensor). These agents sniff the behavior data of the subcomponent of Thing and record it as a variable. Since there are multiple subcomponents, hence we record every subcomponent as a variable. Attaching all these recorded variables gives us a concrete dataset to study the behavior of the Thing as a whole. All the agents send the recorded data to raspberry pi. The raspberry pi has an internal storage of 1 GB to store the daily sensor recorded data locally as we can see in Fig. 1. The scheduled batch job runs periodically to upload the data to Hadoop cluster for batch analysis. Once the data is uploaded to the Hadoop cluster, it is pushed to the analyzer which has an R Engine to identify the relationship between the recorded variables and create the hypothesis. The hypothesis created helps in modeling the sentiment of the health of the product. There are various subcomponents of AC such as compressor, condenser, evaporator, capillary tube, indoor fan, and outdoor fan. Now our goal is to identify:

- If the compressor of the Air conditioner will be faulty in the near future.
- Predicts the date for maintenance, contacts the manufacturer, books the calendar and informs the present health status to the owner and requests to enter the credit card details to finalize the maintenance booked by making the payment.

Here we have a dataset of various subcomponents of air conditioner (AC). For each variable, we have corresponding variable in the dataset as follows:

1. Compressor temperature
2. Condenser
3. Evaporator
4. Amount of Oil.

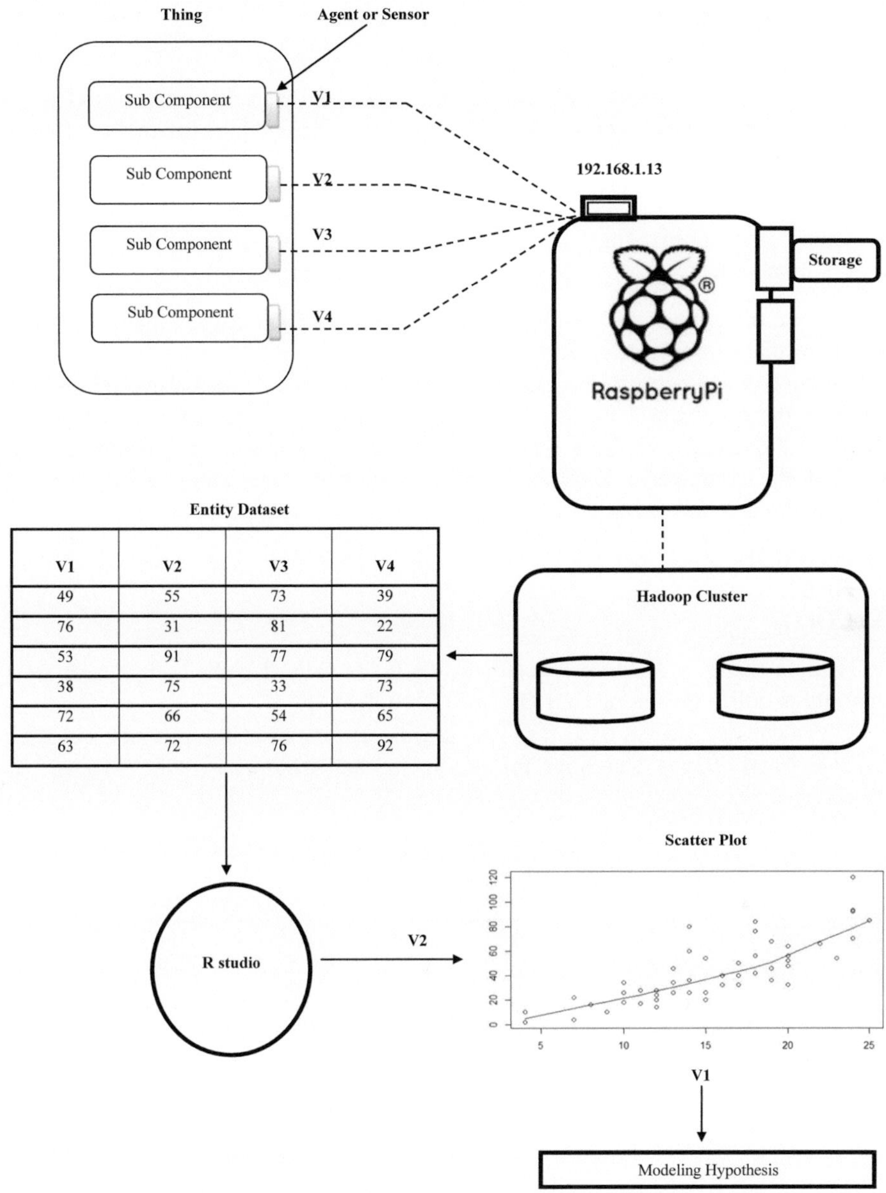
Thing
Agent or Sensor
Sub Component
Sub Component
Sub Component
Sub Component
V1
V2
V3
V4
192.168.1.13
Storage
RaspberryPi
Entity Dataset
V1 V2 V3 V4
49 55 73 39
76 31 81 22
53 91 77 79
38 75 33 73
72 66 54 65
63 72 76 92
Hadoop Cluster
Scatter Plot
R studio
V2
0 20 40 60 80 100 120
5 10 15 20 25
V1
Modeling Hypothesis

Fig. 1

3 Results

Now, we import the dataset and explore the variables (as in descriptive models for Internet of Things) to check the dependency or the relationship, so now we need to check if the compressor will be faulty in near future. So for this, our variables of interest are:

- Compressor temperature
- Amount of Oil.

And we draw the scatterplot to identify the relationship between them as we can see as results of the relationships in Fig. 2.

As we can see here, as the amount of oil in compressor increases, the temperature of the compressor decreases and possess the indirect relationship between them. In the dataset, we have a target variable using which we can categorize the state of the compressor and see if the compressor temperature is in the three classifications listed below:

1. NORMAL
2. HEAT
3. COLD.

Here, is Faulty is a Boolean vector which holds value 1 if the compressor_state variable is either HEAT or COLD else 0 if NORMAL.

The vector isFaulty is used for checking the sentiment of the product. For this, we use Naive Bayes Classifier for predicting the sentiment of the "Thing" as follows:

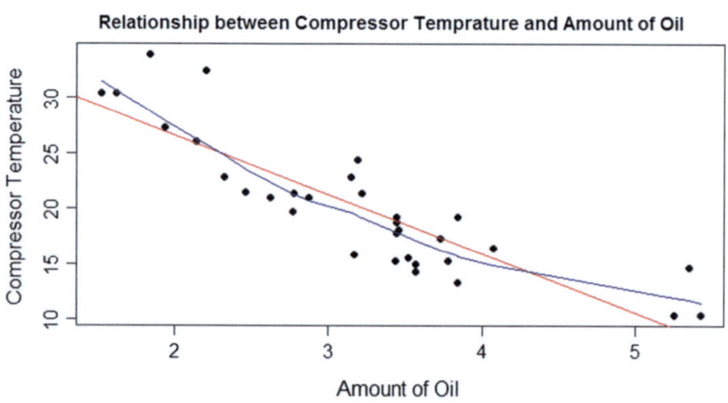

Fig. 2

Sentiment Classification:

Category	Sentiment
NORMAL	Positive
HEAT	Negative
COLD	Negative

CODE:

```
isFaulty <- NULL
#calculates the tempature difference
temprature_difference <- Compressor_temperature - tartemp


#initializing the initial state of vector as NULL
compressor_state <- NULL


#checking if the value of temprature_difference > = < 5
for(temp in temprature_difference){
if(temprature_difference > 5){
 compressor_state <- c(compressor_state, "HEAT")
 isFaulty <- c(isFaulty, 1)
}else if(temprature_difference < 5){
 compressor_state <- c(compressor_state, "COLD")
 isFaulty <- c(isFaulty, 1)
}else
 compressor_state <- c(compressor_state, "NORMAL")
 isFaulty <- c(isFaulty, 0)
}
```

Now, once we get the sentiment of the Thing, the Thing also has a social sensor attached to it. By the term social sensor we mean the "Thing" has the capability to tweet its sentiment, state of health, and also the hypothesis on the social platforms like Twitter and also the human beings. Now as we can see in the Fig. 3, we have a correlation engine. The correlation engine takes the input component sentiment analyzer and the Thing social sensor and also the tweets done by people saying:

"I hate this Thing, since this is not working." The engine will correlate all the sentiments (Sentiment of Thing and Person) and will infer the actionable telling:

What and Why the Thing is not good or something is broken. Next we have a module called Automated Maintenance Recommender. Once it sees that the

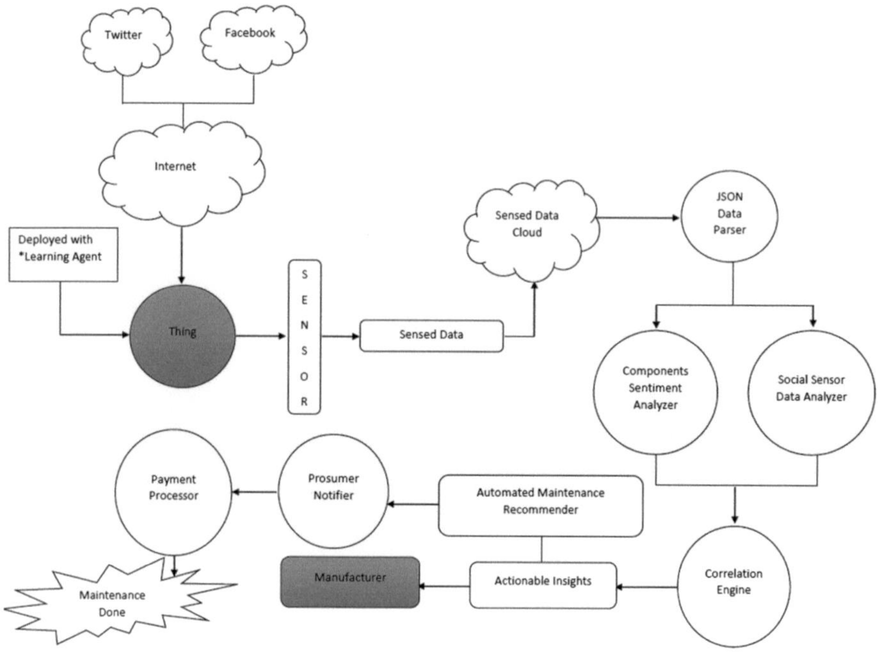

Fig. 3

sentiment of the product is negative, it then automatically books the calendar for maintenance and informs the Prosumer about the details of the payment being requested to book the appointment for maintenance of the air conditioner. Once the Prosumer makes the payment, the Thing finalizes the appointment and drops the e-mail to the Prosumer of the confirmation.

4 Limitation and Future Scope

Recording the variables as properties of the "Thing" and exploring the relationships between them is still a manual process which needs exporting the data from the "Thing" into R Studio and applying the exploratory techniques in order to model a hypothesis and test this hypothesis using confirmatory data analysis to model a prediction equation. The future scope of the present technique is, if we can devise a way, we can automate the exploratory techniques applied on the real-time data on the fly.

5 Conclusion

The current system helps in automated "Thing" maintenance where the thing can automatically keep its health check and request for maintenance from the manufacturer if required. And it also helps the manufacturer to look-understand-react on the problems being faced by the Thing giving them actionable insights.

References

1. Tan, L., Wang, N.: Future internet: the internet of things. Comput. Sci. Technol. Department of East China Normal University, Shanghai, China
2. Shi, Z., Liao, K., Yin, S., Ou, Q.: Design and implementation of the mobile internet of things based on TD-SCDMA network. Chongqing Communication Institute, PLA, Chongqing, China
3. Huang, Y., Li, G.: Descriptive models for internet of things. Inf. Sci. Technol. Coll., Dalian Maritime University, Dalian, China
4. Burange, A.W., Misalkar, H.D.: Review of internet of things in development of smart cities with data management & privacy. Department of Information Technology, PRMIT&R, Badnera, India
5. Yu, Z., Tie-Ning, W.: Research on the visualization of equipment support based on the technology of internet of things. Academy of Armored Forces Engineering, Beijing, China
6. Coetzee, L., Eksteen, J: The internet of things—promise for the future? An introduction. Meraka Institute, CSIR, Pretoria, South Africa
7. Bari, N., Mani, G., Berkovich, S: Internet of things as a methodological concept. George Washington University, Washington, DC, USA

An Innovative Approach of Web Page Ranking Using Hadoop- and Map Reduce-Based Cloud Framework

Dheeraj Malhotra, Monica Malhotra and O.P. Rishi

Abstract In this era of Big Data, Web page searching and ranking in an efficient manner on WWW to satisfy the search needs of modern-day user is undoubtedly a major challenge for search engines. In this paper, we propose an innovative algorithm based on Hadoop–Map Reduce-supported cloud computing framework that can be implemented in the form of Meta Search and Page Ranking Tool to efficiently search and rank Big Data available on WWW which is increasing in the scale of megabytes to terabytes per day. An extensive experimental evaluation shows that the average ranking precision of proposed algorithm and Meta tool is better than other popular search engines.

Keywords Cloud computing · Hadoop · Map Reduce · Big data analysis · Meta search tool · Cluster page ranking algorithm · HDFS · Web page ranking

CSI-2015, 50th Golden Jubilee Annual Convention on **Digital Life** (02nd–05th December, 2015), Delhi, India.

D. Malhotra (✉)
VSIT, Vivekananda Institute of Professional Studies, Delhi, India
e-mail: dheeraj.malhotra@vips.edu

M. Malhotra
IIIST, Delhi, India
e-mail: monicamalhotra777@gmail.com

O.P. Rishi
CSI, University of Kota, Kota, Rajasthan, India
e-mail: dr.oprishi@uok.ac.in

V.B. Aggarwal et al. (eds.), *Big Data Analytics*, Advances in Intelligent Systems and Computing 654, https://doi.org/10.1007/978-981-10-6620-7_40

1 Introduction

Cloud computing is one of the popular technologies among Web developers and SEO industry due to its low-cost infrastructure requirement with highly reliable, parallel, and scalable computing capabilities. However, due to limitations of conventional data mining approaches to mine useful patterns from WWW for reliable page ranking process, a term called Big Data analytics is introduced. Big Data is usually unstructured in nature and is defined as "A huge and complex collection of data sets, difficult to be processed using conventional database management tools." However, Big Data analysis on WWW can be easily accomplished by employing Hadoop- and Map Reduce-based distributed cloud computing framework. Hadoop is a robust, scalable, and open-source platform for processing Big Data [1, 2]. MapReduce programming model may be used to process data in Hadoop cluster with the help of two data processing primitives known as mapper and reducer in (Key, Value) pair format [3]. In this research paper, we worked on enhancing the capabilities of our previously published SNEC algorithm [4] to work with cloud framework using HDFS model.

2 Research Problem and Objectives of Research

The availability of Web data on WWW is quite huge. Such a huge repository of data may be termed as Big Data. In this scenario, it becomes very difficult for the user to find relevant information from the Internet. One of the approaches is to use search engine. However, none of the search engines can completely solve the problem of complete relevant information retrieval as each search engine can index only a subset of information available on WWW due to gigantic size and dynamic nature of Web. Hence, user may be required to query several search engines to achieve the desired level of precision and recall of search results. Moreover, traditional page ranking computation system has been processor bound and hence lacks storage and processing capabilities required for handling Big Data available on the Web. Some of the objectives of present research work are (i) to develop page ranking algorithm using Hadoop and Map Reduce model based on distributed cloud framework, (ii) to implement Meta Search and Page Ranking tool to evaluate the effectiveness of the proposed algorithm.

3 Research Methodology

This research work aims to handle processing at middle layer for service level agreement in a public cloud. This approach first search for user-specified query on each of the back-end search engine for retrieving relevant clusters. Parametric matches such as accessibility, security, and response time will be considered for shortlisting clusters. The first level of ranking will be implemented by determining content relevancy vector (CRV) in two-phase programming model called Map and Reduce to support Hadoop distributed cloud architecture. The second level and third level of ranking are based on calculation of Time Relevancy Vector (TRV) and Semantics Relevancy Vector (SRV) [4]. Finally, all of these vectors with their weighted contribution as required by user lead to ranking formula to determine rank of each of the clusters of Web pages as discussed in the following CPR algorithm in Sect. 3.1. Map and Reduce code to be used by the proposed algorithm is as follows:

```
Map (Integer Cluster_ID, String Cluster_Log) {
      List<String> L = tokenize (log)
        For each token_link in L {
extract ((String) KWL, (Integer) 1)
        }}

Reduce (String token_link, List <Integer> count)
                Integer found = 0
               For each word in KWL {
                      Found = Found + 1
                }
  extract ((string) token, (Integer) found)}
```

3.1 CPR: Cluster-Based Page Ranking Algorithm

```
• Accept & split search string to store keywords in
   KWL list data structure.
•Execute search query on each backend search engine to
   obtain relevant clusters i.e. Cluster(1,…,N)
•For x=1 to N do              // Filtering of Web pages
   {
      o Accessibility Vector, AV[i]=0; if (Cloud =
         Public) { AV[i] =1; }
      o Privacy vector, PV=0; If (strprivacy = priva-
         cy(Cluster(i))  set  PV[i]=1;
      o Reply Time Vector, RTV[i]=0
      o If (strresponse > Reply Time(Cluster(i))
      o {RTV[i] = strresponse - ReplyTime(Cluster(i) }
   } // End of for loop

•Ignore all the clusters for which either of AV=0,
   PV=0 or RTV= 0

   // determine content relevancy
•For x=1 to L
   {
      o Call Map(Cluster_ID, Cluster_Content)
      o Call Reduce(Token_Link, Count)
      o CR_P= FOUND_P
•Store CR_P in content relevancy vector CRV[x] for Clus-
   ter[x]
   }

•Determine timestamp T_S of creation and average time
   spent by previous user T_P to calculate Time rele-
   vancy TR_p to store in time relevance vector TRV[x]
   for Cluster[x]
•Identify navigation session by comparing user search
   query with each of the search query present in user
   profile database using Longest Common Subsequence
   (LCS)to calculate proximity and hence Semantic Rank
   SR_p to be stored in semantic relevance vector SRV[x]
   for cluster[x].

•Rank (Cluster(i)) = AV[i]*((CRV[i]*W1 + TRV[i]*W2 +
   SRV[i]*W3 +PV[i]*W4+ RTV[i]*W5)
```

3.2 *System Design and Meta Page Ranking Tool*

HDFS or Hadoop distributed file system is used for handling distributed storage system. In order to evaluate CPR algorithm discussed in this paper, we implemented it in the form of Meta Search and Page Ranking Tool using ASP.NET framework. The interface of tool is shown in Fig. 1.

Architecture of Proposed System

Various important components are shown in Fig. 2 and are discussed as follows:

Name Node (NN): In this architecture, NN is considered as master that directs commands to all data nodes (DN) which are considered as slaves. NN handles all bookkeeping tasks of HDFS.

Secondary Name Node (SNN): SNN is not a backup of NN, but it does some housekeeping tasks for NN. SNN maintains *Journaling* or *Edit log* where incremental modifications are made to metadata for minimizing the downtime or loss of data.

Cloud Cluster Manager: It is supervisor of Meta Search tool architecture and is responsible for Web page distribution, Web page storage, inter-cluster communication, etc. Its design is crucial for efficient performance of Meta Search tool.

Data Node (DN): HDFS file is broken down into blocks to store in data nodes. DNs are constantly reporting to the NN. Upon initialization, each of the DNs informs the NN regarding blocks it is currently storing.

Meta Search and Page Ranking Tool			
Select Search Engine Tabs for Intermediate Document Retrieval			
GOOGLE	YAHOO	BING	ASK
Enter Search String: HDFS and Map Reduce			
	Search	Reset	
Ranking Box………			
Rank	**Web Links**	**Security**	**Response**
1	https://en.wikipedia.org/wiki/Apache_Hadoop	**HTTPS:**	00:00:00:10ms
2	www.cloudera.com/content/cloudera/hdfs-	**N/A**	00:00:00:25ms
3	www.gttibm.org/software/datacom/infospher/ma	**SSL**	00:00:00:33ms

Fig. 1 Interface of meta search and page ranking tool

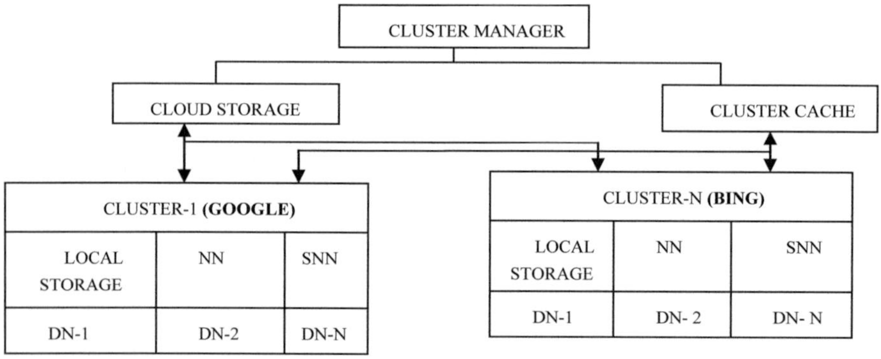

Fig. 2 Architecture of proposed system

3.3 Experimental Verification and Graphical Analysis of Result

In order to evaluate the effectiveness of our proposed algorithm and tool, we took two query sets and assumed top 30 results of search are important as user usually like to check only first two or three pages returned in response to his search query. We first calculated parameters of precision for each of the top 30 Web pages retrieved through tool. These parameters include page freshness to ensure latest updated content delivery, Web site reliability to deliver page within required response time and page size. All of these parameters are important for the Internet user, especially those with slow or unstable Internet connections as they directly affect user satisfaction level [5]. In the second step, we normalized the values of all parameters using

$$Y_{IJ} = (\mathrm{UPR}(X_{IJ}) - X_{IJ})/(\mathrm{UPR}(X_{IJ}) - \mathrm{LOW}(X_{IJ})),$$

where X_{IJ} = value of J_{th} precision parameter of I_{th} Web page; Y_{IJ} = normalized value of J_{th} precision parameter of I_{th} Web page; LOW, UPR = lowest and highest value of each of precision parameter.

In the third step, we calculated the overall weighted precision of each Web page as $\mathbf{Z_I = \sum W_J.Y_{IJ}}$, where Z_I = weighted precision of I_{th} Web page; W_J = weight assigned to J_{th} parameter by user; $0 \leq W_J \leq 1$. We will find out the minimum value of precision obtained among these 30 values and may consider this value as precision of our tool; i.e., **Precision (Tool) = MIN ($\mathbf{Z_I}$)**. Meta tool reports better precision when compared with popular search engines as shown in Fig. 3.

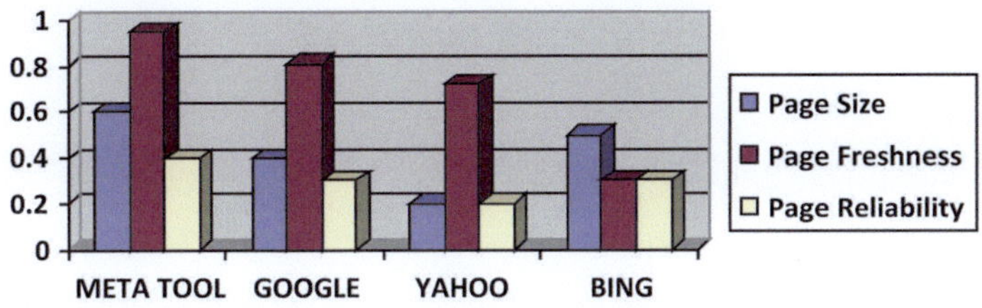

Fig. 3 Precision comparison of meta page ranking tool with popular search engines

4 Conclusion and Future Work

This research work presents a HDFS and Map Reduce-based cloud computing framework to develop an improved CPR page ranking algorithm for implementation of Meta Search and Page Ranking Tool. The effectiveness of proposed algorithm is shown by precision comparison with popular search engines. The proposed work can be further extended to assist retail businesses by deriving useful patterns from Big Data stored in customer databases using cloud technology where conventional data mining techniques are inadequate to mine useful patterns.

References

1. Son, J., Ryu, H., Yi, S., Chung, Y.: SSFile: a novel column-store for efficient data analysis in hadoop-based distributed systems. Inf. Sci. **316**, 68–86 (2015)
2. Feller, E., Ramakrishnan, L., Morin, C.: Performance and energy efficiency of big data applications in cloud environments: a Hadoop case study. J. Parallel. Distrib. Comput. **79**, 80–89 (2015)
3. Lam, C.: Hadoop in Action. Dreamtech Press, New Delhi (2013)
4. Verma, N., Malhotra, D., Malhotra, M., Singh, J.: E-commerce website ranking using semantic web mining and neural computing. In: International Conference on Advanced Computing Technologies and Applications. Elsevier Procedia Computer Science, vol. 45, pp. 42–51. Elsevier, Mumbai, India, 26–27 Mar 2015
5. Chen, X., Ding, C.: QoS based ranking for web search. In: IEEE/WIC/ACM International Conference on Web Intelligence and Intelligent Agent Technology, pp. 747–750. IEEE Computer Society, 9–12 Dec 2008
6. Singh, A., Velez, H.: Hierarchical multi-log cloud-based search engine. In: 8th IEEE International Conference on Complex, Intelligent and Software Intensive Systems, pp. 212–219. IEEE CPS, Birmingham, UK, 2–4 July 2014
7. Iordache, A., Morin, C., Parlavantzas, N., Feller, E. Riteau, P.: Resilin: elastic map reduce over multiple clouds. In: 13th IEEE/ACM International Symposium on Cluster, Cloud and Grid Computing, pp. 261–268. IEEE Computer Society, Delft, Netherlands, 13–16 May 2013
8. White, T.: Hadoop: The Definitive Guide. O'Reilly Media, USA (2010)
9. Shou, G., Bai, H., Chan, K., Chen, G.: Supporting privacy protection in personalized web search. IEEE Trans. Knowl. Data Eng. **26**(2), 453–467 (2014)

SAASQUAL: A Quality Model for Evaluating SaaS on the Cloud Computing Environment

Dhanamma Jagli, Seema Purohit and N. Subhash Chandra

Abstract Cloud computing is a technology that has come out in the last decade and that is transforming the IT industry in huge. The cloud computing is playing a vital role as a backbone component of the Internet of Things (IoT). In a cloud computing scenario, cloud services are accessible via Internet. Cloud computing is providing on-demand resources like infrastructure, platform, and software as it does not pay to possess the software itself but rather to use it. Pay for use concept is very attractive, hence many organizations are adopting the SaaS model drastically. Even though, each customer is unique and leads to unique variation in the requirements of the software. The SaaS is generally pressed into service, and it yields advantages to service providers and service customers. More and more SaaS services are emerging, how to select qualified service is key problem for customers. Present quality models are not sufficient to evaluate SaaS selection on the cloud due to its tremendous increase in the use. A quality model can be used to represent, evaluate and differentiate the quality of the SaaS providers. In this paper, a new quality model proposed and named SAASQUAL for cloud software services. This model is based on different attributes of quality software, quality service and metrics that measure software quality and service quality in order to evaluate potential software as a service on the cloud.

D. Jagli (✉) · S. Purohit · N.S. Chandra
JNTU Hyderabad, Hyderabad, Telangana, India
e-mail: dsjagli.vesit@gmail.com

S. Purohit
e-mail: supurohit@gmail.com

N.S. Chandra
e-mail: subhashchandra_n@yahoo.co.in

D. Jagli
V.E.S. Institute of Technology, University of Mumbai, Mumbai, India

S. Purohit
Kirti College, University of Mumbai, Mumbai, India

N.S. Chandra
Holy Mary Institute of Technology, JNTU Hyderabad, Hyderabad, India

V.B. Aggarwal et al. (eds.), *Big Data Analytics*, Advances in Intelligent Systems and Computing 654, https://doi.org/10.1007/978-981-10-6620-7_41

Keywords Software as a service (SaaS) · EM clustering · Model-based clustering

1 Introduction

The cloud computing has been growing as an essential and leading computing platform for sharing resources like infrastructure, platform, software. Cloud computing has emerged as a new paradigm in the field of network-based services within many industries and application domains. The major benefits that it provides in terms of IT efficiency and business agility represent a huge competitive advantage for an organization. This has proven to be an essential requirement for extending many existing applications. The cloud computing is a latest way of computing and providing several scalable resources dynamically as well as virtualizing often those resources as a service over the Internet. There are three main service models available on the cloud computing environment such as Infrastructure as a Service (IaaS), Platform as a service (PaaS) and Software as a Service (SaaS).

The SaaS is a model that provides several uses to service consumers without installing any application locally. In order to use all advantages of SaaS model efficiently and effectively, there should be proper quality model to evaluate SaaS quality. The customers do not pay to possess the software itself but rather to use it, this concept of pay per use is very attractive and commonly used by many users and it had several advantages. In order to make use of the best of SaaS, it is required to examine the possible quality of SaaS. In fact, service providers have to evaluate their services against needs of service users in order to increase their service. Hence the available SaaS quality evaluation models are lacking to focus on all aspects of quality and services together. However, each customer is unique, which leads to a very large variation in the requirements of the software. Therefore, this paper presents a method to help customers to choose a better SaaS product satisfying most of their conditions and alternatives. This is also known that a good method of adaptive selection should be based on the correct definition of the different parameters of choice. For that reason, the proposed work states that extraction and analysis the various parameters involved in the process of the selection of a SaaS Application.

2 Related Work Towards SaaS Evaluation

The cloud computing will be in need of several numbers of interactions with varying quality requirements. Service quality has become a significant differentiator amid of cloud providers. In order to discriminate between service providers from various competitors and other cloud service vendors, there should be some measure to know superiority of services. Any standard quality model can be used to represent, measure and compare the quality of the software services on the cloud. The work has been done many researchers towards SaaS evaluation is comparatively very less till 2005, afterwards work have been improved towards SaaS evaluation till today and many methods were introduced as follows.

Jae Yoo Lee, Jung Woo Lee, Du Wan Chen, "A Quality Model for Evaluating Software as a Service in Cloud Computing" proposed a quality method that will help to examine the quality aspect of SaaS, based on the SaaS key features derived from primary SaaS features. They also described some standards to measure quality of SaaS based on the quality attributes. They validated and assessed their proposed quality model for evaluating SaaS' quality; they used the standard EIRE 1061 and examined their work. Manish Godse, Shrikant Mulik, "An Approach for Selecting Software as a Service (SaaS) Product", published and presented a new model based on Analytic Hierarchy Process (AHP) approach intended for ranking the SaaS features like functionality, vendor reputation, architecture, usability and cost. Qian Tao, Huiyou Chang, Yang Yi, Chunqin Gu, "A TRUSTWORTHY MANAGEMENT APPROACH FOR CLOUD SERVICES", published work, the authors proposed trustworthy management for all cloud services based on non-functional QoS attributes like reputation, reliability, security, time, cost and availability. They also applied Data Mining PAM (Partitioning Around Medians) clustering algorithm for trustworthy management of all types cloud services. Chen Yiming, Zhu Yiwei, "SaaS Vendor Selection Basing on Analytic Hierarchy Process", published work and they proposed a model for selecting Best SaaS vendor based on the same principles applicable to vendors rather than selecting SaaS Product. This model was analysed by using Analytic Hierarchy Process. Qiang He, Jun Han, Yun Yang and John Grundy Hai Jin, "QoS-Driven Service Selection for Multi-Tenant SaaS", published and proposed a criterion for selecting a SaaS based on QoS parameters like cost, response time, availability and throughput. This method for service, selection was multi-tenant oriented. Pang Xiong Wen, Li Dong, " Quality Model for Evaluating SaaS Service", published and proposed, an advanced quality model measures the security, software quality of the SaaS and quality of service from the perspective view of a service provider and service user independently. Based on this proposed an evaluating model which classify the SaaS service into four levels, including basic level, standard level, optimized level and integrated level. By using the quality model and evaluating model, the customer can evaluate the provider and the provider can use it for quality management. Again, this model was based on key feature of SaaS. Xianrong Zheng, "CLOUD QUAL: A Quality Model for Cloud Services", published in the proceedings of IEEE TRANSACTIONS ON INDUSTRIAL INFORMATICS. In this paper, the author has been considered a service perspective and initiates a quality model called as *CLOUDQUAL* for all type of cloud services. In this model, authors proposed quality model with set of dimensions and metrics that are applicable to all services on the cloud. *CLOUDQUAL* contains six set of dimensions for quality are security, elasticity, usability, availability, responsiveness and reliability. Out of all six dimensions usability is considered as subjective and all others have been considered as an objective. The author demonstrated with the help of Azure Blob, Aliyun OSS and Amazon S3, cloud storage services.

The above-described research work has been proposed for SaaS selection, and SaaS evaluations are based on different attributes, but many authors have been contributed based on key features and quality attributes in order to measure the quality of SaaS on the cloud computing. Even though there are some limitations and restrictions and challenges have been found. In order to face few challenges, the new model is proposed for SaaS evaluation inspired by the SERVQUAL and CLOUDQUAL for measuring general cloud services. The proposed model in this paper is focusing only on the software services on the cloud computing environment, and it is termed as Software as a Service Quality model (SAASQUAL).

3 Address Challenges and Concerns of SaaS

The new quality model is proposed to evaluate Software as a Service (SaaS) on the cloud. The cloud computing software service is completely different from conventional software services. For conventional software services, the standard mode is given to measure the internal characteristics and characteristics of software quality that is called as ISO/IEC 9126 Quality model. This standard was more helpful for conventional software service providers in order to measure their software product quality to fulfil service user requirements and also service user to identify the potential service as per their requirements. The ISO/IEC 9126 Quality model is explained in the following sections.

3.1 ISO/IEC 9126 Quality Model for Conventional Software Services

The standard quality model intended for software products is ISO/IEC 9126 standard. This standard describes the software quality in the form of characteristics. The first part of standard ISO/IEC 9126 presented a classification of software quality in a form of structured set of characteristics and sub-characteristics as shown in Fig. 1. All quality sub-characteristics is classified into several attributes. An attribute is a property that can be certified or evaluated in the software product.

3.2 SaaS Development Life-Cycle (SaaS DLC)

The service development on cloud computing is in need of a different approach than conventional software development life-cycle, because SaaS development life-cycle becomes a significant success feature of the whole project for cloud providers. Within conventional software development surroundings, further prominence is to

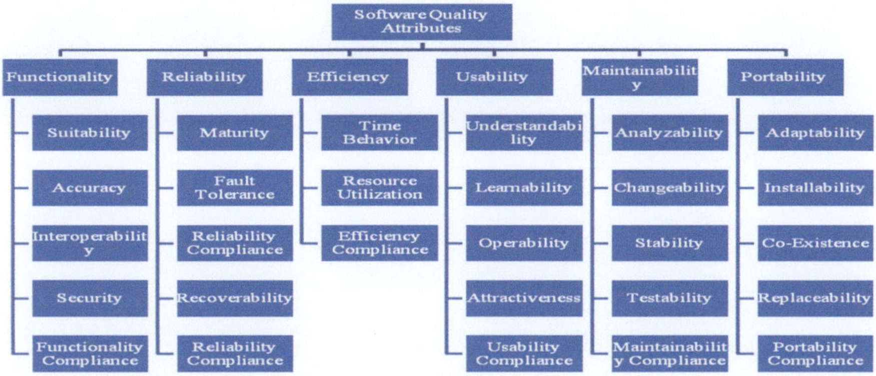

Fig. 1 ISO/IEC 9126 conventional software quality model

settle on the functional characteristic. Since it is situated on an on-premise infrastructure with strong inherent security, dominance, operational simplicity, conformity and alleged service magnitude requirements. An additional significant issue is the cost of operations. It has been repeatedly taking back seat, particularly at cost centres, due to the drop cost and straight payment models. The foremost objective of SaaS-DLC section is intended to achieve centre of attention on the life-cycle features of SaaS service development. This section also describes the inputs, motivation and deliverable of all phases of life-cycle. Cloud services have built for inside utilization as well as for disposing to outside customers. In order to develop cloud services for outside consumption, these development life-cycle needs meticulous architecture implementations to incorporate the service creed mandatory for a victorious business model for services. Therefore, the SaaS (Software as a Service) Development Life Cycle demonstrated here is to asses scope at outmost facing services. The process can simply adopted to inside and private cloud-based applications that aim at internal users. It has been suggested that every IT enterprise have to begin glancing at themselves as service providers and take step correspondingly. The SaaS Development life-cycle is different from traditional SDLC as depicted in Fig. 2.

3.3 Cloud Service Principles

In order to use cloud services effectively to meet the requirement goals and specific targets in economically feasible manner, it is necessary for cloud services to be implemented on strong base. The strong foundation exhibits definite principles of cloud services. The principles have been identified for cloud services are different than conventional services and described as discoverable, detachable, economics, scalability, and supportability. about all these mentioned principles are discussed in the below section.

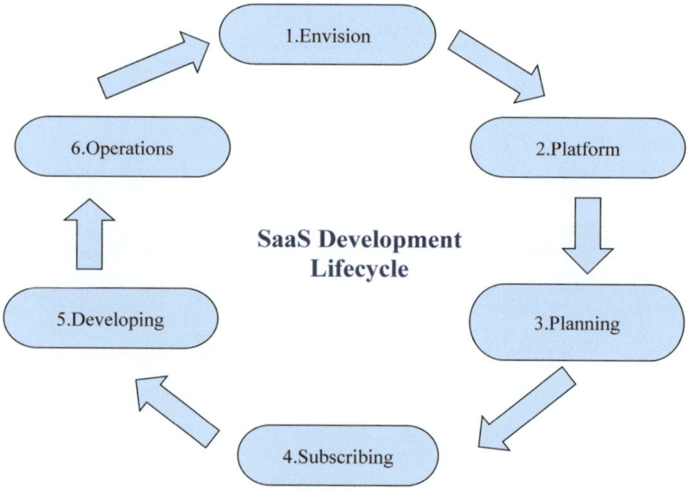

Fig. 2 SaaS development life-cycle (SAAS-DLC)

- *Discoverability*: It is a service that can be taken care by service users with less human interaction on the part of the service provider throughout complete service lifecycle. This principle gives direction to service users by minimizing the gap between deployment and its vision. The major advantage of service discoverability is that it is minimizing the price of deal considerable expected to network outcome generated through the automation engines assist by service architecture.
- *Reachability*: This principle is available for all and helps to service users bridge bigger enterprises and small business similar way. On the cloud platform, choosing service provider and suitable service architecture will entertain significant role in activating reachability of SaaS.
- *Economic Feasibility*: This principle will help to measure consumer usage of service on the cloud at different scales. Any cloud service has to be affordable to operate and use. The service subscription amount should be higher than the grand total of the cloud service utilization cost both direct and indirect. Cloud service providers required to assist SaaS architects with cost-oriented service architecture (CSA) methods that include economical assets utilization as the fundamental principle.
- *Scalability*: This principle demonstrates that cloud services have to supply the multi-tenant platform, which component needed to convey constant performance throughout various conditions of use. In a cloud deployment, all virtualized storage components are not supporting scalability constraints. The same considerations are verifiable for network and compute resources.
- *Supportability*: This principle helps frequently to take a back respective to functionality in applications. The cloud service architecture should take care of suitability as one of underlying creed that gives direction towards designing

solution and implementation. Incorporation to application subjects, supportability of SaaS should provide peak priority to availability, recovery, performance and disaster recovery because of the outward hosting environment.

4 SAASQUAL: Proposed Quality Model

The cloud computing provides many services. Every cloud service should possess some features. The general features of cloud services are shown in Fig. 3.

On the cloud computing environment, there are some key features mostly associated with software services. The essential trademark of SaaS is to recognize an evaluating quality model for SaaS as shown in Fig. 4, and it has become a essential to point SaaS essential features. From several meticulous evaluation quality methods proposed by many researchers [1, 2, 7, 9], the SaaS Key features are recognized as *Reusability, Availability, Scalability, Pay for use, Customizability, Data Managed by Providers.*

4.1 Model-Based Clustering Method

The proposed model is using clustering technique consists of forming groups of objects that possess similar characteristics. Clustering is the method that describes about similar objects in the intra-cluster and dissimilar objects in the inter-clusters. Attention towards clustering has been increased due to its many applications in various knowledge domains. There are so many clustering algorithms in data mining, out them the *Model based Clustering* algorithm hypothesize a model intended for every object belongs the clusters also identifies the foremost suitable of the data. A model-based clustering technique will discover clustering using a density function that considers the data items sparsity in each cluster. It also gives direction to find

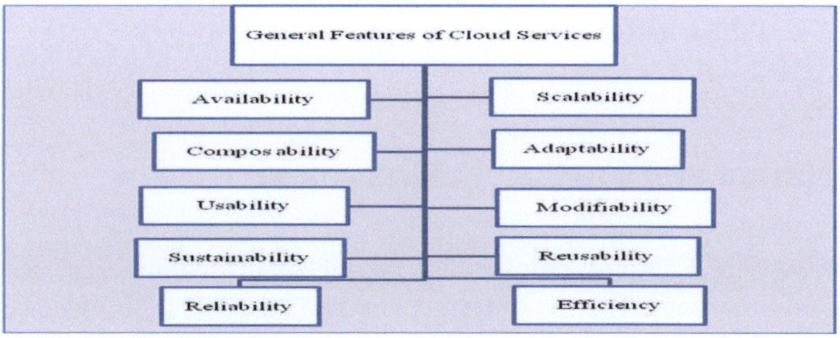

Fig. 3 General features of cloud services

number of clusters depending on standard statistics automatically. One of the significant methods under model-based is EM clustering algorithm. EM clustering works based on the principle of maximum likelihood of unnoticed variables.

4.2 The EM Clustering

The EM algorithm is a type unsupervised learning clustering algorithm, that doesn't need any training data stage. This algorithm is working rely upon mixture models of data mining clustering algorithms. It has been following an iterative process and sub-optimal method to identify the parameters within the probability distribution that have highest chance for its elements. The steps of EM clustering are

- Given data set "x" is input to algorithm.
- The complete number of clusters represented by "M".
- "e" is the acceptable error for the maximum number of iterations.

For every iteration, initially, the E-Step (E-expectation) is executed that gives estimation on the probability of each and every point suited to which cluster. Secondly, the M-step (Maximization) is executed that helps to re-estimates the parameter vector of the probability distribution of every cluster. Finally the EM clustering method stops when the distribution converge is met or stretch out the highest number of specified rotations or iterations.

The proposed quality model used to evaluate software as a service on the cloud. Initially, the data related to software service should be collected from various SaaS users with respect their feedback about product quality and stored in the form of relations. Then separate the SaaS key features data given on the scale of 1 to 10 rating so that the details available as a numeric data. Next, apply the EM model-based clustering algorithm on SaaS data and form a cluster. The clusters will form based on key features of SaaS. Each cluster quality can be measured by using some standard methods for quality measuring of clustering. The quality cluster will help to decide cloud user to select the most desirable features of SaaS, and SaaS providers can improve their product as per the clustering results suggestion to achieve enhancement of their product in order to retain customers in the competitive world. The workflow of SAASQUAL is shown in Fig. 4.

5 Conclusion and Further Enhancement

This paper described about a new quality model for evaluating SaaS on the cloud computing environment. The SAASQUAL model is useful for service users as well as service providers in the cloud to select SaaS and to provide SaaS as per user requirements. Further, it is proposed to use R tool for EM clustering and show

Fig. 4 .

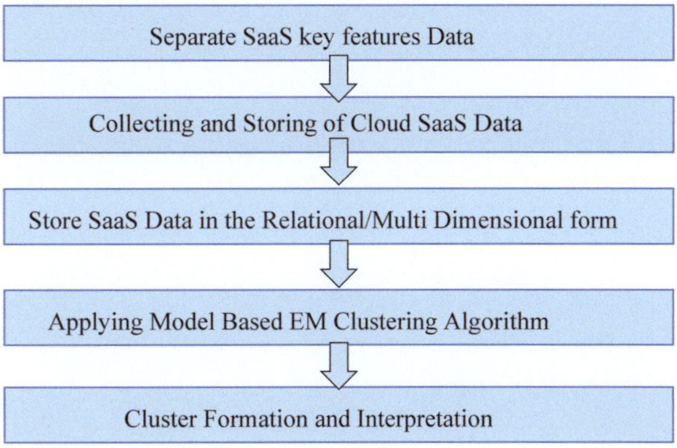

different clusters based on the key features of SaaS [1] and associated metric to measure each quality attributes. In the future i has been intended that the proposed model can be implemented as automated tool for evaluating SaaS Quality.

References

1. Lee, J.Y., Lee, J.W., Cheun, D.W.: A quality model for evaluating software-as-a-service in cloud computing. In: 2009 Seventh ACIS International Conference on Software Engineering Research, Management and Applications (2009)
2. Wen, P.X., Dong, L.: Quality model for evaluating SaaS service. In: 4th International Conference on Emerging Intelligent Data and Web Technologies (2013)
3. Tao, Q., Chang, H., Yi, Y., Gu, C.: Trustworthy management approach for cloud services. In: Proceedings of the 9th International Conference on Machine Learning and Cybernetics, Qingdao (2010). He, Q., Han, J., Yang, Y., Grundy, J., Jin, H.: QoS-driven service selection for multi-tenant SaaS. In: IEEE 5th International Conference on Cloud Computing (2012)
4. Yiming, C., Yiwei, Z.: SaaS vendor selection basing on analytic hierarchy process. In: 4th International Joint Conference on Computational Sciences and Optimization (2011)
5. Godse, M., Mulik, S.: An approach for selecting software-as-a-service (SaaS) product. In: IEEE International Conference on Cloud Computing (2009)
6. Karim, R., Ding, C., Miri, A.: An end-to-end QoS mapping approach for cloud service selection. In: IEEE 9th World Congress on Services (2013)
7. Burkon L.: Quality of service attributes for software as a service in 2003. J. Syst. Integr.
8. Zheng, X.: Cloud qual: a quality model for cloud services. In: IEEE Transactions on Industrial Informatics, vol. 10, No. 2 (2014)
9. Khatibi, A., Hashemi, S.M.: QoS metrics for cloud computing services evaluation. In: I.J Intelligent Systems and Applications (2014)
10. Jagli, D., Mahajan, S., Subhash Chandra, N.: CBC approach for evaluating potential SaaS on the cloud. In: Conference Proceedings of International Technological Conference-2014 (I-TechCON) at VESIT, Mumbai, India, Jan 03–04 (2014)

Scalable Aspect-Based Summarization in the Hadoop Environment

Kalyanasundaram Krishnakumari and Elango Sivasankar

Abstract In the present-day scenario, selecting a good product is a cumbersome process. The reviews from the shopping sites may confuse the user while purchasing the product. It becomes hard for the customers to go through all the reviews, even when they read they may get into a baffling state. Some consumers may like to buy the best product based on its features and its extra comfort. Meanwhile, the size of the datasets for analysis process is huge which cannot be handled by traditional systems. In order to handle the large datasets, we are proposing a parallel approach using Hadoop cluster for extracting the feature and opinion. Then by using online sentiment dictionary and interaction information method, predict the sentiments followed by summarization using clustering. After classifying each opinion words, our summarization system generates an easily readable summary for that particular product based on aspects.

Keywords Sentiment summarization · Aspect · Hadoop · Mapreduce

1 Introduction

Sentiment analysis is the area where sentences, words, or documents are categorized as positive, negative, or neutral based on the opinions expressed in the text. Many online companies wanted to increase their purchase rate by increasing the standards of positively reviewed products and tried to reduce the problems faced by

K. Krishnakumari (✉)
Department of Computer Science and Engineering,
A.V.C. College of Engineering, Mannampandal,
Mayiladuthurai 609305, TamilNadu, India
e-mail: krishna.41999@gmail.com

E. Sivasankar
Department of Computer Science and Engineering,
National Institute of Technology, Tiruchirapalli 609015, TamilNadu, India
e-mail: sivasankarelango@gmail.com

V.B. Aggarwal et al. (eds.), *Big Data Analytics*, Advances in Intelligent Systems and Computing 654, https://doi.org/10.1007/978-981-10-6620-7_42

the products which are negatively reviewed. People share their experiences immediately through social networks, blogs, short messages, and many more means. The reviews given by each and every person is taken into consideration for further development of businesses. The contents like blogs, tweets, product reviews reflect the opinions of users depending upon the context. Most of the shopping sites are requesting for the reviews whenever they purchase the product. The interested people may share their experiences about the product purchased. People want to know the opinion of naïve users before purchasing any product. But it is difficult for any person to read all the reviews from a large number of reviews. People are also not satisfied with only a few good reviews. With the increase in the frequency of the reviews, even the product manufacturer cannot understand the overall opinion of the customers. Accordingly Opinion Mining or Sentiment Analysis followed by sentiment summarization plays a vital role in online shopping. It extracts the customers' opinion on each product and identifies the overall opinion along with a report telling experiences about the product. It is customary to summarize the opinion of all the reviews [2]. Kavita et al. [7] reviewed the study of a generation of concise and meaningful digest of a large number of opinions as Opinion Summarization. This summarization task involves other areas of research including text clustering, text mining, sentiment analysis, natural language processing.

There are two ways of summarization of corpus which includes extractive summarization and abstractive summarization. Extractive Summarization is the strategy of concatenating extracts taken from a corpus into a summary, while abstractive summarization involves paraphrasing the corpus using novel sentences [4, 16]. This type of summarization is applicable for sentiment corpus too. Yuan et al. [29] did an extensive study on effective presentations styles of Opinion Summarization. From this study, it is understood that people are most affinitive toward aspect-based sentiments. However, the authors are not concentrated on sentiments classification. Wang and Liu [27] proposed opinion summarization on spontaneous conversations. The authors identified the importance of pronoun in sentiment summarization. Hamid and Taru [10] advocated methods for handling sentences with noticeable negative comments. The negative keywords like neither, never, but are also considered in our paper.

In the summarization task, many words have the similar kind of orientation irrespective of their positions used. For example, the lexicons like "good," "excellent," "great," "worst" have the same polarity as positive or negative based on the usage called as context-free words. But some other words are context-based because they have different meaning in different places of usage. For example, "The phone is tiny to handle" and "The book is tiny which covers fewer contents." In the first sentence, *tiny* gives positive meaning *of easy to handle,* but in the second sentence *tiny* gives negative meaning of *small book with fewer contents*. The sentiment polarity of context-based words can be identified by knowing the domain knowledge which is not an easy task to know the details about large number of domains. Here, we propose an effective approach for identifying the contextually dependent words. Before sentiment prediction, preprocessing tasks are applied over the raw dataset for reducing the noise.

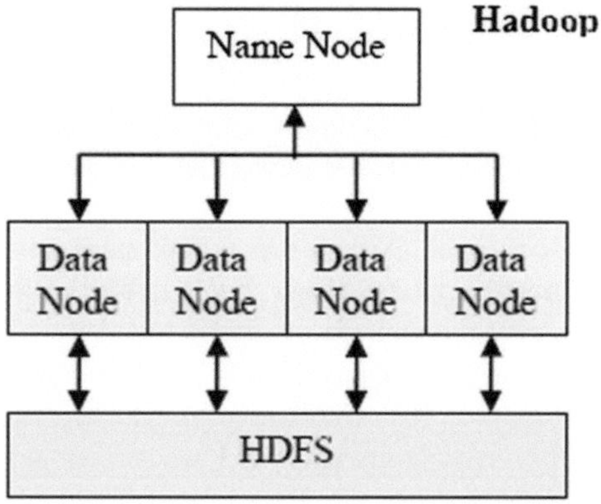

Fig. 1 Hadoop framework [Liu et al.]

In 2011, Kim et al. [13] simplified the task of aspect-based summarization in three steps as (i) Aspect/Feature Identification, (ii) Sentiment Prediction, (iii) Summary Presentation. The authors [17, 18, 21, 24] performed aspect-based sentiment summarization form the sentiment collection. For example, to summarize the phone domain, the aspects to be considered are "Camera," "Battery," "Sound," "Touch panel," etc. The datasets required for sentiment analysis and summarization are very huge. Mining information from a massive dataset cannot be handled by traditional database systems. The Hadoop Mapreduce framework [5] is used to process large datasets using a cluster of commodity hardware. In the proposed work, the parallel environment is used to summarize the opinions based on the co-occurrence of words using point-wise mutual information (PMI) method. The sentiment bar chart and sentiment table are considered in this paper as embedded interfaces. The parallel approach on this summarization gives a structured summary based on the aspects with its positive and negative opinions. Here, we used the Amazon[1] datasets which contain reviews for different domains and results show that our method gives good accuracy for sentiment prediction of aspect opinion pair and provides effective summarization results.

The Hadoop Distributed File System (HDFS) maintains the file system distributed across different machines as shown in Fig. 1. The data collected from the large datasets are collected in the HDFS for identifying the features and opinions in each sentence. After applying the classification algorithm, the features and its opinions are retrieved for each sentence. The data node is responsible for storing the data in a distributed manner, and name node is having the metadata of the data nodes. The tasks given to the Hadoop environment are performed in parallel using Map reduce programming. We follow the similar system of Liu et al. [15] with few modifications in the Job execution.

[1]http://www.cs.jhu.edu/~mdredze/datasets/sentiment/.

2 Related Work

An objective sentence explains the factual information about the product, whereas a subjective sentence depicts the personal feelings, views, or beliefs [14]. The sentiment analysis can be performed at a document level, sentence level, or at the aspect level. Aspect-based sentiment analysis identifies sentiments on aspects of items. It can be either frequency-based where it searches for frequent nouns to identify the aspects or model-based where it searches for model parameters.

Sentiment analysis can be performed in different ways as (i) Supervised approach, (ii) Semi-supervised approach, or (iii) Un-supervised approach. Supervised learning is the process of learning performed by mapping of labeled instances to output. The authors [9, 11, 22, 23] and many authors used supervised learning approaches for sentiment analysis by using machine learning algorithms like Naïve Bayes, SVM, Maximum Entropy, SVM. But supervised approaches need large amount of training data which consumes more time for manual annotation.

In the semi-supervised classification approaches, some amount of labeled data from the domain is considered for training the system. In the un-supervised approach, all the attributes are considered equal and independent where it groups the data based on some measure of resemblance. The semi-supervised and un-supervised approaches use the sentiment lexicon dictionaries like WordNet, SentiwordNet, SentiFul. But these approaches are not suitable for identifying the context of the opinion words. For recognizing the context, the co-occurrence retrieval methods like mutual information (MI) [25], point-wise mutual information (PMI) [23], revised mutual information (RMI) [26] use the relatedness among the lexicons. The polarity of the lexicon gets changed depending on the context. For example, "The battery lasts long for many hours" and "Images take long time to open." The lexicon "long" takes two different orientations in these two sentences. By using conditional mutual information (CMI), [26] is the mutual information of two random variables (opinion and polarity) conditioned on a third one (feature), the context-based opinion words can be identified. Ganesan et al. [6] proposed a graph-based summarization framework called Opinosis which generates an abstractive summary of redundant opinions. Opinosis-based summary contains short sentences and conveys the essential information. Zhu et al. [30] used graph-based method for opinion summarization and detected the leaders of sentences to generate summaries.

In 2011, Kim et al. [13] provide a comprehensive review on Opinion Summarization. The authors identified different techniques used for the opinion summarization and provide a detailed survey about those techniques. In this survey, several ways of aggregating the results are shown as a statistical summary, aggregated ratings, and summary as a timeline. In 2013, Carenini et al. [4] proposed different approaches for summarizing evaluative text which describes the distribution of opinions over the entity and features. However, summary generated by humans were compared which is not scalable. In 2014, Gerani et al. [8] proposed abstractive summarization of product reviews based on discourse structure. The authors used graph model for content selection and product independent template for the summary generation. However, the graph-based approach is not suitable for summarizing from large datasets.

In 2014, Kansal and Toshniwal [12] constructed the training data automatically based on a domain and computed the polarity of opinion words grouped at aspect level using interaction information. In this system, the authors used only nouns for identifying the aspect-based opinions. In our proposed system, we used nouns, verbs, adverbs, and adjectives for finding the opinions. In 2015, Moghaddam [20] proposed a technique to extract actionable information from customer feedback. However, the author is looking only for defect or improvement. In the proposed work, we performed preprocessing, feature extraction using Hadoop, feature-opinion pair formation, opinion analysis, and aspect-based summarization. The summary can be presented in the form of opinion Table and opinion bar charts.

3 Proposed Work

Our summarization system handles context-based opinion words in a scalable manner. We used aspect-based clustering method for summarization. We divide the entire tasks into five subtasks as

1. Preprocessing,
2. Aspect Extraction in Hadoop Environment,
3. Feature-Opinion pair formation in Hadoop Environment,
4. Opinion Analysis,
5. Aspect-based Summarization.

The architecture of the proposed model shown in Fig. 2 describes the entire process of aspect-based summarization.

3.1 Preprocessing

Amazon review dataset[2] is given as input to the preprocessing stage where misspelling handling,[3] POS tagging [19] and lemmatization [3], and stop-word removal are done. In the next step, we tag the words in the sentences using a Stanford POS tagger [23]. In this step, each lexicon in the review document is tagged with their respective part-of-speech (POS) tags. In the third step, lemmatization is performed where the root word of the lexicon is identified. We collect only the nouns, verbs, adjectives, adverbs, and conjunctions for further processing.

---

[2]http://snap.stanford.edu/data/.

[3]http://introcs.cs.princeton.edu/java/44st/misspellings.txt.

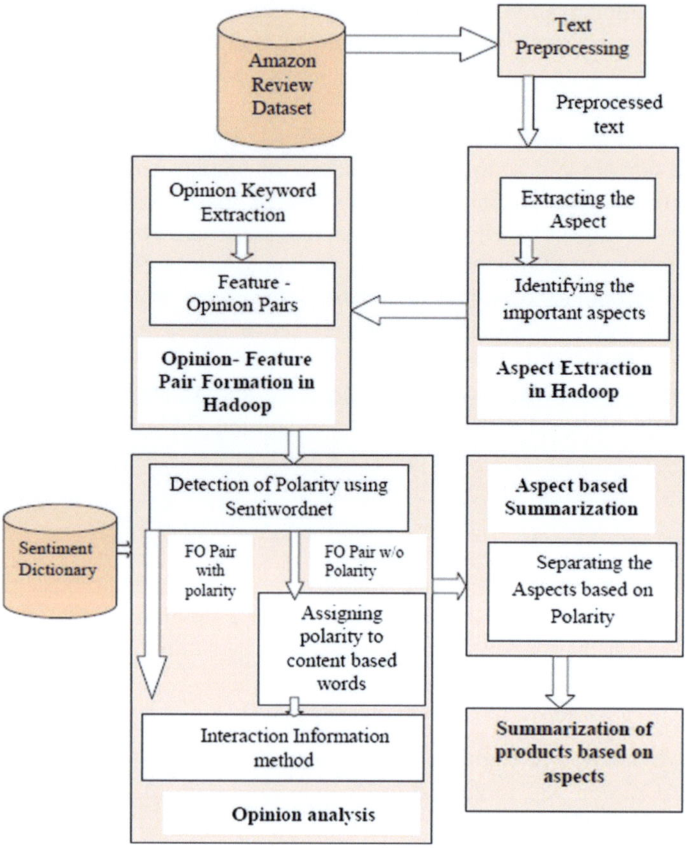

Fig. 2 Flow diagram of proposed work

3.2 Aspect Extraction in Hadoop Environment

From the POS tagged reviews, the aspects are extracted and the important aspects such as nouns and noun phrases are identified using aspect ranking algorithm by means of aspect frequency followed by Yu et al. [28]. After this the opinion, keywords such as adjectives and verbs are extracted from the POS tagged reviews and the formation of feature-opinion pair takes place by mapping each opinion keyword with the nearest feature noun. We map each opinion word to the nearest feature noun and form the pair.

3.3 Feature-Opinion Pair Formation in Hadoop Environment

Based on the observations that most of the users give their review for important aspects and the reviews on important aspects influence the overall opinion of the product to a larger extent, aspect ranking can be done using aspect frequency. This can be done in Hadoop map Reduce environment to achieve scalability. Before going to map the opinion word with the nearest noun, we should handle the negation words because negation words may flip the polarity of the opinion word.

The map and reduce processes of Mapreduce framework take a key/value pair and output a key/value pair [5]. Then construct the feature-opinion pair with the polarity obtained from SentiwordNet [1]. For the classification of remaining feature-opinion pair, we use the interaction information method for finding the co-occurrence between the aspect, opinion, and the polarity. After classifying each opinion word, the system provides aspect-based ranking for each feature in the product. The important features and its opinion words extracted from the Mapreduce framework are listed in Table 1.

3.4 Opinion Analysis

To identify the polarity of the context-based words, we use the linguistic rules of keywords like "and," "or," "neither," "nor". The proposed approach uses Eq. (1) for calculating polarity of feature-opinion pair. The contextual information (CI) for both positive and negative label is identified where the most relevant one is assigned as the label for the Feature-opinion pair.

$$CI(W,O,F) = \log_2 \frac{P(W,O)P(O,F)P(W,F)}{P(W)P(O)P(F)P(W,O,F)}, \quad (1)$$

Table 1 Top features in a sample of 145 reviews of phone domain

Feature	Number of opinion words
Phone	208
Apps	92
Battery	70
Screen	64
Camera	37
Interface	33
Gaming	29
Software	25
Flash	14

where

W is the Opinion word,
O is the sentiment orientation label,
F is the feature associated with the opinion word.

Similarly $P(W, O)$ represents total number of times W and O occur together, $P(O, F)$ represents total number of times O and F occurs together, $P(W, F)$ represents total number of times W and F occurs together, $P(W)$, $P(O)$, $P(F)$ represents total occurrence of W, O, and F in the document.

3.5 Aspect-Based Summarization

After classifying all feature-opinion pairs, we use aspect-based clustering method for summarization. In which we used "2*n*" clusters for "*n*" feature. For each aspect, we create two clusters, one for positive and another for negative to separate positive and negative reviews. We extract the respective aspects based on the feature-opinion pair and put it in their respective cluster and count the number of reviews for positive and negative category. We calculate the star rating of each aspect by dividing all the positive reviews by a total number of reviews represented by the feature. The final output will be the rating along with the top reviews of that product's feature.

4 Experimental Results

We performed the preprocessing, aspect extraction, and feature opinion in the Windows Intel Core Quad 2 CPU, 4 GB RAM with 1 Gbps Network Speed against the Amazon datasets on phone domain in a two node cluster. For a large number of reviews, our system provides good performance. To show the scalability of feature extraction, we change the number of reviews slowly in increasing order and repeat the process a few number of times.

The performance of the system increases gradually when increasing the number of reviews as shown in Fig. 3. The file size ranges from 20 MB to 100 MB. The features and its opinions are extracted and then form the nearest pairs of each sentence of review documents. The top features for positive reviews to appreciate are shown in Table 2 and in Fig. 4.

After clustering the reviews into two major groups as positive and negative, the consumers can get the summary information based on their respective aspects listed.

A sample extractive summary is listed in Fig. 5 for the aspect *Apps*. When the user is interested to go through the complete review, they can then proceed with the links.

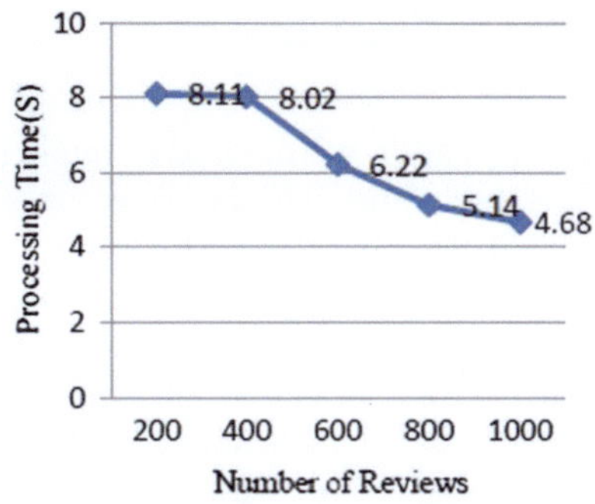

Fig. 3 Performance of Hadoop cluster

Table 2 Positive feedbacks

iPhone 4S	Rating	No. of positive reviews
Camera	4	145
Battery	3	132
Screen touch	3.5	138
Sound	4	142
Apps	4.5	146

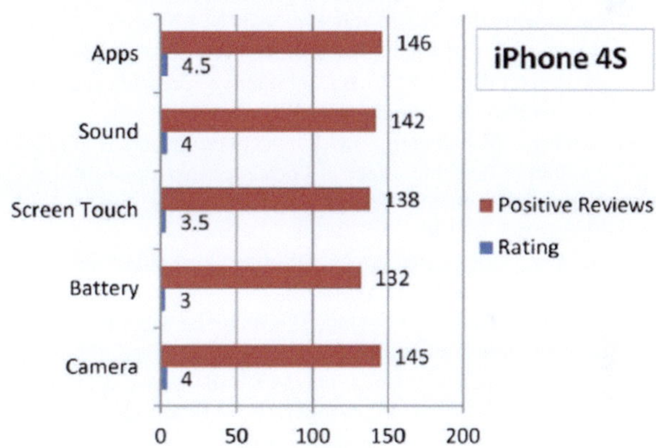

Fig. 4 Positive feedback chart

Fig. 5 Summary of the project

Sample summary for the aspect apps

it is super cool to get all the apps and the phone works great it fits in my purse nicely……

big bright screen accurate multitouch unlimited flexibility through the app store…….

much faster than the original iphone great apps movies videos look fantastic…….

5 Conclusion

In this paper, we provide a simple and effective solution for scalable aspect-based summarization. The co-occurrence framework (RMI) provides better results for identifying the context-based words. The Hadoop cluster works well for feature-opinion extraction with large number of reviews. Our method provides an effective evaluative summary of those reviews without affecting the originality of the reviews. In future, an effective sentiment prediction method can be applied irrespective of their domains and then applying the summarization in the scalable environment with various presentation styles with the help of machine learning libraries like Mahout.

References

1. Baccianella, S., Esuli, A., Sebastiani, F.: SentiWordNet 3.0: an enhanced lexical resource for sentiment analysis and opinion mining. InLREC **10**, 2200–2204 (2010)
2. Blair-Goldensohn, S., Hannan, K., McDonald, R., Neylon, T., Reis, G.A., Reynar, J.: Building a sentiment summarizer for local service reviews. In: WWW Workshop on NLP in the Information Explosion Era, vol. 14 (2008)
3. Briscoe, T., Carroll, J., Watson, R.: The second release of the RASP system. In: Proceedings of the COLING/ACL on Interactive presentation sessions, pp. 77–80. Association for Computational Linguistics (2006)
4. Carenini, G., Cheung, J.C.K.: Extractive versus NLG-based abstractive summarization of evaluative text: the effect of corpus controversiality. In: Proceedings of the 5th International Natural Language Generation Conference, pp. 33–41. Association for Computational Linguistics (2008)
5. Dean, J., Ghemawat, S.: MapReduce: simplified data processing on large clusters. Commun. ACM **51**(1), 107–113 (2008)
6. Ganesan, K., Zhai, C., Han, J.: Opinosis: a graph-based approach to abstractive summarization of highly redundant opinions. In: Proceedings of the 23rd international conference on computational linguistics, pp. 340–348. Association for Computational Linguistics (2010)
7. Ganesan, K., Zhai, C., Viegas, E.: Micropinion generation: an unsupervised approach to generating ultra-concise summaries of opinions. In: Proceedings of the 21st International Conference on World Wide Web, pp. 869–878. ACM (2012)
8. Gerani, S., Mehdad, Y., Carenini, G., Ng, R.T., Nejat, B.: Abstractive summarization of product reviews using discourse structure. In: Proceedings of EMNLP (2014)
9. Gindl, S., Weichselbraun, A., Scharl, A.: Cross-domain contextualisation of sentiment lexicons (2010)
10. Hamid, F., Tarau, P.: Anti-Summaries: enhancing graph-based techniques for summary extraction with sentiment polarity. In: Computational Linguistics and Intelligent Text Processing, pp. 375–389. Springer International Publishing (2015)
11. Hu, M., Liu, B.: Mining and summarizing customer reviews. In: Proceedings of the 10th ACM SIGKDD International Conference on Knowledge Discovery and data mining, pp. 168–177. ACM (2004)
12. Kansal, H., Toshniwal, D.: Aspect based summarization of context-based opinion words. Proc. Comp. Sci. **35**, 166–175 (2014)
13. Kim, H.D., Ganesan, K., Sondhi, P., Zhai, C.: Comprehensive review of opinion summarization (2011)

14. Liu, B., Zhang, L.: A survey of opinion mining and sentiment analysis. In: Mining text data, pp. 415–463. Springer US (2012)
15. Liu, B., Blasch, E., Chen, Y., Shen, D., Chen, G.: Scalable sentiment classification for big data analysis using naive bayes classifier. In: Big Data, 2013 IEEE International Conference on IEEE, pp. 99–104 (2013)
16. Liu, J., Cao, Y., Lin, C.Y., Huang, Y., Zhou, M. Low-Quality product review detection in opinion summarization. In: EMNLP-CoNLL, pp. 334–342 (2007)
17. Lu, Y., Zhai, C., Sundaresan, N.: Rated aspect summarization of short comments. In: Proceedings of the 18th International Conference on World Wide Web, pp. 131–140. ACM (2009)
18. Marrese-Taylor, E., Velásquez, J.D., Bravo-Marquez, F.: A novel deterministic approach for aspect-based opinion mining in tourism products reviews. Expert Syst. Appl. **41**(17), 7764–7775 (2014)
19. McAuley, J., Leskovec, J.: Hidden factors and hidden topics: understanding rating dimensions with review text. In: Proceedings of the 7th ACM Conference on Recommender Systems, pp. 165–172. ACM (2013)
20. Moghaddam, S.: Beyond sentiment analysis: mining defects and improvements from customer feedback. In: Advances in Information Retrieval, pp. 400–410. Springer International Publishing (2015)
21. Mukherjee, A., Liu, B.: Aspect extraction through semi-supervised modeling. In: Proceedings of the 50th Annual Meeting of the Association for Computational Linguistics: Long Papers, vol. 1, pp. 339–348. Association for Computational Linguistics (2012)
22. Pan, S.J., Ni, X., Sun, J.T., Yang, Q., Chen, Z.: Cross-domain sentiment classification via spectral feature alignment. In: Proceedings of the 19th International Conference on World Wide Web, pp. 751–760. ACM (2010)
23. Pang, B., Lee, L., Vaithyanathan, S.: Thumbs up? Sentiment classification using machine learning techniques. In: Proceedings of the ACL-02 Conference on Empirical Methods in Natural Language Processing, vol. 10, pp. 79–86. Association for Computational Linguistics (2002)
24. Shimada, K., Tadano, R., Endo, T.: Multi-aspects review summarization with objective information. Proc. Soc. Behav. Sci. **27**, 140–149 (2011)
25. Turney, P.D.: Thumbs up or thumbs down? Semantic orientation applied to unsupervised classification of reviews. In: Proceedings of the 40th Annual Meeting on Association for Computational Linguistics, pp. 417–424. Association for Computational Linguistics (2002)
26. Van de Cruys, T.: Two multivariate generalizations of pointwise mutual information. In: Proceedings of the Workshop on Distributional Semantics and Compositionality, pp. 16–20. Association for Computational Linguistics (2011)
27. Wang, D., Liu, Y.: Opinion summarization on spontaneous conversations. Comput. Speech Lang. **34**(1), 61–82 (2015)
28. Yu, J., Zha, Z.J., Wang, M., Chua, T.S.: Aspect ranking: identifying important product aspects from online consumer reviews. In: Proceedings of the 49th Annual Meeting of the Association for Computational Linguistics: Human Language Technologies, vol. 1, pp. 1496–1505. Association for Computational Linguistics (2011)
29. Yuan, X., Sa, N., Begany, G., Yang, H.: What users prefer and why: a user study on effective presentation styles of opinion summarization. In: Human-Computer Interaction–INTERACT 2015, pp. 249–264. Springer International Publishing (2015)
30. Zhu, L., Gao, S., Pan, S.J., Li, H., Deng, D., Shahabi, C.: The Pareto principle is everywhere: finding informative sentences for opinion summarization through leader detection. In: Recommendation and Search in Social Networks, pp. 165–187. Springer International Publishing (2015)

Parallel Mining of Frequent Itemsets from Memory-Mapped Files

T. Anuradha

Abstract Due to digitization of data in different fields, data are increasing in leaps and bounds. Mining of these large amounts of data requires two major issues to deal with. The first is the potential to deal with huge data which can be dealt with parallel algorithms as serial algorithms may take very long time or sometimes may not process. The second is the I/O overhead which can be dealt with memory mapping of files. This chapter brings together both parallelization and memory mapping of files concepts in mining the frequent itemsets. Our experiments proved that there is almost 20% more speedup on parallelizing our frequent itemset mining algorithm with memory mapping when compared to conventional I/O without memory mapping.

Keywords Frequent itemset · Parallel mining · Memory-mapped file · Apriori

1 Introduction

As the dimensions of the real-life data sources are increasing from hundreds of gigabytes to terabytes, data mining methods need to work on large quantities of information. Especially, the running time required for the frequent itemset mining algorithms like apriori [1] is so high as it needs to check the data source a number of times. There is a desperate need for parallelism in data mining algorithms to improve the scalability [2]. There are some parallel mining algorithms proposed [3, 4] for satisfying the need.

T. Anuradha (✉)
Department of ECM, KL University, Guntur, India

V.B. Aggarwal et al. (eds.), *Big Data Analytics*, Advances in Intelligent Systems and Computing 654, https://doi.org/10.1007/978-981-10-6620-7_43

Multi-core processors are the emerging parallel computer architectures [5–7] which made the parallel processing accessible even for normal programmers. Frequent itemset mining from different databases on multi-core processors is experimented by [8] which gave better performance compared to existing parallel algorithms. The concept of memory mapping of files (MMF) is more efficient than regular file read or write operations in the case of large files as it avoids several extra data copy operations [9]. CPU utilization can also be reduced by using MMF I/O when used with large data files [10, 11]. So, this is best suited for the data mining applications. The current research concentrates on parallelizing apriori with and without using memory mapping of files concept on Pentium dual core processor and compares the performance of the algorithm in both cases. Our experiments [12–14] proved that there is a speedup of almost 20% more by using memory mapping of files when compared to traditional I/O.

2 Frequent Itemset Mining

Frequent itemset mining is one of the major functionalities of data mining which deals with finding the frequent itemsets from the given dataset [15, 16] for which apriori is the most famous and widely used algorithm. It takes a transactional dataset representing the set of items purchased by the customers in one visit to the super market as input and finds the sets of items in the given dataset which are occurring frequently [1, 15].

3 Memory Mapping of Files

There are two ways of accessing data from the files. The traditional way using fread() and memory mapping of files using mmap(). Memory mapping of files, the concept used in designing Unix-based operating system's internals, can also be used in the applications whenever there are more I/O operations. Apart from design of Unix internals, usage of memory mapping is tested on various networking applications and on SSD data [17, 18].

With mmap() [19–21], the data can be accessed directly without any context switch from user mode to system mode as it maps the file data to process address space. Hence, it greatly reduces I/O overhead [22]. So, it is best suited for data mining applications.

4 Experimental Work

Intel Pentium Dual-Core-a simple multi-core processor, OpenMP threads for parallelization, Fedora Linux for getting gcc compiler, 5 randomly generated datasets with number of records 2, 4, 6, 8 and 10 lakhs and a standard accident dataset [23] are used for experimentation. For each dataset, experimentation is done by changing the number of threads as 2, 3 and 4 and in each case by changing the minimum support count as 5, 15, 25, 35, 45 [12–14].

1. The algorithm is first implemented in serial and parallel modes, respectively, using fread(), and the results are noted down.
2. The algorithm is again implemented in serial and parallel modes using mmap(), and the results are noted down.

In all the cases, execution times are noted down, and speedup obtained with parallelization is calculated using both fread() and mmap() using the formula

$$\text{Speedup}_{\text{P}} = \frac{\text{execution time of serial algorithm}}{\text{execution time of parallel algorithm}}$$

5 Experimental Results

The following terms are used to demonstrate and explain the results:

SAFD, PAFD—to represent the execution times of serial, parallel apriori with fread()
SAMD, PAMD—to represent the execution times of serial, parallel apriori with mmap()
SPAMD, SPAFD—speedup with mmap(), speedup with fread()
pmsc—percentage of minimum support count
nrl—number of records in lakhs
2TH, 3TH, 4TH—2 threads, 3 threads, 4 threads

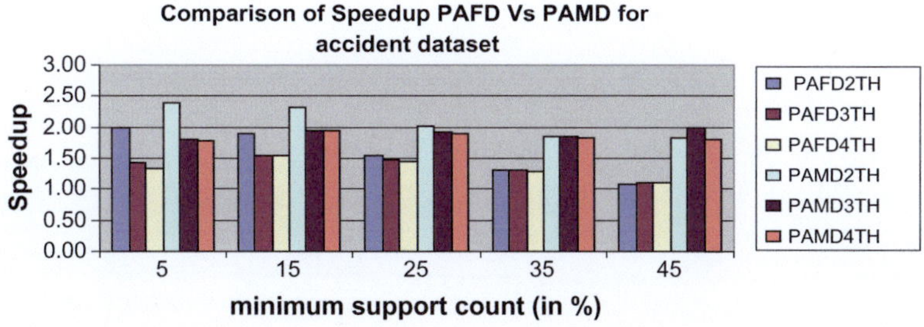

Fig. 1 Comparison of speedup of parallel apriori PAFD versus PAMD for accident dataset

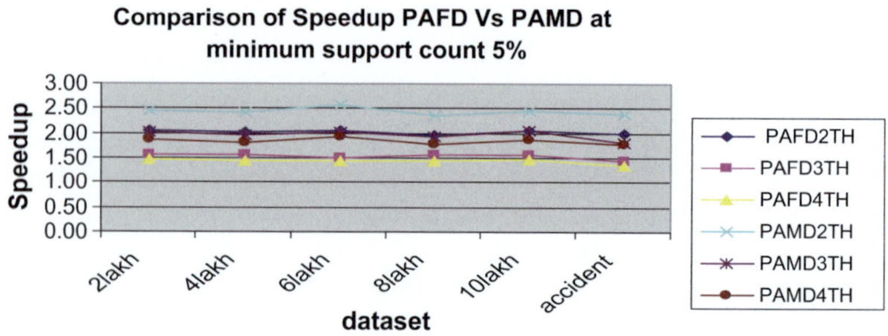

Fig. 2 Comparison of speedup of parallel apriori PAFD versus PAMD for minimum support count 5%

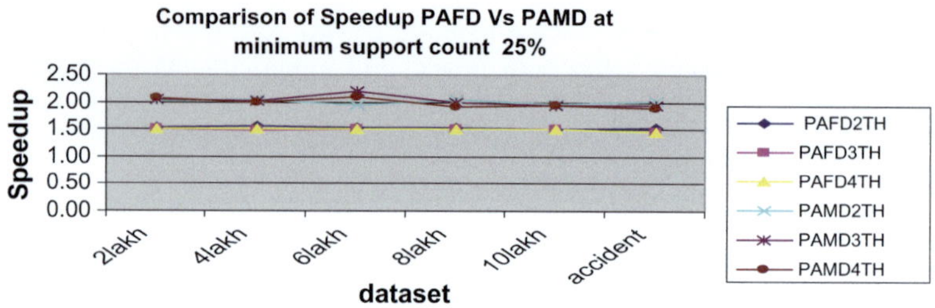

Fig. 3 Comparison of speedup of parallel apriori PAFD versus PAMD for minimum support count 25%

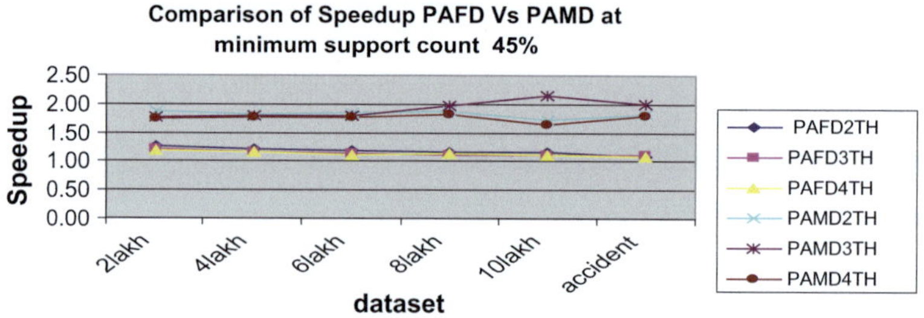

Fig. 4 Comparison of speedup of parallel apriori PAFD versus PAMD for minimum support count 45%

The speedup obtained using PAFD and PAMD compared to serial execution with fread [24, 25] is calculated using the following formulae:

$$\text{Speedup of PAFD} = \frac{\text{SAFD}}{\text{PAFD}} \tag{1}$$

Table 1 Speedup of parallel apriori with mmap() versus fread() with 2 threads

nrl	5%		15%		25%		35%		45%	
	SPAMD	SPAFD	SPAMD	SPAFD	SPAMD	SPAFD	SPAMD	SPAFD	SPAMD	SPAFD
2	2.46	2.04	2.73	2.25	2.01	1.54	1.88	1.35	1.86	1.26
4	2.41	2.01	2.76	2.23	2.03	1.55	1.88	1.4	1.83	1.22
6	2.58	2.05	2.74	2.29	1.94	1.53	1.97	1.38	1.85	1.18
8	2.34	1.95	2.74	2.28	2.04	1.54	1.89	1.37	1.88	1.17
10	2.44	2.04	2.76	2.28	1.96	1.52	1.98	1.39	1.93	1.17
Average	2.45	2.0	2.75	2.27	2	1.54	1.92	1.38	1.87	1.20

$$\text{Speedup of PAMD} = \frac{\text{SAFD}}{\text{PAMD}} \quad (2)$$

The speedup of parallelization using fread() and mmap() was compared at different minimum support counts by keeping datasets fixed (Figs. 1, 2, 3 and 4). An increased speedup of PAMD over PAFD was observed for accident dataset as well as for the taken random datasets for different minimum support counts with different number of threads. Speedup decreased with increase in the minimum support count, and at each minimum support count, speedup decreased with increase in the number of threads.

Figures 2, 3 and 4 represent the comparison of speedup between PAFD and PAMD at a fixed minimum support count, but with changed datasets. The result showed relatively higher speedup of PAMD than PAFD at a constant minimum support count with all the datasets with different number of threads. The speedup of PAMD for all the datasets at a given support count and number of threads was found almost same. A similar trend was also observed with PAFD. Table 1 shows the speedups of PAMD and PAFD with 2 threads at different support counts with different datasets which show the maximum speedups obtained in our experimentation.

6 Conclusions

The experimental results of this study proved that there was a significant performance benefit of mmap() use over fread() with parallelization, especially when number of threads equal to number of cores. We obtained a maximum average speedup of 2.27 with fread() and a maximum average speedup of 2.75 with mmap() using 2 threads. The maximum speedup obtained with mmap() was approximately 20% more compared to the maximum speedup obtained with fread().

References

1. Agrawal, R., Srikant, R.: Fast algorithms for mining association rules. In: Proceedings of the 20th International Conference on Very Large Data Bases (VLDB'94), Santiago, Chile, vol. 1215, pp. 487–499 (1994)
2. Sivanandam, S.N., Sumathi, S.: Data Mining Concepts, Tasks. Techniques Thomson Business Information Pvt. Ltd., India (2006)
3. Radha, T.A., Lavanya, P.: Recent trends in parallel and distributed apriori algorithm. Int. J. Eng. Res. Appl. **1**(4), 1820–1822 (2000)
4. Anuradha, T., Kranthi, M., Saragini, M.: Recent trends in parallel classification and clustering data mining. Glob. J. Comput. Appl. Technol. **1**(4), 617–619 (2011)
5. Barbic, J.: Multi-core architectures—Lecture Notes [Online]. Available http://www.co-array.org/cafvsmpi.Htm (2007)

6. Akhter, S., Roberts, J.: Multi-core Programming, vol. 33. Intel Press (2006)
7. Packirisamy, V., Barathvajasankar, H.: Openmp in Multicore Architectures. University of Minnesota, Tech, Rep (2005)
8. Vu, Lan, Alaghband, Gita: Novel parallel method for association rule mining on multi-core shared memory systems. Parallel Comput. **40**(10), 768–785 (2014)
9. Heidemann, J.: Performance interactions between P-HTTP and TCP implementations. ACM SIGCOMM Comput. Commun. Rev. **27**(2), 65–73 (1997)
10. Tevanian, A., Rashid, R.F., Young, M., Golub, D.B., Thompson, M.R., Bolosky, W.J., Sanzi, R.: A UNIX interface for shared memory and memory mapped files under mach. In: USENIX Summer, pp. 53–68 (1987)
11. Love, R.: Linux System Programming, 2nd edn. O'Reilly Media, Inc (2007)
12. Anuradha, T., Satya Prasad, R., Tirumalarao, S.N.: Parallelizing apriori on dual core using OpenMP. Int. J. Comput. Appl. **43**(24), 33–39 (2012)
13. Anuradha, T., Satya Prasad, R., Tirumalarao, S.N.: Performance evaluation of apriori on dual core with multiple threads. Int. J. Comput. Appl. **50**(16), 9–16 (2012)
14. Anuradha, T., Satya Prasad, R., Tirumala Rao, S.N.: Performance evaluation of apriori with memory mapped files. Int. J. Comput. Sci. Issues 10 **1**(1), 162–169 (2013)
15. Han, J., Kamber, M.: Data Mining: Concepts and Techniques, 2nd edn. Morgan Kaufmann (2006)
16. Bodon, F.: A fast apriori implementation. In: Goethals, B., Zaki, M.J. (Eds.) Proceedings of the IEEE ICDM Workshop on Frequent Itemset Mining Implementations (FIMI'03), pp. 1–10 (2003)
17. Tirumala Rao, S.N., Prasad, E.V., Venkateswrlu, N.B.: A critical performance study of memory mapping on multi-core processors: an experiment with K-means algorithm with large data mining data sets. IJCA 1(9) (2010)
18. Jian, H., Badam, A., Qureshi, M.k., Schwan, K.: Unified address translation for memory-mapped SSDs with FlashMap. In: Proceedings of the 42nd Annual International Symposium on Computer Architecture, ACM, pp. 580–591 (2015)
19. Vahalia, U.: UNIX Internals The New Frontiers, Pearson education, New Delhi, 110 017, India (1996)
20. Venkateswarlu, N.B.: Advanced UNIX Programming. BS publications, Hyderabad (2005)
21. Mmap-memory mapped file support. [online] Accessed on 18 July 2015. Available https://docs.python.org/2/library/mmap.html (2015) (c) Python Software foundation
22. Krieger, O., Reid, K., Stumm, M.: Exploiting mapped files for parallel I/O. In: SPDP Workshop on Modeling and Specification of I/O, pp. 1–11 (1995)
23. Geurts, K., Wets, G., Brijs, T., Vanhoof, K.: Profiling high frequency accident locations using association rules. In: Electronic Proceedings of the 82th Annual Meeting of the Transportation Research Board, Washington, 12–16 January, USA, p. 18 (2003)
24. Anuradha, T., Satya Prasad, R.: Parallelizing apriori on hyper-threaded multi-core processor. Int. J. Adv. Res. Comput. Sci. Softw. Eng. **3**(6), 1072–1082 (2013)
25. Anuradha, T.: Performance of hyper-threading on memory mapped files. Int. J. Appl. Eng. Res. **9**(23), 21421–21431 (2014)

Handling Smurfing Through Big Data

Akshay Chadha and Preeti Kaur

Abstract Money laundering is a worrying term for every country's economy these days. Leading economists of all major developed and developing economies are concerned to devise methods to prevent it. The economy of a country is weakened by the impact of money laundering. Networks created between various banks in different countries facilitate online money transfer, which is turning the process of money laundering into digital money laundering. This promotes money launderers to perform wired transactions from anywhere. People involved in the process of money laundering are efficiently using online banking as their weapon. Evading the anti-money laundering agencies is becoming easier for them because of having online bank accounts. Such people are misusing technology. Therefore, it is restricting one's own country's economic progress. But with the help of recently developed technologies, we are able to prevent such illegal activities. Scrutinizing all the transactions and investigating them manually at financial intelligence units are cumbersome tasks because petabytes of transactions are taking place each day. Advanced technologies like Big Data enable us to detect the suspicious customers possibly involved in money laundering. In this paper, we have proposed a methodology using big data to detect smurfing; based on which, suspicious people involved in money laundering may be identified and appropriate action can be taken against them.

Keywords Money laundering · Smurfing · Cyber threat detection · Anti-money laundering · Terrorism · Counterfeit currency · Hadoop · Big data · Machine learning · Soft computing · Outlier detection · Economic crisis · Hadoop · MapReduce

A. Chadha (✉) · P. Kaur
Department of Computer Engineering,
Netaji Subhas Institute of Technology, New Delhi, India
e-mail: akshaychadha2013@gmail.com

P. Kaur
e-mail: preetikaur1@rediffmail.com

V.B. Aggarwal et al. (eds.), *Big Data Analytics*, Advances in Intelligent Systems and Computing 654, https://doi.org/10.1007/978-981-10-6620-7_44

1 Introduction

Gone are the days when to debit or withdraw money the customer had to stand in long queues in the banks. Technology developed to perform online wired transactions has facilitated end users (customers) of the bank in doing financial transactions through virtual zones. Although it was done for simplifying banking transactions, saving time of end users, and aiding the fluidity of capital in market, money launderers have taken it to their advantage. They can now move both legitimate and illegitimate capital easily by quickly avoiding the involved bank authorities. This is done by making the amount involved in their transaction look like as non-suspicious transaction entity. Electronic funds transfer is facilitated by *SWIFT*, *CHIBPS*, *FEDWIRE*, etc. [1].

Group of G7 countries in 1989 presented a set of 40 recommendations to combat money laundering. These recommendations are taken care of by FATF (Financial Action Task Force). In India, money laundering comes under PMLA Act (Prevention of Money Laundering Act), which enforces liability on financial institutions and other intermediaries to authenticate their clients, maintain records, and provide information required to Financial Intelligence Unit-India. PMLA also includes the provisions under civil procedure court, criminal procedure court, Indian penal code, income tax act, and prevention of corruption act. Prevention of money laundering activities became the central point on the agenda of all the countries as it has been found that terrorist activities of 9/11 attack were majorly funded by money raised from organized crimes [2, 3].

According to the best of our knowledge in literature, there are no proposed or deployed methodologies to identify those users who are channelizing black money into the financial institutions by activities like smurfing [4]. Our proposed technique is scalable because we are using recently developed advanced techniques like big data, which are proven to give appropriate results on large data sets. Deployment of our proposed method will be extremely helpful for all the comparative analysis of the proposed methods in future for detecting people involved in smurfing. If some new methodologies are proposed and deployed to detect smurfing in the near future, then our proposed technique will act as a milestone for the basis of their evaluation.

This paper is divided into four sections. In section I, we provide a brief introduction to the problems raised because of money laundering activities. In section II, we will discuss about money laundering and Big Data in brief, section III discusses the proposed methodology, architecture, and various issues related to the analysis, and finally, we conclude this paper in section IV with some discussion on key ideas about work possibly be done in the future for preventing money laundering activities.

2 Money Laundering and Big Data

Money laundering is the process of transforming the money earned from illegal activities into legal money and simultaneously concealing the source of money. Illegal money, also called black money, is obtained from numerous illegal activities like terrorism, naxalism, bribery, extortion, drug trafficking, human trafficking, and cyber fraud [4, 5]. The illegally obtained money from above-specified illegal activities is again used to support and finance other additional illegal activities. Therefore, the process of money laundering definitely encourages organized crime. According to a recent study, the money laundering activity is annually estimated to account one trillion dollars globally [6]. With such huge capital in flow, it is vital for all the countries whether developing or developed to curb it at the earliest; otherwise, it will definitely restrict the economic progress of any country.

It is very difficult to evaluate the exact effect of money laundering in the economy of a country, but growth of several sectors of the economy is hampered because of it. Financial sector of an economy consists of banks, non-banking financial corporations (NBFC), and equity market. Once black money enters into these institutions through the process of money laundering, then it results into weakening of the roots of financial system of the country. Strong financial systems of any country are crucial for its economic growth and work as an agent of sustainable development.

The process of money laundering is categorized into three steps namely placement, layering, and integrations. In placement stage, the money obtained illegally is integrated back into the economy through banks or other modes, e.g., purchasing luxury items, antiques, gold, art, and jewelry. An individual involved in money laundering tries to place his money into various financial institutions, e.g., bank. However, banks have KYC (know your customer) norms to identify their customer's identity, but many banks still do not have any provisions to verify source of income of their customers, i.e., KYSC (know your source of customer) norms are not there. For large amount of deposits in a single transaction into a bank account, bank authorities could question their customers for the source of money. So to avoid the verification of source of money, the money launderers often divide their single large amount into numerous smaller amount of deposits so that the bank authorities cannot see it as a suspicious transaction amount. This process is called smurfing. It has been observed globally that key stakeholder of illegal wealth opens accounts in name of different customers so that he/she cannot be questioned by the bank for source of his/her source of income. Therefore, it is very often observed in practice that only one person operates all those accounts and easily evades the KYSC (know your source of customer) norms of the banks. So in this way, smurfing introduces an army of malicious users into the banking network. Now, as soon as all those malicious customers who are successful in opening their bank account for the one key person with objective of money laundering gets the facilities provided by the bank like debit card, credit card, and online banking password, they give all the details to the key operating person. Now, the key person can easily make transactions by splitting his large amount of money into such smaller amount that it does not appear as a suspicious transaction to the financial intelligence unit [7]. Once all the accounts are credited with the black money, then this key operating person who has collected all the details like credit/debit card details and online net banking details to perform the wired transfer online can perform wired transactions online. This phenomenon has been observed globally as a common practice that one person is involved in operating all the accounts of many customers. We propose a method to detect such malicious users in the banking system in this paper [8].

Layering involves the process of sending money by various transactions and makes it difficult to follow the anti-money laundering techniques. This is achieved by several bank transactions through various accounts in multiple banks in different countries. Therefore, it is very complex to trace the authenticity of all such transactions. Because of these numerous transactions might also include the malicious key persons performing smurfing by operating different accounts with such a small amount of money so that it does not come into the suspicion of any automated anti-money laundering tool or any bank authority [9]. Therefore, it becomes difficult to differentiate a genuine transaction of an honest customer from a malicious one.

In the step of integration, the money reenters the economy of the country in a legitimate way and appears as if it is coming from a legal source. As once black money is introduced into the banking network, it appears to be coming from a legitimate source to everyone. This is very harmful for any economy as it damages the long-term economic development of the country. Entering of black money into the economy through money laundering activities negatively impacts the productivity. The value of currency also depreciates. It also helps in spreading corruption and encourages crime and therefore, criminals get a chance of having more influence in the system. As the credit and monetary policy announced by the governments or central bank of a country is unable to get its proper results, the rate of inflation also increases in the economy. This weakens the trust of the citizens in the economy. Today, in the era of globalization, foreign investment is used as a major tool in the growth and development of different sectors like infrastructure, power, and telecommunication. In the process of globalization, foreign investment enters into economy through two ways which are in form of Foreign Direct Investment (FDI) and Foreign Portfolio Investment (FII). Due to increase in crime, corruption, and weakening of economy, the foreign investment made in the country also gets negatively affected. From the above points, we can clearly observe the detrimental effects of money laundering.

Different banks have differently defined structures in different formats for the transaction activities performed at them. To combat money laundering and to detect smurfing activities, we would require to gather a single cross data set from all the banks. This would result into big data which might include structured, semi-structured, and unstructured data. Big data is characterized by three Vs, i.e., volume, variety, and velocity [10–12]. The volume obtained in the cross data set obtained from all the bank transactions will definitely include such huge number of transactions. Structured, semi-structured, and unstructured data collected from multiple banks will represent the variety parameter in the single cross bank data set. Various transactions will be added to the data set at a constant rate, e.g., transactions are added at daily, weekly, or monthly basis which represents the velocity of data.

It is beyond the power of traditional database methods to perform a set of operations on this voluminous data set, because petabytes of transactions take place each day. A person involved in smurfing activity will be having his/her bank account in different banks; therefore, any technique which works on only a single-bank data set might not be helpful in identifying malicious customers performing smurfing. Therefore, we require a cross-bank data set, so that the techniques of big data can be used to perform operations for extracting required useful information. This single cross-bank data set will be used to predict the possible outlier customers performing smurfing and therefore involved in the process of money laundering [13]. We can process the large data set using Hadoop on distributed machines.

3 Proposed Approach, Architecture, and Various Issues

We will discuss a technique to identify users involved in smurfing activity using MapReduce of Hadoop in this section [14]. A large amount single transaction is split into multiple transactions to make it look innocent [15]. Numerous transactions take place in the banking environment every day. A bank account may belong to an individual, institution, or a company. In this paper, we propose to detect key malicious individuals who are involved in the smurfing activity and therefore involved in money laundering. There is a high probability that such malicious smurfers will have their accounts in different banks and different branches in different countries. So it is difficult for anti-money laundering authorities to keep track of all of their transactions manually. So we propose to obtain a single cross data set from all the banks across the country so that people involved in smurfing can be detected [16, 17]. The single cross data set will also contain accounts of banks, institutions, individuals, and companies [6].

In our proposed methodology, once we obtain a single cross data set, then we can observe that this database has massive dimensionality in terms of number of transactions each day. This obtained single cross data set should not be anonymized because it will restrict us to compare the details between a set of anonymized random data and it would not yield correct output. Moreover, the online transactions incorporate large amount of metadata with them. This metadata will contain important information to detect smurfing activities like IP address, MAC address, amount debited, amount credited, date, account number, time, branch name, bank name, city, country, and transaction id. Using data science minimization principles, we would maintain bare minimum data required about the customers in the single cross data set.

The single cross data set contains the transaction details of individuals, companies, and banks. Therefore, in order to detect individuals involved in smurfing, we need not involve the transactions of companies and other financial institutions like banks [4]. So we can clearly neglect them by removing them. In our proposed technique, we are able to find those individuals who participate in smurfing either by performing online transactions or by performing cash transactions in the bank.

By sorting the data set on basis of an IP address, we can find out such users who are performing multiple transactions from a single machine. These users are possibly the outlier customers of bank who could be performing smurfing. We can set a threshold on both the amount of transactions and the number of transactions to categorize those customers which possess an abnormal banking behavior than a regular customer of banking institution. Our system can recommend such malicious customers to the anti-money laundering agencies so that their source of income can be questioned by the authorities [16, 17].

In our proposed architecture depicted in Fig. 1, we use the services of Hadoop. Hadoop uses an alternative file system, i.e., Hadoop Distributed File System (HDFS). HDFS is a distributed file system designed to run on commodity hardware. HDFS has several advantages associated with it like it is highly fault tolerant that provides high-throughput rate and it is implemented in low-cost hardware. Hadoop performs extremely well in case of scalability and provides good availability. Another advantage of using Hadoop is that its processes can run on separate Java Virtual Machines (JVMs). JVMs also do not share the state [14].

Hadoop also introduces a programming archetype called MapReduce [14]. MapReduce is a way to think about data problems. Originally, it was devised for indexing the information available on the Internet. It has two parts: Map and Reduce. A HDFS node is by default replicated three times; therefore, the map function will work at all the three nodes. To process large amount of data and to get high accessibility or availability of data, we might have more than three nodes with us so that if a node goes down, the other nodes will be always available. In its first half, Map function gives key value pair as its output on each node. In its second half, Reduce function is executed on some set of data. Reduce function is also executed on some of the nodes of the cluster. Reducer aggregates the set of key-value pairs on some nodes and its output is a single-combined list. For simplification, we take three nodes, but in reality, there may be hundreds of nodes are required to process the real-time data set. Each node may contain different types of data to be processed by the map function. At each node, the data is triple replicated [14].

The output of the MapReduce function is in sorted format. Shuffle and sort functions are also incorporated between the Map and Reduce functions [14]. We can partition the data set in Mapper function according to the data set of the bank, e.g., comma and hash, so the data set can be hash or comma separated. In spite of using default methods already available for the shuffle and sort, we propose to write our own java code for each of the Map and Reduce function. In our java classes written for Map and Reduce, we will take care of applying threshold conditions which will help us to distinguish between a malicious customers performing

Description about Figure A

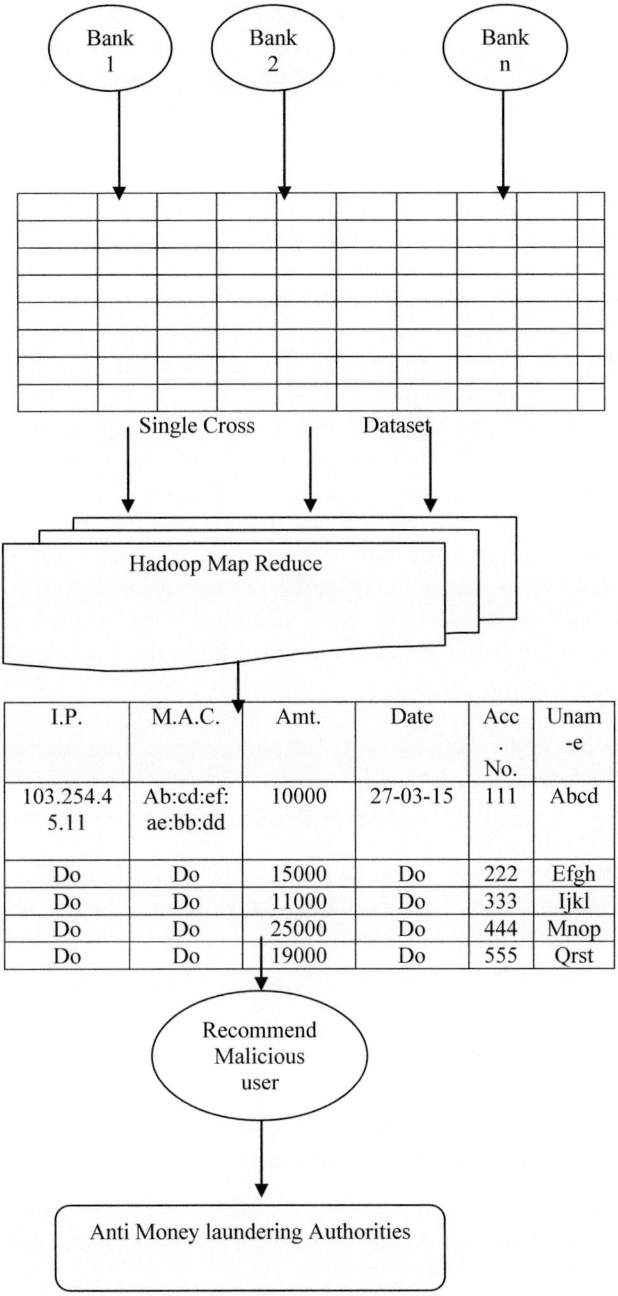

I.P.	M.A.C.	Amt.	Date	Acc. No.	Unam-e
103.254.45.11	Ab:cd:ef:ae:bb:dd	10000	27-03-15	111	Abcd
Do	Do	15000	Do	222	Efgh
Do	Do	11000	Do	333	Ijkl
Do	Do	25000	Do	444	Mnop
Do	Do	19000	Do	555	Qrst

Fig. 1

smurfing from a good customer of the bank. Reduce step will provide us output in the form of all of the suspicious transaction details of the customer performing transactions from a single machine. In Reduce step, malicious customers will only be shown if they fall into the defined range of threshold conditions; in this way, our reduce function is different from the default implementation. Then those transactions can be further scrutinized by the financial intelligence unit. Another advantage of using our proposed technique on the single cross data set is that it is not feasible for a smurfer to open account in several banks and easily evade the tax authorities because our Map and Reduce function will take care of both the IP and MAC addresses used in the transaction. Even if the customer uses bank or an online transaction as a source for channelizing his black money, then we can also fine-tune the Map and Reduce class in such a way that number of transactions and the amount involved in the transactions will be inspected carefully and suspicious transactions could be reported to the concerned authorities.

Reduce function in our logic will clearly be different from its default implementation as it will return a small data set of all suspicious transaction based on the threshold limits instead of simply counting something. In our reduce function, we will sort out the output on the basis of the IP address. Thus, Reduce function will present all the transactions as its output. Because the banking server will only serve the requests coming from public IP addresses and even if a user accesses the network from a private network, his MAC address will be used to identify him. So there is no way out to hide for a customer involved in illicit activity like smurfing.

Pseudo Algorithm for detecting smurfers:

Step 1 Make the single cross data set from all the transactions over all the banks in the country.
Step 2 Apply the data minimization techniques on this data set.
Step 3 Initialize the Map function.
Step 4 Shuffle the transactions on the basis of IP address.
Step 5 Sort the transactions on the basis of amount included in the transaction.
Step 6 Initialize the Reduce function.

The step 6 of the pseudo algorithm will present all the transaction records of the malicious users involved in smurfing. We will show only those users to the concerned financial intelligence units which come under the conditions defined. The condition for such user is like:

IF (No_of_Transaction >= $\prod_1$ || Amt_of_Transaction >= $\prod_2$ ||No_of_Transaction >= $\prod_3$ && Amt_of_Transaction >= $\prod_4$)

THEN show the transactions details of the user by calling MapReduce function.

So for extracting the malicious customers, we have taken three cases into consideration.

Case 1 It may be the case that the amount of transaction may be very low that does not make it suspicious at all but the frequency of the transactions is too high. So there is high probability of this kind of user involved in smurfing activities.

Case 2 It may be the case that the number of transactions made is too low but amount involved in transactions is too high which makes it suspicious. Because it is observed as a common practice that people do perform transactions at regular intervals which makes it difficult to doubt upon for the banking authorities.

Case 3 A smart smurfer may also keep both the amount included in transactions and number of transactions are also less performed at regular intervals.

The value of the thresholds $\prod_1$, $\prod_2$, $\prod_3$, and $\prod_4$ will be fine-tuned by observing the pattern of transaction from the people involved in smurfing and can be changed in consultation with the economists of the financial intelligence unit. Moreover, if a customer of a bank comes under scrutiny because of the above conditions for the first time, then he/she might not be called by the concerned authorities. But if there exists a peculiar pattern of transactions on regular intervals, then he/she definitely depicts malicious behavior. The transaction behavior can be easily analyzed by the results of the Reduce function as the result will be stored in the database separately at regular intervals.

Therefore, the single cross data set is now acting as a digital forensic tool for the anti-money laundering agencies [6, 18]. Using Hadoop's MapReduce function in single cross data set enables us to convert traditional database into a digital forensic tool to combat money launderers. Summarily, big data and Hadoop both help us in detecting those customers too for whom the KYSC norms of the banks are needed to be seriously known to prevent money laundering activities [14]. Once such malicious users are detected, their source of income will be questioned, and if they are not able to provide a fair answer to justify their source of income, then will get punishment under the legal laws of the country. The single cross data set obtained will also work as evidence to the court. Therefore, our method will also help in restricting the channelization of black money back into the economy [4].

Hadoop's MapReduce module can handle very large data sets, and in our proposed methodology, we will be greatly benefited by the parallel processing features of MapReduce [14]. The single cross data set collected from n banks contains all the information about the customer along with his transaction details in form of attributes. We would apply data minimization techniques so that a lot of time can be saved by avoiding unnecessary information. Now the MapReduce function will help us to identify those customers who possess a suspicious transactional behavior determined by the threshold values.

4 Conclusion and Future Work

The banks have privacy issues and are not willing to share data with each other [19]. So the experimental analysis on a real-time data set could not be evaluated by us. But the central bank of a country, e.g., RBI in India, has the power to regulate and direct different public and private banks to share their transaction data. Controlling money laundering helps government in strengthening economy and it is vital for the proper functioning of its financial systems. Anti-money laundering policies are launched by government of India in which the data collected by the central bank helps in its designing, as it is the responsibility of the government only to regulate the economy of the country. We need good governance and willingness of the political parties to implement the use of technology in the fight against money launderers. The channelization of black money can also distort the proper demand and supply ratio, so high chances of inflation are there in such cases.

Our proposed technique will definitely be helpful for banks to detect all the suspicious users involved in smurfing because it is both simple to deploy and scalable in nature. This will help in combating money laundering. Although all the money laundering activities performed on the bank networks cannot be detected, we can certainly detect such fraudulent people around the world who practice smurfing using our proposed approach [4]. Therefore, our proposed method is novel in its application using recently developed technique like Big Data and it is a first effort of such type proposed by us to curb smurfing activities. We propose to use graph mining technique to detect the pattern mining of the nodes involved in smurfing [15]. In this way, many associated criminal networks can also be detected by analyzing their social networks too, because people involved in unorganized crimes do posses black money. Our proposed solution is distributed and scalable, and it is not costly to implement.

References

1. Moser, M., Bohme, R., Breuker, D.: An enquiry into money laundering tools in the Bitcoin ecosystems. In: E-Crime Researchers Summit, pp. 1–14 (2013)
2. Lucian, R.D.: Money laundering economic and legal aspects. In: 2nd IEEE International Conference on Information and Financial Engineering, pp. 713–717 (2010)
3. Tejay, G.P.S.: Introduction to cyber crime in the digital economy minitrack. In: 45th Hawaii International Conference on System Science, pp. 30–40 (2012)
4. Flores, D.A., Angelopoulou, O., Self, R.J.: Combining digital forensic practices and database analysis as an anti money laundering strategy for financial institution. In: 3rd International Conference on Emerging Intelligent Data and Web Technologies, pp. 218–224 (2012)
5. Yang, C.C., Ng, T.D.: Terrorism and crime related weblog social network-link, content analysis and information visualisation. In: Intelligence and Security Informatics, IEEE, pp. 55–58
6. Didimo, W., Liotta, G., Montecchiani, F.: An advanced network visualization system for financial crime detection. In: IEEE Pacific Visualization Symposium, 1–4 Mar 2011, Hongkong, China, pp. 203–210 (2011)

7. Chen, Z., Van Khoa, L.D., Nazir, A., Teoh, E.N., Karupiah, E.K: Exploration of the effectiveness of expectation maximization algorithm for suspicious transaction detection in anti money laundering. In: IEEE Conference on Open System, Subang, Malaysia, 26–28 Oct, pp. 145–149 (2014)
8. Thangiah, M., Basri, S., Suliman, S.: A framework to detect cyber crime in the virtual environment. In: International Conference on Computer and Information Science, pp. 553–557 (2012)
9. Shu, M., Rui, L., Dancheng, L., Shuaizhen, Z.: Anti money laundering system based on main frame and SOA. In: 5th International Conference on Computational Intelligence and Communication Network, pp. 613–616 (2013)
10. Luna Dong, X., Srivastava, D.: Big data Integration. In: 29th International Conference on Data Engineering, pp. 1245–1248 (2013)
11. Leung, C.K., MacKinnon, R.K., Jiang, F.: Reducing the search space for big data mining for interesting patterns from uncertain data. In: IEEE Congress on Big Data, pp. 315–322 (2014)
12. Chen, H., Lin, T.Y., Zhang, Z., Zhong, J.: Parallel mining frequent patterns over big transactional data in extended MapReduce. In: IEEE International Conference on Granular Computing, pp. 43–48 (2013)
13. Tianqing, Z.: An outlier detection model based on cross datasets comparison for financial surveillance. In: Proceedings of th 2006 IEEE Asia Pacific Conference on Services Computing, pp. 601–604 (2006)
14. Patel, A.B., Birla, M., Nair, U.: Addressing big data problem using Hadoop and MapReduce. In: NIRMA University International Conference on Engineering, NUiCONE-2012, 6–8 Dec 2012, pp. 1–5 (2012)
15. Michalak, K., Korczak, J.: Graph mining approach to suspicious transaction Detection. In: Proceeding of the Federated Conference on Computer Science and Information System, pp. 69–75
16. Xuan, L., Pengzhu, Z.: An agent based anti-money laundering system architecture for financial supervision. In: International Conference on Wireless Communications, Networking and Mobile Computing, pp. 5472–5475 (2007)
17. Yang Qifeng, Feng Bin, Song Ping, "Study on Anti-Money Laundering service system of online payment based on Union-Bank mode", International conference on wireless communications, networking and mobile computing, 2007, pp. 49–91
18. Berghel, H.: The Future Of Digital Money Laundering. August 2014, pp. 70–75 (2014)
19. Jutla, D.N., Bodorik, P., Ali, S.: Emerging privacy for big data apps with the unified modeling language. In: IEEE International Congress on Big data, pp. 38–45 (2013)
20. le Khac, N.A., Kechadi, M.T.: Application of data mining for anti money laundering detection: a case study. In: IEEE International Conference on Data Mining Workshops, pp. 577–584 (2010)
21. Bernard, K., Cassidy, A., Clark, M., Liu, K., Lobaon, K., McNeill, D., Brown, D.: Indentifying and tracking online financial services through web mining and latent semantic indexing. In: Proceedings of 2011 IEEE Systems and Information Engineering Design Symposium, University of virginia, 29 Apr 2011, pp. 158–163 (2011)
22. Umadevi, P.M.E., Divya, A.P.E.: Money laundering detection using TFA system. In: International Conference on Software Engineering and Mobile Application Modelling and Development, 19–21 Dec 2012, pp. 1–8 (2012)
23. Wang, S.N., Yang, J.G.: A money laundering risk evaluation method based on decision tree. In: Proceedings of the 6th International Conference on Machine Learning and Cybernetics, Hongkong, 19–22 Aug 2007, pp. 283–286
24. Bastia, S.: Next generation technologies to combat counterfeiting of electronic components. In: IEEE Transaction on Components and Packaging Technologies, vol. 25, No. 1, Mar 2002, pp. 175–176 (2002)

25. Sobolevsky, S., Sitko, I., et. al.: Money on the move: big data of bank card transactions as the new proxy for human mobility patterns and regional delineation. The case of residents and Foreign visitors in Spain. In: IEEE International Congress on Big Data, pp. 136–143 (2014)
26. Demchenko, Y., Grosso, P., de Laat, C., Membray, P.: Addressing big data issues in scientific data infrastructure. In: International Conference on Collaboration Technologies and Systems, pp. 48–55 (2013)
27. Song, Y., Alatorre, G., Mandagree, N., Singh, A.: Storage mining: where IT management meets big data analytics. In: IEEE International Congress on Big data, pp. 421–422 (2013)

A Novel Approach for Semantic Prefetching Using Semantic Information and Semantic Association

Sonia Setia, Jyoti and Neelam Duhan

Abstract Exponential growth of web accesses on the Internet causes substantial delays in providing services to the user. Web prefetching is an effective solution that can improve the performance of the web by reducing the latency perceived by the user. Content on the web page also provides meaningful data to predict the future requests. This paper presents a content-based semantic prefetching approach. The proposed approach basically works on the semantic preferences of the tokens present in the anchor text associated with the URLs. To make more accurate predictions, it also uses the semantic information which is explicitly embedded with each link. It then computes the semantic association between the tokens and links then associates weightage in order to improve the prediction accuracy. This prefetching scheme would be more effective for long browsing sessions and will achieve good hit rate.

Keywords Web prefetching · Content-based prefetching · Semantic prefetching · Semantic information · Semantic association · Prediction

1 Introduction

Today, the number of users accessing the web has increased tremendously, which resulted into the increased traffic in the network as well as load on the web servers. Users are demanding the techniques which can reduce the latencies perceived

S. Setia (✉) · Jyoti · N. Duhan
Department of Computer Engineering, YMCA University of Science and Technology, Faridabad, India
e-mail: setiasonia53@gmail.com

Jyoti
e-mail: justjyoti.verma@gmail.com

N. Duhan
e-mail: neelam_duhan@rediffmail.com

V.B. Aggarwal et al. (eds.), *Big Data Analytics*, Advances in Intelligent Systems and Computing 654, https://doi.org/10.1007/978-981-10-6620-7_45

during web access. To reduce this latency, many techniques have been developed in last few years. One of them is prefetching.

Prefetching is a technique which pro-actively fetches the web pages before the user explicitly demands those pages. To predict the web pages which are likely to be accessed next, content-based prefetching works on the semantic preferences of the pages retrieved in the past. It is found that user surfing is always done by using the anchor texts of URLs. The anchor text provides the description of the links. For example, a user having interest in shopping of a particular brand say 'AMUL' would like to see all the products of 'AMUL.' This is the phenomena of 'Semantic Locality.' This paper works on the similar concept as that of content-based semantic prefetching.

The remainder of this paper is organized as follows: Sect. 2 presents the related work for web prefetching techniques. Section 3 describes the proposed framework. Section 4 discusses the process of proposed technique. Finally, Sect. 5 concludes this paper.

2 Related Work

Many Prefetching techniques are provided in literature. Khan et al. [1] gave a new idea of content-based prefetching. Authors stated that prediction algorithm can give more accurate results if it considers the web space organization. A new prefetching technique is suggested in this paper where predictions are made by analyzing the contents of the current web page. Each web page contains a number of links on it.

Ibrahim et al. [2, 3] introduced a keyword-based semantic prefetching technique where predictions are made based on the semantic preferences of past retrieved web documents. This technique was applied to the Internet news services. This paper motivated the fact that user's surfing is guided by the keywords present in URL anchor text.

Venketesh et al. [4] used the tokens, generated from anchor texts associated with the URLs on the web page, to make effective predictions. Authors applied Naïve Bayes Classifier to compute the probability values of each URL, based on which the preference list is generated to make prefetching more effective.

Sharma and Dubey [5] proposed a semantic-based prefetching scheme which uses decision tree induction to compute the probability of each link to be clicked next. SPRINT-Decision tree induction method [6] is used in the proposed framework. Pruning is also applied on the decision tree so as to improve performance.

Setia et al. [7] provided a review in the area of web prefetching. The paper basically focuses on the various web prefetching techniques. Eight categories of web Prefetching were reviewed with detailed study of each.

Hu et al. [8] proposed a method to organize the multimedia resources on the web. Authors used the semantic link network model to find the associations between multimedia resources. In this paper, social tags and the surrounding text associated with the multimedia resources are used to determine the semantic association between them. The proposed model provides a new method to organize the multimedia resources with their semantics.

There are so many content-based Prefetching techniques in the literature which are using keywords present in the anchor texts of web objects. Existing techniques consider that user surfing is always done by using the anchor texts of URLs where anchor text provides the description of the links. For example, a user having interest in shopping of a particular brand say 'AMUL' would like to see all the products of 'AMUL.' This is the phenomena of 'Semantic Locality.' But these techniques don't consider the semantics of the keywords associated with anchor texts of links as different anchor texts may be used by the web page designer to describe the page. For example, one designer can use 'apple' and other can use 'iphone' for the mobile phone manufactured by 'Apple.' Although these two are different keywords, but if user is interested in the mobile phone manufactured by 'Apple' he would like to see both the pages described by either 'Apple' or 'iphone.' Thus, these two keywords are semantically related to each other. Therefore, it would be more efficient to compute the semantic association between two tokens for better prediction.

3 Proposed Framework for Semantic-Based Prefetching

Proposed framework provides an efficient approach for more accurate predictions of the web pages by resolving the issues discussed above. Proposed approach consists of following components (Fig. 1):

- Semantic Link Analyzer, Token Extractor, Prediction System, Prefetching System, Storage Cache.

A. Semantic Link Analyzer

Semantic Link Analyzer analyzes the links on the web page and determines the priority order of links which should be considered first for evaluation. For this,

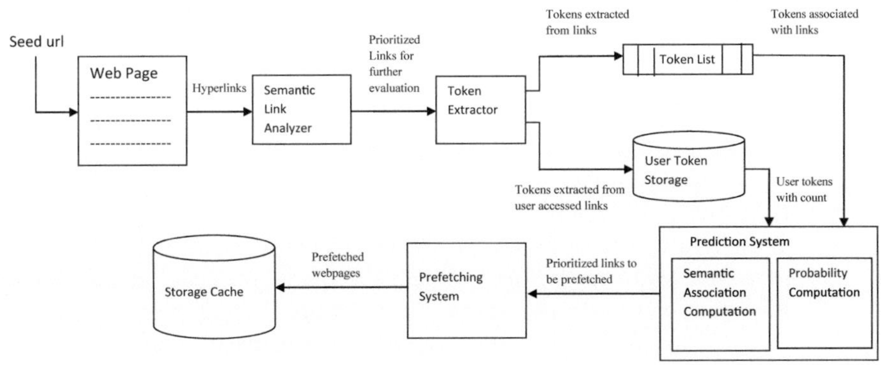

Fig. 1 Components of the system

Semantic Link Analyzer uses the semantic information on a web page that is added while designing the web page i.e., a semantic type is associated with each hyperlink using XML tags. Semantic type reflects a semantic relation between two web pages. Semantic types are defined as follows [9]:

1. Sequential (seq): This type indicates that these two pages should be accessed in a sequence i.e., one after another.
2. Similar (sim): This type indicates that both pages are semantically similar.
3. Cause-Effective (ce): This type indicates that one page is the cause of another.
4. Implication (imp): This type indicates that the semantics of one page implies the other.
5. Subtype (st): This type indicates that one is a part of another.
6. Instance (ins): This indicates that one is an instance of other.
7. Reference (ref): This indicates that one page is a detailed explanation of the other page.

The relative semantic strength orders of these types are as follows:
ref < ins < st < imp < ce < sim < seq

When the user requests for a web page server sends the page with the semantic information associated with each hyperlink on that page. Semantic Link Analyzer extracts the URLs from that page and analyzes all of those links and prioritizes them according to their semantic strength. If more than one link are of same type then relative location of the link on that page is considered for prioritization. This ordered list of links is used by the token extractor for further evaluation.

B. Token Extractor

This component takes the prioritized links as input from the Semantic Link Analyzer. As a large number of links may be there on a web page this can't be examined at a time. Therefore, a fixed '*n*' number of links are considered for further examination. Thus, it takes the first set of links i.e., first '*n*' number of links from the prioritized list of links and extracts the anchor text associated with these links. Further anchor texts are processed to generate the set of tokens. This component maintains two data structures in turn to store the information.

(i) Token List

Token List contains the tokens extracted from the anchor text associated with the URLs on the current page. Based on these tokens, probability of each URL is computed corresponding to the token count is maintained in User Token Storage.

(ii) User Token Storage (UTS)

Whenever user accesses a web page, the tokens generated from the anchor text associated with that page is added to the User Token Storage. Thus, this unit stores the information about the user's interest in a particular topic. With each token, count value is also maintained in User Token Storage. Token count reflects the number of times a token appears in the anchor text associated with the user's requested page. Whenever the token appears in the requested page, its associated count gets incremented by one if it already exists in the storage unit otherwise new entry is created with count value one. These tokens contained in storage unit are used by the prediction system to compute the probability of URLs being accessed in near future.

C. Prediction System

Prediction System is responsible for making predictions of the future web pages. This is being done based on two computations:

(1) Semantic Association Computation [8]

Different anchor texts may be used by the web page designer to describe the page. For example, one designer can use 'apple' and other can use 'iPhone' for the mobile phone manufactured by Apple. Although these two are different keywords, but if user is interested in the mobile phone manufactured by 'Apple' he would like to see both the pages described by either apple or iPhone. Thus, these two keywords are semantically related to each other. Therefore, it would be more efficient to compute the semantic association between token set of a link and each token present in User Token Storage. If any token is found semantically related to the token set of a particular link, then that token will be included in the token set of that particular link. This would give the more weightage to that particular link and will also help in computing the more accurate probability of that link to be accessed in future.

Semantic association is computed between two token sets using following steps:

- Let 'N' be the number of entries in the token list corresponding to N links on the current page, and each entry is a token set $T_i = \{t_1, t_2 \ldots t_m\}$ extracted from the anchor text of a link and $1 \leq m \leq n$; 'n' is a positive integer and $1 \leq i \leq N$.
- Let 'M' be the number of entries in User Token Storage, and S_j represents a token in User Token Storage and $1 \leq j \leq M$.
- $\mathrm{SA}(T_i, S_j)$ is the semantic association between two token sets and it is computed as

$$\mathrm{SA}(T_i, S_j) = \frac{\sum_{\substack{t_k T_i, \\ s_l S_j}} \mathrm{SA}(t_k, s_l)}{|T_i|} \tag{1}$$

where $\mathrm{SA}(t_k, s_l)$ is the semantic association between two tokens and it is computed as follows:

$$\mathrm{SA}(t_k, s_l) = \log\left(\frac{M * M(t_k \cap s_l)}{M(t_k) * M(s_l)}\right) / \log M \tag{2}$$

where

- M is the number of web pages in the search engine.
- $M(t_k)$ denotes the page counts for the token t_k.
- $M(s_l)$ denotes the page counts for the token s_l.
- $M(t_k \cap s_l)$ denotes the page counts for the query $t_k \cap s_l$ which measures the co-occurrence of the tokens t_k and s_l.

If this value is greater than a fixed predefined threshold then tokens will be considered semantically related to that token set and that particular token will be included in the token set associated with a link i.e.

$$T_i = T_i \cup S_j$$

For that particular link, this token set will be considered for further computation.

(2) Probability Computation

Finally, the system computes the probability of each link using Naïve Bayes classifier. Set of tokens associated with a particular link is taken, and the count value corresponding to these tokens is compared to the total tokens count in User Token Storage to determine its probability to be clicked next.

Probability of appearance of a link for a given storage S

$P(T_i/S)$ is computed by taking the product of individual tokens probabilities:

$$P(T_i/S) = \prod_{i=1}^{m} [C + P(t_k/S)] \tag{3}$$

where

- $P(T_i)$ = Probability of appearance of a link
- $P(S)$ = Probability of User Token Storage
- $P(t_k)$ = Probability of individual token associated with a link and $t_k \in T_i$
- $P(t_k/S)$ = Probability of each token for a given storage S which is computed as

$$P(t_k/S) = \frac{\text{Count of } t_k \text{ in } S}{\text{Total count of tokens in } S}$$

- C is a Constant with value '1' which is added to each token probability whether it is present in User Token Storage or not. It is added to avoid two cases:

1. Probability of link to be less than individual token probability
2. To avoid zero probability situation because product value becomes zero if few tokens of a link are not present in User token Storage

Based on these probabilities of links, prediction system generates a priority list of links needed to be prefetched and top priority is given to the links having high probability.

D. Prefetch System

Prefetch System takes the priority list generated by prediction system as input and prefetches the corresponding web pages from the server and stores them in storage cache. When user clicks a link, then any ongoing prefetching will be suspended and system will look for the requested page.

E. Storage Cache

Web pages that are prefetched by the prefetch system are stored in storage cache to satisfy the future requests made by the user. Since the cache is of limited size, replacement of web page would be required when cache gets full. In this paper, Least Recently Used (LRU) algorithm is used as cache replacement algorithm. It removes the web pages from the cache that are not accessed for a long time and makes sufficient space for new pages.

4 Process of Prefetching

The whole process (Fig. 2) involves the following steps:

1. User opens a browser and requests for a page by entering the URL.
2. Server sends the corresponding web page including the semantic information associated with each link on that page which is displayed to the user.
3. Semantic Link Analyzer extracts the links and semantic information associated with each link present in the page and gives a prioritized list of links based on their relative strength and position on the page.
4. Out of these links, first '*n*' set of links are considered for further evaluation.
5. Anchor text is extracted associated with each link. These are further processed to generate the set of tokens where each token refers to single word.
6. These tokens are stored in the Token List.
7. Whenever user clicks a link, tokens generated from the anchor text associated with that link are being added to the User Token Storage with count value '1' if it doesn't exist in storage unit otherwise, count value gets incremented by one each time token appears in user access.
8. Computing the semantic association between the anchor text associated with each link presents in token list and the tokens present in User Token Storage. If it is found greater than the threshold value (in this paper, it is manually computed) then that token is semantically related to the anchor text of a link and it will be added to the token set of the anchor text of that particular link to compute its probability to be accessed in future.

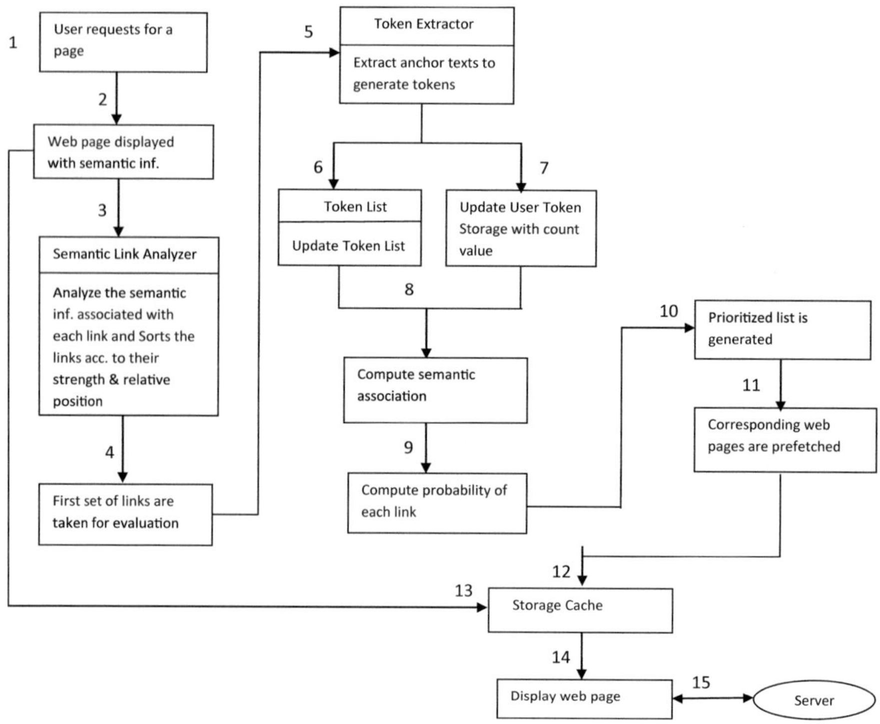

Fig. 2 Process of prefetching

9. Compute the probability of each link to be accessed next using Naïve Bayes classifier.
10. Based on these probability values, priority list of links will be generated.
11. Prefetching will be done based on the priority list.
12. Prefetched web pages are stored in storage cache which is being managed using LRU replacement algorithm.
13. Whenever user clicks a link on the web page, ongoing prefetching will be suspended and system looks for that page in storage cache.
14. If it is present in cache, it is displayed to the user without any delay.
15. Otherwise, it is retrieved from the server and displayed to the user.

5 Conclusion

This paper has presented a novel approach based on semantic prefetching which uses the anchor texts associated with the URLs present on the current page for making effective predictions. Besides this, it also uses the semantic information which is explicitly embedded with each link, to prioritize the links at the first step. This approach basically works on the semantic preferences of the tokens present in the anchor text associated with the URLs. To compute the accurate probability of each link to be prefetched, this approach computes the semantic association between the anchor text of the URLs and tokens present in user token storage so that more accurate weightage can be given to each link if it is found semantically related to any token. The proposed approach helps to minimize the user perceived latency by making more accurate predictions and achieving maximum hits.

References

1. Khan, J.I., Tao, Q.: Exploiting Webspace organization for accelerating Web prefetching. In: Proceedings of the IEEE/WIC International Conference on Web Intelligence, Halifax, Canada (2003)
2. Ibrahim, T.I., Xu, C.: Neural net based predictive prefetching to tolerate WWW latency. In: Proceedings of the 20th International Conference on Distributed Computing Systems (2000)
3. Xu, C.Z., Ibrahim, T.I.: A keyword-based semantic prefetching approach in Internet news services. IEEE Trans. Knowl. Data Eng. **16**(5), 601–611 (2004)
4. Venketesh, P., Venkatesan, R., Arunprakash, L.: Semantic Web prefetching scheme using Naïve Bayes classifier. Int. J. Comput. Sci. Appl. **7**(1), 66–78 (2010)
5. Sharma, N., Dubey, S.K.: Semantic based Web prefetching using decision tree induction. In: Proceedings of 5th International Conference on the Next Generation Information Technology Summit (2014)
6. Shafer, J., Agrawal, R., Mehta, M.: SPRINT- a scalable parallel classifier for data mining. In: Proceedings of 22nd International Conference on Very Large Database, pp. 544–555 (1996)
7. Setia, S., Jyoti, Duhan, N.: Survey of recent Web prefetching techniques. Int. J. Res. Comput. Commun. Technol. **2**(12) (2013)
8. Hu, C., Xu, Z., Liu, Y., Mi, L., Chen L., and Luo, X.: Semantic link network- based model for organizing multimedia big data. IEEE Trans. Emerg. Top. Comput. **2**(3) 2014
9. Pons, A.P.: Object prefetching using semantic links. Database Adv. Inf. Syst. **37**(1) (2006)
10. Venketesh, P., Venkatesan, R.: Adaptive Web prefetching scheme using link anchor information. Int. J. Appl. Inf. Syst. **2**(1) (2012)

Optimized Cost Model with Optimal Disk Usage for Cloud

Mayank Aggrawal, Nishant Kumar and Raj Kumar

Abstract Cloud is a bag full of resources. Using cloud services at an optimal level is required as now cloud is primary technology for deployment over Internet. This is indeed a practice to make use of things efficiently to make cloud a better place. Cloud is providing all computing resources that one may need to compile tasks, but efficiently using of resources can increase the power to accommodate more consumers and also consumer can save on cost for the services subscribed. This paper provides a mechanism to increase or decrease the subscription as per the use.

Keywords Cloud computing · Resource optimization

1 Introduction

Cloud computing refers to the use of computing remotely over network via various ways like as a software, hardware, and platform. It is a big turn in Information technology [1]. This architecture is using the resources to its maximum on a specific cost. There are many ways and parameters to measure cost in cloud. Like Amazon is considering its pricing on the basis of instances time and storage cost is different, bluemix is considering RAM utilization as a parameter of pricing, azure is considering bandwidth for pricing. All giant companies are coming up with cloud data centers and providing service to its customers. Parameters of pricing are based company's policy but all have one thing is common that is Pay-per-use model. All service providers offering this model to their customers at a very affordable price to attract customers to migrate on cloud.

M. Aggrawal (✉)
Department of Computer Science & Engineering, Gurukula Kangri Vishwavidyalaya, Haridwar, India
e-mail: mayank@gkv.ac.in

N. Kumar · R. Kumar
Faculty of Technology, Gurukula Kangri Vishwavidyalaya, Haridwar, India
e-mail: nishant@gkv.ac.in

V.B. Aggarwal et al. (eds.), *Big Data Analytics*, Advances in Intelligent Systems and Computing 654, https://doi.org/10.1007/978-981-10-6620-7_46

Cloud computing is the service-oriented architecture, in which service is the high priority, and cost is another big factor from the consumer side. This paper focusing on a very balanced and optimal use of the resource to accommodate more consumer and to cut in cost of subscription on the basis of Pay-per-use model.

2 Cloud Service Model

2.1 SAAS (Software as a Service)

In SaaS model, the consumer uses an application which is deployed in cloud environment but does not control or know the operating system, hardware or network infrastructure, location which is running the application [5].

2.2 PaaS (Platform as a Service)

In PaaS model, the consumer can hire platform (Operating system with minimal requirements) for its applications or other tasks. It controls the applications that run in the environment but doesn't allow to touch hardware resources over network.

2.3 IaaS (Infrastructure as a Service)

In IaaS model, the consumer can provide the hardware requirements to the service providers. And service providers will give the user the requested hardware resources and then user can install own operating system and can also deploy own applications.

2.4 Storage as a Service

This is the service in which third-party providers rent storage to users. As per the demand, they allocate the storage.

3 Literature Survey

Atar [2] states that if certain amount of cloud resource is not leased by subscribed customers, it makes sense to provide the unused resource to the needy one. This way cloud service provider can accommodate more customers and can increase the revenues.

Kim [3] states on accounting based on power consumption should be also one of the cost factor of cloud. As to run a cloud, a big data centre is consuming a lot of power.

Hsu [4] states that cloud technology adoption is still at initial stage. And the firms with greater IT capability tend to choose the pay-as-you-go pricing schemes. According to [4] there are basic three pricing schemes, pay-as-you-go, License, and Unlimited access with monthly fee.

Yang [6] states that to control cost by using a scheduling algorithm and using market theory to schedule compute resources. According to [6] to get the lowest total price, we need to sort the suppliers for the set of resource requirement. And then as per the requirement increases based on task criticality it chose the supplier.

Li [7] states the dynamic pricing scheme based on real time energy load. According to the [7] dynamic pricing based on energy consumption can save a lot of energy.

There are many cloud service provider like Amazon, IBM, Microsoft etc. All have their own subscription parameters and pricing scheme. With the service, we can compile our tasks online.

IBM's Bluemix is really good with its interface; the best thing about the Bluemix is its user-friendly design and ready to build apps. It gives you a place where apps can be built on cloud directly, no need to know coding. While Microsoft's Azure is providing various ways of use of cloud but mainly concentrated on Bandwidth. IBM Bluemix is offering three pricing schemes for Individuals and Business customers, Pay as you Go, Pay-as-you-go plus extended for individuals, and subscription based for business people. Bluemix has different mechanism of measuring the utilization of the resources. It is using GB-hour mainly focused on RAM usages and providing almost 1 GB space for an application. Let see how GB-Hours work.

$$1 * 24 * 30 = 720 \text{ GB-Hours}$$

An application using 1 GB of RAM and running 30 days and 24 h makes 720 GB-Hours. IBM bluemix is offering 375 GB-Hours in a month, means applications using memory of 512 MB can run on bluemix for free.

Amazon is also providing Pay-as-you-go model. In that a user can sign up for an instance and can pay for the time, the instance was used and the minimum 1vCPU, 0.6 GB memory.

Microsoft's azure is basically focusing on Bandwidth in the free tier of 30 days. It limits the app deployment count. Azure also has the option for Pay-as-You-Go. While using virtual machines, it provides 1 core and 768 MB ram as standard.

4 Proposed Mechanism

This mechanism is described using one resource, storage, it can be applicable on other. As per the queuing theory of optimization the optimum level of utilization can be achieved between 60–80% uses of resources [2]. Above 80 % the graph shows the degrade phase. So, here the same concept is used to optimize the disk usage. This level of optimization could save unused space and money also. As we all know that cloud is famous for its "pay per use" cost model. In this scheme unused space is leading to extra amount paying to cloud services.

This algorithm is to intimate the customer to optimize their disk usage. In this if the usage is lower than 60%, a message will be sent to the customer to cut down your subscribed package as per usage. And if it is 90%, a message will be sent to expand and at 100%, firstly automatic expansion will be done, then a message to expand the storage with in 48 h.

```
per = use*100/sub
per- percentage used.
use- usage of disk.
sub- subscribed usage.
function(use,sub)
{
     per = use*100/sub
     If(per < 60)
     {
          new_sub = use*100/60;
          send_message
("You should subscribe 'new_sub' for the optimal use");
     }
     If(per > 90)
     {
          send_message("please upgrade your plan as the usage is reach-
ing to the maximum");
     }
     If(per > 100)
     {
          automatic_expand("500mb",48 h);
          send_message
("Expansion is done temporarily please upgrade your plan to
meet requirement within 48 h.")
     }
} //FUNCTION ENDS
```

5 Conclusion

Till now there are various cost models are present in the market. In all companies are providing fixe Ram and CPU. There might be situation where the subscribed ram is not being used completely. Suppose a normal static website can run in 64 MB flawlessly, so if the enrolled amount of memory is 600 MB then its the shear waste of the resource 536 MB ram. This is beneficial for the service provider, through this mechanism service provider can accommodate more customers and on the client side, client can save its cost. The proposed mechanism will provide the optimum use of disk or storage and also will save on unused service. Efficient use of cloud services will help in the improvement in quality of service and also will increase the cloud potential to accommodate more end users.

6 Future Work

This work can be extend to the dynamic allocation of the resources by predicting the usage pattern of the application by its client. Resource allocation system functionality is very much similar to human brain. It coordinates with every layer present in cloud environment and allocates resources accordingly [8]; we need to consider it to design dynamic allocation scheme.

References

1. Sindhu, S., Mukherjee, S.: Efficient task scheduling algorithm for cloud computing environment, Springer (2011)
2. Atar, R., Cidon, I., Shifrin, M.: MDP based optimal pricing for a cloud computing queuing model, Elsevier (2014)
3. Kim, N., Cho, J., Seo, E.: Energy-credit scheduler: an energy-aware virtual machine scheduler for cloud systems. Elsevier, Future Generation Computer System (2014)
4. Hsu, P-F., Ray, S., Li-Hsieh, Y-Y.: Examining cloud computing adoption intention, pricing mechanism and deployment model. Int. J. Info. Manage (2014)
5. Buyya, R., Broberg, J., Goscinski, A.: Cloud computing principles and paradigms, pp 13–16 (2013)
6. Yang, Z., Yin, C.: A Cost-based resource scheduling paradigm in cloud computing. In: International Conference on Parallel and Distributed Computing, Applications and Technologies, IEEE (2011), 978–0-7695-4564-6/11
7. Li, X., Lo, J-C.: Pricing and peak aware scheduling algorithm for cloud computing. IEEE (2011) 978-1-4577-2159-50/12
8. Buyya, R., Yeo, C.S., Venugopal, S.: Market-oriented cloud computing: vision, hype, and reality for delivering it services as computing utilities. In: High Performance Computing and Communications, (2008, September), HPCC'08. 10th IEEE International Conference on (pp. 5–13) IEEE, (2011)

Understanding Live Migration Techniques Intended for Resource Interference Minimization in Virtualized Cloud Environment

Tarannum Bloch, R. Sridaran and CSR Prashanth

Abstract Cloud computing is consolidated as an environment which allows concurrent execution of various cloud applications of different organizations via a shared pool of resources. Each cloud user is provided with virtual machine to have further interaction with the cloud architecture components. Effective management of these virtualized machines along with satisfactory level of SLA is major challenge. Due to the resource overbooking over the physical host running, virtual machines need to be migrated from source to destination host. The migrated machine may disrupt other ongoing virtualized machines on destination host which can lead the application performance degradation. This paper provides insight of existing interference-aware live virtual machine migration techniques. As well taxonomy of the resource interference has been introduces. This paper also contains the comparative study of the performance assessment matrix, issues resolved, and mathematical models used by available live migration techniques that can act major key point while making live migration decisions. This paper is useful to cloud architect and the researchers working on automated live VM migration decision support system to achieve higher-level satisfaction of SLA by providing maximum quality-of-service parameters.

Keywords Cloud · Interference · Migration · Performance degradation · Virtual machines

T. Bloch (✉)
RDIC, Wadhwan, Gujarat, India
e-mail: taru.gnd@gmail.com

R. Sridaran
Faculty of Computer Applications, Marwadi Education Foundation's Group of Institutions, Rajkot, Gujarat, India
e-mail: sridaran.rajagopal@gmail.com

C. Prashanth
Head of Computer Science & Engineering,
NHEC, Bangaluru, Karnataka, India
e-mail: drprashanthcsr@gmail.com

V.B. Aggarwal et al. (eds.), *Big Data Analytics*, Advances in Intelligent Systems and Computing 654, https://doi.org/10.1007/978-981-10-6620-7_47

1 Introduction

Virtualization technology provides resource sharing among applications in cloud environment. It supports diverse applications to be executed over a shared pool of resources. This feature provides low-cost IT infrastructure to the organizations. Cloud environment also allows to reserve more resources than the requirement of application on physical host by utilizing resource overbooking characteristic of cloud. Elasticity is another attractive and distinct competence that allows user to increase or decrease resource proportion.

Each physical host runs concurrent applications of different organizations by allocating one virtual machine per application. This scenario overloads the physical machine because of resource overbooking schemes origins basis of migrating running virtual machines to under loaded physical host. This type of migration is called live VM migration.

The performance of cloud applications depends on the availability of the resources such as CPU hours, storage capacity, network bandwidth. The challenging task in such an environment is to guard the VM from its neighbors because the migrated VM may interference the performance of ongoing VMs of physical host. However, this kind of disturbance leads to the degradation of application performance. The minimization techniques to advocate the application performance as per SLA requirements along with interference awareness must be considered in live migration technique.

This paper is aimed to provide the insight of various interferences. The paper is organized as follows: Sect. 2 describes significance of live VM migration. Section 3 presents understanding of interferences occurred because of live VM migrations. Section 4 defines performance assessment matrix to be considered in migration decisions. Section 5 describes available solutions of interference-aware live migration techniques. Section 6 provides comparative study of available solutions, and Sect. 7 presents concluding remarks alluding to future scope.

2 Significance of Live VM Migration

Virtualization can provide efficient and effective use of host resources such as CPU cycles, memory, hard disk, other I/O devices. These resources are handled by kernel of host operating system. To provide virtualized view of these hardware elements, special software called virtual machine monitor (VMM) also known as hypervisor is used. These all elements work together and form cloud environment. Figure 1 shows the alignment of cloud components.

Virtualization means converting hardware base entity into a software component [2]. The resultant entity is an abstraction of this conversion process, and it is known as virtual machine (VM). VMs are also called guest machines which run on physical machine (PM). It is also known as data centers or as host. Per client application one VM is allocated. Each VM has operating system to provide the

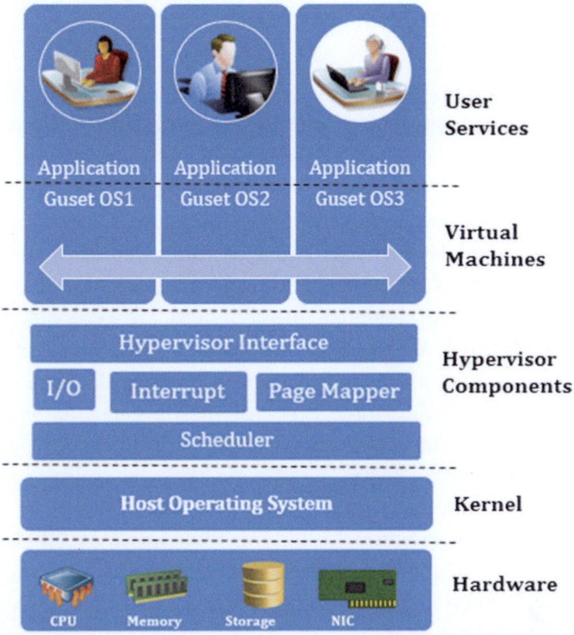

Fig. 1 Alignment of cloud components

interface between user application and allotted virtualized hardware resources. This interface can be any commercial or open-source operating system known as guest OS in cloud environment.

Live VM migration is a method that transfers the all-inclusive OS and its associated solicitation from one physical machine to another physical machine [1, 2]. In other words, VM is transferred to the other PM while executing the cloud application. Memory pages strike as dirty and then move to the new machine. The name of live migration mechanism varies depending on hypervisor (VMM) of each slice of virtualization software. It is called vMotion in VMware, while in Hyper-V and Xen, it is called live migration [3].

Sreenath Acharya et al. have described eleven types of live migrations, named as pre-copy live migration, post-copy live migration, memory management-based live migration, network-aware live migration, energy management-aware live migration, security-aware live migration, application-specific live migration, decentralized approach-based live migration, VM placement-based live migration, business-aware live migration, and stable matching-based live migration. Author has stated that the effectiveness of cloud computing relies on effective workload scheduling, optimized selection of VM to be migrate, efficient memory management, reduction in the number of active physical servers, and minimizing the total migration time and migration downtime [4]. Though live migration plays vital role in cloud environment, it leads to several problems to be taken care while going through it, such as energy management, load balancing after migration over destination host, and minimization of interferences.

3 Inferring Interferences

The major problem that occurs in cloud environments is that the application performance can change due to the presence of other virtual machines on a mutual server. Moreover, the existence of additional applications cannot be controlled by cloud user. As a result, cloud assurances on resource availability and capacity do not guarantee application performance. Cloud service agitating entities in the process of live virtual machine migration lead to performance degradation, and taxonomy of resource interferences are presented in Fig. 2.

Major four types of interferences are co-located: VM interference, inter VM interference, network interference, and application performance interference [5]. Resource interference is one subtype of application performance interference which can have further three types of interferences as shown in Fig. 2; first, CPU contention interference, second memory interference, and third I/O interference.

Migrating VM's workload can be either of one type CPU-intensive, memory-intensive, or I/O-intensive. All the types of workload disrupts the running VMs on destination by having their share in CPU cycles, memory areas, or I/O consumption and thus degrades the application performance. Minimization of the interferences is the burning issue to meet SLA requirements which needs to be taken in consideration while designing live migration techniques.

4 Performance Access Matrix

Performance of live VM migration technique must be capable enough to select VM from host PM to migrate and to choose destination host to place migrated VM. The strength of live VM migration technique depends on the various factors described below:

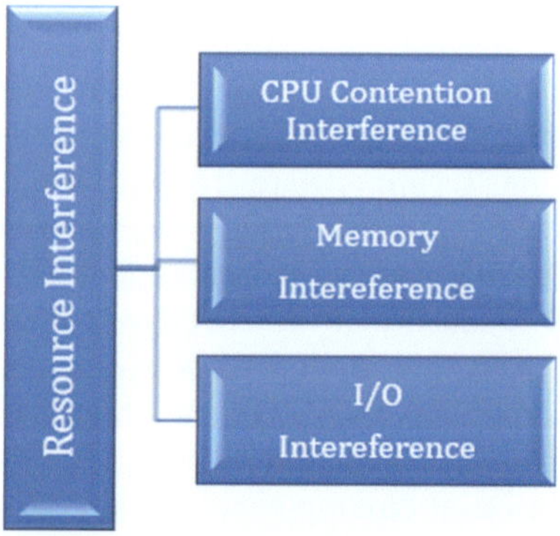

Fig. 2 Taxonomy of resource interference

- **Downtime**: Downtime is period through which performance of VM is paused during live migration process.
- **Throughput**: Number of cloud service request served in given amount of time.
- **Migration Time**: Total migration time is interval occupied by the migration procedure from beginning till completion of the migration procedure.
- **Co-location Interference**: After immigration of virtual machine on other physical host, the other neighbor VMs over destination physical host grieve from the performance lose due to the likely resource consumption. It is called co-location interference.
- **Performance Interference**: Through migration procedure of VM(s), the drifted virtual machine(s) and additional running virtual machine presented on both font and terminus PMs could undertake severe performance degradation is called migration interference.

Live migration technique should be capable enough to minimize co-location interference, and performance interference as well as migration process should reduce downtime and migration time.

5 State-of-the-Art Methods

Various researchers have addressed interferences directly or indirectly in their research work.

A. *iAware: Making Live Migration of Virtual Machines Interference-Aware in Cloud* [6]
   Fei Xu et al. have introduced design and implementation of a lightweight interference attentive live virtual machine migration policy they named it as iAware. iAware uses demand–supply estimation model of VM migration interference and VM co-location interference. Author has addressed various issues such as migration interference, co-location interference, SLA violation, load balancing, and power saving. This research can be further extended for heterogeneous cloud environment, and VM interference with overlapped memory can also be studied.
B. *TRACON: Interference-Aware Scheduling for Data-Intensive Applications in Virtualized Environments* [7]
   Ron C. Chiang et al. have introduced a new **T**ask and **R**esource **A**llocation **CON**trol framework that mitigates the interference possessions from parallel data-intensive applications and greatly progresses whole system performance. TRACON can achieve up to 25% improvement on application throughput on virtualized servers. Author stated that performance degradation occurs due to the adverse inference effects exist in virtualized environment to minimize those adverse effects author has implemented TRACON framework contains three components; first, interference estimation model that concludes application performance from resource consumption detected from different VMs; second,

the interference attentive scheduler that is designed to operate the model for actual resource management and the task; third, resource monitor that gathers application features at the runtime for model alteration. This work can be extended with diverse modeling methods to build a more accurate model and diminish the modeling and profiling overheads. Authors have not considered I/O interference effects. In future, I/O interference effects can also be considered on various storage devices.

C. *VMbuddies: Coordinating Live Migration of Multi-Tier Applications in Cloud Environments* [8]
Haikun Liu et al. have designed and implemented a coordination system VMbuddies that significantly reduces the performance degradation and migration cost of multi-tier applications. VMbuddies implementation contains four elements: (i) use of synchronization protocol for co-related VMs live migration to guarantee that all co-related VM migrations start stop-copy phase at the same time; (ii) a naïve bandwidth allocation method is used for scheduling the VM migrations one by one; (iii) optimal bandwidth allocation for static workload and adaptive bandwidth allocation for dynamic workload; (iv) optimization of VM live migration using two techniques ballooning to evict unused pages from VMs' memory image and an intelligent pre-copying termination to adjust the number of iterations in the pre-copying algorithm. VMbuddies can be further explored for more complex scenario such as workflow, map reduce, and MPI applications that have tree or direct acyclic graph (DAG) topologies.

D. *LVMCI: Efficient and Effective VM Live Migration Selection Scheme in Virtualized Data Centers* [9]
Wei Zhang et al. have presented VM selection method named **L**ive **V**irtual **M**achine migration with less **C**ost and application **I**nterference (LVMCI). LVMCI organism can approximate memory iteration time and downtime with high accurateness. It also guarantees high level of SLAs by lessening performance degradation through migration process and performance interference among co-located VMs at destination PM. LVMCI provides minimization of cost and minimization of performance interference of co-located applications along with automation of detecting migration requirement. LVMCI considers on CPU and disk resources only. Other resources can also be considered.

E. *Pacer: A Progress Management System for Live Virtual Machine Migration in Cloud Computing* [10]
Jie Zheng et al. claim that Pacer is the migration process management system which focuses on inability to trade-off application performance, migration time, and application degradation. Pacer accurately predicts the migration time from very beginning of migration and minimizes performance degradation. The key features of Pacer are as follows: it uses real-time measurements to drive the decisions, it uses detailed analytical models to predict the amount of the remaining data to be migrated according to the application's I/O workload consumption and the migration process, and to predict the completion time of

migration. Pacer adapts the dynamic conditions such as migration speed and targeted migration finish time. Pacer has a fixed adaption interval about 5 s which should be flexible for more accurate prediction.

F. *A Performance Interference-aware Virtual Machine Placement Strategy for Supporting Soft Real-time Applications in the Cloud* [11]
Faruk Caglar et al. have offered machine-learning-based online placement solution named **H**armonious **A**rt of **L**eaving **T**ogether (hALT) that learns from publicly available trace of a large data center owned by Google. Authors have analyzed a trace log of a production data center published by Google. Author has used machine learning to learn algorithm VM placement to predict future performance interference level and used these as a mean of making runtime placement decisions. hALT comprises virtual machine classifier using k-means classifier and silhouette method, back propagation neural network, and choice producer for VM settlement. It has discussed only about the design of the system no implementation discussion presented in the paper. As well only compute-intensive applications have been taken in consideration for other types of application concern more generic performance metric should be designed.

G. *iMIG: Toward an Adaptive Live Migration Method for KVM Virtual Machines* [12]
Jianxin Li et al. have introduced an analytical model named **i**mproved **MIG**ration which delivers better forecasts of migration time and downtime. iMIG primarily evaluates the affiliation between configuration constraints and live migration performance and their agreeing effects. Based on this reflection, iMIG forms model for adaptive control and SLA estimation. Author also resolved few errors in the available **Q**uick **EMU**lator (QEMU)/KVM parameter computation framework. iMig is capable enough to achieve reduction of migration latency and reduction of energy consumption. Author has not carried out investigation of computing techniques for the floating point in the migration progression which can be helpful to attain precise prediction of the migration time and the downtime.

H. *Q-Cloud: Managing performance interference effects or QoS-Aware clouds* [13]
Ripal Nathuji et al. have discussed quality-of-service (QoS)-aware migration technique. Author has modeled VM performance interference to meet QoS requirement to achieve desire SLA. Q-Cloud architecture includes cloud scheduler, interference migration control, and resource control mechanisms. Q-Clouds uses online feedback to build a multi-input multi-output (MIMO) model that records performance interference interactions and uses it to perform closed ring resource management. Q-Cloud improves the cloud utilization by maintaining q-states by allowing the applications to specify multiple levels of QoS. Q-Cloud gives improved cloud efficiency and performance interference-aware control for dynamic placement using live migration techniques. Virtualization issues around application with phased behavior can be addressed to improve the Q-Cloud.

I. *A model of storage I/O performance interference in Virtualized Systems* [14]
Giuliano Casale et al. have given simple performance model to predict the impact of consolidation on the storage I/O performance of virtualized applications. Authors have well-thought-out on distinct characterization of read/write performance attributes on per request level and provide valuable information for parameterization of storage I/O performance models. Author has proposed three classes of linear estimators: (i) for approximation of consolidation mixes, (ii) for approximation of consolidation throughputs, (iii) for approximation of consolidation response time. Heuristic of response time prediction is highly effective for read requests which are most vital to forecast, but the model is inadequate for predicting the write request performance.
J. *Alleviating I/O Interference* via *Caching & Rate-controlled Pre-fetching without Degrading Migration Performance* [15]
Morgan Stuart et al. have performed empirical study of the impact of storage migration offloading and presented live storage migration method named **S**torage **M**igration **O**ffloading (SMO) that decreases I/O interference and preserves lower migration latency and coverage under high dirty rate. SMO is method of live migration that reduces interference without undue sacrifice to migration performance. Author has performed data rate control methodology with buffering. SMO tracks exactly how complete the buffer is in demand to alter where data from the primary storage device should be sent. Author determines what amount of data being relocated directly from primary disk should be moved to destination host. The total data rate that the data is being sent to the estimation host machine is defined. SMO controls runtime cache strategies improved with rate-controlled pre-fetching in order to fill a virtual disk buffer through migration but when the transferring machine subjects very slight I/O to its backing storage co-located with high I/O guest SMO is not performing well.

6 Comparative Study

Various live VM techniques have focused on different parameters. This section gives comparative analysis of all existing solutions. Table 1 gives brief of major cloud issues resolved by existing solutions, namely minimization of migration time, minimization of downtime, throughout, performance interference, and co-location interference. Table 2 gives comparative study of the performance matrix taken into the consideration by existing methods. Table 3 briefs the mathematical models and tools used by existing solution.

Table 1 Comparative performance matrix by existing methods

Topics/References	[6]	[7]	[8]	[9]	[10]	[11]	[12]	[13]	[14]	[15]
Minimization of migration time	✓	✗	✓	✓	✓	✗	✓	✗	✓	✓
Minimization of downtime	✗	✗	✗	✗	✗	✗	✓	✗	✗	✗
Throughput	✓	✗	✓	✓	✗	✗	✗	✗	✓	✓
Performance interference	✓	✓	✓	✓	✗	✓	✓	✓	✗	✗
Co-location interference	✓	✗	✓	✓	✗	✓	✗	✓	✗	✗

Table 2 Issues resolved by existing solutions

Topics/References	[6]	[7]	[8]	[9]	[10]	[11]	[12]	[13]	[14]	[15]
Performance degradation	✗	✓	✓	✗	✓	✗	✗	✓	✗	✓
SLA violation	✓	✗	✗	✓	✗	✗	✗	✗	✗	✗
Load balancing	✓	✗	✗	✗	✗	✗	✗	✓	✓	✓
Power saving	✓	✗	✗	✗	✗	✗	✓	✗	✗	✗
Machine learning	✗	✗	✗	✗	✗	✓	✓	✗	✗	✗
Automatic migration requirement detection	✗	✓	✗	✓	✓	✗	✗	✗	✓	✗

7 Conclusion and Future Scope

Selection of running VM to get migrated is the crucial decision in order to achieve high level of SLA requirements. Various solutions for live migration are available but very few focuses on interference minimization. To have proper resource utilization and to avoid application performance degradation with a negligible downtime and finite dependency on the source machine is must during live migration of VM. This paper presents the comparative analysis of existing solutions. It has been observed that most of the solutions are either compute-intensive or I/O-intensive, whereas cloud applications can be either of compute-intensive, I/O-intensive, or network-intensive. In future, new live migration approach can be provided that takes into account the migration time of VM, downtime, insensitivity of applications, and minimization of interferences to reduce application performance degradation during live migration process.

Table 3 Mathematical models and tools used for implementation

References	Methodology adopted by existing solutions used	Tools used
[6]	•Demand–supply model of VM migration •Demand–supply model for VM co-location interference	Xen cluster
[7]	•Interference prediction model	Xentop, iostat
[8]	•Analytical cost model •Migration cost prediction model	Xen 4.1 with Linux 3.1 Kernel
[9]	•Migration cost model to predict performance degradation •Matrix computational model to calculate interference vector	Xen cluster
[10]	Novel analytical progress model •For predicting remaining data to be migrated •Predicting the finish time of Migration	Quick EMUlator (QEMU)
[13]	•Multiple-input multiple-output (MIMO) model •Linear model	Hyper-V platform
[12]	Systematic model with an adaptive mechanism to increase the migration performance and the success ratio •Static model of migration time •Dynamic model of downtime	Quick EMUlator (QEMU)/ Kernel-based VM (KVM)
[11]	•Virtual machine classifier (k-means classifier and silhouette method) •Back propagation neural network •Decision maker for placement	–
[14]	•Simple linear prediction models for the throughput, response times, and mix of read/write requests	VMware ESX server, network protocol analyzer tshark, block layer I/O tracing tool blktrace
[15]	•Simple mathematical model using min, max functions	Quick EMUlator (QEMU)/ Kernel-based VM (KVM)

References

1. Leelipushpam, P.G.J, Sharmila, J.: Live VM migration techniques in cloud environment-A survey. In: IEEE Conference on Information & Communication Technologies (ICT) pp. 408–413, 11–12 April (2013). ISBN: 978-1-4673-5759-3
2. Upadhyay, A., Lakkdawala, P.: Secure live migration of VM's in cloud computing: a survey. In: 3rd International IEEE Conference on Reliability, Infocom Technologies and Optimization (ICRITO) (Trends and Future Directions) pp. 1–4, 8–10 Oct (2014), ISBN: 978-1-4799-6895-4
3. Matsumoto, Hitoshi, Ezaki, Yutaka: Dynamic resource management in cloud environment. Fujitsu Sci Technol J **47**(3), 270–276 (2011)

4. Acharya, S., D'Mello, DA.: A taxonomy of live virtual machine migration mechnisms in cloud computing environment. In: IEEE International Conference on Green Computing, Communication and Conservation of Energy (ICGCE) (2013), pp. 809–815, 12–14 Dec 2013
5. Bloch, T., Sridaran, R., Prashanth C.S.R.: Analysis and Survey of Issues in Live Virtual Machine Migration Interference. Int. J. Adv. Networking Appl. (IJANA) Nov (2014). ISSN: 0975-0290, 151–157
6. Xu, F., Liu, F., Liu, L., Jin, H., Li, B., Li, B.: iAware: making live migration of virtual machines interference-aware in the cloud, Comput. IEEE Trans. **63**(12), 3012–3025 Dec (2013), ISSN: 0018-9340
7. Chiang, R.C., Huang, H.H.: TRACON: interference-aware scheduling for data-intensive applications in virtualized environments. In: IEEE International Conference on High Performance Computing, Networking, Storage and Analysis, Seattle, Washington, Article 47, pp. 47.1–47.12, 12-18 Nov (2011). ISBN: 978-1-4503-0771-0
8. Liu, H., He, B., VMbuddies: coordinating live migration of multi-tier applications in cloud environments. IEEE Trans. Parallel Distrib Syst. **26**(4), 1045–1205 April (2013). ISSN: 1045-9219
9. Zhang, W., Zhu, M., Mei, Y, et al.: LVMCI: efficient and effective VM live migration selection scheme in virtualized data centers. In: IEEE 18th International Conference on Parallel and Distributed Systems (ICPADS), Singapore (2012), pp. 368–375, 17–19 Dec (2012), ISSN: 1521-9097
10. Zheng, J., Ng, T.S.E., Sripanidkulchai, K., Liu, Z.: Pacer: a progress management system for live virtual machine migration in cloud computing. IEEE Trans. Netw. Serv. Manage. **10**(4) Dec (2013). ISBN: 1932-4537
11. Caglar, F., Shekhar, S., Gokhale, A.: A performance interference-aware virtual machine placement strategy for supporting soft real-time applications in the cloud, Published in Universidad Carlos III de Madrid (2013), ISBN: 978-84-697-1736-3
12. Li, J., Zhao, J., Li, Y., Cui, L., Li, B., Liu, L., Panneerselvam, J.: iMig: Toward an adaptive live migration method for KVM virtual machines. In: Published in The Computer Journal, bxu065 (2014)
13. Nathuji, R., Kansal, A., Ghaffarkhah, A.: Q-Clouds: managing performance interference effects for QoS-Aware clouds. In: EuroSys '10 Proceedings of the 5th European conference on Computer systems ACM press, pp. 237–250 (2010). ISBN: 978-1-60558-577-2
14. Casale, G., Kraft, S., Krishnamurthy, D.: A model of storage I/O performance interference in virtualized systems. In: 31st International IEEE Conference on Distributed Computing Systems Workshops (IDCSW), 20–24 June (2011). ISSN: 1545-0678
15. Stuart, M., Lu, T., He, X.: Alleviating I/O interference via caching & rate-controlled pre-fetching without degrading migration performance. In: Proceedings of the 9th Parallel Data Storage IEEE Workshop, pp. 19–24 (2014). ISBN: 978-1-4799-7025-4

Cloud Security Issues and Challenges

Dhaivat Dave, Nayana Meruliya, Tirth D. Gajjar, Grishma T. Ghoda, Disha H. Parekh and R. Sridaran

Abstract Cloud computing, is open for all from any location of the globe, to utilize the services and resources as per the demand of an individual. Nowadays, any organization can easily migrate its entire system on cloud as it gives the pay-as-you-go service. Cloud has benefits like multi-tenancy, data storage, resource pooling, and a very obvious virtualization. Though there are advantages, cloud computing also has security flaws like loss of subtle data, data escape, cloning, and other security challenges related to virtualization. Because security challenges of cloud are very high, a large area of study is required to signify risks in services and deployment models of the cloud. This study represents the cloud security problems in numerous cloud-related fields and the threats related to cloud model and cloud network. This paper will also mitigate several issues related to virtualization and will be precisely addressed with side effects.

Keywords Virtualization · Network security · Cloud issues · Resource pooling · Cloning

---

D. Dave (✉) · N. Meruliya · T.D. Gajjar · G.T. Ghoda · D.H. Parekh · R. Sridaran
Faculty of Computer Applications, Marwadi Education Foundation's Group of Institutions, Rajkot, Gujarat, India
e-mail: davedhaivat@gmail.com

N. Meruliya
e-mail: nayanameruliya111@gmail.com

D.H. Parekh
e-mail: disha.hparekh213@gmail.com

R. Sridaran
e-mail: sridaran.rajagopal@gmail.com

D.H. Parekh
Computer Science Department, Bharathiar University, Coimbatore, Tamil Nadu, India

V.B. Aggarwal et al. (eds.), *Big Data Analytics*, Advances in Intelligent Systems and Computing 654, https://doi.org/10.1007/978-981-10-6620-7_48

1 Introduction

Cloud computing, as a technology, today is adopted by every organization. It helps in shifting from the traditional approach to cloud computing and is a good choice as it reduces the costs of the organization. In this paradigm shift, in accordance with Parekh et al. [1] stated customers have no need to capitalize on services related to hardware or software. But one can put it on clouds. Wan et al. [2] have stated cloud computing as a very novel model constructed on technologies like service-oriented architecture, virtualization, utility computing, and distributed computing. While Mell [3] defines cloud computing like a prototypical allowing global, a very suitable and a network access as per demand to a communal group of computing assets which can be provided and freed with negligible attempt or interaction of service giver. As per the term used by the NIST, the features of the cloud computing is a service provided on demand, elastic, and pay as per the practice of business models [3]. As per the policy of the cloud, the customers have to pay on the basis of their services usage.

Cloud computing itself is a very broad concept, and its services are transmitted and hosted on the Internet. These are the services that are categorized in 3 ways usually known as Infrastructure as a Service (IaaS), Platform as a Service (PaaS), and Software as a Service (SaaS). Generally, client uses cloud services as per the need, and fare is charged as per the usage of the services which is generally based on the hour rate. This type of cloud-based services is adopted by the clients rapidly and is flexible for them. The clients just have to use the services and need not manage it as the cloud services are administrated by the services provider itself. This makes cloud and its services rapidly accepted by the clients.

Cloud is divided into 3 parts: public, private, and hybrid. As per the Weis et al. [4], when an intermediate between user and provider provides computing resources as a service generally, a public cloud is involved. An official network providing hosted services only to limited individuals involves private cloud [1]. In this type, users shall rent and use the computing resources. On the other hand, the mixture of more than one cloud that remains as unique but is destined jointly in order to give the advantages of multiple deployment models is usually referred as hybrid cloud.

The literature survey, next part in the paper, is based on issues with cloud security and problems associated with cloud. The third chapter of the paper is about security issues and challenges according to the deployment model, service model, as well as other cloud threats which is not related to any type of model. The fourth part is the conclusion and future work of the cloud security issues and challenges.

2 Related Work

Few related work have been found in the literature survey particularly by Parekh et al. [1] where the former research scholar has not considered the issues concerned with database as a service and also not concerned issued for individual deployment model, but in that paper, the discussed issues were common for all deployment model: public, private, and hybrid. From the literature survey, few points were found specifically by Nagaraju and Sridaran [5] were in that paper there is not considered the virtualization related threats and the other issues not related to the deployment model and service model. Ren et al. [6] analyzed several challenges related to cloud security for only public cloud and not on the risks associated with service forms and other cloud threats. Almost all the current research is based on cloud security but from not very specific view. Tsai et al. [7] witnessed different threats on virtualization involved with IaaS, PaaS, and SaaS, but are not efficiently listing the problems with DaaS (Database as a Service). And because virtualization is indispensable field in cloud, the security threats associated with it should be mentioned. This has become the motivation for the development of the proposed survey as it is believed that the database has also become extremely significant in terms of attracting vulnerable.

3 Cloud Security Issues and Challenges

Nowadays, enormous use of the cloud is in the world. Cloud is more flexible and elastic, and it is used for the various purposes in the organization. With that, cloud is not costly as like other resources, so any organization can hire cloud. The most important thing about cloud is cloud security. If cloud is not secure, then the data stored within it is also not secure. So, here Fig. 1 depicts a schematic figure representing the hierarchy of security flaws with challenges on the present cloud computing models, namely deployment and service models.

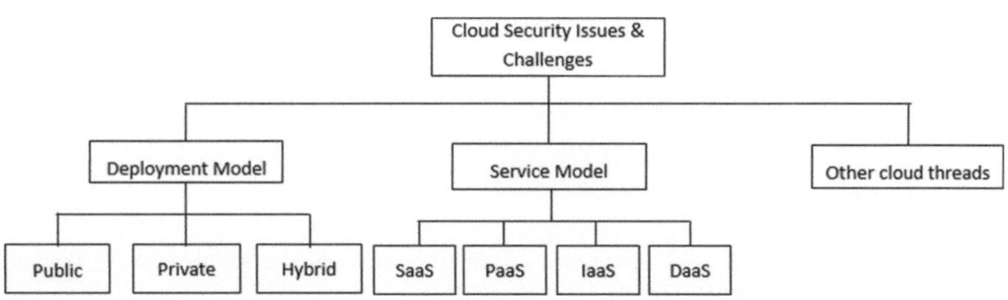

Fig. 1 Categories of cloud security issues—Level 1

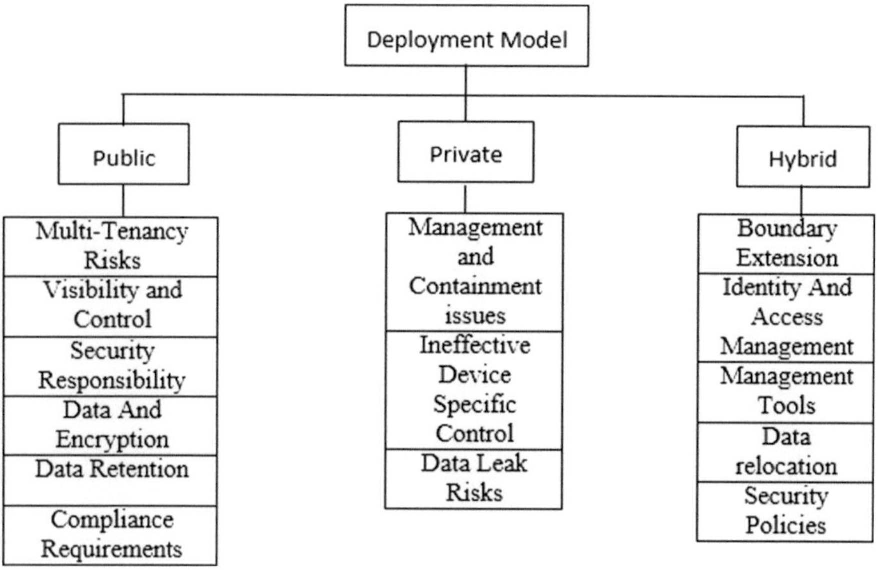

Fig. 2 Threats/issues with public, private, and hybrid clouds

Here is a cloud computing deployment model divided into 3 major clouds: public, private, and hybrid. Each has its separate issues as mentioned in Fig. 2.

Deployment Model Issues and Challenges in Public Cloud Issues
Now, let us look at each in brief to understand issues related to the public cloud.

- Multi-tenancy Risk:

The mutual multi-tenant characteristic of a cloud enhances security problems like illegal access of data by extra residents utilizing the similar infrastructure. AlZain et al. [8] state that multi-tenant nature leaks supply contention problems when any residents use the hardware unequally due to need or any hacks.

- Visibility and Control:

Business nowadays is having imperfect control as the service provider is answerable to the entire management of the infrastructure [7]. This includes security allied with no transparency. Organizations require a dramatic transit as they give the control of IT to an intermediate while utilizing cloud services.

- Security Responsibility:

Sawazaki et al. [9] state that security is collective task of the service provider and the user with changeable types of cloud model.

- Data and Encryption:

If data on cloud is unencrypted [1], it leads to problems of data loss. A possibility for illegal admittance by a reprobate employee on the side of a cloud provider or an intruder is acknowledged at times. This leads to threats of data encryption.

- Data Retention:

Data even after being deleted by the user is retained on cloud during odd times [6]. This leads to access to certain sensitive data on cloud.

- Compliance Requirements:

Countries across globe have regulatory measures on data privacy. As few public cloud service givers offer very less or almost negligible information on location of data, it is essential to consider the regulatory mechanism for the data existence [8].

Private Cloud Issues

Let us now inspect various security issues of private cloud deployment model.

- Management and Suppression Issues:

Resources are kept universally and carried transversely the organizations in private cloud, thus allowing managing security, assessing problems, and putting in place, security errors are diverse and active, partially because of elastic nature. According to Subramanian et al. [10], the fact that numerous departments, clients, and domains lead to data supervision issues is a relevant point.

- Ineffective Device-specific Controls:

Chen [11] states that distinct to conventional IT, relative device controls, like limitations on MAC addresses, will not be effective because virtual machines used are not limited to explicit infrastructure. This truth has almost no control on device.

- Data Leakage:

The cloud environment provides augmented ease of access, particularly to people external the organization when given admission to the computer resources on specific demand. Viega et al. [12] state that not locking the data properly creates a problem important to surplus breaches. Shielding data from leakage becomes dangerous in such a case.

Hybrid Cloud Issues

Described below are the many security issues of hybrid cloud deployment model.

- Boundary Extension:

Hybrid cloud opens up its boundary to a very high range which leads and creates a bigger surface area for hackers to hack with a unit of the infrastructure that is lying with the regulator of the provider [1].

- Identity and Access Management:

In order of solving the problem with identity with hybrid clouds is spreading the organization's identity and entry supervision to the public clouds. Technique involved here gives us the fact of how this advancement will disturb the organization's identity and its force on the enterprise's security.

- Management Tools:

Enterprise achieves multifaceted hybrid cloud utilizing tools of management, may be as a portion of the cloud or as an intermediary tool. According to Wang et al. [13], enterprise should think the security inferences generated by usage of these tools.

- Data Relocation:

With the use of a hybrid cloud environment, the data transfer from a private cloud to a public cloud is carried out at a greater ease [6]. But as a result, the problems with privacy are of a greater concern as the rules of privacy controls are different and variable from private to public cloud environment.

- Security Policies:

Threats related to security policies straddling the hybrid situation like to how encryption keys are attained in a public environment as in relation to the private environment [9].

Service Model Issues and Challenges
The service-oriented architecture promotes "everything as a service," Cloud-computing providers offer "services" according to changed models, which happen to form a stack: software-, infrastructure-, platform- and database-as-a-service. SaaS, IaaS, PaaS, DaaS for this service SaaS, IaaS, PaaS, DaaS for this services security issues and challenges are share in Fig. 3.

Software as a Service (SaaS) Issues
Now, let us discuss the issues of software as a service in brief which as represented in Fig. 3:

- Data Security:

In conventional application, the subtle data in organization endures existence within the organization boundary limits and is focused on its security and admission management policies. Though, in SaaS, the organizational data is saved explicit to the organization boundary. Hence, the SaaS provider has to accept extra security measures to make sure data security. SaaS vendor has to stop break due to security vulnerabilities of applications. It includes the application of robust encryption techniques to switch admission to data. Administrator will form the security and perform the audit operation to safeguard the security of the cloud.

Simple Storage Service (S3) according to Rimal et al. [14] is not in encrypted form by evasion; so, the user has to set up such mechanism to make the data

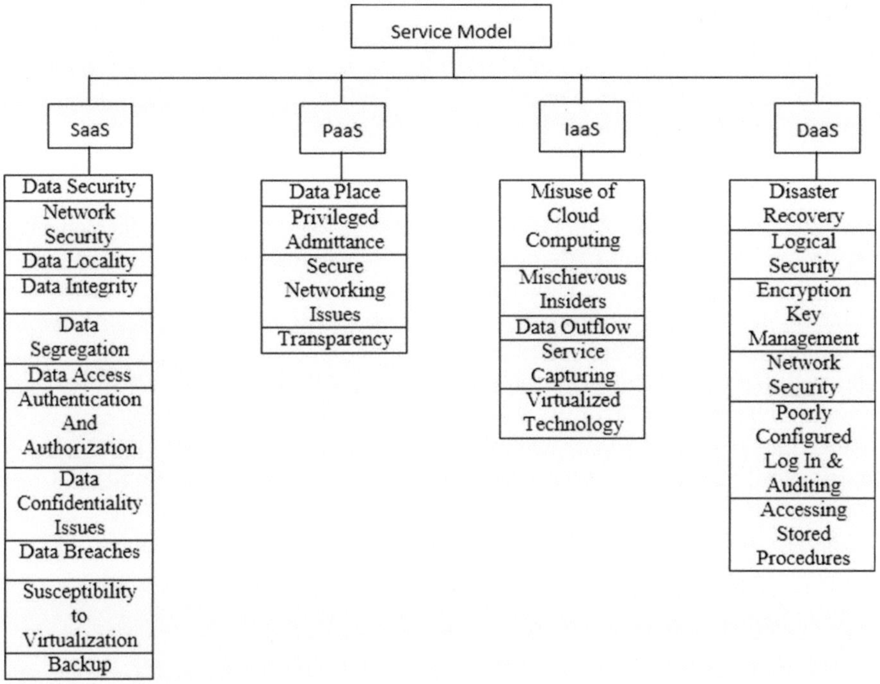

Fig. 3 Issues with SaaS, PaaS, IaaS, and DaaS models of cloud

encrypted. Spiteful user feats weaknesses in security model of data in order to attain illegal entry to achieve data.

- Network Security:

In a SaaS, responsive data is gained from the organization, processed through an application and is saved at the vendor's place. The flow of data on network must be secured to prevent the data leakage of confidential data. This indulges the use of tough network traffic encryption techniques like secure socket layer and the transport layer security.

While considering Amazon Web Services (AWS), Shaikh et al. [15] state that the network provides major protection; as evaluated with conventional network, security risks are far observed In order to enhance the security mechanisms, Amazon S3 is only accessible thru the secure socket layer endpoints. The encrypted endpoints are obtained from both the Internet and Amazon EC2, assuring that information is transmitted securely. However, the intruders can carry out the sniffing and try to obtain the packets which are transmitted over the network and try manipulating the network place.

- Data Locality:

The clients utilize the applications given by the SaaS vendor and route their data. But this leads to problem like a user never knows where the data is located on network, and this creates certain issues and threats at times.

- Data Integrity:

According to Ashktorab et al. [16], data integrity is mainly a very crucial element of the system. Generally, in traditional approach where a single standalone system is there, the data integrity is maintained by use of ACID (Atomicity, Consistency, Isolation, and Durability) properties. In the next phase, if we are talking about the distributed system, multiple databases and multiple applications are there which achieved the data integrity by using central transaction manager. When we enter into the advanced version of the time when cloud came into the picture, most of the applications are multi-tenant and deployed by the intermediates. By the Wayne A. Jansen et al. [17], SaaS uses the XML-based API's with that the application may reside off-premises as compare to the traditional system. One of the very big challenges with Web services is to maintain the transaction management; HTTP is not supporting the secure transaction.

- Data Segregation:

Due to multi-tenancy, a single application can be used by the multiple users at a time, and even they can store their data in the same place. Because of this reason, there are chances that the data of the one user may be merged with the data of the other user [7]. This may happen because of the loop holes of the applications or injecting the data forcefully. In SaaS Web services, when the boundary of the individual user is not defined properly at that time, such kinds of problems arise.

- Data Access:

Data access issues may rely when an individual user is accessing its data. When we consider any small organization which uses the cloud services provided by the third party at that time, the security policies of the cloud and its data access is designed by the provider which may not be suitable to the client. When we consider the case of large organization, it may happen that as per the policy of the organization, only the higher-level person has the access to the certain confidential data, but due to the security policy of the cloud provider, the lower-level employees of the organization can have the access of the same data so at that time it can create an issue for the organization [2].

- Authentication and Authorization:

Nowadays, most of the small-scale industries are chiefly using the cloud and its services [1]. For that these industries are using them for Lightweight Directory Access Protocol types of servers especially for task related to authorization as well as authentication. Many times it may happens that the credentials are stored on the premises of the SaaS provider not on the organization that may lead the organization as due to any of the reason when the cloud is not able to access at that time none of the person is able to maintain its connectivity and authorization to any of the application.

- Data Confidentiality Issues:

Cloud computing indulges services of storage of individual's data on the distant server which may be hosted by any other organization and can be accessed through the network [23]. According to Muthunagai et al. [18], the cloud is adopted by any of the organization, government agency, health care division, educational institutes, etc. When the data is stored in the cloud, the organization or the subscriber of the cloud does not know that where actually a data is stored so this may leads to some confidentiality issues such as:

1. The privacy and confidentiality of the information are varied as per the SLA (Service Level Agreement) established with the cloud provider.
2. Data on cloud can have more than one legal location at a particular instance with contradictory legal consequence.
3. Some of the countries have the law of the country to ask a cloud provider to check the information for crime investigation.

- Data Breaches:

The cloud is adopted by various industrial sectors; all their data lies in the cloud environment; thus, the cloud becomes a elevated price object. Though SaaS providers claim to avail enhanced security to their users data, still few instances are noticed where the access of the stored data is illegally made and thus breaking the security policies. Even this leads to a direct entry to the database of the user [17].

- Susceptibility to Virtualization:

Virtualization is the chief base in the cloud computing, but it encounters many security threats [18]. When the applications are running on the servers, the servers were virtualized to the user, but at the same time, the servers must be isolated with each other too. There are some security issues came in the picture in virtualization software through which the leak can be happened, and the malicious person is able to bypass the certain security restrictions and gains privileges. Microsoft Virtual PC and Virtual Server allow the guest operating system to run its code on the host machine or any other guest operating system [16]. So, a need of some perfection features like inspection, check of data stored, and isolation of data in virtualization is must.

- Backup:

The SaaS provider must acknowledge the backup of sensitive stored data at a periodic interval so that if failure occurs, data can be recovered easily [1]. And, they also need to use strong encryption policy to protect the data from any kind of accidental leakage. The cloud vendor Amazon, the data of S3, is rested in encrypted form by default, so the user needs to encrypt it separately.

Platform as a Service (PaaS) Issues

Now, as per the Fig. 3, let us look at the various issues of the Platform as a Service (PaaS) model.

- Data Place:

PaaS proposes the growth atmosphere not only for software but also for having memory to store result. The rule is to consider not an individual node but a collection of many nodes. According to the Takabi et al. [19], the position of information cannot be distant to a particular segment on a precise host. The deficiency of a solitary place for information appends to the security test, as a sole location informal to secure compared to multiple.

PaaS promises of dropping the price of software improvement by provision of the development apparatus and place, such as software, storage spaces, and the vital work area. The PaaS setting does competence in piece by duplicating information. This creates highly obtainable information for originators as well as buyers. Nonetheless, records are never completely removed; only indicators are removed. The spread information remains. The alteration here is that the precise locality is unfamiliar, generating one more safety issue.

- Privileged Admittance:

A well-admired characteristic in PaaS is "built-in debug" [18]. Creators naturally utilize this to seek troubles in program. This feature allowances contact of information and recall sites, permitting coders to step in their creation and try changes to check several effects. It presents the equal advantage of access making it extremely preferred coders as well as hackers.

The next benefit of using PaaS is freedom from dealing with the harmonizing safety and rights. Frequently, coders request working in the unrestricted atmosphere by requesting complete right to use data. By the PaaS background, an association shifts the sensitive crisis to the provider to solve. Clearly, it is not the best decision for the problem, but it is to be shouldered by provider rather than users.

- Secure Networking Issues:

Due to the insecure usage of networking-related stuffs, such as not properly configured routers, insecure API's, etc., there are chances of data loss as well as data breaching as the connection between the client and the cloud is not as per the international standard and terms. There are also chances of hijacking the service as well as the data, or the malicious user can gain the access to the confidential part of the system or the confidential data [1].

- Transparency:

In the transparency issue, it is always difficult to maintain the transparency in the PaaS. With that, it is always difficult to make an individual's count as per the requirement of client [17]. To make the record of each and every client separately is difficult so in PaaS; the transparency issue required more focus to make it simple and clear in terms of usage and separation.

Infrastructure as a Service (IaaS) Issues

Let us have look at the various security issues of Infrastructure as a Service (IaaS) model as mentioned in Fig. 3.

- Misuse of Cloud Computing:

Cloud suppliers simplify the customers with abundant variants of facilities containing limitless bandwidth and capacity [1]. Some recommend partial trial giving a chance to hackers allowing them to enter the system dishonestly; they can crack passwords, launch potential assault points, and perform bad instructions. Cybercriminals carry out their actions with such authorization, as service providers are besieged for the frail action scheme and limited scam discovery abilities. They utilize affluent contented tools like flashy codes enabling them to conceal their mischievous program exploiting users' to and by installing malware.

- Mischievous Insider:

This can be done by spiteful workers in the organization of either user or provider. They pinch the private information of consumers. This can breakdown the faith of on supplier. The person can effortlessly get all security information. The molestation involves numerous types of cons, destruction or stealing of records, and exploitation of other technical assets. The risks of intruders have augmented because of lack of clearness in cloud supplier's ways and methods. It states that supplier does not disclose how workers are allowed to admittance and how this entrée is judged or how information and policy agreements are studied [12]. In addition, clients have modest visibility for renting services of their supplier that opens up opposite parties, intruders, or trespassers to pilfer trusted facts of the cloud. The height of admittance granted could permit intruders to collect confidential data or to increase entire control to cloud offerings with negligible threat of uncovering.

- Data Outflow:

Loss of data can occur because of the operative breakdowns, undependable storage, and random generation of encrypted keys. Working breakdown means loss or modification of data that does not have any original content to take place deliberately. Untrustworthy storage of data means to save data on independent media which shall lead to no recovery of data if lost [3]. The unpredictable exercise of encryption keys will turn into great loss and limited accesses of data by unauthenticated clients which leads to abolishment of the sensitive data. The available sensitive documents of Twitter were retrieved by hackers and were whipped which were saved actually on Google's online Web office. Google was not considered the responsible for security breaches as the security on the documents stored by Twitter was also not well mannered while the complete data was just a password crack. This makes a sense that data loss can affect a brand, status and cause a defeat that may intentionally shock employee, cohort, and users' confidence and belief.

- Service Capturing:

Service capturing means illegal access of the users' accounts, such as phishing, deception, and utilization of software weaknesses. For instance, an intruder accesses client's authorizations and can keep a check on the transactions carried out by the users. The account of the user is now a platform for the intruders to leverage cloud-based services from the providers, and this leads to several attacks on the cloud service provider's assets. With the illegally gained credentials, intruders often use critical areas of cloud services, availing them to negotiate the confidentiality, integrity, and availability of the services [13]. Confirmation and endorsement through the utilization of roles and password shielding is an ordinary way to carry on contact control when by means of browsers to admittance cloud systems. Though this system is not enough to defend susceptible and critical data.

- Virtualized Technology:

Cloud providers stay on the clientele applications as they use virtual machines in a common structure via virtualization technology. These virtual machines are intended on the physical infrastructure of cloud providers. For enhancing the data security on the virtual machines, providers separate machines so that if any is found malicious or affected, then it will not harm a clear machine. The VMs are organized by a hypervisor for providing virtual memory and the CPU scheduling policies. Because hypervisors are the chief part for organizing cloud policies in virtualization, intruders try to gain control on the hypervisors which reside in between the infrastructure and virtual machine [2]. This attack on hypervisor can injure the VMs and infrastructure. Strong separation must be made effective in order to assure the access of VMs by the authenticated users only and no intruders. Numerous cloud providers, according to Sabahi et al. [20], like Xen and KVM, are providing extensive and highly secured VMs to ensure the total security of the machines, but still certain issues with VMs are compromised.

Database as a Service (DaaS) Issues

Now, the brief look at the issues of Database as a Service (DaaS) as described in Fig. 3.

- Disaster Recovery:

If any kind of data loss is accrued due to any reason, then it is difficult to recover all the data on cloud as some of the data will be lost definitely. To recover that small amount of data; as it's too important to recover it as per the organization's point of view the data is always important [18]. Cloud has no such specific mechanism or the tool through which the recovery of the data can be possible.

- Logical Security:

In the cloud computing, virtualization is one of the key elements, but with the same time, it increases the risk as there are multiple instances, or the application is running on the various but similar kind of machines which are completely isolated from each other [4]. Virtual Machines are organized by the hypervisor to avail and give virtual memory to the virtualized cloud-based platform, the intruders and attackers who always targets to the hypervisor so from that they can easily get the access of virtual machine and physical hardware [14].

- Encryption Key Management:

Only 40% of the cloud service providers have the HTTPS connection to access their clouds. When the HTTP connection is used, the algorithm of encryption which is being used is not that much secure or encrypt a very small bit of encryption which may cause the problem [4]. This may lead the cloud consumer to the risk of being attacked or targeted by the attack of Brute Force, Dictionary Attack, or Rainbow table.

- Network Security:

To interact with cloud, it mainly depends on Internet and server which maintain data for various applications. Security issues are more concerned with networking when we are talking about cloud. Security issues like data deletion, XML signature wrapping, cloud malware injection attack etc.

- Poorly Configured Logging/Auditing:

35% of the databases were not correctly configured for logging or auditing. This is a feature that all databases have in order to track and audit events such as data modifications and access. Not tracking events such as account creation and access or modification to sensitive data on a production system can make it more difficult to discover what has happened if a breach occurs. While this issue is generally considered low-risk, it is still important to include auditing when building a database [17]. This issue also featured in the Top 10 Windows Server Security Misconfigurations, coming in at number two.

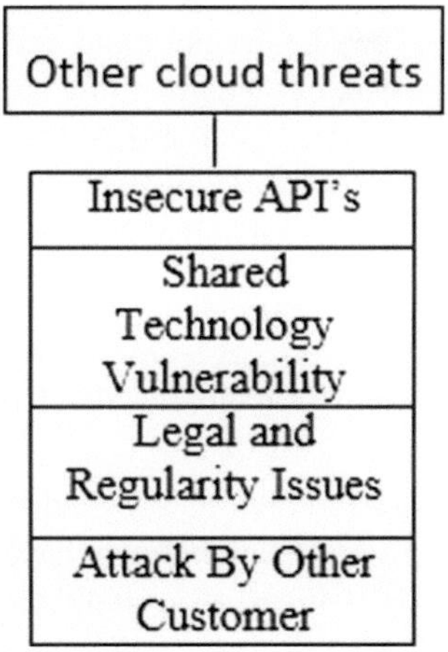

Fig. 4 Other cloud security threats

- Excessive Stored Procedures:

25% of databases were found to have an excessive number of potentially dangerous stored procedures, including those that can run system commands or access files on the underlying operating system [1]. This issue is considered to present a risk to the security posture of a database as stored procedures effectively increase the functionality available which could be leveraged to launch attacks against the underlying operating system of the host and even against other hosts on the network.

Other Cloud Threats
Here, below discussion is about the other cloud threats which are not considered in the deployment model issues and service model issues. So let us look ahead (Fig. 4).

- Insecure API's:

The software which is used by the customer to interact with the cloud service must be very much securely authenticate, controlled with access, encryption with proper and authenticate algorithm, and activity monitoring mechanism especially when it is on the hand of third party [1].

- Shared Technology Vulnerability:

Sharing of the resources is the way of working of IaaS. According to Joshi et al. [21], the components are not based on which the infrastructure is designed; so there must be strong monitoring, and compartmentalization is required.

- Legal and Regularity Issues:

If any organization is going to make its own private cloud, then it must be stand to international standard and norms defined by the international organizations [3].

- Attacks by Other Customer:

As per the current trend, the technology now believes to make such things as open source, but with that, the issues are also arising as the logic of any complex system lies on web, and any of the destructive person can make the reverse mechanism to perform the data leakage or hacking-related activity through an individual's cloud or on individuals cloud [9].

4 Conclusion and Future Work

Cloud computing provides its services to almost all the people nowadays which will help every individual to have their data stored on cloud. Cloud provides a very good facility for storing ample data of the users and also provides with set of extensive services. But users are nowadays highly conscious about security measures and the authorization checks of these stored data on cloud. Users are ready to migrate their data to cloud but only if cloud service providers would ensure a better security and manageability facilities to the data they upload on cloud. This fact is spreading a thrill among various users who are ready to migrate on cloud. This study is focused basically on revealing such cloud security threats prevailing across cloud architecture. There is a very extensive work carried out depending on service, deployment, and other cloud threats associated with network or storage mechanism. The survey will be very helpful to the researchers who are willing to study cloud security threats. The work done in the paper will be enhanced for the structured advancement to find the solutions of the issues lying with the cloud, and we will try to propose a model that ensures a better cloud security.

References

1. Parekh, D., Sridaran, R.: Survey on challenges related to cloud security. IJACSA (2013)
2. Wan, Z., Liu, J., Deng, R.H.: HASBE: a hierarchical attribute based solution for flexible and scalable access control in cloud computing. IEEE Trans. Inf. Forensics Secur. **7** (2012)
3. Mell, P., Grance, T.: The NIST Definition of Cloud Computing, Special Publication 800-145. U.S. National Institute of Standards and Technology (NIST) (2011)
4. Weis, J., Alves-Foss, J.: Securing database as a service, issues and challenges. In: IEEE, pp. 49–55 (2011)
5. Nagaraju, K., Sridaran R.: A survey on security threats for cloud computing. IJERT **1** (2012)
6. Ren, K., Wang, C., Wang, Q.: Security Challenges for the Public Cloud, pp. 69–73. IEEE Press, Illinois Institute of Technology (2012)
7. Tsai, H.-Y., Siebenhaar M., Miede, A., Huang, Y.-L., Steinmetz, R.: Threat as a service? Virtualization's impact on cloud security. IEEE IT Prof. 32–37 (2012)
8. AlZain, M.A., Pardede, E., Soh, B., Thom, J.A.: Cloud computing security: from single to multi-clouds. In: IEEE, pp. 5490–5499 (2012)
9. Sawazaki, J., Maeda, T., Yonezawa, A.: Implementing a hybrid VM monitor for flexible and efficient security mechanisms. In: IEEE, pp. 37–45 (2010)
10. Subramanian, K.: Private, Public and Hybrid Clouds Whitepaper. Trend Micro (2011)
11. Chen, J., Wang, Y., Wang, X.: On demand security architecture for cloud computing. In: IEEE,
DOI 10.1109/MC.2012.120, pp. 1–12; 0018-9162
12. Viega, J.: Cloud computing and the common man. In: IEEE, pp. 106–108; 0018-9162/09
13. Wang, Z., Jiang, X.: Hyper safe: a lightweight approach to provide lifetime hypervisor control flow. In: IEEE, pp. 380–393 (2010)
14. Rimal, B.P., Choi, E., Lumb, I.: A taxonomy and survey of cloud computing systems. In: IEEE, pp. 44–51; 978-0-7695-3769-6/09
15. Shaikh, F.B., Haider, S.: Security in cloud computing. In: IEEE, pp. 214–219 (2010)
16. Ashktorab, V., Taghizadeh, S.R.: Security threats and countermeasures in cloud computing. Islamic Azad University of NajafAbaad, Isfahan, vol. 1, Issue 2, October 2012; ISSN 2319-4847
17. Jansen, W.A.: Cloud hooks: security and privacy issues in cloud computing. NIST, IEEE 1–8 (2011)
18. Muthunagai, S.U., Karthic C.D., Sujatha, S.: Efficient access of cloud resources through virtualization techniques. In: IEEE, pp. 174–178 (2012)
19. Takabi, H., Joshi, J.B.D.: Security and Privacy Challenges in Cloud Computing Environments. University of Pittsburgh, Gail-Joon and Ahn Arizona State University, IEEE Security and Privacy, www.computer.org/security (2010)

20. Sabahi, F., Sabahi, F.: Virtualization-Level Security in Cloud Computing, pp. 250–254. IEEE, Iran (2011)
21. Joshi, B., Vijayan, A.S., Joshi, B.K.: Securing cloud computing environment against DDoS attacks. In: IEEE, pp. 1–5 (2011)

Author Biographies

Mr. Dhaivat Dave is a student of Marwadi College, studying in MCA, Semester 5. He has completed his BCA from Vivekananda College (Bhavnagar University). He has done a certified course of Cyber Security Expert v2.0 from TechDefence, Ahmadabad. His area of interest falls under the field of security-related issues on network and cloud-based systems.

Ms. Nayana Meruliya is a student of Marwadi College, studying in MCA, Semester 5. She has completed her BCA from K. P. Dholakiya InfoTech Mahila College (Saurashtra University). Her area of interest falls under the field of security-related issues on network and cloud-based systems.

Mr. Tirth D. Gajjar is a student of Marwadi College, studying in MCA, Semester 5. He has completed his BCA from Vivekanand College (Saurashtra University). His area of interest falls under the field of Data Center and Network Virtualization and Cyber Security on Cloud Computing

Ms. Grishma T. Ghoda is a student of Marwadi College, studying in MCA, Semester 5. She has completed his BCA from Yadav College (Saurashtra University). Her area of interest falls under the field of Data Center and Network Virtualization.

Ms. Disha H. Parekh MCA, PGDBA (Human Resource), is presently an Assistant Professor of Faculty of Computer Applications at Marwadi Education Foundation's Group of Institutions, Rajkot, Gujarat. She has done MCA from Ganpat University, Gujarat. She has completed PGDBA with specialization in HR from Symbiosis University. She has published 3 papers in the international journal and has presented 1 paper at national conference. She has attended many workshops and seminars. Her areas of interest are Software Engineering and Web Technologies. She is currently pursuing Ph.D in Bharathiyar University.

Dr. R. Sridaran is currently the Dean, Faculty of Computer Applications, Marwadi Education Foundation's Group of Institutions, Rajkot, Gujarat. He did his postgraduation in Computer Applications and Management. He is awarded the Ph.D in Computer Applications in 2010. Having started his career as an entrepreneur, he has offered his consultancy services to various service sectors. He designed and delivered various training programs in the areas of IT and Management. He holds publication of 15 research papers in foremost journals and conferences and is currently guiding five research scholars. He has got 22 years of academic experience and has served in principal educational institutions at diverse capacities.

A Novel Approach to Protect Cloud Environments Against DDOS Attacks

Nagaraju Kilari and R. Sridaran

Abstract Virtualization, which is reflected as the backbone of cloud computing, provides cost-effective resource sharing. Owed to the existence of multiple virtual machines, it passages several challenges. Among the numerous virtualization attacks, the Distributed Denial of Service, widely known as the DDoS attack, is considered to be the momentous. These spells consumes large amount of server resources here after denies access to genuine users. DDoS attacks impact is more in cloud computing as sharing of resources is the innate character of a cloud. At hand are a few kinds of literature dealing with the mitigation of DDoS attacks using single server tactic nonetheless they suffer from poor response time. The proposed model in this paper uses multiple servers to deal with the alleviation of DDoS. An initial test result on the proposed model has provided us with better scalability and protection against further attacks.

Keywords Virtualization · DDoS attacks · Mitigation · Virtual machine and cloud security

1 Introduction

Virtualization knowledge accelerates proficient resource usage at economical costs. Moreover, it guarantees reliability and availability in terms of services. This technology mainly uses virtual machine monitor (VMM), also known as a hypervisor [10]. It works between the hardware and the operating system to run multiple virtual

N. Kilari (✉)
Department of Computer Science—BCA, New Horizon College,
Bangalore, Karnataka, India
e-mail: raju_kilari@yahoo.com

R. Sridaran
Faculty of Computer Applications, Marwadi Education
Foundation's Group of Institutions, Rajkot, Gujarat, India
e-mail: sridaran.rajagopal@gmail.com; sridaran.rajagopal@marwadieducation.edu.in

V.B. Aggarwal et al. (eds.), *Big Data Analytics*, Advances in Intelligent
Systems and Computing 654, https://doi.org/10.1007/978-981-10-6620-7_49

machines (VM) on top of a single physical machine. The top most job of a VMM is to allocate and manage the physical resources among the VMs [4]. Virtualization can also be cast off as a security component as it needs to handle newly occurring problems with safe keeping [5]. Benefits of virtualization are several alongside arises many challenges, especially in the cloud environment. Utmost common security threats associated with virtualized environment in cloud computing is bought out below.

1.1 Overview of Virtualization Threats

Virtualized environments may allow a VM to host an attack which is known as **VM escape**. The attacker can negotiate the hypervisor by running a malicious code which can completely bypass the VMM layer and gets control over the host machine [9]. Likewise, it can access the possessions which are shared by several other VMs. Cloud providers create and configure numerous VMs to extend their facilities and meet certain standards such as SLA (service level agreement) and QoS (quality of service). While creating, VM manager should analyze the need or it may lead to **VM sprawl** attack which can lead to wastage of resources in the cloud environment [4].

An important feature of virtualization is multi-tenancy which allows sharing of physical resources and applications among cloud customers. Coexisting of other VMs on the same physical machine can cause hindrance. If one of the VMs is conceded by an attacker, it can affect other VM's too. This kind of an attack is known as **Client to Client attacks** aka **VM-To-VM attacks** [1].

VM hopping could arise, when an attacker works on one VM to advance control above the other VM [1]. The **Dos (Denial of Service)** attack occurs in VM architecture, while one VM conquers all the physical resources such that the hypervisor cannot offer its services to other VMs. DoS attack leads to unavailability of computer resources to genuine users, by flooding the victim with unwanted traffic. Large amount of resources, such as processing time, bandwidth, are squandered due to this attack. The **DDoS (Distributed Denial of Service)** attack is similar to DoS attack but the impact of this attack is more destructive than the latter. It involves many compromised and distributed systems usually known as botnets. The main objective of the DDoS attack is averting the genuine user to access the resource [5].

2 Related Work

Efforts to mitigate DDoS attacks in cloud environments found in the literature are consolidated here.

Qi et al. [7] approach is based on the correlation patterns and CBF (Confidence-Based Filtering) scores for each incoming packet. The confidence value is calculated to appraise the nominal profile during the non-attack period. During an attack, the CBF uses the nominal profiles confidence value to distinguish the actual user against an attacker. Though this method is fast to detect DDoS attacks, it is not foolproof.

Myung Keun et al. [6] have implemented a VIP list known as a white list for genuine consumers. But a single point of failures can lead to server congestion when multiple requests arise simultaneously from the attacks. The motivation for the development of the proposed N-S model is to eliminate the pitfalls of these models.

3 Objectives of Proposed N-S Model

N-S model's first objective is to mitigate the DDoS attack in the cloud environs and to ensure QoS and SLA in a cloud setting. Virtual Web servers to increase cloud scalability by implementing load balancing is the second impartial. The detached is to protect the actual servers from external world with the aid of HAProxy (High Availability Proxy) that acts as an interface between the users and the actual Web servers.

The various terms associated with the proposed work are listed below:

3.1 Terms Used

(a) **Bloom filter**: This is to check the existence of an object in a data set, by considering only the few bits of an array [15]. With this, the probability of picking false positives is possible but no false negatives [3].

(b) **Bit array**: The operations of Bloom filter such as object membership are implemented using bit arrays [18]. It is an array of bit values which are denoted as 0's or 1's (Booleans). When the object is obtainable in a data set, it returns True (1), else returns False (0).

(c) **HAProxy**: HAProxy is a free and open-source Linux application useful for load balancing by distributing the incoming network traffic across multiple servers [16].

(d) **MonitoriX**: A freeware network monitoring tool collects data from the servers and generates graphs [17]. It divulges spikes in a graph when the system is under DDoS attack, the response status of HAProxy and other virtual servers are cast off in our experiment.

(e) **Threshold**: It delineates a control limit to specify the maximum number of connections that can be made to a server. If this exceeds, an appropriate action has to be taken for the smooth functioning of a server.
(f) **VIP list**: List of genuine users who are allowed to access the cloud services when the system is under attack. This list is generated based on successful logins of the client IPs.
(g) **Netstat**: Network statistics tool ascertains the network-related information such as details of connections, routing tables, and so on [19]. It can produce various network statistics by altering its routes.

The N-S Model's architecture and its associated algorithm are explained in the following section.

3.2 *The Proposed N-S Architecture*

DDoS attacks are often created by a group of widely distributed and compromised systems (Botnet) to disrupt the services of cloud, by consuming a lot of network and system resources such as bandwidth, processing time. The N-S architecture for shielding the cloud environment against DDoS attack is presented in Fig. 1.

At this point, various client machines would try to access the HAProxy server through the Internet (Step 1). When the HAProxy accepts the incoming requests, it increases the total number of connections by 1 and checks whether the connections exceed the threshold. If not, the VIP generator prepares the list of VIP users based on the IP addresses currently logged in (Step 2). This list would be valuable when the system is under an attack. The VIP filter module is activated only when the system is under an attack (Step 3).Through this attack period, the proposed N-S architecture filters the incoming packets based on the VIP list primed earlier (Step 4). In order to improve the scalability and to maintain the load balance, the

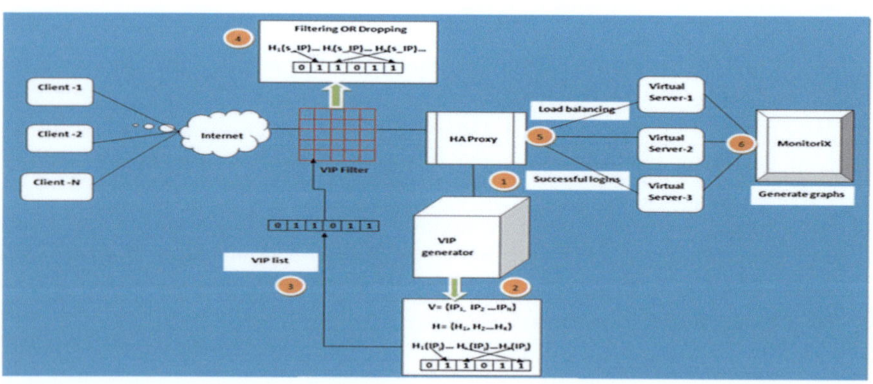

Fig. 1 Proposed N-S architecture of DDoS attack mitigation

incoming network traffic is distributed among the various virtual Web servers in a round-robin fashion, and graphs are generated accordingly (Step 5 & 6). Thus, the major task here is to build the VIP list and carry out filtering the packets whose details are accessible in the next section.

3.2.1 The N-S Algorithm

DDoS threat largely affects the availability of the services in cloud environment [8]. To mitigate this, the N-S algorithm is incorporated into the model (Fig. 2).

This N-S algorithm has been applied in HAProxy. When a user attempts to connect to the server, the statistics of the incoming traffic requests are composed. The requests are populated into the VIP list as given below:

```
1. Bit_array.setall (0).
2. No.of_Connections_Count=0.
3. Out=Popen (netstat –atn | grep: port no|…)
4. IP=split (out.[field number])
5. Count=count+1;
6. If(No.of_Connections_Count<threshold)
     a. If it's true, then hash the connected IPs using and change bit values:
        i.    Sha224 method.
              i=hash_sha224 (IP)
        ii.   MD5 method.
              j=hash_MD5 (IP)
     b. Bit_array[i] =1 and Bir_array[j] =1
Else
          If (No.of_Connections_Count> threshold):
   a. hash the connected IPs using and check in VIP list:
        i.    Sha224 method.
              i=hash_sha224 (IP)
        ii.   MD5 method.
              j=hash_MD5 (IP)
          if (Bit_array[i]==1 and Bit_array[j]==1)
          {
              Allow the user to access the server (Assumed that IP is in VIP list).
          }
          Else
          {
              Block the IP using IP table.
              Popen (iptable –s IP drop)
          }
```

Fig. 2 N-S algorithm

a. If the total numbers of connections are within the threshold, the N-S algorithm will permit the client machines to access the HAProxy. Concurrently, it crafts the VIP list centered on positive IP logins. The login IPs are encoded using two hashing algorithms namely SHA224 [12, 14] and MD5 [12, 14]. Based on the resultant values of two hashing algorithms, the Bloom filter modifies the bit values to ON state (a binary1) from the OFF state (a binary 0) of the bit array.
b. If the total number of network connections exceeds the threshold limit (assuming as DDoS attack), the N-S algorithm checks for the availability of IP in the VIP list. The IP is decoded using the same algorithms (SHA 224 and MD5), which were used while encoding. The decoded values are compared against the bit array values. If the values of the bit array and the decoded are ON state (a binary 1), then the client IP is reflected to be in the VIP list. This IP is allowed access; else considered to have initiated by an attacker. Consequently, if the connected IP does not exist in the VIP list, the client machine is impassable [2,13].

Thus, the first objective has been tackled.

3.3 Load Balancing and Protection of Web Servers—HAProxy

To avoid a single point of failure and maximize the network throughput, the incoming network traffic is distributed among the available servers to cut the load imbalance [11]. HAProxy configuration file (.cfg) comes to rescue. This is achieved by modifying the four back end servers connected to the main server to redirect or distribute the incoming network traffic. This is carried out in round-robin fashion. The third objective of N-S architecture is protecting the actual Web servers from the external world.

4 Performance Analysis

The performances of the N-S architecture and its associated algorithm have been tested in VMW are® work station environment. This environment is a hypervisor that allows creation and running of several VMs on a single physical system. To facilitate this, the HULK.PY simulator was installed in three client machines for the simulation of the DDoS attacks.

The DDoS mitigation using the proposed N-S model involving multiple servers has been compared with an existing approach that involves only a single server. The comparison is presented in three different scenarios namely (A) During the non-attack period, (B) During the attack period, and (C) Period after blocking the attack.

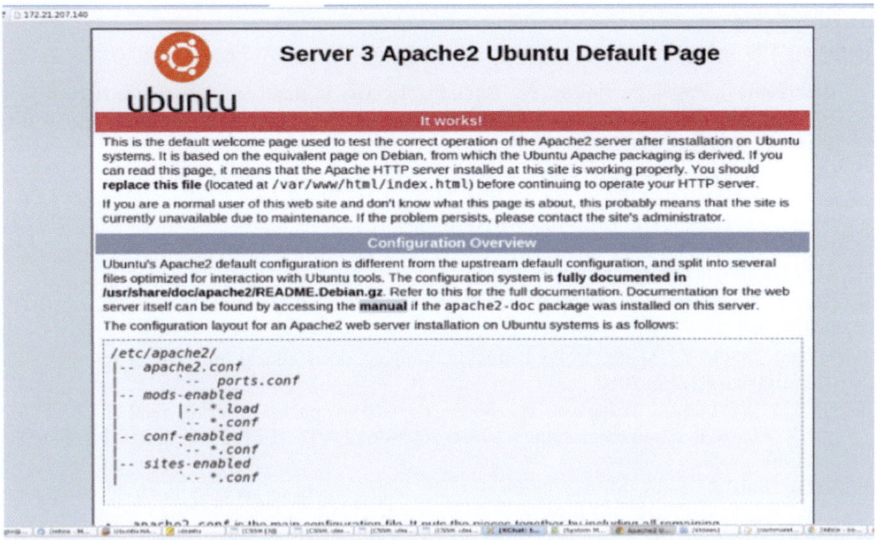

Fig. 3 Client is able to access the server successfully

Here is an implementation of case (A) as follows.

Case A) Non-attack period:
A default Web page has been created in the Apache Web server to demonstrate. As soon as the client issues a request to the server, it responds immediately with the default Web page as shown in Fig. 3. It indicates that the server is not under any attack.

To calculate the response time of a server (HAProxy), **curl** command has been used, and the resultant values are presented later.

5 Conclusion

The N-S model proposed in this paper is found to have many advantages including mitigation of DDoS attack, load balancing, and protection of the server from the attackers. From the three scenarios namely before, during, and after the attacks, the proposed model is found to be consistent. Moreover, the model is proven to be robust and reliable since it provides the services from several Web servers instead of a single server.

References

1. Amarnath, J., Payal, S., Rajeev, N., Ravi, P.: Security in multi-tenancy cloud. 2010 IEEE
2. Bahaa Qasim, M., AL-Musawi.: Mitigating DoS/DDoS attacks using IPtables. Int. J. Eng. Technol. IJET-IJENS **12**(03)
3. Chi, J.: Application and research on weighted bloom filter and bloom filter in web cache. In: Second Pacific-Asia Conference on Web Mining and Web-based Application (WMWA'09), pp. 187–191 (2009). doi:10.1109/WMWA.2009.51
4. Fu, W., Li, X.: The study on data security in cloud computing based on virtualization, 978-1-61284-704-7/11/ IEEE 2011
5. Hsin-Yi, T., Melanie, S., Andre,M., Yu-Lun , H., Ralf, S.: Threat as a service, 1520-9202/12/ IEEE 2012
6. Myung Keun, Y.: Using white listing to mitigate ddos attacks on critical internet sites, 0163-6804/10/ IEEE 2010
7. Qi, C., Wenmin,L., Wanchun, D., Shui, Y.: CBF:A packet filtering method for DDoS attack defense in cloud environment. 978-0-7695-4612-4/11, IEEE 2011, doi:10.1109/DASC.2011.86
8. Ramgovind, S., Eloff, M. M., Smith, E.: The management of security in cloud computing, 978-1-4244-5495-2/10, IEEE 2010
9. Sarfraz Nawaz ,B., Mervat Adib, B., Muhammad Nawaz, B., Rukshanda, K.: Identifying and analyzing security threats to virtualized cloud computing infrastructures, 978-1-4673-4416-6/12/ IEEE 2012
10. Shengmei, L., Zhaoji, L., Xiaohua, C., Zhuolin, Y., Jianyong, C.: Virtualization security for cloud computing service, 978-1-4577-1637-9/11/ IEEE 2011
11. Vinh, P., Erlend, L., Oivind, K., Engelstad, P. E.: Gateway load balancing in future tactical networks. IEEE 1844–1850 (2010)
12. Yang, J., Ding, J., Li, N., Guo, Y.: FPGA implementation of SHA-224/256 algorithm oriented digital signature. In International Conference on Challenges in Environmental Science and Computer Engineering, 978-0-7695-3972-0/10, 2010 IEEE, doi: 10.1109/CESCE.2010.124
13. Most Frequently Used Linux IPTables Rules Examples.htm
14. http://bandwidthco.com/whitepapers/netforensics/crafting/Getting
15. http://www.cs.utexas.edu/users/lam/386p/slides/Bloom%20Filters.pdf
16. http://www.haproxy.org/
17. http://www.monitorix.org/
18. maxburstein.com/blog/creating-a-simple-bloom-filter/
19. www.binarytides.com/linux-netstat-command-examples/

Author Biographies

Mr. Nagaraju Kilari , M.Sc. (Information System) and M.Phil. and is presently working as a senior assistant professor, Department of Computer Science, New Horizon College, Bangalore. He has done M.Sc. Information System from Andhra University and M.Phil Computer Science from Global University, Nagaland. He has participated and presented various papers in national conferences. His areas of interest are object-oriented languages and Web technologies.

Prof. R. Sridaran has done his post-graduation in computer applications, management and a doctoral degree in computer science. As an entrepreneur, he has offered his consultancy services to various service sectors. He is having 18 years of academic experience and currently associated with Marwadi Education Foundation's Group of Institutions, Rajkot, Gujarat, as Dean. His research interests include design pattern, cloud computing, HCI & business intelligence.

An Approach for Workflow Scheduling in Cloud Using ACO

V Vinothina and R Sridaran

Abstract Clouds have emerged as a new model for service provisioning in heterogeneous distributed systems. In this model, users can achieve their Quality of Service from service providers through service level agreements. In addition to that, cloud resources are heterogeneous in nature. Workflow is made up of heterogeneous tasks in terms of their length, runtime, input, and output data. Hence, cloud is the best computing environment for scientific workflow. Workflow scheduling problem by considering the parameters of makespan, cost, and resource utilization is one of the interesting problems in cloud. In this paper, we propose steps to map workflow tasks to cloud resources using ACO (Ant Colony Optimization) that attempts to minimize the makespan, resource cost and maximize the resource utilization.

Keywords Task scheduling · Cloud computing · Ant colony optimization

1 Introduction

Workflow applications are common in science and engineering and their structure/composition is known in advance [1]. Workflow may be a service, application, or a module. The resource requirement of each task in the workflow depends on its functional capacity and data input. Cloud provides virtual servers to reduce the users' cost in purchasing, operating and maintaining a physical computing infrastructure [2]. Moreover, virtualization technology enables the use of

V. Vinothina (✉)
Bharathiar University, Coimbatore, India
e-mail: rvvino@yahoo.com

R. Sridaran
Faculty of Computer Applications, Marwadi Education Foundation's
Group of Institutions, Rajkot, Gujarat, India
e-mail: Sridaran.rajagopal@gmail.com

V.B. Aggarwal et al. (eds.), *Big Data Analytics*, Advances in Intelligent
Systems and Computing 654, https://doi.org/10.1007/978-981-10-6620-7_50

multiple virtual machines on one physical machine. This results in more optimization of sharing and better utilization of physical resources [3].

The deployment models such as Infrastructure as a Service (IaaS), Platform as a Service (PaaS), and Software as a Service (SaaS) permit the users to deploy their own applications in the cloud using the policy of pay-per-use. Since cost involved in cloud usage, users have to utilize the cloud efficiently. Workflow scheduling is the problem of scheduling tasks in workflow and mapping each task to suitable resources based on some performance impact factors [4]. The factors such as makespan, resource cost, and resource utilization mainly depend upon the algorithm and practices used for scheduling and allocation of resources to the tasks.

This paper suggests certain basic steps for computing scientific workflow using Ant Colony Optimization (ACO) in cloud. Ant Colony Optimization (ACO) algorithms are probabilistic models inspired by the social behavior of ants. Initially, ACO has been applied for traveling salesman problem. Since then, it has been successfully applied to NP-hard combinatorial problem [5]. This paper is organized as follows: A few similar works have been discussed in Sect. 2. The proposed scheduling system has been explained under Session 3. The steps for scheduling workflow have been furnished in Sect. 4.

2 Related Work

Many researches on task scheduling in various environments such as single processor system, multiprocessor homogeneous system, multiprocessor heterogeneous system, homogeneous distributed system, and heterogeneous distributed system are found in the literature. In this section, some related works which have been carried out for task scheduling are discussed in short.

The PBTS (Partitioned Balanced Time Scheduling) algorithm proposed by Byun et al. [6] schedules the tasks based on the performance criteria of cost and execution budgets. The proposed algorithms, however, focus on parallelizable workflow tasks with precedence constraint, for which much fine-grained time information is needed. The algorithms based on critical path method have been proposed in grid system for scheduling scientific workflow applications [7, 8] without considering the resource utilization and cost. Achar et al. [1] proposed an optimal scheduling algorithm for computational task which used the tree-based data structure of virtual machine tree (VMT). The simulated results provide better results than traditional algorithm.

Yuan et al. [9] have proposed the DET algorithm which uses dynamic programming approach and an iterative procedure to distribute deadline for critical tasks and non-critical tasks, respectively. Then, a local optimization procedure is used to minimize the execution cost. The study made by Wen et al. [10] on resource scheduling first found out the several groups of solutions using ACO algorithm according to the updated pheromone and then got more effective solution using

PSO algorithm to do crossover operation and mutation which improved the resource utilization ratio.

Zhou et al. [11] addressed resource-constrained project scheduling problem using ACO but the algorithm lacks in making comprehensive use of several priority rules. Hybrid algorithm using ACO and Cuckoo search for job scheduling has been proposed by Babukartik et al. [12] minimizes the makespan but does not discuss about resource cost and resource utilization. PACO (Period ACO)-based scheduling algorithm in cloud computing is proposed by Weifeng Sun et.al [13] that has a good performance in makespan and load balance of whole cloud cluster, but this is designed for independent task scheduling. In this paper, makespan has been considered as heuristics data for the proposed approach. The same approach can be applied for independent task scheduling since tasks in each level are independent.

3 Scheduling System Model

The workflow is modeled by directed acyclic graph G (T, E) where T is a set of n tasks $(t_1, t_2,\ldots,t_n)$ and E is a set of directed edges $(e_1, e_2, e_3,\ldots,e_n)$. Edge from e_i to e_j represents a precedence constraint that indicates that task$_i$ should complete execution before task$_j$ can start. Figure 1 depicts the basic structure of workflow.

The set of VMs are used for processing the workflow, and the speed of each VM is represented in MIPS (million instructions per second). Execution time and communication time define the cost of the workflow. Execution cost is calculated

Fig. 1 Workflow structure

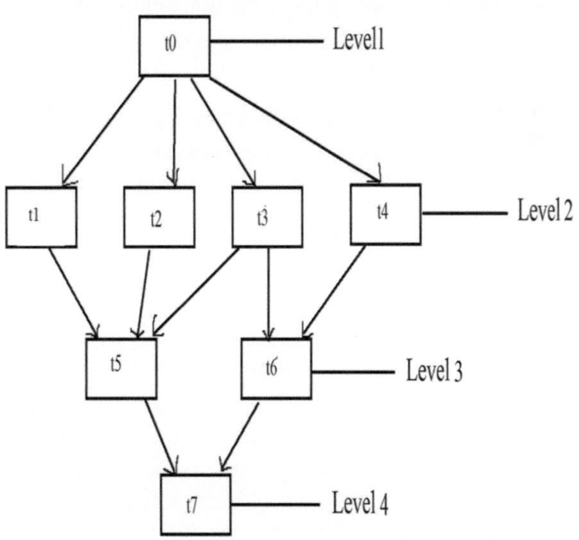

using completion time of workflow and cost per second of resource used for computation. The communication cost is calculated using transfer time and bandwidth cost per second.

The objective of this paper is to minimize the completion time (makespan) of the workflow. However, usage of cloud is based on pay-per-use. Therefore, resource cost and resource usage are also considered as important factors affecting the performance.

4 Improved Workflow Scheduling Using ACO

ACO (Ant colony optimization) was proposed by Dorigo [14] which is based on the social food seeking behavior of ants having the objective of finding the shortest path between two points. Since then, it has been successfully applied to several NP-hard combinatorial optimization problems [5]. The proposed approach uses ACO for mapping of tasks to resources so that all the tasks can complete its computation within minimal time.

This approach is designed for public cloud environment due to heterogeneity nature of computational resources in a cloud datacenter and heterogeneity natured tasks in the workflow. Each task in the workflow differs in terms of the amount of input data taken by it, amount of output data sent by it, its size, its runtime, number of its parent tasks, and number of its child tasks. Moreover, each workflow has different number of tasks at various levels. Hence, the proposed approach dynamically changes the number of VMs and its capacity at each level of the workflow. Even the traditional algorithm HEFT (Heterogeneous Earliest Finish Time) [15] used heterogeneous resources to schedule computational tasks.

The steps are described as follows.

1. Initially, the submitted workflow as directed acyclic graph is parsed and based on precedence constraint the tasks are arranged level wise. Once the tasks in first level are computed, then tasks in next level are submitted for computing.
2. The number of ants is constantly set to 4 in order to assign the tasks in each level in four different ways: Topological order, Longest task first, Shortest task first, and Random manner.
3. To get the optimal solution, the ants try scheduling tasks with different number of VMs in each iteration. Hence, the number of iteration is equal to the number of VMs that are created from the available computing capacity (in mips) in a host.
4. The pheromone and heuristics value of each VM is initialized. The proposed approach lets the pheromone τ_j is the computing capacity of VM_j (in mips) and heuristics (η_j) is inversely proportional to the completion time of last task assigned to that VM_j. Initially, the pheromone value $\tau_j = Mips_j$ and heuristics value $\eta_j = 1$.

5. The transition probability (TP) of assigning a $task_i$ to a VM_j by an ant is calculated using Eq. 1.

$$\mathrm{TP}_{ij} = \frac{(\tau_j)^{\alpha} * (\eta_j)^{\beta}}{\sum_{j \in n} (\tau_j)^{\alpha} * (\eta_j)^{\beta}} \tag{1}$$

Where n is set of available VMs, α represents the importance of computing capacity and β represents the importance of completion time of task in our algorithm. Initially, both parameters are set to the same value.

6. After an ant chooses a VM, the pheromone and heuristics value is updated on selected VMs using the following Eqs. 2 and 4, respectively, so that other task will not choose the selected VM till the completion of the assigned task.

$$\tau_{j+1} = (1 - \rho)\tau_j + \Delta\tau_j \tag{2}$$

To prevent infinite accumulation of pheromone, the pheromone trail decay coefficient $\rho \in [0, 1]$ is used . $\Delta\tau_j$ is local pheromone updating factor and the value of $\Delta\tau_j$ is given by Eq. 3.

$$\Delta\tau_j = 1 - \left(\left(\mathrm{CT}_{ij} - \mathrm{vm}_{\mathrm{avg}}\right)/\mathrm{vm}_{\mathrm{sum}}\right) \tag{3}$$

Where CT_{ij} is the completion time (makespan) of last $task_i$ being assigned to vm_j, vm_{avg} is the average completion time of all vms and vm_{sum} is the sum of makespan of all vms. The heuristics value is updated as follows

$$\eta_j = 1/\mathrm{CT}_{ij} \tag{4}$$

7. The pheromone value for non-selected vms is set using Eq. 5.

$$\tau_{j+1} = \tau_j * \Delta\tau_j \tag{5}$$

8. When an ant completes assigning of all the tasks to VMs, their pheromone and heuristics values are reset. The ant keeps mapping tasks to VMs to get the optimal schedule till the number of VMs reach to n.
9. When all ants complete mapping of the tasks assigned in VMs, the best schedule with minimal time is selected.

As per the best schedule, the tasks are mapped to VMs. The resource cost can be calculated using makespan, cost of computational resource and bandwidth per second. The resource usage can be estimated by finding the idle time slot in each virtual machine. The same approach is applied for the subsequent levels in the workflow.

5 Conclusion

The approach presented in this paper for workflow scheduling using ACO minimizes the makespan and in turn the resource cost as pay-per-use nature of the cloud. First, tasks in each level of the workflow are scheduled and mapped to resources using ACO. To minimize the makespan, pheromone levels are updated for each machine, based on transition probability. The comparison of empirical results of the approach with that of other existing algorithms is being worked out. The future work will be aimed at implementing the approach in one of the public cloud simulated environment.

References

1. Achar, R., Thilagam, P.S., Shwetha, D., Pooja, H., Andrea, R.: Optimal scheduling of computational task in cloud using virtual machine tree. In Third International Conference on Emerging Applications of Information Technology, (pp. 143–146) 2012
2. Lin, X., Wu, C. Q.: On scientific workflow scheduling in cloud under budget constraint. In: 42nd International Conference on Parallel Processing, pp. 90–99 (2013)
3. Hoffa, C., Mehta, G., Freeman, T., Deelman, E., Keahey, K., Berriman, B., Good, J.: On the use of cloud computing for scientific workflows. In: Proceedings of the 4th IEEE International Conference one Science, Washington DC, USA, pp. 640–645 (2008)
4. Abrishami, S., Naghibzadeh, M., Dick, H., Epema, J.: Cost-driven scheduling of grid workflows using partial critical paths. IEEE Trans. Parallel Distrib. Syst. **23**(8) (2012)
5. Tang, R., Qin, Y., Zhang, L.: Research on heuristics logistics distribution algorithm based on parallel multi-ant colonies. J. Softw. 612–619 (2011)
6. KByun, E., Kee, Y. S., Kim, J.S., Maeng, S.: Cost optimized provisioning of elastic resources for application workflows. Future Gener. Comput. Syst. **27**(8), 1011–1026 (2011)
7. Ma, T., Buyya, R.: Critical path and priority based algorithms for scheduling workflows with parameter sweep tasks on global grids. In 17th International Symposium on Computer Architecture and High Performance Computing, IEEE Computer Society
8. Rahman, M., Venugopal, S., Buyya, R.: A dynamic critical path algorithm for scheduling scientific workflow applications on global grids. In: 3rd International Conference on e-Science and Grid Computing, pp. 35–42
9. Yuan, Y., Li, X., Wang, Q., Zhu, X.: Deadline division-based heuristic for cost-optimization in workflow scheduling. Inf. Sci. **179**(15), 2562–2575 (2009)
10. Wen, X., Huang, M., Shi, J.: Study on resource scheduling based on ACO algorithm and PSO algorithm in cloud computing. In: 11th International Symposium on Distributed Computing and Applications to Business, Engineering & Science, pp. 219–222, (2012)
11. Zhou, Y., Guo, Q.,Gan, R.: Improved ACO algorithm for resource—constrained project scheduling problem. International conference on Artificial Intelligence and Computational Intelligence, pp. 358–365 (2009)
12. Banukartik, R.G., Dhavachelvan, P: Hybrid algorithm using the advantage of ACO and Cuckoo search for job scheduling. Int. J. Inf. Technol. Convergence Serv. **2**, 25–34 (2012)

13. Sun, W., Zhang, N., Wang, H., Yin, W., Qiu, T.: PACO: A period ACO_based scheduling algorithm in cloud computing. In: International Conference on Cloud computing and Big Data, pp. 482–486, (2013)
14. Dorigo, M., Blum, C.: Ant colony optimization theory: A survey. Theor. Comput. Sci. **344** (2–3), 243–278 2005
15. Topcuoglu, H., Hariri, S., Wu, M.: Performance-effective and low-complexity task scheduling for heterogeneous computing. IEEE Trans. Parallel Distrib. Syst. **13**(3), 260–274 (2002)

Data Type Identification and Extension Validator Framework Model for Public Cloud Storage

D. Boopathy and M. Sundaresan

Abstract Cloud online storage is one of the sensational and more sensitive topics among the cloud users and cloud service providers. The cloud users can store and retrieve their data in different file formats like document, audio, video, image, and compressed files. Most of the cloud service providers are not providing basic level of encryption service to the data stored in online, so the cloud service providers are not taking care of file format issues. Some of the users may store the files without the file extension and that type of data file may raise the privacy issues for users. This paper discusses and proposes a Data Type Identification and Extension Validator (DTI&EV) framework model for cloud storage to avoid the privacy issues and other regulatory issues related to data file.

Keywords Data identification · Online storage · Cloud storage · Cloud services · Cloud data security · File extension validator

1 Introduction

Cloud computing is one of the buzz words in today's information technology world. The cloud computing services are accessed through browsers and thin clients. The applications which are running on cloud computing are neither language dependent nor operating system dependent.

D. Boopathy (✉) · M. Sundaresan
Department of Information Technology,
Bharathiar University, Coimbatore, Tamil Nadu, India
e-mail: ndboopathy@gmail.com

M. Sundaresan
e-mail: bu.sundaresan@gmail.com

V.B. Aggarwal et al. (eds.), *Big Data Analytics*, Advances in Intelligent Systems and Computing 654, https://doi.org/10.1007/978-981-10-6620-7_51

Cloud computing models are of two types; they are service models and deployment models. The service model includes Software as a Service (SaaS), Platform as a Service (PaaS), and Infrastructure as a Service (IaaS). The deployment model includes Private Cloud model, Public Cloud model, Community Cloud model, and Hybrid Cloud model [1–3].

The most cloud service providers are concentrating on providing the cloud storage-related services. The cloud storage services are also named as online storage, cloud drive, sky drive, and on-demand storage.

The data stored in online has three states; they are data in transit, data in process, and data at rest. Most of the service providers are not providing encryption method for data at rest state.

The cloud service providers (CSPs) are working on the concept of increasing their profit earnings ratio using the number of services acquiring clients and end-level cloud users.

2 Literature Review

A file format is a standard way that information is encoded for storage as a file in a computer. It defines how bits are used to encode information in a digital storage medium. The file formats may be free or either proprietary and may be either unpublished or open [4].

File format identification is the process of figuring out the format of a sequence of bytes. The operating systems typically do this by file type extension or by embedded MIME information of a file. Forensic applications need to identify file types by its content [5].

Most file formats begin with a "header," a few bytes that describe the file format type and its version. Because there are many incompatible file formats with the same extension (e.g., ".doc" and ".cod"). The header gives a program enough additional information to see if this file is one of the formats that program can handle [6].

Every file has a particular defined format. The system stored files are either binary or ASCII. Normally, common ASCII files would be in simple text or more complicated formatted text such as PDF or XML. Common binary files are compressed files or images. But the file formats can be layered as DOCX or PPTX [7]. File types often have an associate explicit format [8]. Limited abilities of the present available tools of forensic examiners working on the certain case have to manually analyze the data one by one method only [9].

3 Objective of Research

When a user uploads a file into online storage, the file type format was not verified by the CSP. Some online file type verification services are also available, but it reads only the extension of the file and gives the extension results to the users. The content of the uploading file was not verified by any online file type identifier. If the service provider reads the contents to verify whether the extension and its contents are same, it will affect the user's privacy and also the mismatched file type will affect the cloud service providers, so it will result in security breach.

The online cloud storage service providers are not taking care of what types of data are stored by user. The user can store any kind of information without the knowledge of cloud service provider (CSP).

For example, the users are not allowed to send the executable files through a mail due to some viruses and worms-related threat issues. The user can simply change the extension of the file into some other text format or document format. After changing the executable file format into different file formats, the service provider server will allow him to send that executable file through the mail.

The file type and file format identifiers are identifying the file only by using the file format extensions and magic numbers. The user can easily change both the file extension formats and the magic numbers. This method needs to make user data vulnerable and will raise privacy issues in cloud computing. The proposed method will overcome these issues.

4 Data Type Identification and Extension Validator Model

To avoid this issue, this paper proposed a model named as Data Type Identification and Extension Validator. It identifies the file types using its file format extensions only. After the file type or file format identification, it will declare some data as sensitive and remaining data as non-sensitive. After identifying the sensitive and non-sensitive data, the identified data will be forwarded to the next level of process.

If the data is sensitive, it will be forwarded to the digital watermark allocation process else if the data is non-sensitive, that data will be forwarded to the encryption and decryption process. So the next level of process will avoid the mismatched extension data uploading.

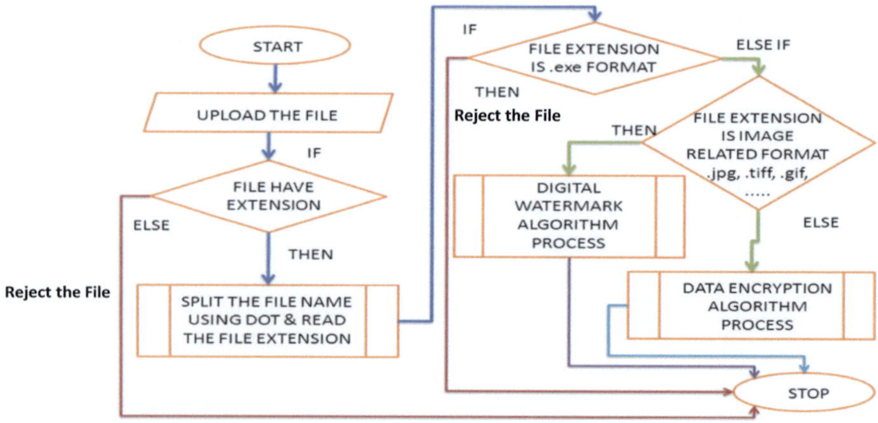

Fig. 1 Data type identification and extension validator flowchart

The Data Type Identification and Extension Validator model is used to identify the file types at the time of uploading on online storage or cloud storage. In this DTI&EV model, all types of image format files are declared as sensitive data type and remaining files are declared as non-sensitive data type (Fig. 1).

The Data Type Identification and Extension Validator (DTI&EV) model is coupled with next process. The output of the DTI&EV will be the input for the further processes, so the results of the DTI&EV model will not store any information at any concern. The DTI&EV just reads the file extension and identifies the data type and forwards that data to the encryption process or digital watermark allocation process.

Procedure for Data Type Identification (DTI&EV) Model

1. Get the input file from the user.
2. Read the file name and its extension.
3. Check whether the file has extension or not.
4. If the file has extension, move that file to the next process else terminate the process.
5. Reverse the file name and then split the file name and extension using dot.
6. Validate the file extension, if it is executable or compression-related extension then terminate the process else move file to the next step.
7. Validate the extension, if it is image file; declare it as a sensitive data and forward to digital watermark allocation process (DWA).
8. Otherwise declare as non-sensitive data and forward it to Encryption and Decryption Gateway Server (E&DGS).
9. Stop the process.

Pseudo Code

```
Create File Object as N, N1, N2
Get the file name from the user with N
Read the Nth file extension
        If (N Contain Dot)
                Move N to Reverse
        Else
                Reject that N
Reverse the Nth file name
Split N using DOT and Store in N1 and N2
Compare the Nth file extension with file format extensions
        If N1 equals execution or compressed file type then
                Reject N
        Else if N1 equals image type then
                Declare N as Sensitive and transfer file to image encryption
        Else
                Declare N as Non-sensitive and transfer file to text encryption
```

5 Results and Discussion

The existing file format identification method verifies only the file extension with their database or by reading the header and content of the file. Whether the file extension is available in database it identifies the file type or else it is not able to identify the file type. The mail attachment screenshot is shown in Fig. 2. The file with malfunctioned extension was allowed to upload and sent to another person easily via electronic mail without any huddles. This shows two thing, one is the extension are not taking care seriously in online storage and second thing is the file which was sent and stored in online is not encrypted.

The DTI&EV model pseudocode was implemented using core Java language platform. The process first reverses the file name. Then, the file name and extension were split using dot operator and stored in two variables. The first variable contains extension, and the second variable contains file name. The extension variable is taken into verification and validation process.

Figure 3 is an image file format. The program processes are executed in that figure, and it was identified that input data type is related to image format. Figure 4 is a document file format. Figure 5 shows that inputted file format is executable, so it was not allowed to upload. Figure 6 shows that user input file name does not contain any extension, so it was unable to process due to lack of file extension. This file was declared as invalid file to upload.

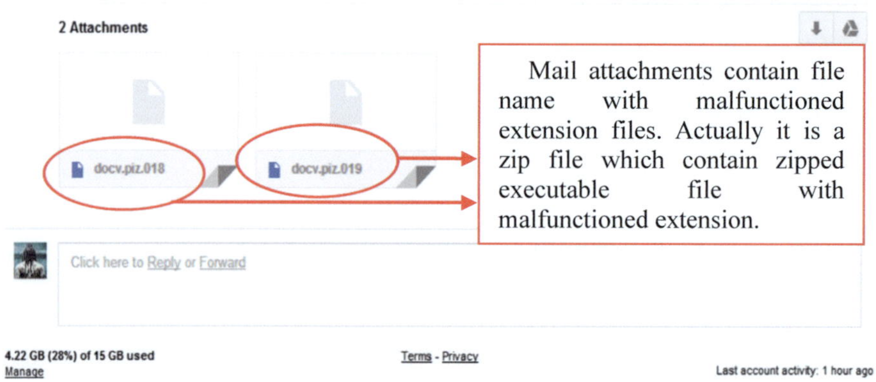

Fig. 2 Existing method was not able to identify and terminate the malfunctioned file extension—A mail sent with malfunctioned extensions

Fig. 3 Data type identified as image file

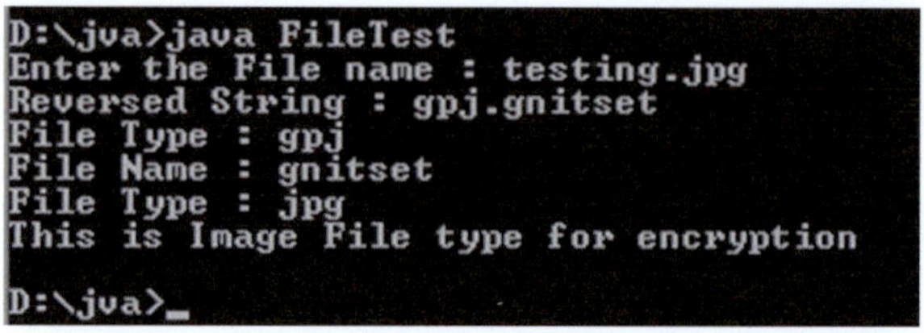

Fig. 4 Data type identified as document file

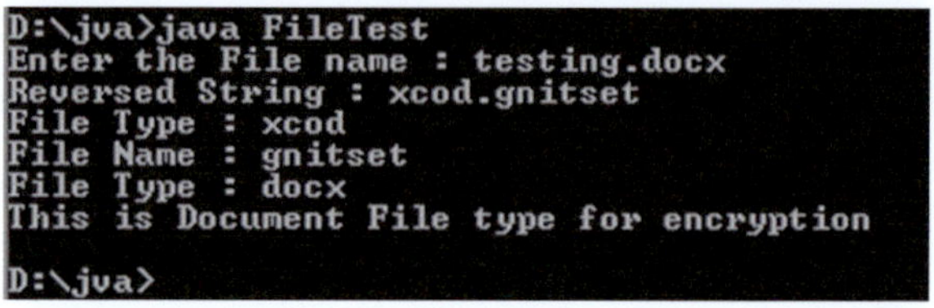

Fig. 5 Data type identified as executable file

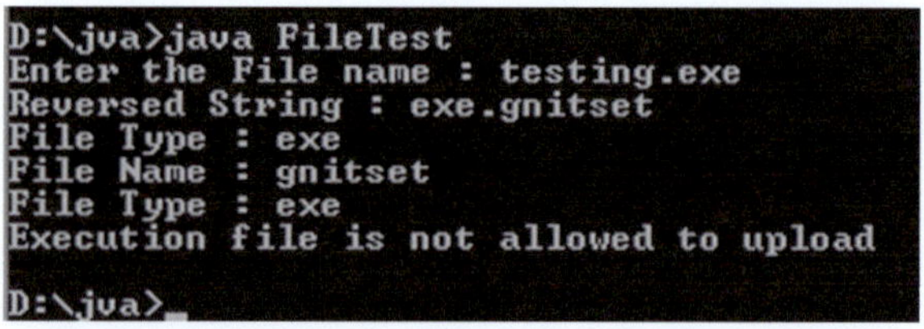

Fig. 6 Data type identified as invalid file

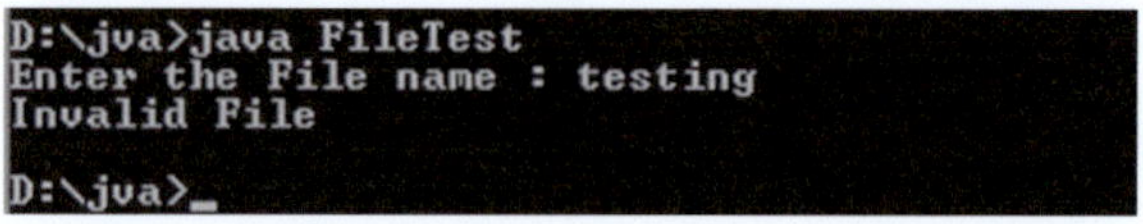

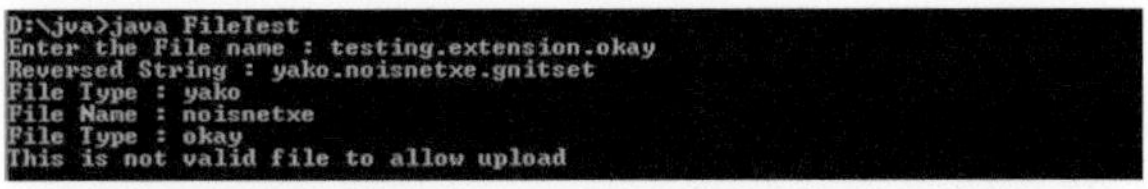

Fig. 7 Data type identified multiple dots file as invalid file

Sometimes, file name may contain multiple dots. Such type of file name is also processed accurately in the DTI&EV model. Figure 7 screen shot is shows that file name contain multiple dots. It was also processed, and if file name does not contain extension with multiple dots, it was declared as an invalid file.

The existing method MIME (Multipurpose Internet Mail Extension) is used to figure out the file type using its extension, but it failed to identify and reject the files which contain malfunction extensions. For example, zip and exe files are not allowed to send via mails. But the user can change the file extension and then send the same file. If that extension is related to permit format or it may malfunctioned like.piz and .ex. (shown in Fig. 2).

It is not possible to verify each and every file by CSP at the time of file uploading to the cloud storage by the cloud user, due to the limited resources allocated for this specific purpose.

But DTI&EV model will act as a data type identifier before the file upload to the cloud storage by using its file extension, and it requires very less resource compared to existing models. The content-based data identification will raise privacy issues in cloud due to reading the content of the file to identify the file type. DTI&EV model is used to identify the file format using its extension and also without reading the file content. It will avoid the privacy-related issues indirectly in cloud and maintains the confidentiality of data.

The time taken to identify the file format is needed to consider because of online uploading. If the method took more time to identify the format means, it will result in lack of performance on cloud service provider. Table 1 and Fig. 8 show the comparison of time taken by DTI&EV and other model to identify the file formats. Thus, the Fig. 8's A–H explanations are shown in Table 1.

Table 1 Time taken to identify the file in milliseconds (ms)

File type and its refers		Existing method (ms)	Proposed method (ms)
Image file	A	15.863748	1.471137
Document file	B	12.684852	1.464152
Execution file and other file formats	C	12.372801	1.493206
File without extension	D	12.471138	0.338311
Image file with more dots with extension	E	12.697704	1.521702
Document file with more dots with extension	F	12.652725	1.54433
Execution file with more dots with extension	G	12.650769	1.491251
File name with more dots without extension	H	12.691837	1.549359

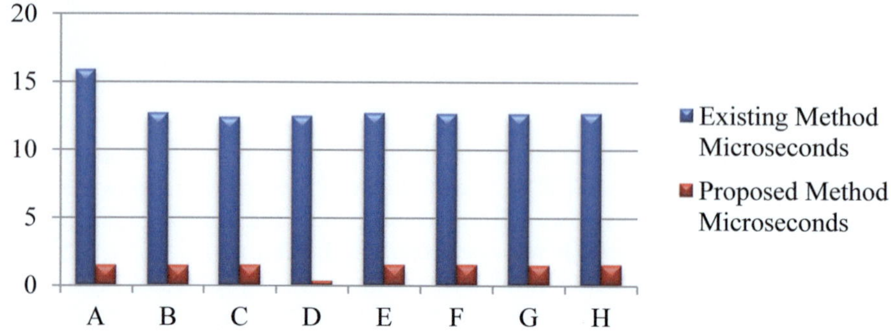

Fig. 8 Time taken by DTI&EV model to identify the data type in milliseconds (ms)

Table 2 Extension types identified by MIME and DTI&EV

File type extension identification	MIME	DTI&EV
Image type format (Png, jpg, jpeg, bmp…)	Yes	Yes
Document type format (Doc, docx, ppt, xls, pptx, etc.)	Yes	Yes
Compressed file formats (rar, zip)	Yes	Yes
Executable file format (Exe)	Yes	Yes
Mismatched file or malfunctioned file format (ra, zi, ex, dx, zi, xe, etc.)	No	Yes
Non-extension file format (file names without extension)	No	Yes

Table 2 explains about the different types of file formats identified by the MIME and DTI&EV. The proposed DTI&EV is able to identify the mismatched file format and malfunctioned file format. In the mean time, the DTI&EV avoids the file name which does not contain extension.

The data type identification processing time was reduced in proposed DTI&EV model. Thus, the resource utilization cost is reduced, and in the mean time, CSP will utilize that reduced resource for other purpose and they can gain profit in that too. So the reducing time in DTI&EV model process will give benefit to both CSP and its cloud user. Thus, the cloud user will upload their data to online cloud storage in rapid speed with safe manner and the uploaded data never became vulnerable.

6 Conclusion and Future Work

The file identification method identifies the file format by its extension only. Some file content may be irrelevant to its file extension.

The data type identification model identifies the data type by its extension only. After that data type identification, that data will be forwarded to the next level of process. And DTI&EV model will avoid the privacy issue and cloud data security breach.

The next level data processing model will confirm that whether file extension contains its format contents or not, at the time of encryption process. If the file format contains its relevant contents, it will automatically process and store that file in the cloud storage, else the file will be rejected with error message.

The data identification model is one of the modules of secured cloud data storage framework model. The output of the data type identification model is declared as input to the two different modules. They are digital watermark allocation process module and data encryption & decryption process module. The remaining two modules are in the process.

References

1. http://csrc.nist.gov/publications/nistpubs/800-145/SP800-145.pdf
2. Boopathy, D., Sundaresan, M.: Data encryption framework model with watermark security for data storage in public cloud model. In: Proceedings of 2014 IEEE eighth international conference on computing for sustainable global development (INDIACom-2014), pp 1040–1044, ISSN 0973-7529, ISBN 978-93-80544-11-3, 05–07 March 2014
3. Boopathy, D., Sundaresan, M.: Policy based data encryption mechanism framework model for data storage in public cloud service deployment model. In: Proceedings of 2013 Elsevier fourth international joint conference on advances in computer science (AET 2013), pp 423–429, 13–14 December 2013
4. http://en.wikipedia.org/wiki/File_format
5. http://www.forensicswiki.org/wiki/File_Format_Identification
6. http://en.wikibooks.org/wiki/Reverse_Engineering/File_Formats
7. http://www.checkfiletype.com/
8. http://www.library.yale.edu/iac/DPC/FileIDandValidate.pdf
9. Karresand, M., Shahmehri, N.: File type identification of data fragments by their binary structure. In: Proceedings of the 2006, IEEE, workshop on information assurance, United States Military Academy, West Point, NY, pp 140–147 (2006)

Robust Fuzzy Neuro system for Big Data Analytics

Ritu Taneja and Deepti Gaur

Abstract Big Data is the name given to relationship of data size and its processing speed. These days, it is a high challenge to construct architecture to take out information economically from huge, diverse volume of data at significant rate. So, there is a need to find cost-effective and time-efficient solutions for the major challenges of fast growing volume and uncertainty. Through this paper, we can become skilled in big data analytics, its tools, and application areas. It also presents uncertainty issues related to Big Data for which the solution we provided by combining fuzzy and neural network concepts to assemble a new intelligent system ANFIS that has accumulated characteristics to get the results by relating knowledge representation, uncertainty, and modeling the key feature of big data to provide an optimal solution. Combined intelligent system is proposed to solve complex problems in the domain of big data to give superior modeling and computation to tackle uncertainty issues.

Keywords ANFIS · Fuzzy system · Membership function · Neural system · Uncertainty

1 Introduction

Over the last two decades, we can find repertoire of data to be generated digitally on the Web, social networking sites, from mobile devices, or online transactions. Data is complex, and making it useful information is the main concern to make it

R. Taneja (✉) · D. Gaur
NCU (Formerly ITM University), Gurgaon, India
e-mail: ritu.taneja@gmail.com

D. Gaur
e-mail: deeptigaur@ncuindia.edu

V.B. Aggarwal et al. (eds.), *Big Data Analytics*, Advances in Intelligent Systems and Computing 654, https://doi.org/10.1007/978-981-10-6620-7_52

presentable and understood by users or learners. Processing the huge data sets to make meaning out of it is the major concern in big data. These large amounts of data sets are increasing with passage of time at a much bigger scale that are generally petabytes and zettabytes to exabytes [1] thus termed as Big Data [2]. The 5V's constituents the characteristics of Big data, namely volume, velocity, variety, value, and veracity. Data is generated from different sources in a huge volume and flowing continuously generating some useful business insights in a safe manner.

This massive volume is categorized into 3 categories, namely

- Structured data having SQL databases that can be text or numerals values that are specific to them [3]. All SQL-based relational data for performing operations.
- Unstructured data cannot be fixed into relational database schemas. WebPages, PDF files, PowerPoint presentations, emails, document files are some of the examples that fall into this category.
- Semi-structured data comprises of both the structured as well as unstructured data, word processing software, NoSQL databases, weblogs and social media feeds.

It is difficult to store and analyze huge datasets using usual software tools. Now, these days' new technology is available to manage this Big Data. Big Data handling is now a challenging technology for new generation. Data is often distributed or decentralized, and replicas are made on each system to prevent failure, but it increases duplicacy. It was Google who recognized the significance of Big data. The motive of this program is to mine the relevant information from huge load data sets efficiently, removing storage, fault tolerance [4], and scalability issues and thus managing it to use in the market for profit making. Encapsulating heterogeneous and complex data from different areas and getting the quality of data for performing required operations by machines is an important factor. Data is exploding in a massive order, and this high-frequency data needs to be analyzed and put into use [5].

2 Big Data Analytics

Big data analysis is defined to be a channel of acquisition, extraction, cleaning, integration, aggregation and visualization, analysis and modeling, and interpretation as shown in Fig. 1.

Earlier, all the work in big data analytics was based on transactional database which has been shifted to unstructured or semi-structured datasets based on data mining and machine learning techniques.

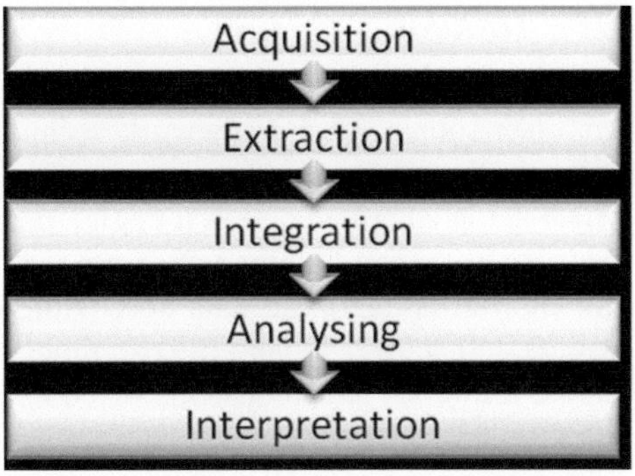

Fig. 1 Phases of big data analysis [21]

3 Application Areas

There are many implications of Big data in day-to-day life that has made innovations and inventions grown in this real world. It is implied on researchers, patients, business tycoons, government, and stakeholders.

In health department, there is huge amount of data stored regarding patient's medical data including test reports, prescriptions, follow ups that are recorded by the medical practitioners [2]. Correlating the medical history of patients with the drug manufacturing companies is complex. In security, activities related to criminal activities can be predicted using big data analysis by detecting fraud transactions in banks and to halt terrorists [6] plans by various security agencies [3]. Net surfing, online shopping, making social networks [7] on Web is a big source for big data analytics. It provides maximum utilization of data on the web these days and thus creating issues for managing it. By using real-time traffic information, there will be ease of traffic management and optimized route can be profound using advanced analytics. Anything that includes transaction in result of various operations conducted on Web takes the picture of trading. Along with that taking log of all the transactions and maintaining it requires analytics. There are various big data algorithms driven for trading for the benefit of financial traders [8]

4 Tools

To cope with the situation, various technologies are introduced namely Hadoop, MapReduce which again follows distributed file system.

4.1 Hadoop

An open-source Java framework technology and library proposed by Apache Software Foundation were created by Goug Cutting [9] and Mike Cafarella in 2005 which act as distributed search engine project named as Hadoop (Highly Archived Distributed Object Oriented Programming) [10]. The technology is built with the aim of processing large data sets with several servers to work in a distributed manner and achieve benefit of cost, time, and storage efficiency. It is a tool that can handle hundreds and thousands of computers with fault tolerance and scalability detection [2].

A single cluster of Hadoop contains one master node and multiple slave nodes [11]. The master node consists of data node, name node, job tracker, and task tracker where slave node acts as both a tasktracker and data node, each having their tasks for handling structured as well as unstructured data.

Hadoop distributed file system is a file system which is highly fault tolerant and works on low-cost hardware. The size of node ranges from 64 MB to GB values. With high bandwidth clustered storage, architecture reduces data loss. But it has the risk of data access, theft as the data is replicated on several nodes, so security aspects were increased to protect it from breaches [10].

4.2 Map Reduce

A simple parallel programming model for computation on large clusters for substantial scalability of thousands of servers and processing huge data sets. The working is signified by its name "MapReduce" where first mapping is done and then reducing the data sets. The basic idea is to divide the clusters into subclusters and after applying MapReduce combining them to get the results. It has master/slave architecture [12] with one master node and several slave nodes managed by it. Each node of cluster is broken down into key/value pairs [1]. The different phases included in it are

- sorting,
- partitioning, and
- combining values.

Different ways have been implemented by Google for possessing work in the field of Big data. Usage of thousand bunch of machines for scalability has not work as it was supposed due to malfunctioning of machines [13–15]. Programs are robotically parallelized due to the abstraction designed for simplifying the untidy representation of the computation because of the huge complications faced by the system [16]. So, the idea of key/value pairs was anticipated which worked well for even large amount of data.

In Map—Two defined tuples act as input which generates intermediate values by emitting each value individually after that acts as input for reduce stage.

Map(key,value) → list(key,Intermediate(values))
Emit Intermediate(value,“1”) [15]

In Reduce—All the values which are output of map stage in list form are processed in parallel, and combined values are generated

List (key,Intermediate(value)) → list(values)(Fig. 2).

5 Uncertainty and Heterogeneity of Big Data

Uncertainty is the term for inappropriate and abnormal data which may lead to incorrect classification of system. There are various factors involved for its existence and in a variety of forms as of dimension errors, noise, processing issues, or faulty data management. In big data, uncertainty can be caused due to large volume of data, miscellaneous and ever changing sources of data, and unstructured and different data formats [17]. Anything below 100% is uncertain for scientists and researchers so it is vital to toil uncertainty for decision making. Veracity plays an important role in dealing with uncertainty aspect. Monte Carlo sampling is one of the ways to deal with uncertainty in spatial. Different ways to tackle uncertainty are to construct optimized algorithms and use advanced mathematics for calculation of probabilistic distributions [18].

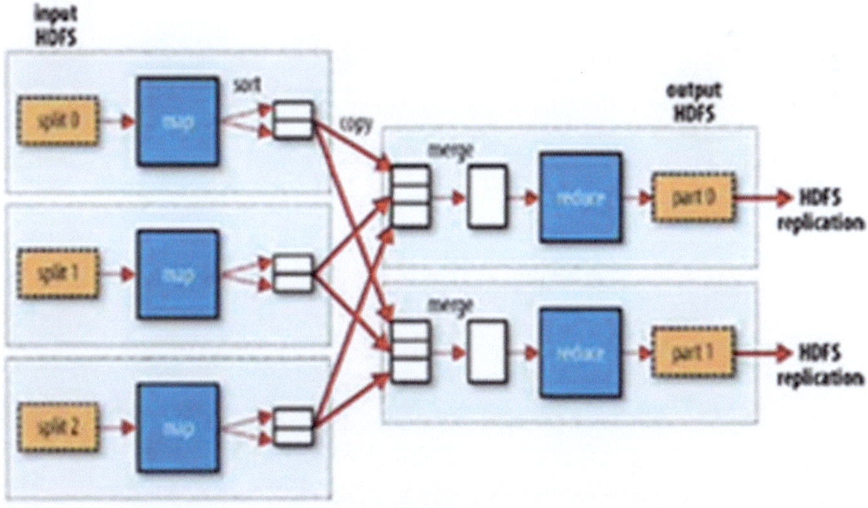

Fig. 2 Map reduce data flow with multiple reducer

To solve complex machine learning problem, a technique of combining fuzzy system neural network for big data came into existence named as ANFIS. This collective intelligence system plays crucial role by combining feature of both system and removes some of the limitations of each other by using few artificial intelligence technique and algorithm which makes system performance very well.

In Table 1 it is understandable that neural network have the learning capability, fault tolerance, and uncertainty tolerance while fuzzy inference systems are very apt for information representation, interpretability, as well as explanation and analysis of data. But they both give good results in uncertainty tolerance, adaptability, and imprecision tolerance. It is completely human network with set of rules and contains multiple layers. Its motive is to borrow learning capability from neural network and put it into fuzzy system, that is, superimposition of fuzzy over neural network so the fuzzy inference system behaves similar to neural network and thus good modeling and computation is achieved. The ANFIS architecture is shown in Fig. 3.

6 Results

Expert knowledge and fuzzy systems to represent big data, neural network for making if and then rules and change input/output membership function to progress the overall performance of the system. Reference [19] to analyze output by adaptive

Table 1 Comparison between neuro and fuzzy logic

	Fuzzy system	Neural network
Interpretable	Yes	No
Fault tolerance	No	Yes
Knowledge depiction	Yes	No
Learning capability	No	Yes
Explanation capability	Yes	No

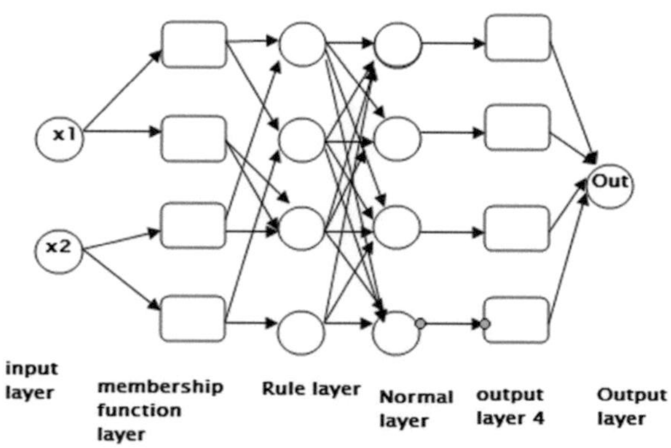

Fig. 3 Architecture of ANFIS

neurofuzzy inference system (ANFIS) in MATLAB by using the datasets in which 3 inputs are applied and one output is produced where ANFIS perform as a classifier with inputs Uncrtn, Krep,Mod, respectively, (Figs. 4 and 5).

Here, uncertainty and modeling are provided with values. Yes, if the value is taken, else No. And knowledge representation has three levels designated by poor, good, and excellent.

The data sets are applied with rules to generate neurofuzzy output that will give result 1, only if uncertainty and Modeling gives input as Yes.

Membership function plots are produced from the training data set as an important role in the network. An inappropriate choice of membership functions can lead to erroneous descriptions [20]. The learning algorithm works in off-line mode to check the error rate. We have used a supervised learning system that is Mamdani neurofuzzy system. The membership function plots are shown in Fig. 6. Here, membership functions are plotted w.r.t each input and its corresponding output (Fig. 7).

Figure 8 shows the surface view of the output generated by applying fuzzy neurologic on Uncertainty, Knowledge Representation and Modeling.

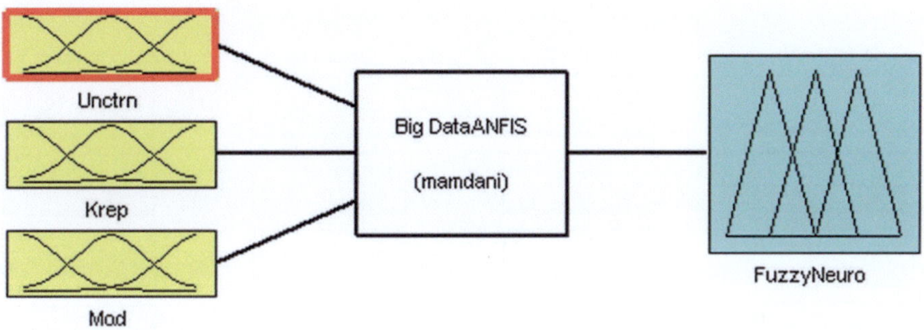

Fig. 4 Generating fuzzy neurooutput

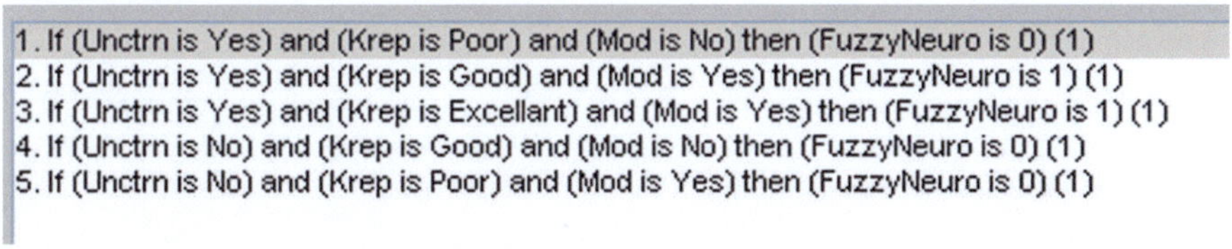
1. If (Unctrn is Yes) and (Krep is Poor) and (Mod is No) then (FuzzyNeuro is 0) (1)
2. If (Unctrn is Yes) and (Krep is Good) and (Mod is Yes) then (FuzzyNeuro is 1) (1)
3. If (Unctrn is Yes) and (Krep is Excellant) and (Mod is Yes) then (FuzzyNeuro is 1) (1)
4. If (Unctrn is No) and (Krep is Good) and (Mod is No) then (FuzzyNeuro is 0) (1)
5. If (Unctrn is No) and (Krep is Poor) and (Mod is Yes) then (FuzzyNeuro is 0) (1)

Fig. 5 Using dataset to prepare rules

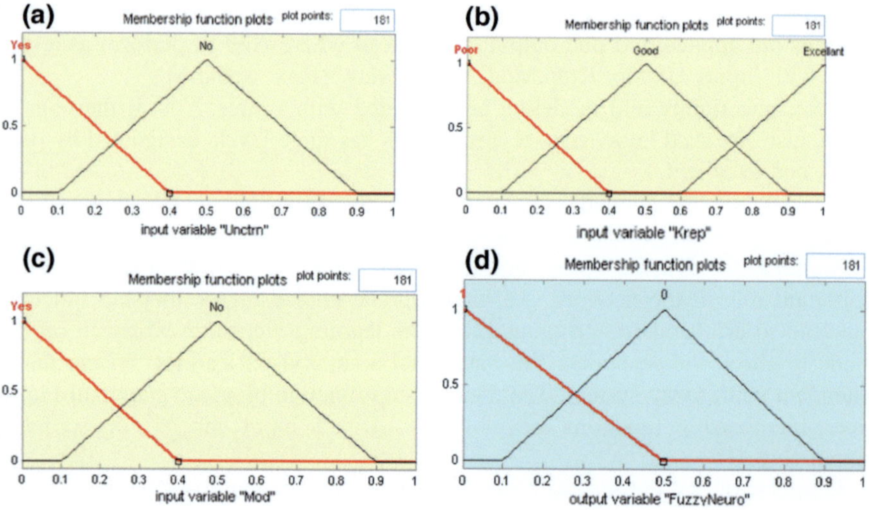

Fig. 6 Membership function plots **a** uncertainty **b** knowledge representation **c** modeling **d** fuzzy neuro

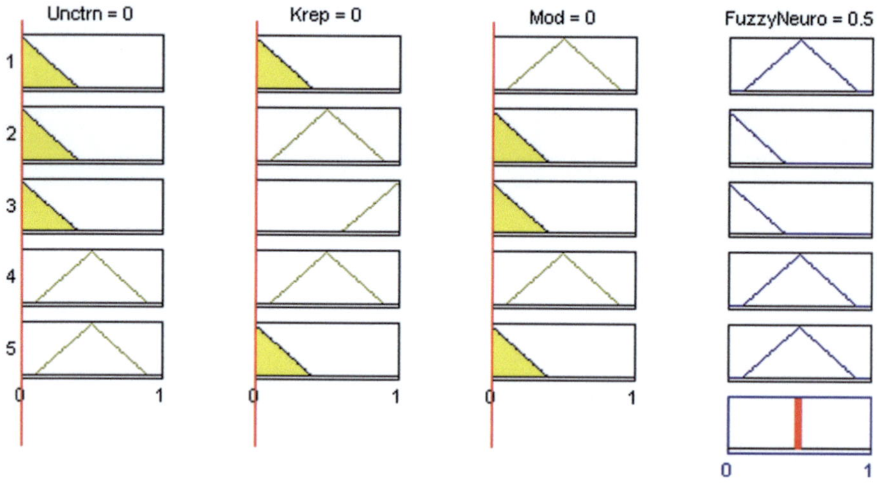

Fig. 7 Rule viewing with inputs [0 0 0]

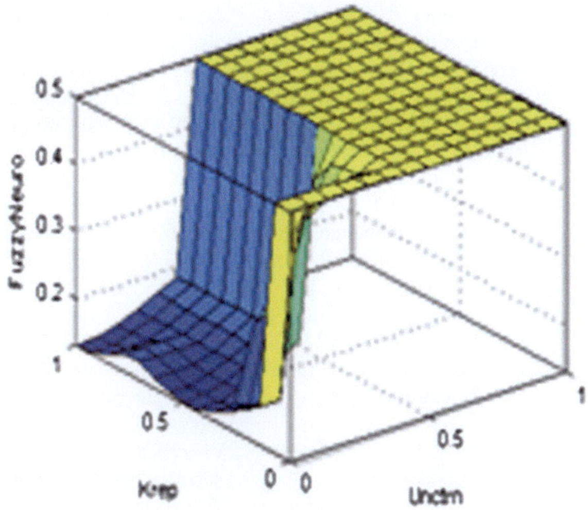

Fig. 8 Surface viewing of adaptive fuzzyneuro system

7 Conclusion

Fuzzy inference system is a framework based on if-then rules and fuzzy reasoning. Neural network is based on feed forward and approximation method. The combination of fuzzy inference system and soft computing techniques like neural network provides a good solution for solving big data problems.

The experimental results show that fuzzy rules are implemented on training set to eradicate uncertainty and resolve complex machine learning algorithm. Keeping this thing in mind, we have provided an adaptive supervised learning Mamdani type of fuzzy inference system as a solution in this paper by taking the benefit of learning capability with the power of fault tolerance and explanation competence. Membership function plots generated from training data sets play an important role to represent different parameters and generate its surface view. The expert knowledge In future, we can think about constructing high performance and accurate computational model of Sugeno-type for big data and we can also compare our system with the proposed model.

References

1. Qin, X., Kelley, B., Saedy, M.: A fast map-reduce algorithm for burst errors in big data cloud storage. In: 10th System of Systems Engineering Conference (SoSE) (2015). 978-1-4799-7611-9/15/$31.00 ©2015 IEEE
2. Vijayalakshmi, M.: Big data analytics frameworks Parth Chandarana. In: International Conference on Circuits, Systems, Communication and Information Technology Applications, (CSCITA). doi: 10.1109/CSCITA.2014.6839299

3. Fazal-e-Amin, A.K., Alghamdi, A.S., Ahmad, I., Hussain, T.: Big data for C4I systems: goals, applications, challenges and tools. In: Fifth International Conference on Innovative Computing Technology, 978-1-4673-7551-1/15/$31.00© 2015 IEEE
4. Ghemawat, S., Gobioff, H., Leung, S.-T.: The Google file system. In: 19th Symposium on Operating Systems Principles, pages 29.43, Lake George, New York (2003)
5. Gandomi, A., Haider, M., Rogers, T.: Beyond the hype: big data concepts, methods, and analytics. Int. J. Inf. Manage, 0268–4012/©2014
6. Fazal-e-Amin, A.K., Alghamdi, A.S., Ahmad, I., Hussain, T.: Big data for C4I systems: goals, applications, challenges and tools. In: Fifth International Conference on Innovative Computing Tech(INTECH 2015) 978-1-4673-7551-1/15/$31.00© 2015 IEEE
7. Mousanif, H., Sabah, H., Douiji, Y., Sayad, Y.O.: From big data to big projects: a step-by-step roadmap. In: 2014 International Conference on Future Internet of Things and Cloud 978-1-4799-4357-9/14 $31.00 © 2014 IEEE DOI 10.1109/FiCloud.2014.66(OSER)
8. Sangeetha, S., Sreeja, A.K.: Science no humans, no new technologies no changes "Big Data a Great Revolution". (IJCSIT) Int. J. Comput. Sci. Inf. Technol. **6**(4), 3269–3274 (2015)
9. Apache hadoop. http://en.wikipedia.org/wiki/ApacheHadoop
10. Saraladevia, B., Pazhanirajaa, N., Victer Paula, P., Saleem Bashab, M.S., Dhavachelvanc, P.: Big data and Hadoop-A study in security perspective. In: 2nd International Symposium on Big Data and Cloud Computing (ISBCC'15)
11. Yahoo Hadoop Tutorial. http://public.yahoo.com/gogate/hadooptutorial/starttutorial.html
12. Hadoop Distributed File System (HDFS). http://hortonworks.com/hadoop/
13. Selvi, U., Pushpa, S.: A review of big data and anonymization algorithms, Int. J. Appl. Eng. Res. **10**(17) (2015) ISSN 0973-4562
14. Manoharan, S.: Effect of task duplication on the assignment of dependency graphs. Parallel Comput. **27**, 257–268 (2001)
15. Siddaraju, D., Sowmya, C.L., Rashmi, K., Rahul, M.: Efficient analysis of big data using map reduce framework. Int. J. Recent Dev. Eng. Technol. **2**(6). ISSN 2347-6435 (Online) (2014)
16. Dean, J., Ghemawat, S.: Mapreduce: simplified data processing on large clusters. Commun. ACM **51**, 107–113 (2008)
17. Abraham, A.: Adaptation of fuzzy inference system using neural learning, Chapter 3. http://ajith.softcomputing.net
18. Khadse, S.G.: A survey of data uncertainty in face recognition. Int. J. Comput. Sci. Inf. Technol. **5**(6), 7623–7625 (2014)
19. http://in.mathworks.com/matlabcentral/fileexchange/29043-neuro-fuzzy-classifier
20. Barouni, F., Moulin, B.: An intelligent atial proximity system using neurofuzzy classifiers and contextual information. In: The International Archives Of The Photogrammetry, Remote Sensing And Spatial Information Sciences, Vol. Xl-2, 2014 Isprs Technical Commission Ii Symposium, 6–8 October 2014
21. Tulasi, B.: Significance of big data and analytics in higher education, Int. J. Comput. Appl. **68** (14), 0975–8887 (2013)

Deployment of Cloud Using Open-Source Virtualization: Study of VM Migration Methods and Benefits

Garima Rastogi, Satya Narayan, Gopal Krishan and Rama Sushil

Abstract Cloud computing has become a buzz word in the field of Information Technology today. It increases the machine potential in terms of computing using virtualization as a core technology. Virtualization is a core of cloud computing in which creation of virtual machines provides the scalability and portability by hosting the components of different applications. Requirements in the cloud environment are dynamic; therefore, there is always a need to move virtual machines within the same cloud or in different clouds. The goal of this paper is to conduct the experiment for deployment of cloud using open source and show the virtual machine (VM) migration between different hosts within a cloud in different scenarios. For secure migration of VM, we have used secure shell method and compared open-source virtualization with other technologies available in the market. The experiment for this study was conducted in the computer service center of IIT Delhi on their private cloud "Baadal."

Keywords Virtualization · Virtual machines · Scalability · Portability · Migration · Secure shell

1 Introduction

The cloud computing has gained great focus in Information Technology today. This is happening due to its ability to meet the dynamic demands of industry with reduced investment on infrastructure and maintenance. Cloud computing provides the shared pool of computing resources such as CPU, storage, applications,

G. Rastogi (✉) · R. Sushil
CSE Department, DIT University, Dehradun, India

S. Narayan
CSE Department, Government Engineering College, Ajmer, India

G. Krishan
Computer Service Center, IIT, Delhi, India

V.B. Aggarwal et al. (eds.), *Big Data Analytics*, Advances in Intelligent Systems and Computing 654, https://doi.org/10.1007/978-981-10-6620-7_53

software, and services and works on pay-per-use model wherein a user can pay only for services that he/she avails without making him/her invest in hardware and software.

There are five essential features of cloud computing given by NIST (National Institute of Standard Technology): rapid elasticity, resource pooling, on demand self-service, broad network access, and measured services. In this, resources are pooled at the centralized places called as data centers that are accessible from everywhere on demand. For implementing cloud computing, virtualization is a core technology that creates an abstract layer over the actual hardware and software [1]. It can also be referred as emulating a physical machine in software or running multiple operating systems on single machine hardware [2]. The main purpose of virtualization is to utilize resources to their full capacity.

In this paper, we are going to deploy a simple cloud using open-source KVM (Kernel Virtual Machine) and will conduct an experiment for VM migration between different hosts in different scenario using secure socket shell for secure communication. The remaining paper is organized as follows: Sect. 2 gives the overview of related studies, Sect. 3 an introduction about virtualization technologies, its type, and hypervisor, Sect. 4 includes implementation of experiment and results with detailed discussion, and Sect. 5 explains the benefits of using KVM in comparison with other popular hypervisors with conclusion discussion at the end of the paper.

2 Related Studies

In cloud computing virtualization, various studies have been conducted with researchers proposing variety of models and techniques discussed as below.

Graziano [3] in a study on "performance analysis of Xen and KVM hypervisors for hosting the Xen world's project" did an analysis of two open-source platforms and conducted some evaluations for overall performance and throughput. In their study, Rabiatul et al. [4], the migration of VM in load balancing was shown. They proposed a method to minimize the VM migration using load balancing which could further provide the efficient utilization of resources. Alexander et al. [5] carried out a study on "testing VM interoperability at an Operating System and Application Level" to suggest a methodology for interoperability. They also conducted surveys of different hypervisors.

In their study, Sharma et al. [6] have developed a migration assessment toolkit for PaaS cloud and named it as MAT (Migration Assessment Toolkit). The approach that they used was static analysis on two rich set of repositories named red list and blue list. The result was presented through a dynamic interface. Using this tool, a user can get the detailed view of migration assessment for different services.

Wu et al. [7] have done performance modeling of VM live migration by conducting several experiments using Xen as hypervisor. They used statistical methods to design the performance model and concluded that the number of resources at the time of live migration has an impact on the migration time.

Feng et al. [8] have done a performance study of live VM migration technologies. They compared the performance of major live migration technologies VMotion and XenMotion of vendors VMware and Citrix, respectively. After conducting the experiment, they concluded that XenMotion outperformed VMotion in total migration time.

LeVasseur et al. [9] have done a study on virtualization to conclude that if we combine performance of para-virtualization and virtualization, then it becomes more useful. They showed how to use both together and also their approach they were able to reduce the burden of implementation and maintenance of para-virtualization.

Leelipushpam et al. [10] have done survey on live VM migration techniques in cloud environment to brief about the VM migration techniques like energy efficient VM migration, load balancing VM migration, and fault tolerant VM migration.

In their study, Aidan et al. [11] explained about the pre-copy and post-copy VM migration techniques for memory intensive application. They discussed several techniques to provide better support for migration.

3 Virtualization Technology

Virtualization is a technology used to divert the industry perspective from the utilization of resources physical to logical [1]. The main goal of virtualization is to utilize the maximum capacity of resources whether it is processor, storage, network, or anything. This is achieved by collaborating multiple unutilized resources into a shared resource pool and utilize them by creating virtual machines to perform different tasks simultaneously to fulfill demands. These resources can be scaled on virtual machines i.e., allocated dynamically.

3.1 Type of Virtualization

- Application Virtualization—The applications including operating system of host machine is moved to the virtual environment. It is a technology in which the application is present somewhere else but is accessed by the client computer. The application behaves same as the local application on the client system, for example, VMWare Thinapp, Oracle secure Global desktop, etc.
- Storage Virtualization—It provides a virtual storage environment by collecting or combining various physical storages. Through this, distributed storage is managed in such a way as it is one consolidated storage. After this virtualization, the availability of storage increases because now the applications do not

have limited or specific resource. The storage can be updated any time without affecting the performance of the application [4].

- Server Virtualization—In this, existing server is moved into a virtual environment i.e., hypervisor, which is hosted on a physical server [1]. The resources of server will be hidden from clients, and physical server is divided into multiple virtual environments. Web server virtualization is one of the most popular examples of this technology used for providing low-cost Web hosting services.
- Hardware Virtualization—Making hardware components of real machine as virtual components. This technology hides all the physical components and details of actual computing platform from end users.

3.2 *Hypervisors*

A software which acts as an intermediator between virtual machine and physical hardware. It is used to create virtual machines. The hypervisor manages virtual hardware and guest operating system on said hardware with on-virtual platform. Hypervisor can be native (Type-1) or hosted (Type-2). Figure 1 is showing the placement of hypervisor, and Table 1 is a list of some hypervisors used nowadays.

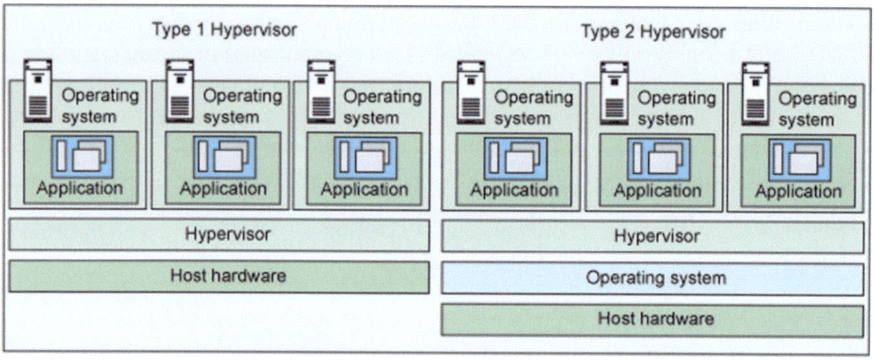

Fig. 1 Type-1 and Type-2 hypervisor

Table 1 Some hypervisors and their type

Name of hypervisor	Company	Payed	Type-1	Type-2
Xen Citirix	Linux	Partially	Yes	–
VMWare	VMWare Inc.	Yes	Yes	
KVM	Red Hat	No	Yes	–
Hyper-V	Microsoft	Yes	Yes	–
VMWare Workstation	VMWare Inc.	Yes	–	Yes

Type-1
These hypervisors include itself with operating system. It runs on hardware directly and manages the guest operating system [1]. This type of virtualization is called as full virtualization.

Type-2
These hypervisors require host operating system to run. Guest operating system is managed by the hypervisor. This type of virtualization is called as para-virtualization.

4 Implementation and Results

Virtual machine migration is a process of moving virtual machine running on one physical host to some other physical host. Migration is required due do several reasons such as energy saving. If the system is not having much load, then migration of VM to some other host having some more tasks can save energy of host. Whenever any changes in host hardware are required, then it is better to migrate VM from the host to some other host so that VM is not down, and host can be easily upgraded. More importantly, it can be used for load balancing like VMs on one host are under loaded due to less tasks, and other host VMs are overloaded. The migration of under loaded VM to overloaded host can help in load balancing [10].

We have conducted this experiment as shown in Fig. 2 in the computer service center laboratory of IIT Delhi. We have used host machines of their data center created for private cloud Baadal. The configuration of host was—2 × 4 core Intel ® Xeon ® CPU E5540 @ 2.53 GHz and 12 GB RAM. We have used two hosts at

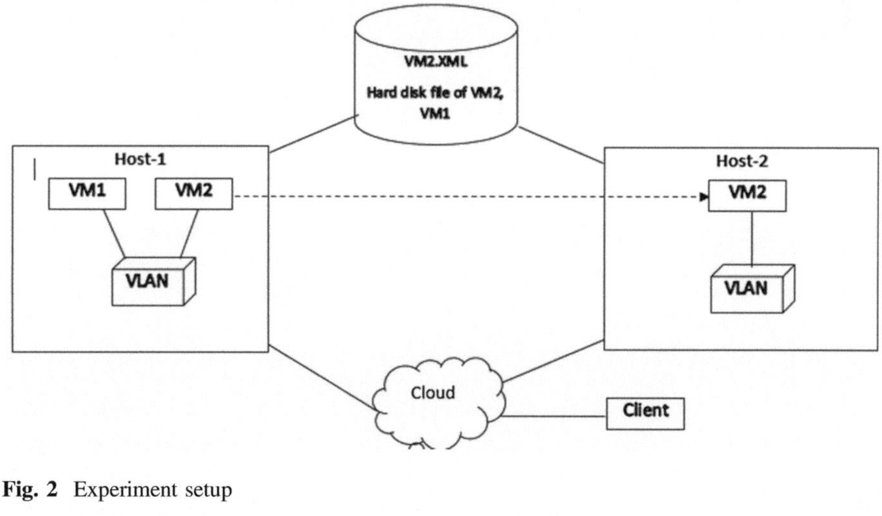

Fig. 2 Experiment setup

the start. All the host servers could access the shared storage 50 TB based on NetApp 3210 V NAS and HP EVA6400 SAN with FC disks. For virtualization, we have used KVM (Kernel Virtual Machine) as an open source [2].

4.1 Experiment

For migration of VM between hosts, we have used remote management using secure shell (SSH). It is a network protocol which allows data exchange between two hosts on the network through a very secure channel. Earlier protocols like FTP and POP were not secure because with them, we could transfer information in the form of plain text, which made it easily accessible to hackers. By using this scheme, we restrict hackers and attackers and thus transfer information in a more secure way.

Figure 2 is our experiment setup. We have followed below-mentioned steps to implement the KVM, creation of VM, and performing Migration.

1. We configured the operating system on the host machines.

   # apt-get update
   # apt-get install kvm, etc.

2. Created two Virtual machines on host1, allocated 1 GB RAM and 14 GB hard disk to each VM. Figure 3 is showing VM status.

   # ssh root@10.16.171.23 virt-install –virt-type kvm —name vm1 –ram 1024 –cdrom =/home/garima/downloads/ubuntu.iso –disk/var/lib/libvirt/images/vm1. qcow2, size = 14, format = qcow2,bus = virtio – network bridge = br0, model = virtio, mac = 52:54:00:10:55:ef –graphics vnc, port = 5901, listen = 0.0.0.0, password = abc –noautoconsole –os-type = linux

3. Made changes in the network interface file of the host1 and added bridge port into it. Figure 4 is network configuration used for VM.
4. We used two scenarios for VM Migration.

   (a) Migrated VM from one host to another when VM was not running

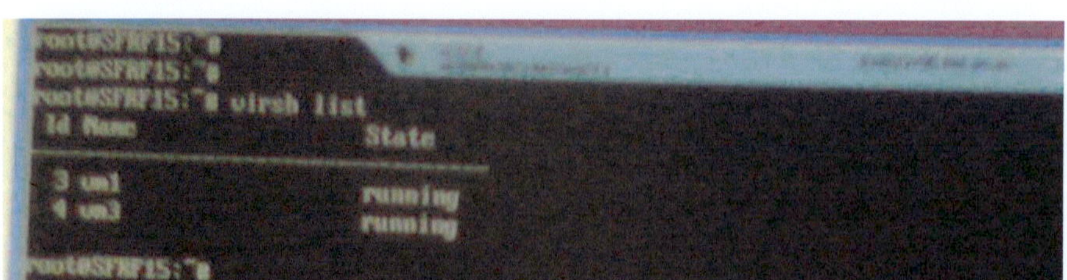

Fig. 3 VM status

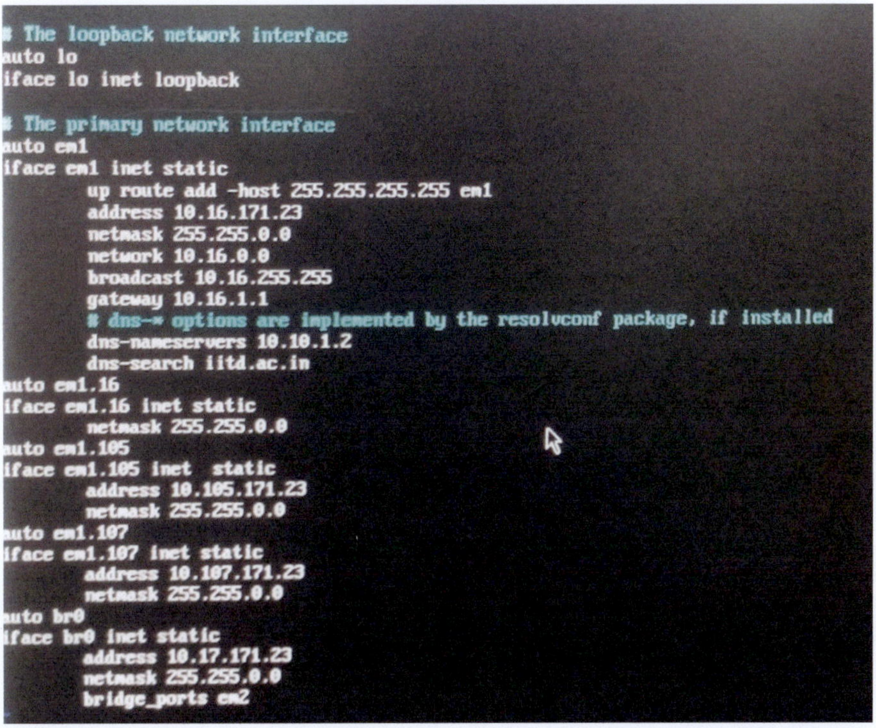

Fig. 4 Network configuration

(b) Migrated VM from one host to another when VM was running called as Live VM migration.

(a) Migration of VM from one host to another when VM was not running

virsh -c qemu + ssh://10.16.171.25 define/etc./libvirt/qemu/vm1.xml
virsh undefine vm1

(b) Live Migration of VM

ssh root@10.16.171.23 virsh migrate –live 10.16.171.23 qemu + ssh://10.16.171.25/system

In VM migration, the memory migration is one of the most important aspects. There are number of ways through which memory of the VM moves from one physical state to other. There are three methods used for memory migration: stop and copy, pre-copy, and post-copy.

Stop and copy method is used when the VM is migrated offline. In this technique, three steps are involved: 1. Stop the virtual machine on source, 2. Copy all its memory contents to destination, and 3. Start the VM at destination host.

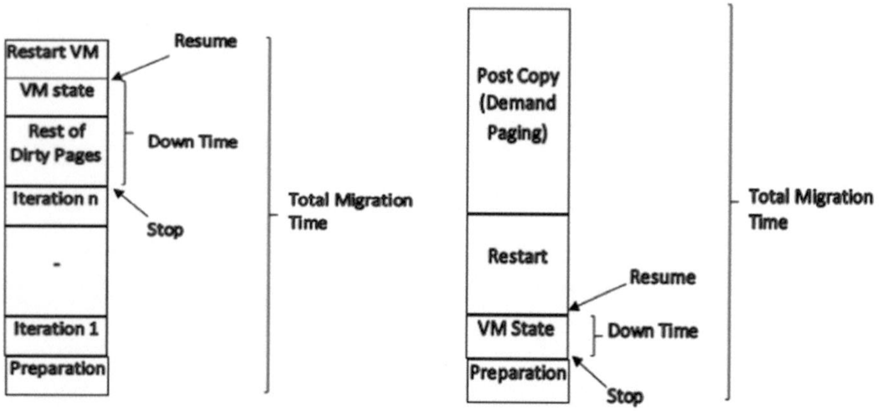

Fig. 5 **a** Pre-copy migration, **b** post-copy migration

Pre-copy and post-copy approaches are used while VM is migrated live. In the pre-copy approach (Fig. 5a), series of iterations is involved for transferring the memory. When migration is started, only dirty pages keep copying. If the number of dirty pages is under threshold, the source VM will stop and will copy all remaining dirty pages after this; at last, VM at destination is resumed. This technique can take longer downtime which depends on the writable set.

In the post-copy approach (Fig. 5b), first source VM will be stopped, and all VCPUs and states will be copied to destination. Now, the execution of VM at destination will be resumed. If in case the VM tries to access some pages which are not currently available, then network page fault occurs, and page will be transferred to destination VM.

4.2 *Metrics for VM Migration*

Two metrics were used for migration.

1. Total Migration Time—Total time when all states, CPU, and memory are transferred.

$$\text{TMT (Precopy)} = \text{TI} + \text{OV} \tag{1}$$

$$\text{TMT (Postcopy)} = \text{OV} \tag{2}$$

2. DownTime—time between VM resume and stop state.

$$\text{TDT (Precopy)} = \text{DM} + \text{V S} \tag{3}$$

$$\text{TDT (Postcopy)} = \text{V S} \tag{4}$$

where
TI—total time of all iterations, OV—Overhead, DM—Dirty Memory, and VS—VM State Time.

5 KVM and Other Hypervisors

XEN and VMWare are the most established hypervisors used for full virtualization. According to a survey by openvirtualizationalloiance.com, the analysis showed that KVM is almost 60 to 70% less expensive than other hypervisors with same functionalities i.e., it is a good option for those organizations that want to reduce cost on licensing. The survey further showed that KVM performance is better than VMWare. It is built on the top of Linux and is implemented as a kernel module, when loaded convert the kernel into a type-1 hypervisor [12]. Since KVM is the part of Linux Kernel, KVM utilizes the security capabilities of Linux, and VM is same as other program running on Linux. Administrator can set parameters according to requirements to guarantee QoS for VM. Use of other hypervisors like Hyper-V gives vendor lock-in. Various big companies like IBM, HP, and Intel are promoting KVM to avoid vendor lock-in.

6 Conclusion

Cloud computing has gained increased focus in Information Technology. This is happening due to its ability to meet the dynamic demands of industry with reduced investment on infrastructure and maintenance. Creation of virtual machines can provide the scalability and portability by hosting the components of different applications. Requirements in the cloud environment are dynamic; therefore, there is always a need to move virtual machines within the same cloud or in different clouds. There can be various reasons for VM migrations like migration is required for saving energy of host which is less in use, can be required for fault tolerance if some host is not working properly, or can be required for load balancing among all hosts.

This work was conducted in the private cloud "Baadal" in computer service center at IIT Delhi. In this work, we discussed the concept of virtualization technology, hypervisors, and its different types. We used KVM as an open-source hypervisor and conducted experiments on VM Migration from one host to other host within cloud in two scenarios—online and offline. We also discussed the memory migration techniques while VM migration. At last, we compared KVM with other hypervisors in the market and tried to find out benefits to use KVM by organizations. This work will help organizations and researcher to decide KVM is a better option if they have less budget and want all the facilities of cloud computing environment. In future, we will propose a hybrid pre-copy migration technique as there is a chance to reduce live migration time.

Acknowledgements We want to offer our sincere thanks to all the members of computer service center of IIT Delhi and especially to Dr. Gopal Krishan for his extraordinary support and guidance.

References

1. Durairaj, M., Kannan, P.: A study on virtualization techniques and challenges in cloud computing. Int. J. Sci. Technol. Res. **3**(11), 147–151 (2014)
2. Gupta, A., Kumar, J., Mathew, D.J., Bansal, S., Banerjee, S., Saran, H.: Design and implementation of the workflow of an academic cloud. In: Proceedings of the 7th International Conference on Databases in Networked Information Systems Springer Lecture notes in Computer Science, pp. 16–25 (2011)
3. Graziano, C.D.: A performance analysis of Xen and KVM hypervisors for hosting the Xen worlds project. Graduate Thesis Iowa state University, (2011)
4. Razali, R.A.M., Rahman, R.Ab., Zaini, N., Samad, M.: Virtual machine migration implementation in load balancing for cloud computing. In: Proceedings of IEEE Conference Intelligent and Advanced Systems, pp. 1–4. Kuala Lumpur (2014)
5. Lenk, A., Katsaros, G., Menzel, M., Revelant, J.R., Skipp, R., Leon, E.C., Gopan, V.P.: TIOSA: Testing VM interoperability at an OS and Application Level- A hypervisor testing method and interoperability survey. In: Proceedings of IEEE International Conference on Cloud Engineering, pp. 245–252 (2014)
6. Sharma, V.S., Sengupta, S., Nagasamudram, S.: MAT: A migration assessment toolkit for PaaS clouds. In: Proceedings of 6th International Conference on Cloud Computing, pp. 794–801 (2013)
7. Wu, Y., Zhao, M.: Performance modeling of virtual machine live migration. In: Proceedings of IEEE 4th International Conference on Cloud Computing, pp. 492–499 (2011)
8. Feng, X.J., Tang, J., Luo, X., Jin, Y.: A performance study of live VM migration technologies: VMotion versus XenMotion. In: Proceedings of IEEE Conference Communications and Photonics, Shinghai, pp. 1–6 (2011)
9. LeVasseur, J., Uhlig, V., Yang, Y., Chapman, M., Chubb, P., Leslie, B., Heiser, G.: Pre-virtualization: Soft layering for virtual machines. In: Proceedings of IEEE Conference Computer Systems Architechture, Hsinchu, pp. 1–9 (2008)
10. Leelipushpam, P.G.J., Sharmila, J.: Live VM migration techniques in cloud environment–A survey. In: Proceedings of IEEE Conference on Information and Communication Technologies, Je Ju Island, pp. 408–413 (2013)
11. Shribman, A., Hudzia, B.: Pre-copy and post-copy VM live migration for memory intensive applications. Springer Lecture Notes in Computer science, vol. 7640, pp. 539–547 (2013)

12. Red Hat Inc. Kvm—kernel based virtual machine. Technical report, Red Hat Inc., (2009)
13. Sugerman, J., Venkitachalam, G., Lim, B-.H.: Virtualizing I/O devices on VMware workstation's hosted virtual machine monitor. In: Poceedings of the USENIX Annual Technical Conference, pp. 1–14. Boston, Massachusetts, USA (2001)

Implementation of Category-Wise Focused Web Crawler

Jyoti Pruthi and Monika

Abstract The size of the World Wide Web is increasing rapidly and has reached a point where it is difficult to handle and manage such amount of information. Search engines are used to gather, index and make available the information across the web for the users. A web crawler is an important part of search engine that finds all the information. As the size of the web is beyond our imaginations, a user needs and focuses only on relevant information available on the web. Focused crawler is a crawler that gives only relevant information to the users and discards the information that is not relevant. The objective of the paper is to implement category-wise focused web crawler so that the user will be able to get focused and relevant information.

Keywords Category-wise focused crawler · Relevant page · Page relevance · Search

1 Introduction

In today's scenario, the information on the WWW has increased enormously and it leads to the great demand of the system that helps to retrieve the relevant information. When searching the web, the ultimate goal of the user is to get the information that is relevant. Typing "Delhi" on Google gives us 3.49 million results, and similarly, typing on Yahoo gives us 0.63 million results. Most of them are useless for the users as no one will check millions of results. So, there rises a key issue that how to retrieve most relevant web pages for the user. A traditional crawler traverses all the hyperlinks from the web page; it requires computing resources and time. To overcome this problem, a crawler has been designed that is focused to retrieve the

J. Pruthi (✉)
Department of Computer Science and Technology,
Manav Rachna University, Faridabad, India

Monika
Department of Computer Science and Engineering,
Manav Rachna College of Engineering, Faridabad, India

V.B. Aggarwal et al. (eds.), *Big Data Analytics*, Advances in Intelligent
Systems and Computing 654, https://doi.org/10.1007/978-981-10-6620-7_54

desired information from the pool of web. This focused crawler crawls the boundary to find the relevant links and discard the irrelevant web pages [1].

2 Related Works

In 1999, Soumen Chackrabarti introduced focused crawling [1]. The ultimate objective of a focused crawler was to seek out the selective pages that are related to already define sets of various topics. P.M.E De Bra introduced the fish-search algorithm to collect topic-specific web pages or links [2]. To improve the fish-search algorithm, shark-search algorithm was proposed by Hersovici et al. [3]. It was an improved version of FSA.

Martin Ester, Matthias Grob and Hans-Peter Kriegel proposed the generalized version of focused crawler [4]. The framework is comprised of two major components. The first component concerned about the interest of the user and therefore measured the relevancy of the web link. The second component was to arrange the links in an order of relevancy score.

Mohsen Jamali, Hassan Sayyadi, Babak Bagheri Hariri and Hassan Abolhassani introduced the link structure approach [5]. The approach proposed to create a link structure of pages and metric to measure the similarity of pages. But this approach was not proved to be successful to distinguish between the irrelevant and relevant pages. To improve the relevancy of retrieved pages, Safran and Althagafi [6] proposed a naïve Bayesian approach to be used with base prediction model. Sampat and Mistry [7] also discussed the various approaches related to focused crawler.

We also contributed in this direction and proposed the detailed design of category-wise focused web crawler [8].

3 Architecture and Algorithm

According to the proposed architecture of category-wise focused crawler [9], the system crawls the various websites as per the choice of category and gives relevant web pages as a result. The architecture has two modules.

- The first module crawls the web links and applies focused approach to store the relevant result in the database.
- The second module is related to search the crawled data. The search interface is provided for the user to submit the query. The user also chooses the specific category for searching and will get the most relevant web links (Fig. 1).

The above system recursively crawls the various web pages and stores the best matched data in the database. It saves the information related to the web pages like title, keywords and meta-description. When the user submits the query to the search engine, it searches the already stored data and shares all the relevant links as per the query.

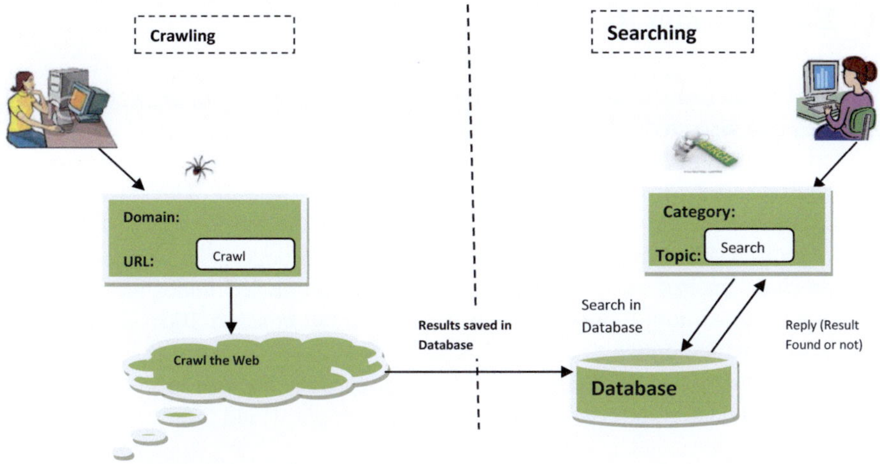

Fig. 1 Proposed architecture [9]

We proposed the design of the category-wise focused crawler in [8], wherein we have proposed the basic design of focused crawler which includes UML diagram, ER diagram and flow chart.

The proposed algorithm for the above-said system is initialized with domain, URL and category. Page relevance is calculated. For stopping the crawl, we can keep a count of maximum number of web pages to visit and maximum depth up to which to crawl. The crawler will stop crawling if any of the conditions is met.

Algorithm

Step 1: Initialize with a starting URL, crawl it with focusing on the specified Category.
Step 2: Calculate Page Relevance by:
R = Number of Occurrences of C in P
Where,
R: - Page Relevancy
P:-webpage under investigation
C: - Category
Step 3: Add URL, Category, Page Relevance and level to the URL Queue.
Step 4: Repeat until, **visitedpages<=Max AND depth <= Variable d**, where d =depth.
a) Select URL with maximum score from URL Queue.
b) Extract all the internal links of URL.
c) Repeat for all internal Links
i. Crawl the link.
ii. Calculate Page Relevance.
iii. If page is relevant then insert URL, Category, Page Relevance and level in the URL Queue.
iv. If page is not relevant then discard the page.
v. Visitedpages= visitedpages + 1;
d) Visitedpages= visitedpages + 1;
Step 5: Stop

4 Experimental Results

We have implemented the focused crawler that is consisting of crawl and search modules and also study the results of the same. Both the modules are implemented in Asp .net using C# in Manav Rachna University Laboratory. We have crawled different websites according to category and domain of website. The crawled URLs saved in the database according to the category for the purpose of searching the information. Table 1 contains the total no. of crawled pages, no. of relevant links and precision rate of various websites that we have crawled under different categories. Our maximum number of web pages to crawl is set to 100 and maximum depth up to which crawler can crawl is set to 3.

To compare the performance of the category-wise focused web crawler, the formula of precision rate [6] is used, which is (Graphs 1 and 2):

$$\text{Precision Rate} = \frac{\text{No. of relevant Page}}{\text{No. of Downloaded Pages}}[6]$$

Crawl Module
For crawling, we pick the website www.makemytrip.com. Initially, URL queue has only one URL, i.e. starting URL. So it is taken as root node and status is set "Done" and the URL is explored further. After exploring this URL, we get internal links of this URL, and we initially set status of all the internal links as "Pending". On this next level, the best URL, i.e. URL with maximum value, is www.makemytrip/bus-tickets/neeta-travels-booking.html, with relevance score 104. So, this best URL is

Table 1 Websites crawled under various categories with precision rate

Category	URL	Total crawled pages	Relevant pages	Precision rate
News	Zeenews.india.com	291	285	0.97
	Ibnlive.in.com	113	101	0.89
	Abpnews.abplive.in	145	128	0.88
	www.bbc.com	20	18	0.9
Travel	www.makemytrip.com	78	68	0.87
	www.tripadvisor.in	88	80	0.9
	www.travelandleisure.com	44	42	0.95
Education	w3schools.com	84	75	0.89
	www.mrce.ac.in	119	100	0.84
	www.codeproject.com	121	99	0.81
Entertainment	Timesofindia.indiatimes.com	87	40	0.45
	www.bollywoodnews.org	80	57	0.71
Sports	Timesofindia.indiatimes.com	56	30	0.53

Graph 1 Graph of travel category

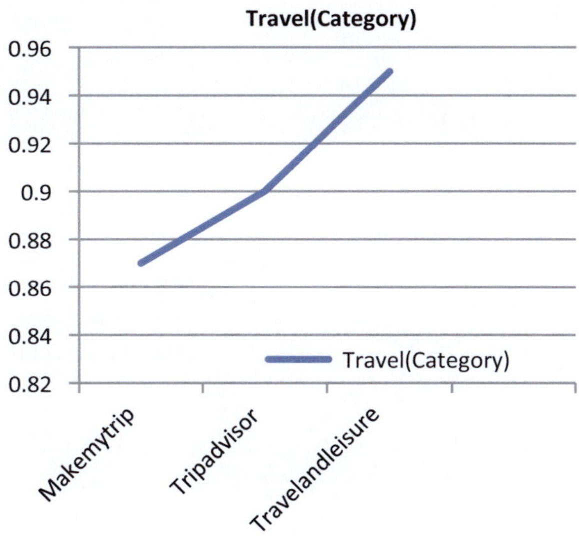

Graph 2 Graph of news category

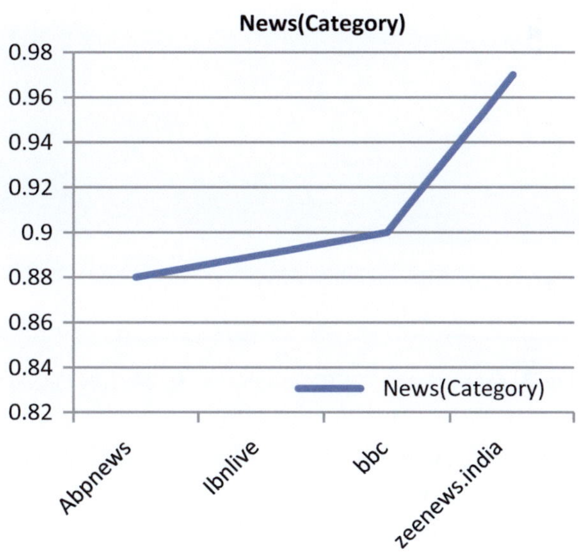

picked and status is set as "Done", and this URL is explored further. This process is followed and stops when the stopping condition is matched. The movement is also shown in Fig. 2.

Implementation Snapshots:

The crawling module screen is shown in Fig. 3. The Crawler is taking 3 inputs from the user, i.e. domain, URL and category.

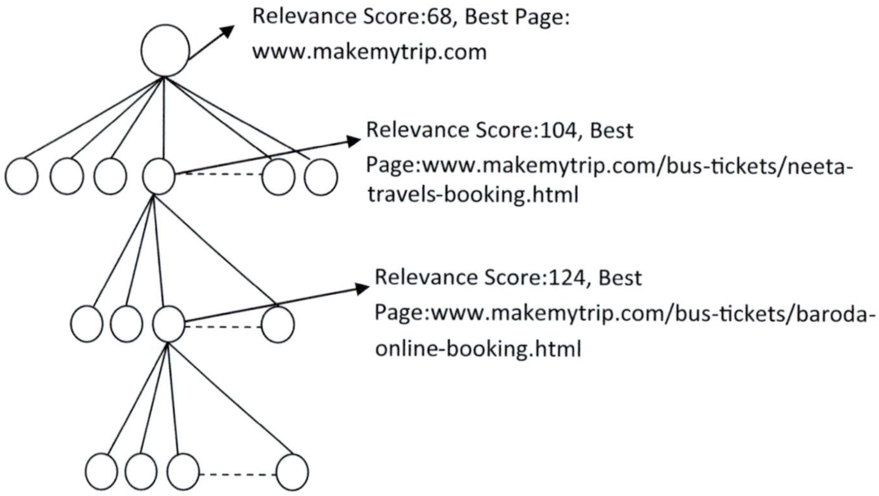

Fig. 2 Crawling movement

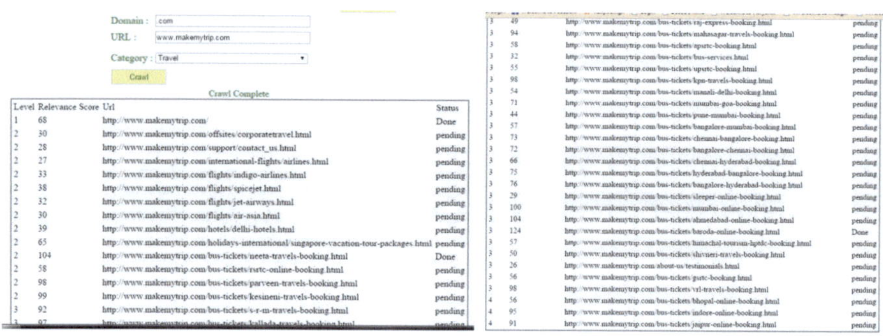

Fig. 3 Crawl results of URL searched under category "travel"

In this way, the crawled results saved in the database under the category chosen, for example, Travel in this crawl.

In the testing of the crawl module, we have ensured that:

1. The crawler will crawl the web according to the given category and domain.
2. Validations are appropriate according to the requirement of the module, for example, textbox in the page must be filled (null check) by the user and entered URL must belong to the domain.

3. If already crawled, website is crawled again. It should update the database with new web pages.

Search Module

In the search module, we search query in a specified category. First, we choose a category under which search will be focused and then any user query. The search will search for the query in the database, and if the result is found, it will be displayed to the user; otherwise, dialog box (No results found) will be displayed.

5 Comparison

Let us take a query "Delhi", when this query is searched in traditional search engine, it will give all results. The result will contain all categories it can belong to, for example, search results for "Delhi" may contain any News of it or any travelling information about it (Fig. 4).

But if we want information about a specified category only, other extra information is of no use to us. Instead of getting combined results, we want to search only News about Delhi. As our crawler has crawled the web page category-wise, we can search them category-wise. In Fig. 5, the query "Delhi" is searched under category Travel, and in Fig. 6, the query "Delhi" is searched under category News. Both results are different in spite of same user query (Graph 3).

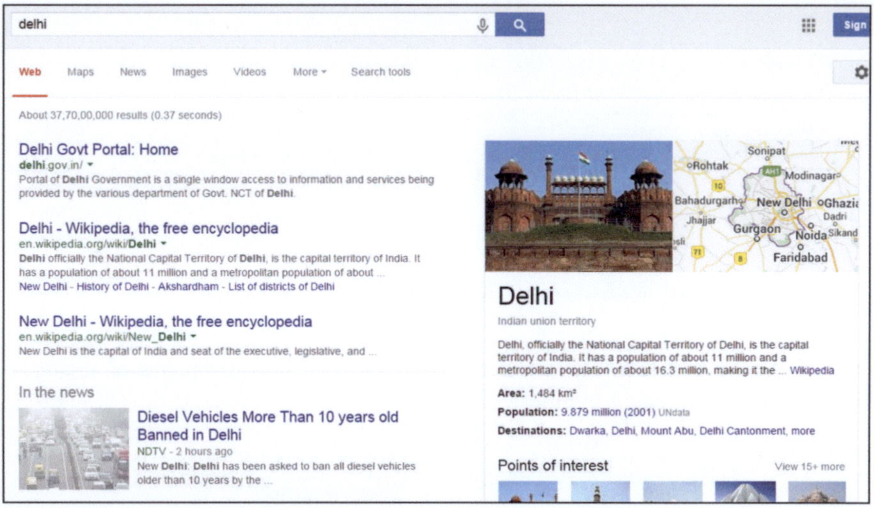

Fig. 4 Query searched in traditional search engine

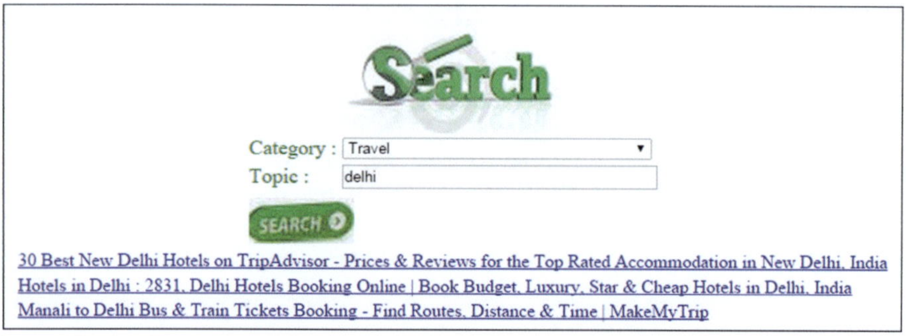

Fig. 5 Query searched in category travel

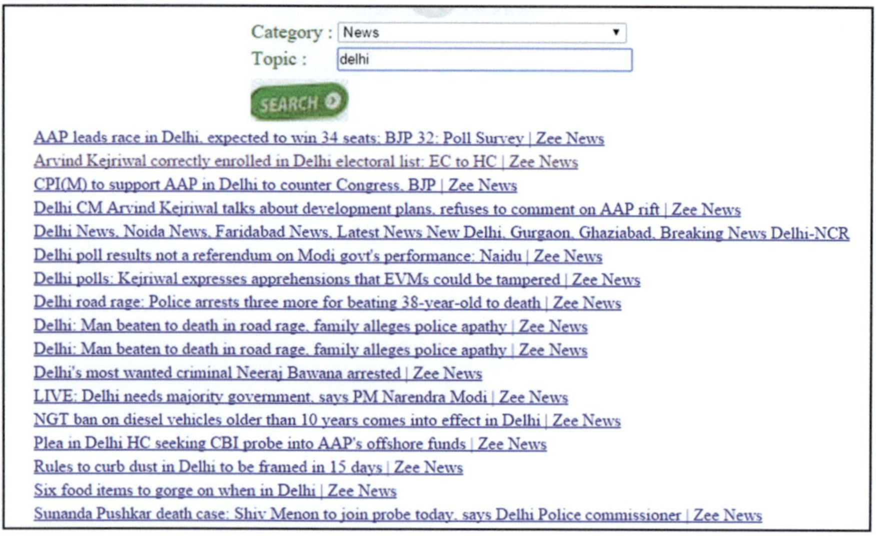

Fig. 6 Query searched in category news

5.1 *Comparing Relevancy Percentage*

Graph 3 shows that how our search engine has more relevant pages as results as compared to other search engines:

$$\text{Relevant Pages Percent} = \frac{\text{Relevant Results}}{\text{Total Results}} \times 100.$$

Graph 3 Comparison of search engine

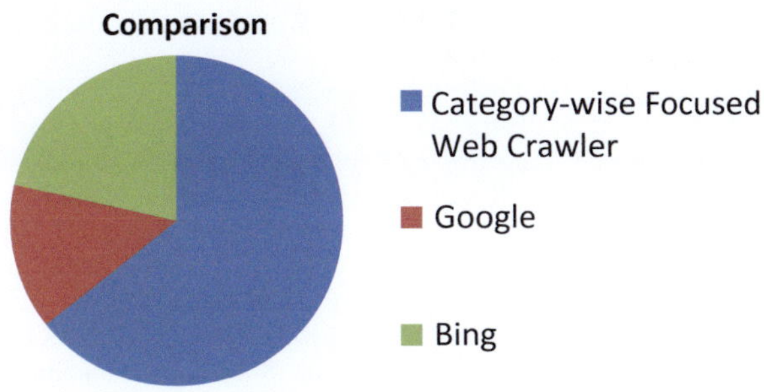

6 Conclusion

As the web is evolving, we should place our crawling and searching. As a result, the user will be able to find relevant and useful information in less time. So, focused crawlers can be used to categorize more relevant results. In the crawl module, focused crawler is focusing on the category specified by the user; while crawling, the crawler chooses the best web page to explore further, and in the search module, the topic is searched only among the category specified by the user. With this implementation, we have achieved our objective. With the help of this focused crawler, the user is able to find the most relevant information.

References

1. Chakrabarti, S., M. van den Berg, Dom, B.: Focused crawling: A new approach to topic-specific Web resource discovery. In: 8th International WWWConference (1999)
2. De Bra, P.M.E., Post, R.D.J.: Information retrieval in the world wide web: making client-based searching feasible. Comput. Networks ISDN Syst. **27**(2), 183–192 (1994)
3. Hersovici, M., Jacovi, M., Maarek, Y.S., Pelleg, D., Shtalhaim, M., UR, S.: The sharksearch algorithm—An application: tailored web site mapping. In: 7th International World-Wide Web Conference (1998)
4. Ester, M., Grob, M., Kriegel, H-.P.: Focused web crawling: A generic framework for specifying the user interest and for adaptive crawling strategies. In: 27 International Conference on Very Large Databases, VLDB pp. 633–637 (2001)
5. Jamali, M., Sayyadi, H., Hariri, B.B., Abolhassani, H.: A method for focused crawling using combination of link structure and content similarity. In: IEEE International Conference on Web Intelligence, pp. 753–756 (2006)
6. Safran, M.S., Althagafi, A., Che, D.: Improving relevance prediction for focused web crawlers. In: IEEE 11 International Conference on Computer and Information Science, (2012)
7. Sampat, J., Jain, A., Mistry, D.: Focused web crawler and its approaches. Int. J. Curr. Eng. Technol. **4**(5) (2014)
8. Monika, Pruthi, J.: Design of category-wise focused web crawler. IJARSE **4**, March 2015, Impact Factor- 1.1
9. Monika, Pruthi, J.: Focused web crawler: proposed architecture. In: 2nd International Conference on Innovation and Sustainability: Managing for Change, pp. 433–437 (2015)

10. Ahuja, M.S., Bal, J.S., Varnica.: Web crawler: Extracting the web data. Int. J. Comput. Trends Technol. **13**(3) (2014)
11. Kaur, M., Dhaliwal, Y.K.: Focused crawler: A review. IJARCSSE **4**(5) (2014)
12. Bastakis, S., Petrakis, E.G.M., Milios, E.: Improving the performance of focused web crawlers. J. Data Knowl. Eng. **68**(10), 1001–1013 (2009)
13. Pal, A., Tomar, D.S., Shrivastava, S.C.: Efficient focused crawling based on content and link structure analysis. Int. J. Comput. Sci. Inf. Secur. **2**(1) (2009)
14. Qu, C., Wang, B., Wei, P.: Efficient focused crawling strategy using combination of link structure and content similarity. IEEE (2008)
15. Peshave, M., Dezhgosha, K.: How search engine works and a web crawler application. (2005)
16. Menczer, Filippo, Pant, Gautam, Srinivasan, Padmini: Topical web crawlers: Evaluating adaptive algorithms. ACM Trans. Internet Technol. **4**(4), 378–419 (2004)
17. Pant, G., Srinivasan, P., Menczer, F.: Crawling the web. In: Levene, M., Poulovassilis, A. (eds.) Web Dynamics, Springer, New York (2003)

MAYA: An Approach for Energy and Cost Optimization for Mobile Cloud Computing Environments

Jitender Kumar and Amita Malik

Abstract Mobile Cloud Computing (MCC) is the latest paradigm shift to cope up the inherent limitations of SMDs (smart mobile devices). Various strategies have been proposed by the research community to counter these limitations, but current solutions focus mainly on energy and resources optimization and price benefits are still not explored. This paper presents a three-tier Cloud model, MAYA (mobile agility augmentation), to optimize energy and costs savings for MCC users, whereas at the same time it also reduces monetary cost for service providers. It categorizes the users in different price paying categories viz., maximum price paying users, medium price paying users, and low price paying users, based on the remaining battery and focuses on augmenting execution of compute intensive mobile workflow applications using Cloud resources, more profoundly known as *offloading*. This paper also presents two scheduling techniques for the realization of such system and shows the effectiveness of the MAYA system in minimizing the SaaS (Software as a service) provider's monetary cost as well as service user's cost.

Keywords MCC · Augmented execution · SMDs

1 Introduction

Current technology landscape and its ever-evolving nature has led to a new era of computing where SMDs with sophisticated operating systems are seamlessly being used for performing day-to-day activities. Besides this, the inherent challenges of mobile computing viz. limited battery; limited resources are still hindering its further growth. One of the key issues with SMD is battery life [1]. In fact, many

---

J. Kumar (✉) · A. Malik
Computer Science and Engineering Department,
DCRUST Murthal, Sonepat, Haryana, India
e-mail: jitenderkbhardwaj@gmail.com

A. Malik
e-mail: amitamalik.cse@gmail.com

V.B. Aggarwal et al. (eds.), *Big Data Analytics*, Advances in Intelligent Systems and Computing 654, https://doi.org/10.1007/978-981-10-6620-7_55

solutions are being proposed to overcome this limitation by using Cloud resources as remote resources due to their on-demand availability feature like [2–5].

However, the key challenge lies in mapping the individual mobile device demands on Cloud resources and how Cloud service providers manage these services. Pricing model is also a big concern as Cloud VMs are available for fixed time quanta. In case if an instance is used for less than an hour, charging users for complete one-hour duration would prove to be costlier for users. If per instruction pricing model is used and VM instance remains intact till the application finishes, then it would be costlier for service provider because during the execution of local executable component VM instance will remain unutilized. So the intermediate option like COSMOS [3] prevails which advocates for re-obtaining VM instance for each component of the application. However, the problem with COSMOS [3] is that it uses per instruction pricing model due to which penalties cannot be imposed on service providers for unnecessary queuing delays.

This paper chronologically investigates all such issues and presents a three-tier Cloud model, mobile agility augmentation (MAYA) which solves two key issues: (1) It solves the key problem of deciding which set of components would execute at Cloud so that customers would get the maximum energy saving in the required price paying category and (2) how the execution of Cloud 'offloadable' components can be carried out seamlessly on Cloud resources without paying the same prices for uneven energy savings due to unnecessary queuing delays. The optimization framework is completely placed on middleware server, so partitioning the framework does not impose extra overheads on the mobile device. It uses homogeneous size VMs so that the pricing as well as penalty policy would be uniform for all service users. However, at the same time, it also offers heterogeneity according to individual mobile demands.

The rest of the paper is organized as follows: Sect. 2 covers related work, Sect. 3 covers problem statement, Sect. 4 contains performance evaluation, Sect. 5 covers results and discussions, and Sect. 6 covers the conclusion and future scope.

2 Related Work

Kumar and Lu [6] proposed a framework whether computation offloading saves energy or not. Similarly, Cuervo et al. [1], Kovachev et al. [7], Shiraz and Gani [4], and Bohez et al. [5] proposed a distributed framework to enhance the compute resources of SMDs with the objective to minimize energy consumption and increase the responsiveness. But their work is limited to local Cloud, and the pricing and scheduling policies are not discussed. Yang et al. [8] exclusively assumed that the Cloud has abundant resources and the computation time at Cloud is negligible. But in practice, the computation time at Cloud side can never be negligible. Ferber et al. [2] exclusively assumed that an application has a single compute intensive component which needs to be executed remotely, but in practice an application may have more than one 'offloadable' component. Chun et al. [9] proposed partitioning

Table 1 Simulation parameters and values

Parameter	Value	Unit	Meaning
$P_{\mathrm{h}}^{\mathrm{m}}$	0.4	W	Power consumption by SMD processor when busy
$P_{\mathrm{l}}^{\mathrm{m}}$	0.05	W	Power consumption by SMD processor when idle
$P_{\mathrm{c}}^{\mathrm{m}}$	0.6	W	Power consumption by 3G connection of SMD
$P_{\mathrm{d}}^{\mathrm{m}}$	0.9	W	Power consumption by SMD display
$\mathrm{Bw}_{\mathrm{up}}$	300	KB/s	Upload bandwidth of SMD
$\mathrm{Bw}_{\mathrm{down}}$	400	Kb/s	Download bandwidth of SMD
$C_{\mathrm{speed}}^{\mathrm{m}}$	1.2	GHz	CPU clock speed of SMD
$C_{\mathrm{speed}}^{\mathrm{m}}$	2.5	GHz	CPU clock speed of c1.medium VM [11]
$C_{\mathrm{per\ minute}}^{\mathrm{vm\ cost}}$	0.024	$	Per minute CPU cost of c1.medium VM [11]

framework for offloading part of unmodified mobile phone application's execution from mobile device to the device clones. But such strategy requires exclusive VM for each request which is beneficial for either service providers or for service users. COSMOS [3] provides details of both scheduling and scaling, but it uses per instruction price policy due to which penalties cannot be imposed on the service providers, so all service users whether they suffered queuing delays or not have to pay same amount of price with uneven amount of computation speed ups. However, if the pricing model of COSMOS is changed from per instruction pricing to per minute pricing for accommodation of penalty model, then the execution cost on m1. medium instance would dominate the execution cost on c1.medium instance in just 5 min of execution, e.g., if the execution time on m1.medium instance with 2 GHz CPU core is 5 min, then the execution time on c1.medium instance with 2.5 GHz CPU core would be (5 * 2)/2.5 = 4 min (assuming that c1.medium instance is having only one core of 2.5 GHz). So according to the figures of Table 1 of COSMOS [3], the customer getting m1.medium instance would be paying $0.01, whereas customers getting c1.medium instance would be paying $0.0096.

3 Problem Statement

Let the sample workflow application represented by data flow graph is modeled as a set of components denoted by $s = \{C_0, C_2 \ldots C_{n+1}\}$where execution order is C_1 then C_2, and so on, and every component is a candidate for remote execution except the first and last one or more formally C_0 and C_{n+1}. A component is equivalent to a mobile service and is modeled as a 3-tuple $C_i = \{S_i, \mathrm{MI}_i, R_i\}$, where S_i denotes the amount of input data, R_i denotes the amount of output data, and MI_i denotes the amount of CPU workload required by the service and is measured in million instructions (MI). A mobile device is modeled as a 6-tuple $M_{\mathrm{config}} = \left\{C_{\mathrm{speed}}^{\mathrm{m}}, P_{\mathrm{h}}^{\mathrm{m}}, P_{\mathrm{l}}^{\mathrm{m}}, P_{\mathrm{c}}^{\mathrm{m}}, P_{\mathrm{d}}^{\mathrm{m}}, R_{\mathrm{battery}}^{\mathrm{m}}\right\}$, where $C_{\mathrm{speed}}^{\mathrm{m}}$ denotes the clock speed of SMD (in GHz), $P_{\mathrm{h}}^{\mathrm{m}}$ is the average power consumption by the SMD for local execution, $P_{\mathrm{l}}^{\mathrm{m}}$ is the average power consumption by the SMD when its CPU is idle, $P_{\mathrm{d}}^{\mathrm{m}}$ is the average power consumption by the display of the SMD and $P_{\mathrm{c}}^{\mathrm{m}}$ is the power consumption by the SMD during communication i.e., for upload/download of data. $R_{\mathrm{battery}}^{\mathrm{m}}$ denotes the remaining battery in the mobile device at the starting of a workflow application. A service provisioner is modeled as 3-tuple $\mathrm{Vm} = \left\{C_{\mathrm{speed}}^{\mathrm{vm}}, V_{\mathrm{comp}}^{\mathrm{vm}}, V_{\mathrm{data}}^{\mathrm{vm}}\right\}$ where $C_{\mathrm{speed}}^{\mathrm{vm}}$ is CPU clock speed of Cloud VM (in GHz) hosting the software service, $V_{\mathrm{comp}}^{\mathrm{vm}}$ is the computation cost at a particular VM leased from an IaaS provider, $V_{\mathrm{data}}^{\mathrm{vm}}$ is the cost of input and output data transferred from a particular VM instance. A variable x_i is introduced for each component C_i, which indicates whether the component C_i is to be executed locally (for $x_i = 1$) or remotely (for $x_i = 0$). The application partitioning problem is being formulated as 0/1 integer linear programming problem along with the objective to provide optimum energy savings in the required price paying category. The resulting solution $(x_1, x_2, \ldots x_n)$ represents the required partitioning of the application and is assumed to remain intact till the application finishes.

However, for scheduling, two policies are used, namely static scheduling and dynamic scheduling, and it is assumed that the corresponding component's code is available on the Cloud VMs exclusively as like SaaS services. Fully qualified names of remote methods can be attached by the middleware dynamically at run time or statically at application partitioning time. MAYA system contains three entities, namely client devices, trusted middleware, and service provisioner. Whenever an application starts on the mobile device, a signal is sent to the middleware server along with the information of amount of input data to the first component. The middleware then first categorizes the user in the corresponding price paying category. The initial categorization is based on the simple heuristics, i.e., if $R_{\mathrm{battery}}^{\mathrm{m}} \leq 60$, then the user is kept in maximum price paying category, if $60 < R_{\mathrm{battery}}^{\mathrm{m}} \leq 80$, then the user is kept in medium price paying category, if $R_{battery}^{\mathrm{m}} > 80$, then the user is kept in minimum price paying category.

The optimization solver in middleware tries to maximize energy savings (Eq. 1) within the required budget.

$$\max_{i \in n} \sum_{i=0}^{n} E_i^s * x_i \leq E_{\mathrm{req}}^{\mathrm{s}} \tag{1}$$

Such that

$$\sum_{i=0}^{n} V_i * x_i \leq \mathrm{Price}_{\mathrm{req}} \tag{2}$$

where

$$\text{Price}_{\text{req}} = \frac{\text{Price}_{\text{max}} * \text{cat}_{\text{req}}}{100} \quad (3)$$

And V_i is the sum of computation cost, input data cost, and output data cost. $\text{Price}_{\text{max}}$ is the cost of all 'offloadable' components. Input and output data cost can be calculated easily using the simple heuristic of comparison with per GB cost. E_i^{s} is the energy saving achieved by offloading the execution of C_i to Cloud and can be calculated similar to the work of Kumar and Lu [6].

4 Performance Evaluation

For the simulation purpose, we have extended the state of art Cloud Simulator CloudSim [10] with additional 10,000 added lines of code. A sample application containing 10 'offloadable' is used as workflow job. Output metrics collected for each scenario is VMs total price. COSMOS scaling policy is used for resource scaling. As no such application and its load characteristics are available, the framework has been evaluated with a synthetic workload. The requests arrive according to Poisson distribution with mean 3 per minute during the peak hours from 8:00 AM to 8:00 PM and 1.5 per minute during off-peak hours from 8:00 PM to 8:00 AM, respectively, with overall total 3272 requests. We first evaluate the effect of CCR (Communication to Computation time ratio) on the percentage of components transferred to Cloud, and percentage of energy saving achieved in different price paying categories. Sample readings of parameters $P_{\text{h}}^{\text{m}}, P_{\text{l}}^{\text{m}}, P_{\text{c}}^{\text{m}}, P_{\text{d}}^{\text{m}}$ are obtained from an HTC desire 500 phone using the work of [11]. These values are shown in Table 1.

5 Results and Discussions

Figure 1a shows the effect of communication to computation ratio (CCR) for different price paying categories. It shows that for medium price paying category all components start running on mobile device after the CCR reaches to 1.24. This is because for CCR greater than 1.24 only one component is available for execution at Cloud side yielding lesser than 5% energy saving. Also at CCR = 1.24, if the VM speed is changed from 2.5 to 2.0 GHz then only 0.096% energy saving is achieved which is too low. So like heterogeneous size VMs concept, homogeneous size VMs concept can also offer demand-based computing, but unlike heterogeneous size VMs, the use of homogeneous size VMs results in uniform pricing policy and customers getting m1.medium instance shall not have to pay higher prices. Figure 1b shows the effect of CCR for the percent of components transferred.

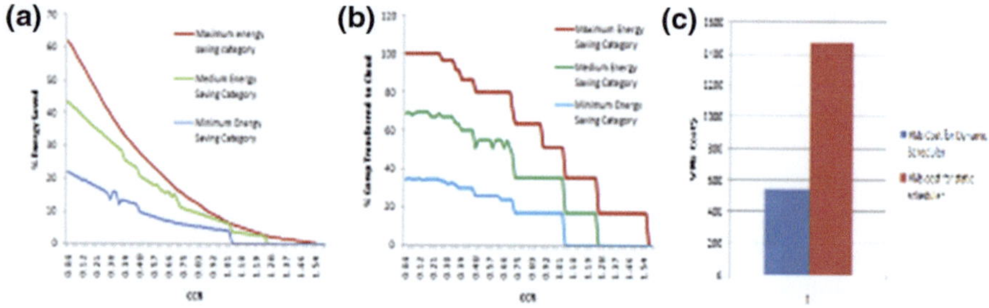

Fig. 1 **a** Impact of variation in CCR on % energy savings, **b** impact of variation in CCR on components transferred to cloud, **c** cost analysis of dynamic scheduler and static scheduler

However, Fig. 1c shows the price paid by SaaS provider for all VMs in static scheduler and dynamic scheduler. Although, static scheduler imposes lower overhead for service users but results in huge loss to the service provider in terms of VMs cost.

6 Conclusions and Future Work

Although adoption of Cloud platforms as software service provisioning environments has several benefits, there are still complexities hindering the opportunistic and uniform delivery of application services in such environments.

To counter those issues related to application provisioning over Clouds, this paper presented an improved mechanism for delivery of software service to users which resolves the individual mobile demands as well as compensates the price benefits in case of uneven delivery of service due to queuing delays.

As future work, the dynamic scheduler will be improved to further minimize monetary costs for service providers and extensive evaluation study will be carried out for all other parameters like VMs utilization, queuing delays, and penalty losses.

References

1. Cuervo, E., Balasubramanian, A., Cho, D.K., Wolman, A., Saroiu, S., Chandra, R., Bahl, P.: MAUI: Making Smartphones Last Longer with Code Offload. ACM MobiSys (2010)
2. Ferber, M., Rauber, T, Torres, M.H.C., Holvoet, T.: Resource allocation for cloud-assisted mobile applications. In: Proceedings of 5th IEEE Conference on Cloud Computing (CLOUD 2012), pp. 400–407
3. Shi, C., Habak, K., Pandurangan, P., Ammar, M., Naik, M., Zegura, E.: COSMOS: computaion offloading as a service for mobile devices (MobiHoc'14), Philadelphia, PA, USA, 11–14 Aug 2014. doi:10.1145/2632951.2632958

4. Shiraz, M., Gani, A.: A lightweight active service migration framework for computational offloading in mobile cloud computing. J. Supercomput. **68**, 978–995 (2014). doi:10.1007/s11227-013-1076-7
5. Bohez, S., Coninck, E.D., Verbelen, T., Simoens, P., Dhoedt, B.: Enabling component-based mobile cloud computing with AIOLOS middleware. In: ARM'14, Bordeaux, France, 9 Dec 2014. doi:10.1145/2677017.2677019
6. Kumar, K., Lu, Y.-H.: Cloud Computing for Mobile Users: Can Offloading computation saves Energy? IEEE Computer Society (2010)
7. Kovachev, D., Yu, T., Klamma, R.: Adaptive computation offloading from mobile devices into the cloud. In: Proceedings of 10th IEEE International Symposium on Parallel and Distributed Processing with Applications (ISPA 2012), pp. 784–791
8. Yang, L., Cao, J., Tang, S., Li, T., Chan, A.T.S.: A framework for partitioning and execution of data stream application in mobile cloud computing. In: IEEE Fifth International Conference on Cloud Computing (2012)
9. Chun, B.G., Ihm, S., Maniatis, P., Naik, M., Patti, A.: CloneCloud: elastic execution between mobile devices and Cloud. In: EuroSys, pp. 301–314 (2011)
10. Calheiros, R.N., Ranjan, R., Beloglazov, A., De Rose, C.A.F., Buyya, R.: CloudSim: a toolkit for modeling and simulation of cloud computing environments and evaluation of resource provisioning algorithms. Softw. Practice Exper. (SPE) **41**(1), 23–50 (2011). ISSN: 0038-0644
11. Zhang, L., Tiwana, B., Qian, Z., Wang, Z., Dick, R.P., Mao, Z.M., Yang, L.: Accurate online power estimation and automatic battery behavior based power model generation for smartphones. In: CODES + ISSS'10, Arizona, USA (2010). ACM 978-1-60558-905-3/10/10, 2010

Load Balancing in Cloud—A Systematic Review

Veenita Kunwar, Neha Agarwal, Ajay Rana and J.P. Pandey

Abstract Cloud computing is an upcoming technology, which has been recently introduced in the field of IT for delivering services that are hosted over the Internet. It is an amalgamation of Grid computing, Utility computing, Autonomic computing, and utilizes the concept of virtualization. It provides on demand service to the users for accessing resources, information, and software as per their needs. With increased popularity, there has been a tremendous increase in the demands of services by the users, which can be fulfilled by effective load balancing techniques. Load balancing allows even distribution of workload across various nodes in the cloud and aims to provide efficient utilization of resources, improving the system performance, minimizing the resource consumption resulting in low energy usage. In this paper, load balancing techniques proposed by researchers have been discussed and studied and a comparative analysis is being provided based on certain parameters.

Keywords Cloud computing · Load balancing · Virtualization

V. Kunwar (✉) · N. Agarwal · A. Rana
Amity University Uttar Pradesh, Noida, Uttar Pradesh, India
e-mail: veenitakunwar@gmail.com

N. Agarwal
e-mail: agarwalnehajain@gmail.com

A. Rana
e-mail: ajay_rana@amity.edu

J.P. Pandey
KNIT, Sultanpur, India
e-mail: tojppandey@rediffmail.com

V.B. Aggarwal et al. (eds.), *Big Data Analytics*, Advances in Intelligent Systems and Computing 654, https://doi.org/10.1007/978-981-10-6620-7_56

1 Introduction

In the modern era, the Internet technology is developing at a faster rate, which has led to increase in the number of user requests for various services, which needs to be fulfilled in minimum possible time. For this, faster processing of servers is required in order to respond to various client requests. Thus, cloud computing comes into the picture.

Cloud computing is an evolutionary outgrowth of prevailing technologies that provides hosting and storage services on the Internet. It is an on demand, virtualized, location independent, pay peruse pricing model, which aims to achieve optimal resource utilization and higher throughput. But there are also certain issues involved like security, privacy, load balancing, fault tolerance, server consolidation. This paper addresses the load balancing issues.

Load Balancing is one of the prime challenges in the cloud, which distributes the tasks among multiple nodes evenly to provide proper resource utilization improving the overall system performance. It also provides low energy usage and less rate of carbon emission, which helps to achieve green computing.

In this paper, we have discussed and compared various load balancing algorithms developed in the cloud. The rest of the paper is organized as follows: Sect. 2 gives the overview of the cloud. Section 3 describes load balancing and its types. In Sect. 4, we discuss various load balancing algorithms with pros and cons. Finally, Sect. 5 concludes the paper showing areas of improvement in load balancing algorithms for the future scope.

2 Cloud Computing Overview

As defined by NIST [1] *Cloud computing is a model for enabling ubiquitous, convenient, on-demand network access to a shared pool of configurable computing resources (e.g.,* networks, servers, *storage, applications, and services) that can be rapidly provisioned and released with minimal management effort or service provider interaction.* It provides various benefits like low hardware and maintenance cost, accessibility, flexibility, scalability, high reliability, multi-tenancy, quick response, faster deployment, location independence. It uses virtualization concepts, which are the key technology used in the cloud that hides the details of physical machines and provides virtualized resources to various applications. It can of two kinds, namely full and paravirtualization. In full virtualization, the whole system is installed on another system while in para, multiple operating systems execute on a single system providing only partial services.

Cloud has four deployment models named as private, public, hybrid, and community. Private cloud is used by a single organization and offers highest degree control over performance, security, maintenance, reliability, deployment, and use. They are more secure and expensive than public clouds. Public clouds on the other hand are hosted by cloud vendors and can be used by anyone but lack control over data, network, and security settings. Users need to pay depending on the service used. Its benefits are low cost, on demand scalability, flexibility, location independence, efficiency in shared resources. Hybrid cloud is a combination of public and private cloud offering improved flexibility, scalability, and security. Community cloud is shared among several organizations and managed internally or by third-party service providers and are secure and cost effective.

Cloud offers three service models named as IaaS, PaaS, and SaaS. In Infrastructure as a Service, the resources like servers, network, storage, virtual machines, data centers, load balancers are made available by cloud providers, which can be accessed by applications and operating systems. Examples include Amazon EC2, GoGrid. Platform as a service provides a platform including operating system, software development framework, database, and Web server, which makes the development, testing, deployment, and installation of applications in a quick and cost effective manner. Examples include Google App Engine, Microsoft Azure. Software as a service delivers various applications over the Internet, which are managed by a third party vendor. The users can get rid off installing and running applications on individual systems. Google Apps is an example.

3 Load Balancing in Cloud Computing

Load Balancing is a mechanism that plays a vital role in the cloud by distributing workload from overloaded nodes to under loaded nodes in an efficient manner to achieve optimal utilization of resources. The load can be of any kind like load on CPU, memory usage, delay, or load on the network. It aims to achieve maximum resource utilization, higher throughput, minimum response time, and increased user satisfaction. Its objective is to minimize energy consumption, enhance system performance, accommodate future modifications, build a fault-tolerant system, and maintain the stability of the system.

Load Balancing can be broadly classified as static and dynamic. Static algorithms do not take into account the current state of the system and aforementioned knowledge about system applications and resources is required to assign tasks at compile time and to process new requests. They are easy to implement and well suited for homogeneous environments. Dynamic algorithms are based on the current state of the system. The tasks are assigned to processors at runtime. They are complex to implement, but provide better fault tolerance and performance. They provide efficient load balancing, but may face runtime overheads and communication delays. Dynamic algorithms can be distributed or non-distributed. The distributed algorithm involves all the nodes of the system while in non-distributed one or some of the nodes perform load balancing. Further the distributed dynamic algorithms can be classified as cooperative and non-cooperative. In cooperative, the nodes try to achieve a common objective while in non-cooperative nodes work independently toward individual goals. The non-distributed dynamic algorithms can be classified further as semi-distributed and centralized. In semi-distributed, system nodes are divided into clusters performing load balancing of centralized kinds in each cluster. In centralized, the central node performs the balancing of workload.

3.1 Load Balancing Measurement Parameters

1. *Throughput*—It is used to estimate the number of tasks successfully completed in a given amount of time.
2. *Overhead Associated*—It tells the number of overheads associated while implementing an algorithm.
3. *Fault Tolerance*—It is the ability of an algorithm to perform well even after failure.
4. *Performance*—It checks the overall efficiency of the system.
5. *Scalability*—The algorithm should perform well with the increase in the number of nodes as per needs.
6. *Response Time*—It is the time interval between request sent and the response received.
7. *Resource Utilization*—It keeps the track of utilization of resources.
8. *Migration Time*—It is the amount of time taken for migrating tasks from one node to another.

4 Literature Review

4.1 Decentralized Content-Aware Load Balancing

A policy was given by Mehta et al. [2] known as workload and client aware policy (WCAP), which has a unique and special property (USP) that is used to define the property of the service provider's nodes as well as the user's requests for information. It enables the scheduler to decide an apt node that can process these requests. Its implementation is being done in a decentralized manner with minimum overheads.

4.2 Server-Based Load Balancing for Internet Distributed Services

This solution was proposed by Nakai et al. [3] for balancing load that decreases the service response time by sending requests to the nearest server avoiding their overload. A middleware is defined that implements it.

4.3 Join-Idle-Queue

The technique was suggested by Lua et al. [4] for distributed load balancing in large systems. Initially, the load is balanced on idle processors across dispatchers and then, jobs are assigned to processors in order to minimize the length of the queue at each processor. It minimizes system load and response time is decreased.

4.4 A Lock-Free Multiprocessing Solution for LB

Liu et al. [5] proposed a technique that avoids shared memory usage, unlike other multiprocessing load balancing techniques that require shared memory and lock to manage sessions. The performance is boosted.

4.5 A Task Scheduling Algorithm Based on Load Balancing

It was suggested by Fang et al. [6]. A two-level task scheduling mechanism is provided in which tasks are mapped to VMs and VMs to host resources. It effectively improves the response time and system performance.

4.6 Scheduling Strategy on Load Balancing of Virtual Machine Resources

This strategy was described by Hu et al. [7], which is based on genetic algorithm. It considers previous data and present state of the system. It avoids dynamic migration. It attains optimal resource utilization.

4.7 Central Load Balancing Policy for Virtual Machines

The algorithm has been suggested by Bhadani and Chaudhary [8] and in this load is balanced evenly across virtual machines. It makes the system function well.

4.8 LBVS: Load Balancing Strategy for Virtual Storage

The strategy described by Liu et al. [9] makes an available model for data storage and storage as a service model. A three-layered architecture is used to obtain storage virtualization, and two load balancing modules are required for balancing the load on the system. It improves the efficiency of concurrent access, minimizes the response time, and boosts disaster recovery. It offers flexibility and robustness.

4.9 Two-Phase Load Balancing Algorithm (OLB + LBMM)

This algorithm was suggested by Wang et al. [10] that integrates OLB (opportunistic load balancing) and LBMM (Load Balance Min-Min) scheduling algorithms to have better execution. The tasks are stored in a queue, which are performed by the manager. OLB scheduling manager assigns the job to the service manager. LBMM algorithm chooses the apt service node, which will execute the subtasks. OLB keeps every node in working state to accomplish the goal of load balancing, and LBMM is utilized to curtail the runtime of each task on a node, which helps to minimize the overall completion time. This combined approach helps in obtaining proper and efficient resource utilization and boosts the working efficiency of the system.

4.10 Compare and Balance

This distributed load balancing algorithm was suggested by Zhao et al. [11], which is based on sampling to attain an equilibrium solution. A model has been implemented to decrease the VM migration time using shared storage and to achieve the zero-downtime relocation of VM by changing them as Red Hat cluster services. Implementation is being provided by adaptive live migration of VMs.

4.11 Honeybee Foraging Behavior

A decentralized honeybee solution was investigated by Randles et al. [12], which is based on bee's behavior for finding and reaping food. Scout bees forage for food sources and advertise this through waggle dance, which helps to know about the quality, quantity, and distance of food from the beehive. They are followed by forager bees to the food location to reap it. The tasks are considered as honeybees, which are removed from overloaded VMs and submitted to under loaded VMs. VMs act as food sources. The task which is removed updates the remaining tasks about the status of the VM and gives an idea about the assignment of tasks to other VMs based on the VM availability and load. It improves the overall throughput and reduces waiting time of the task.

4.12 Biased Random Sampling

A distributed and scalable approach was explored by Randles et al. [12], which uses random sampling to realize self-organization. The server load is shown by its connectivity with each node in a virtual graph. Each server node represents a node in the graph, in which each in-degree is mapped to the free resources of the server. When a node starts a new job, an incoming edge is removed, which indicates that the resources available are decreased. When the node finishes a job an inward edge is created, which indicates that the resources available are increased. The addition and deletion process are executed by random sampling. The walk starts from a particular node and moves to a randomly chosen neighbor. The final node in the walk is chosen for the allocation of the load. When a job is received by the node, it will get executed if the job's present walk length is more than or equal to the threshold of walk length. Otherwise, the walk length of job, which is under consideration, will be incremented and will be sent to a random neighbor. On job completion, an edge is generated from the initiating node allocation process to the executing job node. A directed graph is obtained at last.

4.13 ACCLB (Load Balancing Mechanism Based on Ant Colony and Complex Network Theory)

This procedure was suggested by Zhang et al. [13]. It takes the characteristic of complex network into account. It has excellent fault tolerance, good scalability, and enhances system performance.

4.14 Ant Colony Optimization

Nishant [14] proposed an algorithm, which is a modified version of *ACCLB* and makes use of ant's behavior to collect information about nodes to assign the task. He tries to resolve the issue of synchronization in ACCLB by the addition of "suicide" feature to the ants. When a request is made the ant's movement starts from the "head" node. A forward movement indicates the ant's movement from one overloaded node in search of the other node. If an under-loaded node is found by ants, it will keep on moving to check the next node. If next node turns out to be overloaded, then ant will return back to the prior node. Ant commits suicide if the target node is found.

4.15 MapReduce

MapReduce [15] takes two major tasks: mapping of tasks and result reduction. It involves three methods known as part, comp, and group. Initially, the part method is executed for mapping the tasks. The request entity is divided into parts using map tasks. The hash key table saves the key of each part and comp method compares the parts. The group method combines the parts of similar entities through the reduce tasks. Reduce tasks may get overloaded due to parallel reading and processing of entities by map tasks. One more level is added, which decreases the load on the tasks. The large tasks are divided into smaller tasks, which are sent to the Reduce tasks.

4.16 Dual Direction FTP

The technique proposed by Al-Jaroodi and Mohamed [16] is a dual direction algorithm from FTP servers. It splits m sized into m/2 parts. Each and every server node processes the assigned task that depends on certain patterns. For instance, a server starts from block 0 and downloads incrementally while some other server begins from block m and keeps downloading decrementally. Both these servers work independently and download the complete file to the client on best time given the properties as well as the performance of these servers. The task is considered to be complete when two servers download two conservative blocks and remaining tasks are assigned to servers. It minimizes communication needed between client and nodes and hence reduce network overhead. Load on node, network, and speed are taken into account. It does not require any runtime monitoring.

4.17 LBMM

This algorithm has three level framework of load balancing [17]. It makes use of OLB, which is static in nature and might cause slower processing of tasks. LBMM enhances OLB by providing three-layer architecture. The request manager receives the tasks and assigns it to the service manager, which divides the tasks into subtasks to boost the processing of that request. The subtask is assigned to the service node based on CPU space, memory.

Table 1 Existing load balancing algorithms

Algorithm	Observations
Decentralized content aware [2]	Searching performance is enhanced with minimum idle time
LB for internet distributed services [3]	Service response time is reduced
Join-Idle-Queue [4]	No Communication overhead but power consumption is more
Lock-free multiprocessing [5]	Performance is improved
Task scheduling based on LB [6]	Improved response time and proper resource utilization
Scheduling strategy on LB of VM resources [7]	The issue of load imbalance is resolved, but migration cost is high
Central LB policy for VMs [8]	Improvement in overall performance but no fault tolerance
LBVS [9]	Provides flexibility, robustness, and data storage
Two-phase scheduling (OLB + LBMM) [10]	Enhanced work efficiency with optimal resource utilization and better execution time. It is suitable for static environment
Compare and balance [11]	Load is balanced among servers, and equilibrium is attained faster
Honeybee foraging behavior [12]	Performs well under heterogeneous resources
Biased random sampling [12]	Performance is better but does not suit a dynamic environment
ACCLB [13]	Suitable for dynamic environments and provides excellent fault tolerance, scalability
Ant colony optimization [14]	It is decentralized. Network overhead occurs. Provides fault tolerance
MapReduce [15]	Less number of overheads with high processing time. It has high implementation complexity
DDFTP [16]	The calculation is faster. It provides reliable file download. Full replication of data files requiring high storage. No network overheads. Provides fault tolerance. Low implementation complexity
LBMM [17]	Load unbalance of Min-Min is improved and reduces the execution time. Node selection for complex tasks is not specified
ESCE	Enhances response time and processing time but no fault tolerance
Throttled	Current load on the node is not considered
Modified throttled [18]	Provides better response time. The index table state may change

4.18 Equally Spread Current Execution (ESCE)

In this, VMs are scanned. If an available VM can handle the request, then request is assigned to it. If a VM is overloaded then some of its tasks are distributed to VM having minimum load. It faces single point failure.

4.19 Throttled

In this, state of each VM is recorded. On arrival of the request, a table is searched. If a match is found, then the request is accepted else -1 is returned and the request lies in the queue. It increases the response time.

4.20 Modified Throttled

In this, a table is maintained containing a list of VMs and their states. The first VM is selected in the same way as in throttled. On arrival of a subsequent request, VM which is next to already assigned VM is selected and steps are followed. It provides better response time in comparison with throttled [18] (Table 1).

5 Conclusion and Future Work

Cloud computing is a very vast domain. It is used widely in present times, and therefore load balancing has become a huge challenge to overcome. Load balancing is used to evenly distribute the workload among various nodes. Numerous techniques proposed by the researchers have been discussed in this paper, and a comparative analysis has been done. Each technique differs from the other and covers some of the parameters. There is a need to develop new techniques, which can satisfy all the parameters. In future, we will try to create new algorithms, which will maintain trade offs among various different performance parameters. Also, there is a requirement of energy efficient techniques that provide maximum resource utilization and reduce energy consumption which will contribute toward green computing.

References

1. Mell, P., Grance, T.: The NIST definition of cloud computing. National Institute of Standards and Technology, Computer Security Resource Center. www.csrc.nist.gov
2. Mehta, H., Kanungo, P., Chandwani, M.: Decentralized content aware load balancing algorithm for distributed computing environments. In: Proceedings of the International Conference Workshop on Emerging Trends in Technology (ICWET), pp. 370–375 (2011)
3. Nakai, A.M., Madeira, E., Buzato, L.E.: Load balancing for internet distributed services using limited redirection rates. In: 5th IEEE Latin-American Symposium on Dependable Computing (LADC), pp. 156–165 (2011)
4. Lua, Y., Xiea, Q., Kliotb, G., Gellerb, A., Larusb, J.R., Greenber, A.: Join-idle-queue: a novel load balancing algorithm for dynamically scalable web services. Int. J. Perform. Eval. **68**, 1056–1071 (2011)
5. Liu, S., Pan, L., Wang, C.-J., Xie, J.-Y.: A lock-free solution for load balancing in multi-core environment. In: 3rd IEEE International Workshop on Intelligent Systems and Applications (ISA), pp. 1–4 (2011)
6. Fang, Y., Wang, F., Ge, J.: A task scheduling algorithm based on load balancing in cloud computing. In: Web Information Systems and Mining. LNCS, vol. 6318, pp. 271–277 (2010)
7. Hu, J., Gu, J., Sun, G., Zhao, T.: A scheduling strategy on load balancing of virtual machine resources in cloud computing environment. In: Third International Symposium on Parallel Architectures, Algorithms and Programming (PAAP), pp. 89–96 (2010)
8. Bhadani, A., Chaudhary, S.: Performance evaluation of web servers using central load balancing policy over virtual machines on cloud. In: Proceedings of the Third Annual ACM Bangalore Conference (COMPUTE) (2010)
9. Liu, H., Liu, S., Meng, X., Yang, C., Zhang, Y.: LBVS: a load balancing strategy for virtual storage. In: International Conference on Service Sciences (ICSS), pp. 257–262. IEEE (2010)
10. Wang, S., Yan, K., Liao, W., Wang, S.: Towards a load balancing in a three-level cloud computing network. In: Proceedings of the 3rd IEEE International Conference on Computer Science and Information Technology (ICCSIT), Chengdu, China, pp. 108–113 (2010)
11. Zhao, Y., Huang, W.: Adaptive distributed load balancing algorithm based on live migration of virtual machines in cloud. In: Proceedings of 5th IEEE International Joint Conference on INC, IMS and IDC, Seoul, Republic of Korea, pp. 170–175(2009)
12. Randles, M., Lamb, D., Taleb-Bendiab, A.: A comparative study into distributed load balancing algorithms for cloud computing. In: Proceedings of 24th IEEE International Conference on Advanced Information Networking and Applications Workshops, Perth, Australia, pp. 551–556 (2010)
13. Zhang, Z., Zhang, X.: A load balancing mechanism based on ant colony and complex network theory in open cloud computing federation. In: Proceedings of 2nd International Conference on Industrial Mechatronics and Automation (ICIMA), Wuhan, China, pp. 240–243 (2010)
14. Nishant, K., Sharma, P., Krishna, V., Gupta, C., Singh, K.P., Nitin, N., Rastogi, R.: Load balancing of nodes in cloud using ant colony optimization. In: Proceedings 14th International Conference on Computer Modelling and Simulation (UKSim), pp. 3–8. IEEE (2012)
15. Kolb, L., Thor, A., Rahm, E.: Load balancing for MapReduce based entity resolution. In: Proceedings 28th International Conference on Data Engineering (ICDE), pp. 618–629. IEEE (2012)
16. Al-Jaroodi, J., Mohamed, N.: DDFTP: dual-direction FTP. In: Proceedings 11th IEEE/ACM International Symposium on Cluster, Cloud and Grid Computing (CCGrid), pp. 504–503. IEEE (2011)
17. Wang, S.-C., Yan, K.-Q., Liao, W.-P., Wang, S.-S.: Towards a load balancing in a three-level cloud computing network. In: Proceedings 3rd International Conference on Computer Science and Information Technology (ICCSIT), vol. 1, pp. 108–113. IEEE (2010)
18. Domanal, S.G., Ram Mohana Reddy, G.: Load balancing in cloud computing using modified throttled algorithm. In: IEEE, International conference on CCEM (2013)

Cloud-Based Big Data Analytics—A Survey of Current Research and Future Directions

Samiya Khan, Kashish Ara Shakil and Mansaf Alam

Abstract The advent of the digital age has led to a rise in different types of data with every passing day. In fact, it is expected that half of the total data will be on the cloud by 2016. This data is complex and needs to be stored, processed, and analyzed for information that can be used by organizations. Cloud computing provides an apt platform for big data analytics in view of the storage and computing requirements of the latter. This makes cloud-based analytics a viable research field. However, several issues need to be addressed and risks need to be mitigated before practical applications of this synergistic model can be popularly used. This paper explores the existing research, challenges, open issues, and future research direction for this field of study.

Keywords Cloud-based big data analytics · Big data · Big data analytics · Big data cloud computing

1 Introduction

With the advent of the digital age, the amount of data being generated, stored, and shared has been on the rise. From data warehouses, Web pages, and blogs to audio/video streams, all of these are sources of massive amounts of data. The result of this proliferation is the generation of massive amounts of pervasive and complex data, which needs to be efficiently created, stored, shared, and analyzed to extract useful information.

S. Khan (✉) · K.A. Shakil · M. Alam
Department of Computer Science, Jamia Millia Islamia, New Delhi, India
e-mail: samiyashaukat@yahoo.com

K.A. Shakil
e-mail: shakilkashish@yahoo.co.in

M. Alam
e-mail: malam2@jmi.ac.in

V.B. Aggarwal et al. (eds.), *Big Data Analytics*, Advances in Intelligent Systems and Computing 654, https://doi.org/10.1007/978-981-10-6620-7_57

This data has huge potential, ever-increasing complexity, insecurity and risks, and irrelevance. The benefits and limitations of accessing this data are arguable in view of the fact that this analysis may involve access and analysis of medical records, social media interactions [1], financial data, government records, and genetic sequences. The requirement of an efficient and effective analytics service, applications, programming tools, and frameworks has given birth to the concept of Big Data Processing and Analytics.

Big data analytics has found application in several domains and fields. Some of these applications include medical research, solutions for the transportation and logistics sector, global security, and prediction and management of issues concerning the socioeconomic and environmental sector, to name a few. Apart from standard applications in business [2] and commerce and society administration, scientific research is one of the most critical applications of big data in the real world [3].

According to O'Driscoll et al. [4], one of the main future applications of big data analytics and cloud computing lies in life sciences. Some of the identified high-impact areas include systems biology, structure and protein function prediction, personalized medicine, and meta-genomics. Besides this, one of the most relevant applications of big data analytics is to improve the existing business models for efficiency and customer satisfaction.

Big data, by definition, is a term used to describe a variety of data— structured, semi-structured, and unstructured—which makes it a complex data infrastructure [5]. The complexity of this infrastructure requires powerful management and technological solutions. One of the commonly used models for explaining big data is the multi-V model. Figure 1 illustrates the multi-V model.

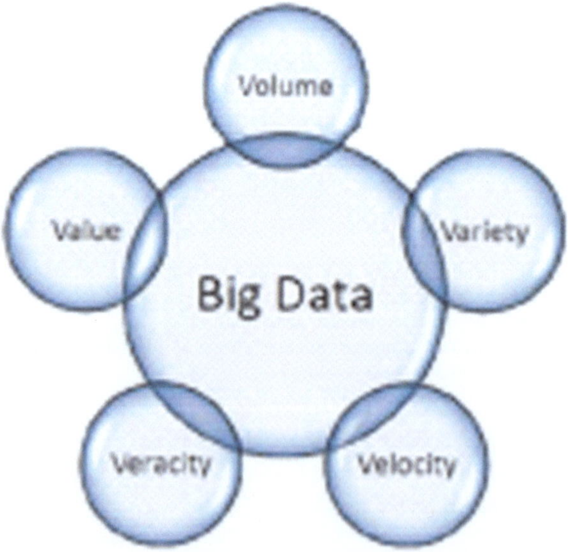

Fig. 1 Big data characteristics [37]

Some of the V's used to characterize big data include variety, volume, velocity, veracity, and value [6]. The different types of data available on a dataset determine variety while the rate at which data is produced determines velocity. Predictably, the size of data is called volume. The two additional characteristics, veracity and value, indicate data reliability and worth with respect to big data exploitation, respectively.

In addition, Wu et al. [7] proposed another characterization called the HACE theorem. According to this theorem, big data has two main characteristics. Firstly, it has a large volume of data that comes from different and heterogeneous sources, which is complex in nature. Secondly, the data is decentralized and distributed in nature.

Data is the central element of communication and collaboration in Internet and all the applications that are built on this platform. The immense popularity of data-intensive applications like Facebook, LinkedIn, Twitter, Amazon, eBay, and Google + contributes to the increasing requirement of storage and processing of data in the cloud environment. Schouten [8] used Gartner's estimation to predict that by the year 2016, half of the data will be on the cloud.

Moreover, the data mining algorithms used for Big Data analytics possess high computing requirements. Therefore, they require high-performance processors to do the job. The cloud provides a good platform for big data storage, processing, and analysis, addressing two of the main requirements of big data analytics, high storage, and high-performance computing.

The cloud computing environment offers development, installation, and implementation of software and data applications 'as a service.' Three multi-layered infrastructures, namely platform as a service (PaaS), software as a service (SaaS), and infrastructure as a service (IaaS), exist [9]. Infrastructure as a service is a model that provides computing and storage resources as a service. On the other hand, in case of PaaS and SaaS, the cloud services provide software platform or software itself as a service to its clients.

The cost of storage has considerably reduced with the advent of cloud-based solutions. In addition, the 'pay-as-you-go' model and the concept of commodity hardware allow effective and timely processing of large data, giving rise to the concept of 'big data as a service.' An example of one such platform is Google BigQuery, which provides real-time insights from big data in the cloud environment [10]. Shakil et al. [11] demonstrated the application of cloud for management of Big Data in educational institutions which specially focus on university-level data.

However, there have not been many practical applications of big data analytics that make use of the cloud. This has led to an increasing shift of research focus toward cloud-based big data analytics. An issue that is evident in this arrangement is information security and data privacy. As part of the cloud services, trust in data is also defined as a service. There shall be a considerable decrease in trust in view of the fact that the chances of security breaches and privacy violation will significantly rise upon implementation of big data strategies in the cloud. In addition, another important issue of ownership and control will also exist.

However, the potential of cloud-based big data analytics has compelled researchers to look into the existing issues to explore solutions. This paper discusses the different facets and aspects of data mining techniques/strategies adoption in the cloud environment for big data analytics. Moreover, it also looks into the existing research, identified challenges, and future research directions in cloud-based big data analytics.

2 Background

Traditional data management tools and data processing or data mining techniques cannot be used for Big Data analytics for the large volume and complexity of the datasets that it includes. Conventional business intelligence applications make use of methods, which are based on traditional analytics methods and techniques and make use of OLAP, BPM, mining, and database systems like RDBMS.

It was in the 1980 s that artificial intelligence-based algorithms were developed for data mining. Wu et al. [12] mentioned the ten most influential data mining algorithms k-means, C4.5, Apriori, Expectation Maximization (EM), PageRank, SVM (support vector machine), AdaBoost, CART, Naïve Bayes, and kNN (k-nearest neighbors). Most of these algorithms have been used commercially as well. Alam and Shakil [13] proposed an architecture for management of data through cloud techniques.

One of the most popular models used for data processing on cluster of computers is MapReduce [14]. Jackson et al. [15] provided a survey on the programming models that support big data analytics. It identifies MapReduce/Hadoop as the most productive model for Big Data analytics yet mentions that languages and extensions like HiveQL, Latin, and Pig have overpowering benefits for this use.

Hadoop is simply an open-source implementation of the MapReduce framework, which was originally created as a distributed file system. According to Neaga and Hao [16], the evolution of Hadoop as a complete ecosystem or infrastructure that works alongside MapReduce components and includes a range of software systems like Hive and Pig languages, a coordination service called Zookeeper and a distributed table store called HBase.

For cloud-based big data analytics, several frameworks like Google MapReduce, Spark, Haloop, Twister, Hadoop Reduce, and Hadoop++ are available. Figure 2 gives a pictorial representation of the use of cloud computing in big data analytics. These frameworks are used for storing and processing of data. In order to store this data, which may be of any structure, databases like HBase, BigTable, and HadoopDB may be used. When it comes to data processing, the Pig and Hive technologies come into the picture.

Some of the recent research breakthroughs and milestones in cloud-based big data analytics are discussed here. Lee et al. [17] elaborated on the advantages and limitations of MapReduce in parallel data analytics. A Hadoop-based data analytics system, created by Starfish [18], improves the performance of the clusters

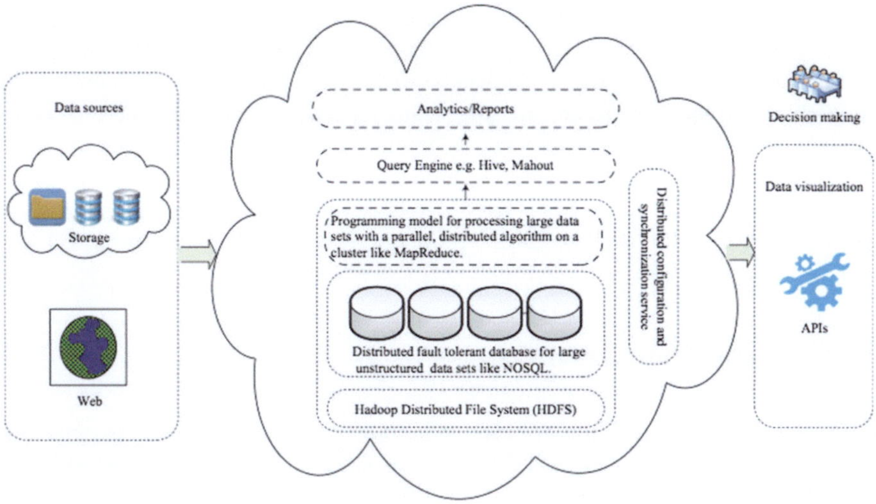

Fig. 2 Use of cloud computing in big data [38]

throughout the cycle of data analytics. Moreover, the users are not required to understand the configuration details.

In recent times, lack of interactivity has been identified as a major issue, and several efforts have been made in this area. Borthakur et al. [19] optimized the HBase and HDFS implementation for better responsiveness. Strambei [20] evaluated the viability of OLAP Web Services for cloud-based architectures, with the specific objective to allow open and wide access to web analytical technologies.

Research efforts have been made to create a big data management framework for the cloud. Khan et al. [21] proposed a data model and provided a schema for big data in the cloud and attempted to ease the process of querying data for the user. Moreover, performance and speed of operation have been important subjects of research. Ortiz et al. [22] explored the use of a proposed integrated Hadoop and MPI/OpenMP system and how the same can improve speed and performance.

In view of the fact that data needs to be transferred between data centers that are usually located distances apart, power consumption becomes a crucial parameter when it comes to analyzing the efficiency of the system. A network-based routing algorithm called GreeDi can be used for finding the most energy efficient path to the cloud data center during big data processing and storage [23]. There are several practical simulation-enabled analytics systems. One such system is given by Li et al. [24], which is a direct acrylic graph (DAG) from analytical application used for modeling and predicting the outbreak of Dengue in Singapore.

Online risk analytics and the need for an infrastructure that can provide users the programming resources and infrastructure for carrying out the same have also appeared in the form of Aneka [25] and CometCloud [26]. Chen et al. [27], and

Demirkan and Delen [28] investigated the concept of CAAAS or continuous analytics as a service, which is used for predicting the behavior of a service or a user.

The last topic under Big Data Analysis that has caught the attention of the research community is Real-time Big Data Analysis. Many commercial cloud service providers are providing solutions for real-time analysis. AWS based-solution for real-time stream processing is AWS Kinesis [29]. Many frameworks and software systems have also been introduced for this purpose, some of which are Apache S4 [30], IBM InfoSphere Streams [31], and Storm [32].

3 Challenges and Issues

In order to move beyond the existing techniques and strategies used for machine learning and data analytics, some challenges need to be overcome. NESSI [33] identified the following requirements as critical.

- In order to select an adequate method or design, a solid scientific foundation needs to be developed.
- New efficient and scalable algorithms need to be developed.
- For proper implementation of devised solutions, appropriate development skills and technological platforms must be identified and developed.
- Lastly, the business value of the solutions must be explored just as much as the data structure and its usability.

It is paradoxical that the tools and software to be developed for analyzing the huge and complex data are expected to be simple and uncomplicated. Additionally, these solutions must be naturally inclined toward parallel and distributed computing and must be based on foundations of computational paradigms. This is what that gives rise to the need for newer and better simulation and visualization technologies and tools. A summary of the issues and challenges pointed out by Assuncao et al. [6] is given in Table 1.

In view of cloud-based big data analytics, additional challenges like adoption and implementation of effective big data solutions using cloud architecture and mitigating the security and privacy risks also exist. One of the biggest concerns while using big data analytics and cloud computing in an integrated model is security. This is perhaps the reason why this aspect of cloud-based big data analytics and its practical usage, and implementation has attracted immense attention.

Liu et al. [34] provided a summary, analysis, and comparison of authenticator-based data integrity verification techniques on cloud and Internet-of-things data. This paper suggests that any future developments in this area need to look at three main aspects, namely efficiency, security, and scalability/elasticity.

A G-Hadoop-based security framework is proposed by Zhao et al. [35], which makes use of solutions like SSL and public key cryptography for ensuring security

Table 1 Summary of identified issues and challenges

Category	Issues/challenges
Data management	• Handling ever-increasing volumes and varieties of data • Storing data more efficiently • Integration and porting of data between different data centers • Data integration for data coming from different sources and of diverse types • Optimization of energy consumption and resource usage
Model building and scoring	• Exploring the elasticity and scalability potential of the cloud
Visualization and user interaction	• Finding better data processing techniques for real-time visualization • Exploring options that can lead to more cost-effective devices, particularly for large scale visualization
Business value-related and others	• From the perspective of business-related applications, striking a balance between generality and usefulness is a challenge • Finding techniques for better interactivity in the cloud to improve usability of the solution from the data analysts' point of view • Debugging and checking the validity of the developed solutions • Other non-technical challenges also exist, which include lack of staffing, skills, and business support

of big data resident on distributed cloud data centers. In addition to several security mechanisms, this framework also aims to simplify the processes of submitting job and authenticating users. Talia [36] suggested further research and development in the following areas:

- Programming abstracts or scalable high-level models and tools.
- Solutions for data and computing interoperability issues.
- Integration of different big data analytics frameworks.
- Techniques for mining provenance data.

4 Future Research Directions

Several open source data mining techniques, resources, and tools exist. Some of these include R, Gate, Rapid-Miner, and Weka, in addition to many others. Cloud-based big data analytics solutions must provide a provision for the availability of these affordable data analytics on the cloud so that cost-effective and efficient services can be provided. The fundamental reason why cloud-based analytics are such a big thing is their easy accessibility, cost-effectiveness, and ease of setting up and testing. In view of this, some of the main research directions identified by Neaga and Hao [16] include:

- Evolution of analytics and information management with respect to cloud-based analytics.

- Adaptation and evolution of techniques and strategies to improve efficiency and mitigate risks.
- Formulate strategies and techniques to deal with the privacy and security concerns.
- Analysis and adaptation of legal and ethical practices to suit the changing viewpoint, impact, and effects of technological advances in this regard.

With this said, the research directions are not limited to the above-mentioned points. The main goal is to transform the cloud from being a data management and infrastructure platform to a scalable data analytics platform.

5 Conclusion

This is an age of big data and the emergence of this field of study has attracted the attention of many practitioners and researchers. Considering the rate at which data is being created in the digital world, big data analytics and analysis have become all the more relevant. Moreover, most of this data is already on the cloud. Therefore, shifting big data analytics to the cloud framework is a viable option.

Moreover, the cloud infrastructure suffices the storage and computing requirements of data analytics algorithms. On the other hand, open issues like security, privacy, and the lack of ownership and control exist. Research studies in the area of cloud-based big data analytics aim to create an effective and efficient system that addresses the identified risks and concerns.

References

1. Chen, H., Chiang, R.H.L., Storey, V.C.: Business intelligence and analytics: from big data to big impact. Bus. Intell. Res., MIS Quarterly. Special Issue (2012)
2. GigaSpaces: Big data survey. http://www.gigaspaces.com/sites/default/files/product/BigDataSurvey_Report.pdf
3. Chen, C.L.P., Zhang, C.Y.: Data-intensive applications, challenges, techniques and technologies: a survey on Big Data. Inf. Sci. **275**, 314–347 (2014)
4. O'Driscoll, A., Daugelaite, J., Sleator, R.D.: 'Big data', hadoop and cloud computing in genomics. J. Biomed. Inform. **46**(5), 774–781 (2013)
5. Manekar, A., Pradeepini, G.: A review on cloud-based big data analytics. ICSES J. Comput. Netw. Commun. (IJCNC) **1**(1) (2015)
6. Assuncao, M.D., Calheiros, R.N., Bianchi, S., Netto, M.A.S.: Big data computing and clouds: trends and future directions. J. Parallel Distrib. Comput. **79–80**, 3–15 (2015)
7. Wu, X., Zhu, X., Wu, G., Ding, W.: Data mining with big data. Retrieved from: http://www.cs.umb.edu/~ding/papers/TKDE2013.pdf. (2013)
8. Schouten, E: Big data as a service. http://edwinschouten.nl/2012/09/19/bigdata-as-a-service/ (2012)
9. Agarwal, D., Das, S., Abbadi, A.: Big data and cloud computing: current state and future opportunities. ACM 978-1-4503-0528-0/11/0003 (2011)

10. Google Cloud Platform: Big query. https://cloud.google.com/bigquery/
11. Shakil, K.A., Sethi, S., Alam, M.: An effective framework for managing university data using a cloud based environment. In: 2nd International Conference on Computing for Sustainable Global Development (INDIACom), vols. 1262, 1266, pp. 11–13 (2015)
12. Wu, X., Kumar, V., Quinlan, J.R., Ghosh, J., Yang, Q., Motoda, H., McLachlan, G.J., Ng, A., Liu, B., Yu, P.S., Zhou, Z.H., Steinbach, M., Hand, D.J., Steinberg, D.: Top 10 algorithms in data mining. Knowl Inf. Syst. **14**:1–37
13. Alam, M., Shakil, K.A.: Cloud database management system architecture. UACEE Int. J. Comput. Sci. Appl. **3**(1), 27–31 (2013)
14. Dean, J., Ghemawat, S.: OSDI 2004, http://static.googleusercontent.com/media/research.google.com/en//archive/mapreduce-osdi04.pdf
15. Jackson, J.C., Vijayakumar, V., Quadir, M.A., Bharathi, C.: Survey on programming models and environments for cluster, cloud and grid computing that defends big data. In: 2nd International Symposium on Big Data and Cloud Computing (ISBCC'15), pp. 517–523 (2015)
16. Neaga, I., Hao, Y.: A holistic analysis of cloud based big data mining. Int. J. Knowl. Innov. Entrepreneurship. **2**(2), 56–64 (2014)
17. Lee, K.H., Lee, Y.J., Choi, H., Chung, Y.D., Moon, B.: Parallel data processing with MapReduce: a survey. SIGMOD Rec. **40**(4), 11–20 (2011)
18. Herodotou, H., Lim, H., Luo, G., Borisov, N., Dong, L., Cetin, F.B., Babu, S.: Starfish: a self-tuning system for big data analytics. In: Proceedings of the 5th Biennial Conference on Innovative Data Systems Research (CIDR 2011), pp. 261–272 (2011)
19. Borthakur, D., Gray, J., Sarma, J.S., Muthukkaruppan, K., Spiegelberg, N., Kuang, H., Ranganathan, K., Molkov, D., Menon, A., Rash, S., Schmidt, R., Aiyer, A.: Apache Hadoop goes real-time at Facebook. In: Proceedings of the ACM SIGMOD International Conference on Management of Data, ACM, New York, USA, pp. 1071–1080 (2011)
20. Strambei, C.: OLAP services on cloud architecture. J. Softw. Syst. Develop. (2012). doi:10.5171/2012.840273
21. Khan, I., Naqvi, S.K. Alam, M. Rizvi, S.N.A.: Data model for Big Data in cloud environment. In: 2nd International Conference on Computing for Sustainable Global Development (INDIACom), pp. 582–585 (2015)
22. Ortiz, J.L.R., Oneto, L., Anguita, D.: Big data analytics in the cloud: spark on hadoop vs MPI/OpenMP on Beowulf. P2015 INNS Conference on Big Data, vol. 53, 121–130 (2015)
23. Baker, T., Al-Dawsari, B., Tawfik, H., Reid, D., Nyogo, Y.: GreeDi: an energy efficient routing algorithm for big data on cloud. Ad Hoc Netw. **000**, 1–14 (2015)
24. Li, X., Calheiros, R.N., Lu, S., Wang, L., Palit, H., Zheng, Q., Buyya, R.: Design and development of an adaptive workflow-enabled spatial-temporal analytics framework. In: Proceedings of the IEEE 18th International Conference on Parallel and Distributed Systems (ICPADS 2012), pp. 862–867. IEEE Computer Society, Singapore (2012)
25. Calheiros, R.N., Vecchiola, C., Karunamoorthy, D., Buyya, R.: The Aneka platform and QoS-driven resource provisioning for elastic applications on hybrid Clouds. Fut. Gener. Comput. Syst. **28**(6), 861–870 (2012)
26. Kim, H., Abdelbaky, M., Parashar, M.: CometPortal: a portal for online risk analytics using CometCloud. In: 17th International Conference on Computer Theory and Applications (ICCTA2009) (2009)
27. Chen, Q., Hsu, M., Zeller, H.: Experience in continuous analytics as a service (CaaaS). In: Proceedings of the 14th International Conference on Extending Database Technology, ACM, New York, USA, pp. 509–514 (2011)
28. Demirkan, H., Delen, D.: Leveraging the capabilities of service-oriented decision support systems: putting analytics and big data in cloud. Decis. Support Syst. **55**, 412–421 (2013)
29. Amazon Kinesis: Developer resources. http://aws.amazon.com/kinesis/developer-resources/
30. Apache S4: Distributed stream computing platform. http://incubator.apache.org/s4/
31. IBM InfoSphere Streams: InfoSphere Streams. http://www.ibm.com/software/products/en/infosphere-streams

32. Storm: Apache Storm: Distributed and fault-tolerant real-time computation. http://storm.incubator.apache.org
33. NESSI: Big data: a new world of opportunities. http://www.nessi-europe.com/Files/Private/NESSI_WhitePaper_BigData.pdf (2012)
34. Liu, C., Yang, C., Zhang, X., Chen, J.: External integrity verification for outsourced big data in cloud and IoT: a big picture. Futu. Gener. Comput. Syst. **49**, 58–67 (2015)
35. Zhao, J., Wang, L., Tao, J., Chen, J., Sun, W., Ranjan, R., Kołodziej, J., Streit, A., Georgakopoulos, D.: A security framework in G-Hadoop for big data computing across distributed cloud data centers. J. Comput. Syst. Sci. **80**, 994–1007 (2014)
36. Talia, D.: Clouds for scalable big data analytics. Published by IEEE Computer Society (2013), http://scholar.google.co.in/scholar_url?url=http://xa.yimg.com/kq/groups/16253916/1476905727/name/06515548.pdf&hl=en&sa=X&scisig=AAGBfm12aY-Nbu37oZYRuEqeqsdslzKfBQ&nossl=1&oi=scholarr&ved=0CCYQgAMoADAAahUKEwi3k4Hymv7GAhUHUKYKHdToBCM
37. Elragal, A.: ERP and big data: the inept couple. Procedia Technol. **16**, 242–249 (2014)
38. Hashem, I.A.T., Yaqoob, I., Anuar, N.B., Mokhtar, S., Gani, A., Khan, S.U.: The rise of "big data" on cloud computing: review and open research issues. Inf. Syst. **47**, 98–115 (2015)

Fully Homomorphic Encryption Scheme with Probabilistic Encryption Based on Euler's Theorem and Application in Cloud Computing

Vinod Kumar, Rajendra Kumar, Santosh Kumar Pandey and Mansaf Alam

Abstract Homomorphic encryption is an encryption scheme that allows different operations on encrypted data and produces the same result as well that the operations performed on the plaintext. Homomorphic encryption can be used to enhance the security measure of un-trusted systems which manipulates and stores sensitive data. Therefore, homomorphic encryption can be used in cloud computing environment for ensuring the confidentiality of processed data. In this paper, we propose a fully Homomorphic Encryption Scheme with probabilistic encryption for better security in cloud computing.

Keywords Homomorphism · Cloud computing · Fully homomorphic encryption · Security

1 Introduction

Cloud computing enables sharing of services and focuses on maximizing the effectiveness of the shared resources. In the Cloud computing the user data place their data in the cloud, and any computation on the stored data will be performed on the cloud. The Cloud computing has privacy issues because the service provider can access, alter or even delete the data intentionally. Some of the cloud service providers share the information with third parties to provide the effective services. The

V. Kumar
Department of I.T, Centre for Development of Advanced Computing Noida, Noida, India

R. Kumar · M. Alam (✉)
Department of Computer Science, Jamia Millia Islamia, New Delhi, India
e-mail: malam2@jmi.ac.in

S.K. Pandey
Department of Electronics and Information Technology, Ministry of Communication and Information Technology, New Delhi, India

V.B. Aggarwal et al. (eds.), *Big Data Analytics*, Advances in Intelligent Systems and Computing 654, https://doi.org/10.1007/978-981-10-6620-7_58

third party can also access the user private data and modifies the information to make it beneficial to himself. Therefore, security is major thing over the cloud. To protect the private information from cloud service provider or third party—encryption is needed. But it is not enough to protect the computation done on the cloud because to perform computation, decryption of stored data is needed on the cloud.

To protect such computation on the cloud, we need an encryption scheme that enables us to perform the computation of encrypted data. The Fully Homomorphic encryption is the technique that can be used to perform computation on encrypted data [1]. Homomorphic encryption is the encryption scheme that allows to perform some computations on message without decrypting the message [2]. Therefore, using Fully Homomorphic scheme we can perform any computations on the cloud stored data without any obstruction by cloud provider [3].

Here, we propose an Euler's Theorem-Based Fully Homomorphic Encryption Scheme with probabilistic Encryption to solve the issues of third-party control and data security of Cloud computing.

The Remaining part of the paper is organized as follows. Section 2 describes the related work. Section 3 provides the details of proposed scheme and proof of correctness of scheme. Section 4 presents a working example. Finally, Sect. 5 describes concluding remarks of contributions.

2 Related Work

In 1978, the concept of Homomorphic encryption introduced by Ronald Rivest, Leonard Adleman, and Michael Dertouzos. In 1982, Shafi Goldwasser and Silvio Micali invented an additive Homomorphic encryption that can encrypt only single bit. In 1999 Pa Paillier also given an additive Homomorphic encryption. In 2005, a security system that can compute only one multiplication and an unlimited number of additions proposed by Dan Boneh, et al. In 2009, the first fully Homomorphic encryption system that computes an arbitrary number of additions and multiplications proposed by Gentry and Halevi [4], Gentry [5]. Gentry [3] also proposed ideal lattices hardness based a fully homomorphic encryption in 2009. In 2010, A Fully homomorphic encryption scheme based on integers given by Van Dijk et al. [6]. In 2012, Xiang Guangli, Cui Zhuxiao proposed Fermat's Little Theorem Based, Algebra Homomorphic Encryption Scheme that works for rational number [7].

3 Fully Homomorphic Encryption with Probabilistic Encryption

Our proposed scheme is fully homomorphic scheme with probabilistic Encryption, which supports both additive and multiplicative homomorphism property. It is also based on Euler's theorem that can be thought of as a generalization of Fermat's little theorem. The Fermat theorem uses prime modulus, and the modulus in Euler's theorem is an integer. Two versions of Euler theorem are as follows:

1. If a and n are co-prime, then $a^{\varnothing(n)} \equiv 1 (\bmod n)$.
2. It removes the condition that a and n should be co-prime. If $n = p \times q, a < n$, and k an integer, then $a^{k \times \varnothing(n) + 1} \equiv a (\bmod n)$.

The Euler's theorem sometimes is helpful for quickly finding a solution to some exponentiations. The proposed Homomorphic encryption scheme consists three phases which are as follows:

- Key generation
- Message Encryption
- Message Decryption

Phase-I: Key Generation

1. Select two prime numbers p and q
2. Calculate $n = p \times q$ and $\varnothing(n)$
3. Select another prime number z such that $\gcd(n, z) = 1$
4. Calculate $x = n \times z$

Phase-II: Messages Encryption

1. Messages addition $(M_1 + M_2)$ and multiplication $(M_1 * M_2)$ should be less than $< n.$, therefore, M_1 & M_2 will always be less than n
2. Select two random integer k_1 and k_2 for probabilistic encryption
3. $C_1 = M^{k_1 \times \varnothing(n) + 1} \bmod x$ and $C_2 = M^{k_2 \times \varnothing(n) + 1} \bmod x$
   Here, C_1 and C_2 are cipher texts
4. Evaluate result C_3 after performing operations on cipher texts C_1 and C_2

Phase-III: Message Decryption

1. $M = C_3 \bmod n$, Where C_3 is cipher text after performing operations on C_1 and C_2, n is private key and M is plain text

Proof of Correctness of scheme

$$\begin{aligned} C &= M^{k \times \varnothing(n)+1} \bmod x \\ D &= C \bmod n \\ &= \left(M^{k \times \varnothing(n)+1} \bmod x\right) \bmod n \\ &= \left(M^{k \times \varnothing(n)+1} \bmod n\right) \bmod x \end{aligned}$$

Now by second version of Euler's theorem, we know that $\left(a^{k \times \varnothing(n)+1}\right) \equiv a (\bmod\, n)$
$= (M) \bmod x = M, M < x$ *(Hence proved)*

Homomorphism

For message M_1 and M_2, we have the corresponding cipher texts as C_1 and C_2, and random integer's k_1 and k_2 used for deciphering, respectively. The multiplicative and additive Homomorphic property and their proof are presented below.

Multiplicative homomorphism

Multiplicative homomorphism property is stated as:

$$M_1 \times M_2 = \mathrm{DEC}[\mathrm{ENC}(M_1) \times \mathrm{ENC}(M_2)]$$

DEC represents Decryption function, and ENC represents Encryption function.

Proof

$$\begin{aligned} C_1 &= \left(M_1^{k_1 \times \varnothing(n)+1} \bmod x\right), \\ C_2 &= \left(M_2^{k_2 \times \varnothing(n)+1} \bmod x\right) \\ C_1 \times C_2 &= \left(M_1^{k_1 \times \varnothing(n)+1} \bmod x\right) \times \left(M_2^{k_2 \times \varnothing(n)+1} \bmod x\right) \\ D(C_1 \times C_2) &= (C_1 \times C_2) \bmod n \\ &= \left[\left(M_1^{k_1 \times \varnothing(n)+1} \bmod x\right) \times \left(M_2^{k_2 \times \varnothing(n)+1} \bmod x\right)\right] \bmod n \\ &= \left[\left(M_1^{k_1 \times \varnothing(n)+1} \bmod x\right) \bmod n \times \left(M_2^{k_2 \times \varnothing(n)+1} \bmod x\right) \bmod n\right] \\ &= \left[\left(M_1^{k_1 \times \varnothing(n)+1} \bmod n\right) \bmod x \times \left(M_2^{k_2 \times \varnothing(n)+1} \bmod n\right) \bmod x\right] \end{aligned}$$

Now, we know that $\left(a^{k \times \varnothing(n)+1}\right) \equiv a (\bmod\, n)$ so

$$= [(M_1 \bmod x) \times (M_2 \bmod x)] = M_1 \times M_2$$

Additive Homomorphism:

Additive homomorphism property is stated as:

$$M_1 + M_2 = \mathrm{DEC}[\mathrm{ENC}(M_1) + \mathrm{ENC}(M_2)]$$

Proof

$$\begin{aligned}
C_1 &= \left(M_1^{k_1 \times \varnothing(n)+1} \bmod x\right), \\
C_2 &= \left(M_2^{k_2 \times \varnothing(n)+1} \bmod x\right) \\
C_1 + C_2 &= \left(M_1^{k_1 \times \varnothing(n)+1} \bmod x\right) + \left(M_2^{k_2 \times \varnothing(n)+1} \bmod x\right) \\
D(C_1 + C_2) &= (C_1 + C_2) \bmod n \\
&= \left[\left(M_1^{k_1 \times \varnothing(n)+1} \bmod x\right) + \left(M_2^{k_2 \times \varnothing(n)+1} \bmod x\right)\right] \bmod n \\
&= \left[\left(M_1^{k_1 \times \varnothing(n)+1} \bmod x\right) \bmod n + \left(M_2^{k_2 \times \varnothing(n)+1} \bmod x\right) \bmod n\right] \\
&= \left[\left(M_1^{k_1 \times \varnothing(n)+1} \bmod n\right) \bmod x + \left(M_2^{k_2 \times \varnothing(n)+1} \bmod n\right) \bmod x\right]
\end{aligned}$$

Now we know that $\left(a^{k \times \varnothing(n)+1}\right) \equiv a(\bmod n)$ so

$$= [(M_1) \bmod x + (M_2) \bmod x] = M_1 + M_2$$

4 Working Example

Example Let we take two prime number $p = 5$ and $q = 7$, then

$$n = p \times q \rightarrow n = 5 \times 7 \rightarrow n = 35$$

Now calculate $\varnothing(\mathrm{n})$ according to the Euler Totient function, $\varnothing(35) = 24$,
Now select a prime number z such that $\gcd(n, z) = 1$
Let $z = 31$, and calculate $\gcd(35, 31) = 1$,
Now, calculate $x = n \times z \rightarrow x = 35 \times 31 \rightarrow x = 1085$
Now take two random integer $k_1 = 3$ and $k_2 = 2$, and two messages $m_1 = 2$ and $m_2 = 4$, such that $(m_1 + m_2)$ and $(m_1 * m_2)$ less than n
Now $c_1 = {m_1}^{k_1 \times \varnothing(n)+1} \bmod x$

$$c_1 = 2^{3 \times \varnothing(35)+1} \bmod 1085 \rightarrow c_1 = 2^{3 \times 24+1} \bmod 1085 \rightarrow c_1 = 597$$

And $c_2 = {m_2}^{k_2 \times \varnothing(n)+1} \bmod x$

$$c_2 = 4^{2 \times \varnothing(35)+1} \bmod 1085 \rightarrow c_2 = 4^{2 \times 24+1} \bmod 1085 \rightarrow c_2 = 39$$

Additive Homomorphism:

Let the addition of two encrypted messages is c_3 then

$$c_3 = c_1 + c_2 \rightarrow c_3 = 597 + 39 \rightarrow c_3 = 636$$

Now decryption of this message is m_3 then

$m_3 = c_3 \bmod n \rightarrow m_3 = 636 \bmod 35 \rightarrow m_3 = 6$, this is equal to $m_1 + m_2$ (i.e., 2 + 4 = 6)

Multiplicative homomorphism:

Let the multiplication of two encrypted messages is c_4 then

$$c_4 = c_1 \times c_2 \rightarrow c_4 = 597 \times 39 \rightarrow c_4 = 23,283$$

Now let the decryption of this message is m_4 then
$m_4 = c_4 \bmod n \rightarrow m_4 = 23{,}283 \bmod 35 \rightarrow m_4 = 8$, this is equal to $m_1 \times m_2$ (i.e. 2 × 4 = 8).

5 Conclusion

In this paper, a Fully Homomorphic encryption scheme was applied to Cloud computing with different computations on cipher text without decryption. The Homomorphic encryption schemes are used in secure electronic voting, searching over encrypted data, securing biometric information etc. The operations on small numbers are supported by Fully Homomorphic encryption scheme till now. In future, we can develop a fully Homomorphic encryption scheme that support a large number of circuits.

References

1. Chen, L., Gao, C.M.: Public key homomorphism based on modified ElGamal in real domain. In: 2008 International Conference on Computer Science and Software Engineering. IEEE Computer Society, Wuhan, Hubei, China, pp. 802–805 (2008)

2. Smart, N.P., Vercauteren, F.: Fully homomorphic encryption with relatively small key and ciphertext sizes. In: Public Key Cryptography—PKC'10, vol. 6056 of Lecture Notes in Computer Science, pp. 420–443. Springer, 2010
3. Gentry, C.: Fully homomorphic encryption using ideal lattices. In: Symposium on the Theory of Computing (STOC), pp. 169–178 (2009)
4. Gentry, C., Halevi, S.: Implementing gentry's fully-homomorphic encryption scheme. Adv. Cryptol EUROCRYPT 2011, pp. 129–148 (2011)
5. Gentry, C.: A fully homomorphic encryption scheme. PhD thesis, submitted to the department of computer science and the committee on graduate Stanford University, September (2009)
6. Van Dijk, M., Gentry, C., et al.: Fully homomorphic encryption over the integers. In: Advances in Cryptology EUROCRYPT 2010
7. Xiang, G., Cui, Z.: The algebra homomorphic encryption scheme based on Fermat's little theorem. In: International Conference on Communication Systems and Network Technologies (CSNT), pp. 978–981, 11–13 May 2012 (2012)
8. Goldwasser, S., Micali, S.: Probabilistic encryption and how to play mental poker keeping secret all partial information. In: Proceedings of the 14th ACM Symposium on the Theory of Computing (STOC '82), pp. 365–377, New York, NY, USA (1982)
9. Okamoto, T., Uchiyama, S.: A new public-key cryptosystem as secure as factoring. In: Advances in Cryptology (EUROCRYPT '98), vol. 1403 of Lecture Notes in Computer Science, pp. 308–318. Springer, New York (1998)
10. Van Dijk, M., Gentry, C., Halevi, S., Vaikuntanathan, V.: Fully homomorphic encryption over the integers. In: Advances in Cryptology EUROCRYPT 2010, p. 24-4 (2010)
11. Yu, Y., Leiwo, J., Premkumar, B.: A study on the security of privacy homomorphism‖, Nanyang Technological University, School of Computer Engineering. In: Proceedings of the Third International Conference on Information Technology: New Generations (ITNG'06), IEEE (2006)

Big Data: Issues, Challenges, and Techniques in Business Intelligence

Mudasir Ahmad Wani and Suraiya Jabin

Abstract During the last decade, the most challenging problem the world envisaged was big data problem. The big data problem means that data is growing at a much faster rate than computational speeds. And it is the result of the fact that storage cost is getting cheaper day by day, so people as well as almost all business or scientific organizations are storing more and more data. Social activities, scientific experiments, biological explorations along with the sensor devices are great big data contributors. Big data is beneficial to the society and business but at the same time, it brings challenges to the scientific communities. The existing traditional tools, machine learning algorithms, and techniques are not capable of handling, managing, and analyzing big data, although various scalable machine learning algorithms, techniques, and tools (e.g., Hadoop and Apache Spark open source platforms) are prevalent. In this paper, we have identified the most pertinent issues and challenges related to big data and point out a comprehensive comparison of various techniques for handling big data problem.

Keywords Big data · Business intelligence · Online social networks · Big data analytics · Hadoop MapReduce · Apache Spark

1 Introduction

Data is growing exponentially as it is being generated and recorded from everyone and everywhere, for example, online social networks, sensor devices, health records, human genome sequencing, phone logs, government records, and professionals such as scientists, journalists, and writers [1]. Formation of such huge amount of data from multiple sources with high volume and velocity by variety of

M.A. Wani (✉) · S. Jabin
Department of Computer Science, Jamia Millia Islamia, New Delhi 110025, India
e-mail: mudasirwanijmi@gmail.com; wani@iiitb.org

S. Jabin
e-mail: sjabin@jmi.ac.in

V.B. Aggarwal et al. (eds.), *Big Data Analytics*, Advances in Intelligent Systems and Computing 654, https://doi.org/10.1007/978-981-10-6620-7_59

digital devices gives birth to the term *big data*. As the big data grows with high velocity (speed), it becomes very complex to handle, manage, and analyze by using existing traditional systems. Data stored within the data warehouses is different from the big data. The former one is cleaned, managed, known, and trusted, and the latter one includes all the warehouse data as well as the data in which these warehouses are not capable to store [2]. The big data problem means that a single machine can no longer process or even hold all of the data that we want to analyze. The only solution we have is to distribute the data over large clusters. An example of a large cluster is one of Google's data centers that contain tens of thousands of machines.

1.1 Big Data: Definition

Big data can be described as the ample amount of data which differs from the traditional warehouse data in terms of size and structure. It can be viewed as the mixture of unstructured, semi-structured, and structured data, and its volume is considered in the range of exabytes (10^{18}). Different authors have given different definitions to the big data, e.g., [2] used variety, volume, velocity, variability, complexity, and value to define the big data. Authors in [1] defined the big data as volume of data in the range of exabyte for which the existing technology is not capable to effectively hold, manage, and process. According to [3], big data refers to the explosion of information. Analysts at Gartner [4, 5] described the characteristics of big data as huge volume, fast velocity, and diverse variety, also termed as 3Vs. Most commonly, big data is the ample amount of data (mostly semi-structured or unstructured data) for which various technologies and

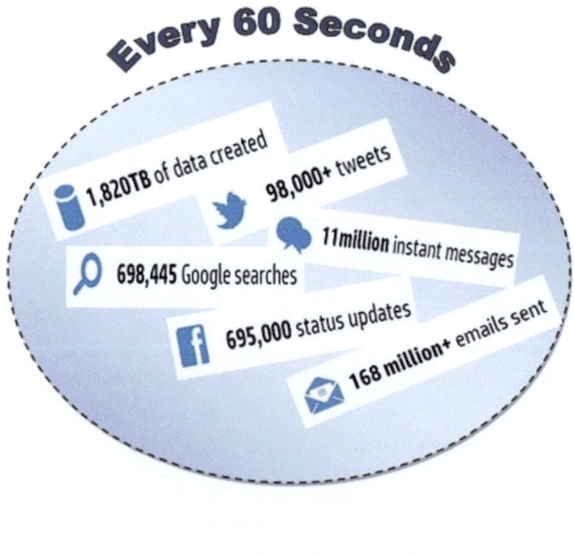

Fig. 1 Some big data ingredients

architectures are needed to mine the valuable information. Online social media networks (Facebook, Twitter, LinkedIn, Quora, and Google+) are the main contributors of big data. Sharing of information, status updates, videos, photographs, etc., all have never been the same. Following Fig. 1 shows a snip of some big data contents generated in one minute. According to a study, more than 80% of the data today on the planet got populated in last couple of years only [3].

Along with different varieties of data, huge quantity of data is also getting populated every second and requires organizations to make real-time decisions and responses [6]. But the existing analytical techniques can hardly extract the useful information in real time from the huge volume of data with various verities. If the data has reached terabytes (10^{12}) or petabytes (10^{15}) in size or a single organization does not have enough space to store it, it is considered as big [7]. Also according to Lenay [8], big data has three key characteristics those are high variety, huge volume, and greater velocity. Various other studies have introduced the fourth V as one more dimension of big data and all the four Vs are shown in Fig. 2.

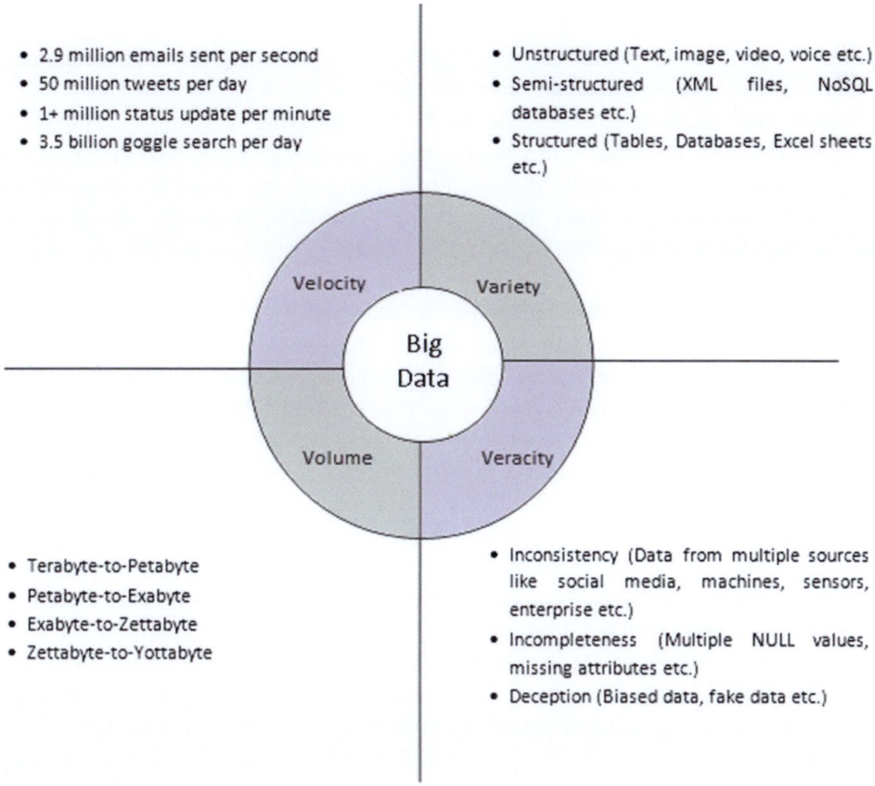

Fig. 2 Four Vs of big data

1.2 Business Intelligence and Big Data

Business intelligence (BI) relates to a technology-oriented process for analyzing data and presenting actionable information to help scientists, corporate executives, business managers, and other end users make more informed business decisions. BI covers a number of tools, applications, and methods that help business firms to gather data from internal as well as external sources, make it ready for analysis, create and execute queries in order to gain valuable information from the data, generate reports and charts for data visualizations so that the analytical results generated will help the organizations to make accurate and quick decisions. Business intelligence usually includes methods like statistical/quantitative analysis [9], data mining and analytics [10, 11], predictive modeling/analytics [12], big data analytics, and text analytics [13–15] for effective decision making. The process of analyzing the large amount of data sets (big data) containing different variety of data types in order to reveal unseen patterns, unknown relations, customer interests, new marketing strategies, and other important information about business is called *big data analytics*. This big data analytics plays an important role in making business more effective, helping to achieve for more customer satisfaction, and enhancing outputs and other business profits. Actually, the key objective of big data analytics is to aid data scientists, analysts, and other business professionals to make effective and accurate business decisions by analyzing the ample amount of transactional data and other forms of data which was not possible with conventional business intelligence. Business organizations are taking the advantage of analytical tools and techniques to gain the profit from the data available, also they are employing data scientists who are adept in managing big data and bringing useful insights into big data. Big data is going to change the way we think, make decisions, and do our business. Managing big data usefully has the potential to help companies to take faster and more intelligent decisions.

The most prevalent method of storage and management of data has been relational database management system (RDBMS). But RDBMSs can be used for structured data only, and it cannot deal with semi-structured or unstructured data. Also RDBMSs cannot handle large amount of data as well as heterogeneous data. Capability to analyze big data effectively is considered as one of the reasons for the success and popularity of any business organization. The question arises here is how companies tackle the situation while dealing with the ever-increasing amount of data. According to [16], the main problem why companies are losing competitiveness is not analyzing the information in a systematic manner. According to [17], it will be more beneficial for the companies to store and analyze the large datasets with MapReduce [18] instead of traditional databases. Mining of big data has unwrapped many new opportunities and challenges in the business [19]. Even though the big data contains the greater value (ability to analyze data to develop actionable information [1]), it encounters many challenges in extracting the hidden valuable information from big data because the traditional database systems and data mining techniques are not scalable for big data. The existing systems and technology need to have immense parallel processing architectures and distributed storage systems to cope up with the big data. NoSQL and distributed file systems (DFS) [20] can be the choices to store and manage large datasets, but their capacity is also limited. Some of the most popular techniques Hadoop MapReduce [18] and Apache Spark [21] have been introduced and compared to the solution toward big data analytics in Sect. 4.

No doubt, big data analytics is one of the effective ways to identify business opportunities, and the firms lacking in it would not gain the competitive advantage. For any business organization, what is actually important is to convert the data into information and extract the valuable and deep understanding of things from this information. In the present paper, we put an effort to congregate the issues, challenges, and techniques of big data all at one place. Section 2 precisely reviews the issues of big data. Section 3 addresses some emerging challenges of big data from business intelligence perspective. And, the Sect. 4 provides a comparative discussion on two most widely used big data processing techniques Hadoop MapReduce and Apache Spark, then finally Sect. 5 concludes the discussion.

2 Issues of Big Data

Many researchers have discussed and suggested various big data issues in the literature; we have tried to summarize most relevant big data issues in this section.

2.1 Management Issue

Unmanaged data is always treated as unwanted data. Since the big data is formed by multiple heterogeneous sources with different formats, representations, etc., [22], so managing the big data requires high-performance and multidimensional management tools, otherwise, we are likely to get unacceptable results. As one of the characteristics of big data is its variety [3], therefore to manage the data with heterogeneous formats and structures, business organizations need to have more sophisticated data stores with the feature of elasticity and scalability as well.

For better marketing strategies, business professionals often need relevant, cleaned, accurate complete, and managed data to perform analysis. Management of data includes tasks like cleaning, transforming, clarification, dimension reduction, and validation. Firms can make the use of business intelligence to manage a large amount of data; for example, quantum computing and in-memory database management systems allow economically effective and quick management of large datasets [23]. But the existing businesses are already established on traditional platforms, moving the whole business to the new platform can be very expensive and time-consuming. As the big data is not in the managed form, it becomes very complex for business organizations to analyze and extract meaningful information from it. There is still need to upgrade the existing big data management techniques and/or tools and deployment of scalable data management tools and techniques since the beginning for setting up a new business.

2.2 Storage Issue

The more the information we have, the more accurate decisions (marketing strategies) we can make [2]. Also according to the big data professionals, a good amount of the world's information exists within the massive, unstructured big data [19]. From the above statement and observation, we can realize that how much important is big data for any business organization to grow. But unfortunately, we lack the devices which can store this ample amount of data; as a result, our decisions, marketing strategies, recommendation systems, etc., seem to be very poor.

Our existing systems have the storage capacity up to 4 terabytes per disk [1], and big data is usually populated in exabytes. So, to store 1 exabytes, we need 25,000 disk spaces and it could be very complex, almost not feasible task to attach such huge number of disks to a single system. One possible solution could be to store the data onto the cloud. But storing the big data onto a cloud (or any storage place) is like filling a swimming pool with a drinking straw. It would take very long time to transfer data from multiple data sources to the cloud and back from cloud to processing point. To overcome this transferring issue, two methods have been proposed [2]. First, just process the data at the same place where it is stored and only transfer the required information. More specifically, bring the processing code to the stored data instead of transferring the stored data to the processing code, known as MapReduce algorithm [24]. Second, transfer only the part of data which seems more critical for analysis [2].

Since the data is populated in terabytes (Fig. 2 shows a scale of data in bytes) and the existing storage capacity is very limited, it is quite confusing for the business organizations to choose the part of the data that can be skipped, and the part of the data is of greater value or which optimal set of attributes can represent the whole dataset. So, there is a pertinent need of tools and methods which can help different firms to identify optimal features (or principal components) out of thousands of attributes to understand customers in depth.

2.3 Processing Issue

Nowadays, the on-time results really matter a lot especially for business organizations. If the results are not generated accurately and timely, they will be of least use [19]. In the current scenario, most of the organizations have transferred their mode of business from "brick and mortar" mode to online mode in order to grab the customers and boost the sales globally which results in storm of data. Our existing infrastructure, machinery, and techniques are not capable to process such ample amount of data in real time [2] which leaves the business organizations handicapped. Although some advanced indexing schemes (like FastBit) [25] and processing methods like MapReduce [26, 27] are available to boost the processing speed, but processing of zettabytes (10^{21}) and even exabytes (10^{18}) of data is still a challenging task.

As shown in Fig. 2, one of the big data characteristics is the velocity with which it is generated. Data comes from multiple sources in greater speed (Fig. 1) which needs to be processed in real time by business organizations in order to gain the competitive edge in the market. Many organizations are using MapReduce for long-running time batch jobs. For real-time processing of big data, simple scalable streaming systems (S4) have been proposed [28]. Besides the accurate processing of real-time data, organizations are also looking for its fast processing, therefore the conventional data processing systems should be upgraded to become not only accurate but also fast.

Figure 3 shows the growth of data in bytes from a single bit to a yottabyte. For the sake of convenience, we have shown the bytes using exponential power from megabyte to a yottabyte.

From the above figure, it is clearly shown that the data has grown beyond the terabytes and even petabytes. Our advanced machineries (like supercomputers) are capable to store and process the data up to petabytes only. Therefore, organizations dealing with big data need such advanced machines and methods which can store and process the data beyond petabytes.

For glimpse, Table 1 shows the comprehensive conclusion of the above identified issues.

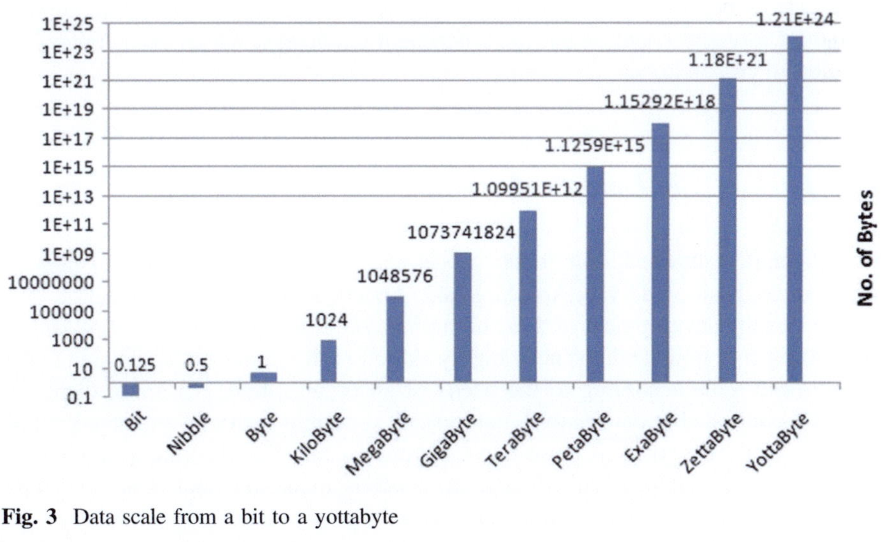

Fig. 3 Data scale from a bit to a yottabyte

Table 1 Summary of issues

Issue	Possible solutions	Limitations
Management	Quantum computing and in-memory database management systems	Moving the whole business to the new platform can be very expensive and time-consuming
Storage	NoSQL, distributed file systems, and cloud computing	Storing one exabyte needs 25,000 no. of disk space which is complex and loading onto cloud is time-consuming
Processing	Advanced indexing schemas, MapReduce and simple scalable streaming systems (S4)	Processing of zettabytes (10^{21}) and even exabytes (10^{18}) of data still seems a matter of concern

Efficient big data processing can be one of the effective ways to identify business opportunities, but in order to gain the competitive edge, the firms certainly need to handle the above summarized issues.

3 Challenges for Big Data

Opportunities and challenges always travel along with each other. Big data from one hand brings various openings for the society and business, but on the other hand, it also brings huge number of challenges [29]. So for various researchers have identified and addressed plentiful challenges faced while dealing with big data like storage and transport, management and processing issues [1], variety and heterogeneity, scalability, velocity, accuracy etc. [19], privacy and security, data accessing and sharing of information, skill requirements, technical or hardware related challenges, analytical challenges [2] etc. On the basis of literature survey, we have addressed some of the most pertinent challenges which need immediate attention of researchers.

3.1 Lack of Big Data Professionals

Most recently devised big data processing tools and algorithms include MapReduce, Hadoop, Dryad, Apache Spark, Apache mahout, and Tableau [22, 29]. But besides the development of these high processing, complex technologies for big data processing, organizations need highly skilled professionals to handle and make use of these tools according to the needs of an organization. No doubt there are experts around the big data as well, but looking at current scenario, a special kind of training should be given to these naïve experts so that they become proficient to deal with the big data from different dimensions including data modeling, data architecture, and data integration [2]. According to a report by McKinesey &

Company [30], the USA might realize the requirement of 140,000–190,000 skilled persons for data analysis as well as more than one million managers and analysts with advanced analytical knowledge and skills to make correct and accurate decisions.

So, finally we can conclude, for the business organizations who are engaged with big data analytics and frameworks, there is huge demand of professionals namely data scientists/engineers to address challenges like data architecture and management for efficient decision making. Every business firm needs to recruit big data analysts in order to stand in the competing market. According to a study [31], every organization should have special data force (SDF) with great analytical skills to deal with the big data. Big data analysts along with the business intelligence have been seen as one of the reasons for the exponential growth of businesses [30].

3.2 Interactiveness (or Designing)

Interactiveness of a data mining system is the capability which allows the users to interact with system efficiently [19] including user feedback, guidance, and suggestions. Coming to the big data mining, interactiveness is considered as one of the critical challenges for the system designers especially in business organizations. Better interactiveness can overcome the challenges found around the 3Vs (volume, velocity, and variety) [1]. Adequate user interaction provides users better way to identify their domain of interest out of huge volume of data which also allow marketing experts to easily obtain the mining results. Since now, the user is concerned with only his or her subspace, which boosts the processing speed (velocity) and also the scalability of the system gets increased. Also, the heterogeneity (or variety) of the big data introduces complexity in the data which may also complicate the mining results. However, the better interactiveness provides the ways to easily visualize the big data processing and mining results.

It can be concluded that mining results of a system with better interactiveness has fairer chance to be accepted by the potential users; lack of interactiveness of the data mining system will likely end up with poor or unacceptable mining results. According to authors in [22, 32], the organization dealing with big data needs to design the systems in such a way that they can understand both the customer needs and the technology to be used to solve the problem. Also, it has been shown that various valuable customers were paid least attention by business organizations because of poor interaction system. Therefore in order to grab valuable customers and understand the needs of each individual customer out of thousands of customers, designers need to take care of interfaces, graphics, conceptual models, user feedback systems, etc., [1].

3.3 Loading and Synchronization

Data loading includes getting data from multiple heterogeneous data sources into a single data repository [33]. Loading process suffers from various issues those need the keen attention of researchers and practitioners; for example, multiple data sources should be mapped onto a unified structural framework, tools and infrastructure which cooperate with the size and speed of big data should be available and should transfer the data in a timely manner.

Along with these loading issues, synchronization across different data sources is also considered as one of the critical challenges. Once the data gets loaded into a big data platform from different data sources, at different time intervals with different velocity, it is likely to get away from synchronization. Synchronization among data sources refers to the process of establishing consistency of data over time between different data sources and common repository. In other words, the data coming from different sources should match with each other in respect of time and sequence [34]. If the big data processing system is unable to guarantee synchronization, it is likely to get inconsistent or even invalid data which leads to poor and/or incorrect mining results. Therefore, a great attention should be paid toward the synchronization among data sources in order to help business organizations to avoid the risks in analysis process and hence draw accurate and appropriate conclusions. Also, the heterogeneous nature of data makes it more complex for businesses to transform and clean before loading them into warehouse for analysis [20]. Hadoop and MapReduce, employed by many firms, provide the different ways to efficiently process the unstructured data.

3.4 Visualization

Data visualization is the process of representing knowledge in an understandable way in order to enable more efficient decision making [35]. As the big data is growing exponentially with unbridled velocity and huge volume, it becomes very difficult to extract the hidden information because of unavailability of scalable visualization tools. There is no doubt that online marketplaces (e.g., eBay) are using big data visualization tools like Tableau [36] and other tools mentioned in Sect. 3.1 for transforming their large, complex datasets into picture formats to make all the data clearly understandable. But as the tsunami of big data is approaching to us with a very high speed [34], these existing visualization tools are likely to be of no use in the near future. So far researchers have paid their attention toward the visualizing challenges of big data in the current scenario, but we must be prepared to face the future challenges of big data as well. In other words, in order to hold and visualize the zettabytes (10^{21}) or even yottabytes (10^{24}) of data or beyond, we should have tools ready. As the data is generated from everywhere by everyone, like online social networks, medical science, geostationary satellites, and sensors [1], the big

Table 2 Summary of challenges

Challenge	Possible approaches	Limitations
Big data professionals	Establishment of special data force (SDF) with advanced analytical skills	Expensive but necessary to survive
Interactiveness	Design of systems by taking user needs and technology under consideration	User interactive designs satisfy customers. And, a satisfied customer is itself an advertisement
Loading and synchronization	Hadoop and MapReduce to load various formats of data in a distributed and synchronous manner	Heterogeneous nature of data is the reason which raised the challenge
Visualization	Tableau, QlikView, etc.	Businesses use visualization tools to increase the throughput over big data

data is becoming “bigger data.” So there are more chances of facing challenges in the future, therefore we should be prepared in advance with the new technologies and tools to deal with challenges which are approaching us horrendously and uninformed.

Big data visualization techniques have the responsibility to visually present the analytical results by using different graphs for decision making [20]. A visual report speaks two times more than a text report, and also the visualization techniques have been proved to be sophisticated for complex customer data. Visualization tools like Tableau and QlikView [36] have been used by businesses to increase the throughput over big data, also provide the visualizations specific to the business and ensure the meaningful data discovery.

For glimpse, Table 2 shows the comprehensive conclusion of identified challenges and their associated solutions applied so far. But still, the shortcomings exist there in the available approaches which need the great attention of researchers.

4 Techniques for Big Data Processing

Keeping processing latency as prime concern, two methods have been suggested and employed for big data processing: *batch-based stored data processing* and *real-time data-stream processing*. The two most promising and upcoming open source methods, Hadoop MapReduce and Apache Spark, have been explored along with a discussion of when to use which in the following subsections.

4.1 Hadoop

Hadoop is a freely available framework and has been used by data analysts, researchers, and other professionals from more than eight years as a big data processing platform [37]. Hadoop MapReduce is a good choice for processing of data which requires all its inputs to be read exactly once (one-pass computation) while it seems very lazy in case of multi-pass computations. Google developed MapReduce with two components to process large datasets. Map and reduce are the two components, a map is used to calculate the key/value pairs for the inputs, and reduce combines the results of map function into a scalar. In order to take the full advantage of Hadoop MapReduce, we need to convert inputs into MapReduce form. Also, this framework is responsible for scheduling, monitoring tasks and execution of failed tasks [38].

Since in the MapReduce framework after every step and before the next step begins, the output data is stored into distributed file system (DFS) which results in slow down of processing speed. Also, it deals with the large amount of clusters which are very complicated and hectic to manage. Furthermore, integration of several approaches is required in many cases of big data processing, like for stream-data processing and to produce machine learning algorithms, we need Storm [39] and Mahout [18], respectively. Hence in order to execute a set of complicated tasks, we would have to run a series of MapReduce jobs to execute them. MapReduce is designed for high-speed jobs to be executed in some specific sequence.

4.2 Apache Spark

Like MapReduce, Spark is also a cluster computing framework with language-integrated APIs and parallel operators [39]. It was developed six years before at AMP Lab, Berkeley, and is open sourced from 2010 as an Apache Project [37]. Spark is more advantageous than Hadoop and Storm (MapReduce technologies) and other big data technologies. It provides a united approach to manage processing requirements of big data along with the enhancement of speed of applications in Hadoop cluster to run 100 times faster in-memory and 10 times faster on the disk. Further, it assists in writing applications (in scala, java, or python language) with more than 75 high-level operators. In addition to map and reduce operations, it also processes SQL queries, streaming data, machine learning, and graph-based data. Direct Cyclic Graphs (DCG) is used in Spark to develop complex, multi-step data pipelines and support in-memory sharing among different jobs.

4.3 Comparison of Hadoop MapReduce and Apache Spark

Spark is designed to run on top of Hadoop, and it is an alternative to the traditional batch MapReduce model. Although Hadoop MapReduce and Apache Spark are developed to deal with big data, still there are some differences between the two [38, 40]. Following Table 3 highlights some of the differences between Hadoop

Table 3 Key differences between Hadoop MapReduce and Apache Spark

Properties	Hadoop MapReduce	Apache Spark
Processing method	After each map task, output is written to a buffer	Output of map tasks is directly written to disk after completion
Time efficiency	A parallel data processing method to process long-running jobs that take minutes even hours to complete	Spark is designed to process real-time stream-data and SQL queries that take few seconds to complete
Error recovery	In order to achieve recovery from errors, Hadoop uses the concept of "replication"	Recovery from errors is achieved by using different data storage models, RDD (resilient distributed datasets), etc., which allows to transparently store data on memory and reconstructs it automatically in case of a failure
Memory requirements	Hadoop does not have any memory issue, but it is not good for iterative algorithms	Spark performs well in case of iterative operations, but has high memory requirements. Spark uses more RAM instead of network and disk I/O. It is relatively fast as compared to Hadoop. But as it uses large RAM it needs a dedicated high-end physical machine for producing effective results

MapReduce and Apache Spark. Although there exist other big data tools as well like GridGain, HPCC, and Storm. But the Hadoop MapReduce and Apache Spark are the most popular and commonly used.

Thus, Hadoop Spark can be recommended as the most suitable choice for the future big data applications that possibly would require lower latency queries, iterative computation, and real-time processing on similar data [21].

5 Conclusions and Future Directions

As we live in the era of big data, here comes the need of modern, high-performance, and capable equipment along with scalable techniques and algorithms to deal with the issues and challenges which must come across while playing with the large datasets. Big data analytics is one of the reasons for the universal success of any business organization. Organizations lagging behind in big data analytics are likely to be visually and physically handicapped as they would suffer from monitory losses in terms of their future customers and better future investments. The birth of big data revealed the shortcomings of existing data mining technologies which in turn raised new challenges. In this paper, we have presented a brief overview of big data along with its key properties, also identified some challenges of big data. A very brief introduction and a comparison for most popular big data processing frameworks, Hadoop MapReduce and Apache Spark, are presented which help young researchers and data scientists to analyze the big data and uncover hidden, unknown patterns.

A rigorous effort from researchers is needed to overcome the existing challenges and to be ready to deal with upcoming challenges in terms of both hardware and software. It can be concluded that Apache Spark is perceived as a better alternative than Hadoop MapReduce as it offers more efficiency for stream processing, e.g., log processing and fraud detection in live streams for alerts, aggregates, and analysis. The most recent and future research in big data analysis includes fake identity detection using online social networks [15, 41, 42], identification and ranking of influential personalities in online social media [43], to gain competitive advantage by enhancing their supply chain innovation capabilities thus helping business economics, understanding the basis of crop diseases from plant genomics data, getting more insights into the human diseases by analyzing human genome [13, 14], and next-generation sequencing data [44].

References

1. Kaisler, S., Armour, F., Espinosa, J.A., Money, W.: Big data: issues and challenges moving forward. In: 2013 46th Hawaii International Conference on System Sciences (HICSS), pp. 995–1004. IEEE (2013)
2. Katal, A., Wazid, M., Goudar, R.: Big data: issues, challenges, tools and good practices. In: 2013 Sixth International Conference on Contemporary Computing (IC3), pp. 404–409. IEEE (2013)
3. Fan, J., Han, F., Liu, H.: Challenges of big data analysis. Natl. Sci. Rev. **1**(2), 293–314 (2014)
4. Beyer, M.A., Laney, D.: The Importance of Big Data: A Definition. Gartner, Stamford (2012)
5. Laney, D.: 3d data management: controlling data volume, velocity and variety. META Group Research Note, 6, 70 (2001)
6. Minelli, M., Chambers, M., Dhiraj, A.: Big Data, Big Analytics: Emerging Business Intelligence and Analytic Trends for Today's Businesses. Wiley, New York (2012)
7. Vossen, G.: Big data as the new enabler in business and other intelligence. Vietnam J. Comput. Sci. **1**(1), 3–14 (2014)
8. Laney, D.: 3D data management: controlling data volume, velocity and variety. META Group Research Note, 6, 70 (2001)
9. Han, J., Kamber, M.: Data Mining: Concepts and Techniques. Morgan Kaumann Publishers, United States of America (2001)
10. Jabin, S., Zareen, F.J.: Biometric signature verification. Int. J. Biom. **7**(2), 97–118 (2015)
11. Jabin, S.: Stock market prediction using feed-forward artificial neural network. Int. J. Comput. Appl. **99**(9), 4–8 (2014)
12. Jabin, S.: Learning classifier systems approach for automated discovery of hierarchical censored production rules. In: Information and Communication Technologies, pp. 68-77. Springer, Berlin (2010)
13. Xiong, H.Y., Alipanahi, B., Lee, L.J., Bretschneider, H., Merico, D., Yuen, R.K., Hua, Y., Gueroussov, S., Najafabadi, H.S., Hughes, T.R., et al.: The human splicing code reveals new insights into the genetic determinants of disease. Science **347**(6218), 1254806 (2015)
14. Kellis, M., Wold, B., Snyder, M.P., Bernstein, B.E., Kundaje, A., Marinov, G.K., Ward, L.D., Birney, E., Crawford, G.E., Dekker, J., et al.: Defining functional DNA elements in the human genome. Proc. Natl. Acad. Sci. **111**(17), 6131–6138 (2014)

15. Tsikerdekis, M., Zeadally, S.: Multiple account identity deception detection in social media using nonverbal behavior. IEEE Trans. Inf. Forensics Secur. **9**(8), 1311–1321 (2014)
16. Schön, D.A., Argyris, C.: Organizational learning: a theory of action perspective. Reis: Revista española de investigaciones sociológicas **77**, 345–350 (1997)
17. Ebner, K., Buhnen, T., Urbach, N.: Think big with big data: identifying suitable big data strategies in corporate environments. In: 2014 47th Hawaii International Conference on System Sciences (HICSS), pp. 3748–3757. IEEE (2014)
18. MAHOUT (2015). http://www.tutorialspoint.com/mahout/
19. Che, D., Safran, M., Peng, Z.: From big data to big data mining: challenges, issues, and opportunities. In: Database Systems for Advanced Applications, pp. 1–15. Springer, Berlin (2013)
20. Hashem, I.A.T., Yaqoob, I., Anuar, N.B., Mokhtar, S., Gani, A., Khan, S.U.: The rise of "big data" on cloud computing: review and open research issues. Inf. Syst. **47**, 98–115 (2015)
21. Spark 0.6.2 (2015). Spark Overview: http://spark.apache.org/docs/0.6.2/
22. Wu, X., Zhu, X., Wu, G.Q., Ding, W.: Data mining with big data. IEEE Trans. Knowl. Data Eng. **26**(1), 97–107 (2014)
23. Buhl, H.U., Röglinger, M., Moser, D.K.F., Heidemann, J.: Big data. Bus. Inf. Syst. Eng. **5**(2), 65–69 (2013)
24. Dean, J., Ghemawat, S.: MapReduce: simplified data processing on large clusters. Commun. ACM **51**(1), 107–113 (2008)
25. Wu, K.: Fastbit: an efficient indexing technology for accelerating data-intensive science. In: Journal of Physics: Conference Series, vol. 16, p. 556. IOP Publishing (2005)
26. Dittrich, J., Quiane-Ruiz, J.A.: Efficient big data processing in hadoop MapReduce. Proc. VLDB Endowment **5**(12), 2014–2015 (2012)
27. Triguero, I., Peralta, D., Bacardit, J., Garc a, S., Herrera, F.: MRPR: a MapReduce solution for prototype reduction in big data classification. Neurocomputing **150**, 331–345 (2015)
28. Neumeyer, L., Robbins, B., Nair, A., Kesari, A.: S4: distributed stream computing platform. In: 2010 IEEE International Conference on Data Mining Workshops (ICDMW), pp. 170–177 (2010)
29. Chen, C.P., Zhang, C.Y.: Data-intensive applications, challenges, techniques and technologies: a survey on big data. In: Information Conference on Cloud System and *Big Data* Engineering, pp. 404–409. IEEE (2013)
30. Manyika, J., Chui, M., Brown, B., Bughin, J., Dobbs, R., Roxburgh, C., Byers, A.H.: Big data: the next frontier for innovation, competition, and productivity (2011)
31. Kim, G.H., Trimi, S., Chung, J.H.: Big-data applications in the government sector. Commun. ACM **57**(3), 78–85 (2014)
32. Stonebraker, M., Hong, J.: Researchers 'big data crisis; understanding design and functionality. Commun ACM **55**(2), 10–11 (2012)
33. Zaharia, M., Chowdhury, M., Franklin, M.J., Shenker, S., Stoica, I.: Spark: cluster computing with working sets. In: Proceedings of the 2nd USENIX Conference on Hot Topics in Cloud Computing, vol. 10, p. 10 (2010)
34. Driscoll, A.O., Daugelaite, J., Sleator, R.D.: Big data, Hadoop and cloud computing in genomics. J. Biomed. Inf. **46**(5), 774–781 (2013)
35. Simoff, S., Bohlen, M.H., Mazeika, A.: Visual Data Mining: Theory, Techniques and Tools for Visual Analytics, vol. 4404. Springer Science & Business Media (2008)
36. Sawant, N., Shah, H.: Big data visualization patterns. In: Big Data Application Architecture Q&A, pp. 79–90 (2013)
37. Apache Software Foundation: The Apache Software Foundation Blog (2014). https://blogs.apache.org/foundation/entry/the_apache_software_foundation_announces80
38. Hadoop: MapReduce Tutorial. http://hadoop.apache.org/docs/current/hadoop-mapreduce-client/hadoop-mapreduce-client-core/MapReduceTutorial.html#MapReduceTutorial
39. Apache Storm (2015). https://storm.apache.org/
40. Gu, L., Li, H.: Memory or time: performance evaluation for iterative operation on hadoop and spark. In: 2013 IEEE 10th International Conference on High Performance Computing and

Communications & 2013 IEEE International Conference on Embedded and Ubiquitous Computing (HPCC EUC), pp. 721–727. IEEE (2013)
41. Zheng, X., Zeng, Z., Chen, Z., Yu, Y., Rong, C.: Detecting spammers on social networks. Neurocomputing **159**, 27–34 (2015)
42. Conti, M., Poovendran, R., Secchiero, M.: Fakebook: detecting fake profiles in on-line social networks. In: Proceedings of the 2012 International Conference on Advances in Social Networks Analysis and Mining (ASONAM 2012), pp. 1071–1078. IEEE Computer Society (2012)
43. Anwar, T., Abulaish, M.: Ranking radically influential web forum users. IEEE Trans. Inf. Forensics Secur. **10**(6), 1289–1298 (2015)
44. McKenna, A., Hanna, M., Banks, E., Sivachenko, A., Cibulskis, K., Kernytsky, A., Garimella, K., Altshuler, D., Gabriel, S., Daly, M., et al.: The genome analysis toolkit: a MapReduce framework for analyzing next-generation DNA sequencing data. Genome Res. **20**(9), 1297–1303 (2010)
45. Addressing five challenges of Big Data. https://www.progress.com/docs/default-source/default-document-library/Progress/Documents/Papers/Addressing-Five-Emerging-Challenges-of-Big-Data.pdf
46. Webpopedia: Unstructured Data. http://www.webopedia.com/TERM/U/unstructured_data.html
47. Marx, V.: Biology: the big challenges of big data. Nature **498**(7453), 255–260 (2013)
48. Assuncao, M.D., Calheiros, R.N., Bianchi, S., Netto, M.A., Buyya, R.: Big data computing and clouds: trends and future directions. J. Parallel Distrib. Comput. **79**, 3–15 (2015)
49. Kambatla, K., Kollias, G., Kumar, V., Grama, A.: Trends in big data analytics. J. Parallel Distrib. Comput. **74**(7), 2561–2573 (2014)
50. Shanahan, J.G., Dai, L.: Large scale distributed data science using apache spark. In: Proceedings of the 21th ACM SIGKDD International Conference on Knowledge Discovery and Data Mining, pp. 2323–2324. ACM (2015)
51. Stich, V., Jordan, F., Birkmeier, M., Oazgil, K., Reschke, J., Diews, A.: Big data technology for resilient failure management in production systems. In: Advances in Production Management Systems: Innovative Production Management Towards Sustainable Growth, pp. 447–454. Springer, Berlin (2015)
52. Agrawal, D., Das, S., El Abbadi, A.: Big data and cloud computing: current state and future opportunities. In: Proceedings of the 14th International Conference on Extending Database Technology, pp. 530–533. ACM (2011)
53. McDaniel, M.A.: Big-brained people are smarter: a meta-analysis of the relation-ship between in vivo brain volume and intelligence. Intelligence **33**(4), 337–346 (2005)
54. Tan, K.H., Zhan, Y., Ji, G., Ye, F., Chang, C.: Harvesting big data to enhance supply chain innovation capabilities: an analytic infrastructure based on deduction graph. Int. J. Prod. Econ. **165**, 223–233 (2015)
55. Chen, M., Mao, S., Liu, Y.: Big data: a survey. Mobile Netw. Appl. **19**(2), 171–209 (2014)

Cloud Computing in Bioinformatics and Big Data Analytics: Current Status and Future Research

Kashish Ara Shakil and Mansaf Alam

Abstract Bioinformatics research involves a huge amount of data which is complex in nature. It also involves analysis of huge data sets. Conventional techniques used in bioinformatics takes a lot of time to get results and also it's difficult to analyze the complex nature of data involved. Therefore, machines having huge processing capabilities are required leading to an escalation in the amount of money which is required do research in bioinformatics field. The problems faced by bioinformatics researchers in order to carry out their research in an economic and fast manner can be solved easily with the help of Cloud computing concepts. Thus, cloud computing is a boon for bioinformatics research. In this paper, we have discussed how the cloud computing will be helpful for bioinformatics researchers ultimately acting as a stepping stone towards big data analytics. It also explains about the current state of the art in bioinformatics and big data analytics and potential future research issues that need to be addressed.

Keywords Cloud computing · Big data analytics · Bioinformatics

1 Introduction

There has been a gradual shift in the interest of researchers towards cloud computing in the past few years [1]. Several researchers have started the use of cloud computing in bioinformatics research. According to [2] researchers who are working in the field of bioinformatics are confronted with analysis of ultra large-scale data sets right now. They have also come up with a problem that growth of data will boost at a shocking velocity in upcoming years and current developments in real-world open-source software, the Hadoop project and associated

K.A. Shakil (✉) · M. Alam
Department of Computer Science, Jamia Millia Islamia, New Delhi 110025, India
e-mail: shakilkashish@yahoo.co.in

M. Alam
e-mail: malam2@jmi.ac.in

V.B. Aggarwal et al. (eds.), *Big Data Analytics*, Advances in Intelligent Systems and Computing 654, https://doi.org/10.1007/978-981-10-6620-7_60

software will provide an establishment for scaling to petabyte-size data warehouses on Linux clusters. Hadoop also provides fault-tolerant parallelized investigations on such data by means of a programming approach called MapReduce. Hadoop-based analysis on Linux clusters also shows an astonishing cost-effectiveness in case when the data was uploaded to cloud vendors who have implemented Hadoop or HBase. They have taken advantage of effectiveness and ease-of-use offered by MapReduce methods such as parallelization of many data analysis algorithms. In [3], the authors have proposed an architecture for management of data in cloud environment. *K*-median clustering [4] technique can also be used for management of huge data sets. Several researchers [5, 6] have also studied production workloads such as Google cluster trace for studying the behaviour of users and data in cloud environment while some have resorted to the use of decision matrix techniques for studying data access patterns in cloud [7, 8].

Cloud BLAST [9] is a work carried out by the researchers where the authors have proposed and evaluated an approach to the parallelization, deployment and management of bioinformatics applications which combine numerous promising technologies for distributed computing. Their approach involves the use of MapReduce model in order to parallelize tools and deal with their implementation. To put in a nutshell, their implementation environment involved machine virtualization and universally used data sets into flexibly deployable virtual machines, and set of connections virtualization to hook up resources behind firewalls or NATs while preserving the essential performance and the communication surroundings. Biodoop: bioinformatics on Hadoop [10] is another application of bioinformatics using Hadoop platform. It provides an intriguing advantage of cloud computing by allowing rapid setups, migration and demolishment of large-scale virtual clusters that are based on utilization of different distributed file system implementations such as MapReduce. In their work, the authors parallelized GenGR-GC because of its higher statistical power [11]. In this method, heritability evaluation is done with the kinship matrix K, whose coefficients are in roll expected from genomic data using the following formula [10]:

$$\begin{aligned} k_{ij} &= \frac{1}{M_{ij}^{*}} \sum_{m=1}^{M} \frac{(g_{im} - p_m)(g_{jm} - p_m)\left[g_{im} \wedge g_{jm}\right]}{p_m(1 - p_m)} \\ M_{ij}^{*} &= \sum_{m=1}^{M} \left[g_{im} \wedge g_{jm}\right] \end{aligned} \qquad (1)$$

where g_{im} and g_{jm} (i = 2, …, N, j = 1, …, i − 1) are the genotypes of the i-th and j-th individual at the m-th SNP, set as 1/2 for heterozygote and 0 or 1 correspondingly for exceptional or frequent allele homozygote, p_m is the occurrence of the most important allele, M and N are in that order the number of SNPs and the number of individuals. Note that sums make longer to SNPs for which both genotypes are non-missing (or “measured”). Cloud Store [12] provides possible improvements on present applications by embracing improved post-processing of

BLAST results and subordinate level parallelization of GRAMMAR's qtscore or empirical p-value working out segment.

Thus, the bioinformatics research community is now finding cloud computing as an important research tool and an answer to all their research hurdles and murky issues which they had to deal with in the past due to lack of proper infrastructure and computing needs. It has also been recognized as a jigger for handling big data and is a probable solution in big data analytics as well. Thus, this paper identifies the applications of cloud computing in bioinformatics and big data analytics. It also explores the potential future research issues that need to be addressed while using cloud computing in bioinformatics and big data analytics research.

The rest of the paper is organized as follows: Sect. 2 provides us with an overview of current status of research in bioinformatics domain using cloud computing while Sect. 3 identifies the applications of cloud computing in bioinformatics. Section 4 gives an overview of current status of using cloud computing in big data analytics. Furthermore, Sect. 5 elaborates the future research potential of using cloud computing in bioinformatics research followed by future research potential of cloud computing in big data analytics in section. Finally, the paper concludes with conclusion in Sect. 6.

2 Cloud Computing in Bioinformatics: Current Status

Traditional bioinformatics research usually involves downloading huge data sets from publicly available data repositories and then analyzing these data sets through in-house infrastructure. The major problem faced by these scientists who are working in the field of bioinformatics is that they need machines having high computation power requirements but such high-power computation machines require a great deal of economies of scale posing as a hurdle to the researchers. It is here that cloud computing comes into picture by providing rescue to researchers facing economic crises. Through cloud computing many high-power machines can be taken on rent basis depending upon the user requirements and usage. Softwares and data required for carrying out research can also be placed in cloud [13] and then accessed as a service as per the usage and requirements. Apart from meeting the infrastructure needs of researchers, it also makes the entire process of installing software's now a redundant task. The biologist needs no longer to develop any expertise for installing software's operating systems etc. They can just log on to the respective cloud and use the software required by them without any initial setups. Thus, saving a lot of money and time required for performing initial laboratory setups.

Cloud computing also has its application in healthcare and biomedicine domain. In [14], the authors have discussed the main cloud-based healthcare and biomedicine applications along with a special focus on bioinformatics solutions and its underlying important issues and problems related to the use of cloud computing environment for the storage and analysis. They have used data of patients in this study. They have also discussed recent studies which show that cloud computing can improve healthcare services and benefit biomedical research [15–17], through proposing innovative solutions and applications. Reduced costs are essential drivers that have led to the recognition of cloud as a technology in the healthcare domain. The cost of basic healthcare conveyance has increased to such a huge amount that government is facing severe funding issues, and several patients are on the verge of remaining unattended to basic medical amenities. The recognition of cloud computing as a technology can enhance patient's care and overall well-being of an individual along with reduced costs which mean that government can move the usually slow healthcare business to a quicker step of acceptance. In [18], the researchers have discussed, Azures pricing model, the price of their cloud-based telemedicine service is based on the amount of CPU utilization. The cost of resource usage is about USD $0.1 per hour and usage of its database price is approximately USD $9.99 per GB for one month. Apart from Azure, several other researchers [19] have confirmed that cloud computing is a sustainable and economical technology that facilitates large-scale incorporation and investigation for training in genomic medicine. Their perspective is based on computational and profitable characteristics of a cloud-based service, with a native institutional cluster.

In [20], the authors have analyzed scalability and load characteristics of cloud computing on six data sets which are available on GEO [21] through a locally based computer, these experiments were later on replicated on Azure cloud. The results obtained in their experiments computed on Azure were identical to the ones on a local computer. Thus, they are self-confident of reproducibility. They have performed full analysis through 576 experiments that were carried on Azure platform.

Therefore, we can conclude that cloud computing is gradually becoming a popular technology in bioinformatics sector. This popularity can be attributed to Hadoop [13] which is an open-source software for meeting high computational requirements. Hadoop works in bioinformatics field because it deals with bringing computation to data rather than moving the entire data to computation thus reducing performance bottleneck characterized with poor network latency and slow computational devices. MapReduce which is a programming framework supported by Hadoop can be used in cloud environment for performing computations in cloud environment in a parallel fashion. Data in Hadoop environment can be stored in Hadoop distributed file system (HDFS) which can be used for storage of data of any volume. HDFS works by storing data in the form of chunks on multiple data nodes. Thus, HDFS can be another characteristic of cloud computing which supports bioinformatics application which usually involves capturing of data, storage of huge amount of data and also analysis of large data sets. Bioinformatics applications use different services offered by cloud computing such as data as a service [22, 23] which involves dynamic on demand data access and also makes available the latest data available. Amazon's AWS makes available data sets such as GenBank, 1000 Genomes, Influenza virus and Unigene [24]. These data sets can be integrated transparently with the existing cloud applications. Bioinformatics application tool can also be accessed through software as a service in cloud. Orthology detection

[25] and peak caller [26] for ChIP-seq data are some of the bioinformatics tools available as a service. Apart from software and data as a service platforms such as Galaxy Cloud [27, 28] for analysis of huge amount of data is also offered through cloud techniques.

Though cloud computing can be an effective technology for meeting the computation needs in bioinformatics research, there are certain issues that can affect the performance of the available cloud platforms. One such hindrance is the speed of data transfer. Usually, the speed of data transfer is slow, and at present, there are not many solutions available for moving the existing physical hard drives to cloud. Therefore, we need cloud solutions for integrating cloud computing with efficient data transfer technologies [13].

3 Applications in Bioinformatics

Bioinformatics research is generally synonyms with high computations, huge data sets and expensive computational equipment. These computational requirements involve high-end laboratories to meet the computational needs of the research personnel's. Thus, this need for an expensive setup is becoming a bottleneck in biological discovery at the computational level [29]. Therefore, cloud computing comes as a handy solution to researchers in the field of bioinformatics. Cloud computing helps in easing down the burden of bioinformatics researchers by reducing the computation time and optimizing costs involved. With the help of cloud computing researcher can get result easily and quickly without wasting time and money involved in laboratory setups.

In [29], the authors have discussed how cloud computing offers vibrant set of resources to small and medium-sized laboratories to quickly adjust their computational capacity depending on their requirements. In this work, the authors have benchmarked two-established cloud computing services, Amazon Web Services Elastic MapReduce and Google Compute Engine (GCE), using widely available genomic data sets and a standard bioinformatics channel based on Hadoop platform.

Marx [30] has discussed in his paper about big data challenges that Biologists are facing. According to them, biologists are joining the big-data club. According to them, with the advent of high-throughput genomics, scientists engaged in life sciences have started grappling with massive data sets. It is also stated that with every transitory year, scientist rotates extra frequently to big data to investigate the whole thing from the regulation of genes and the progression of genomes to why coastal algae bloom, what microbes dwell where in human body cavities and how the genetic composition of dissimilar cancers influences the cancer patients. Some of the bioinformatics platforms based on cloud computing and the technology used by them are given in Table 1.

Table 1 Bioinformatics platforms based on cloud

Platform	Description	Cloud technology
CloudBLAST [9]	Bioinformatics application using a combination of virtualization technology and MapReduce	Hadoop, MapReduce, Blast
Myrna [34]	RNA-sequencing through differential expression analysis	Bio-Linux, Amazon EC2, Galaxy Cloud
CloudBurst [35]	Performs sensitive read mapping and SNP calling through Hadoop MapReduce	Amazon EC2, Hadoop MapReduce
PeakRanger [36]	Peak caller for ChIP-seq data on cloud	Hadoop MapReduce
Rainbow [37]	Whole genome sequence data analysis through cloud computing	MapReduce, SOAPsnp, CrossBow, perl, picard
BioPig [38]	Analytical toolkit for large-scale data analysis using hadoops pig	ApachePig, Hadoop
SeqPig [39]	Analytical toolkit for large sequencing data set analysis using hadoops pig	ApachePig, Hadoop
Galaxy [40]	Scientific workflow system available online for genomic research	Python, SQL database, web server
Galaxy CloudMan [28]	Delivers clusters using cloud computing through Amazon EC2 for bioinformatics application	Amazon EC2, galaxy, Bio-linux

4 Cloud Computing in Big Data Analytics: Current Status

Now day's data generation rate is very high, so it is very difficult to manage such huge amount of data through the use of conventional systems. According to a survey conducted by authors in [30], biological data is growing at an exponential rate. Figure 1 shows the growth of biological data from 2004 to 2012. It also shows that genomic sequencing data increases to almost double its amount within a period of less than a year. The velocity of this data is so high that traditional systems fail to manage it. There is therefore a need to manage, store and process this huge volume of data. This phenomenon is what led to the emergence of a new field in computational sciences referred as "big data analytics". According to NIST [24], big data analytics involve the following characteristics: value: when the data is analyzed and veracity: which measures timeliness, accuracy and quality of data, latency between availability and measurement of data and cleanliness of data.

In [31], the authors have discussed that big knowledge refers to large, heterogeneous, and often unstructured digital content which is difficult to exploit through traditional methods, data management tools and techniques. The term encompasses the complexness, knowledge sorts, period of time for knowledge collection and process desires, and the value which will be obtained by smart analytics of huge data sets. Distributed big-data analytics services can improve performance over a federation of heterogeneous clouds [32]. However, contrary to common intuition, there is always an associated inherent trade-off between the amount of similarity

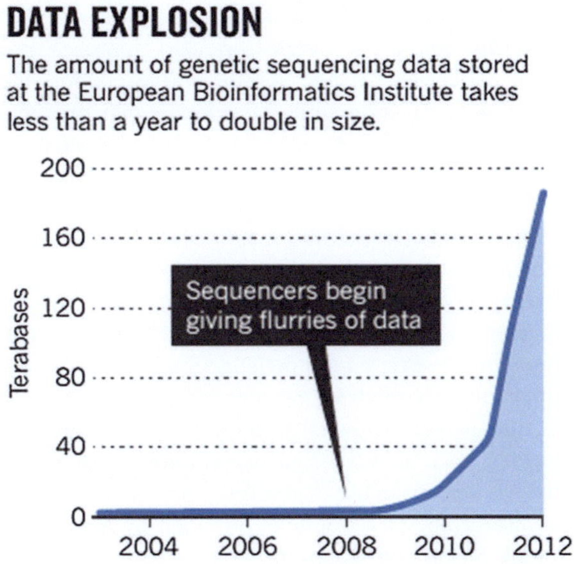

Fig. 1 Growth of biological data [30]

and performance for big-data analytics primarily owing due to a long delay for big-data to be transferred over the network. In [33], the authors have analyzed the current status of supporting tools for small CSE groups to utilize cloud computing. They have also discussed that cloud computing can be perceived as an interesting model and have identified several issues that prevent wide adoption of cloud computing from small CSE research groups. They have also given recommendations for addressing these issues in order to attract small CSE groups to utilize cloud computing. Advanced data processing techniques and associated tools can facilitate extraction of information from giant and complex data sets. This can be helpful in creating sophisticated choices in several business and scientific applications as well as applications such as tax payment collections, market sales, social studies, biosciences and high-energy physics. Combining huge knowledge analytics and data discovery techniques with alleviating computing systems can in turn provide new insights in a short span of time. Although few cloud-based analytics platforms square measures are accessible today, current analysis work anticipates that they are going to become common insight in a few number of years. There are few current solutions that support square measure. They apply the recently enforced knowledge Mining Cloud Framework as a high-level PaaS programming setting and create a collection of SaaS suites for giant data analytics. With this approach, users need not agonize about the cloud platform or other application programming details. Big knowledge analytics workflows developers will use workflows, which carry with it, complicated graphs of many simultaneous tasks, to address the complexness of scientific and business applications. This approach supports knowledge analytics design by providing a paradigm that encompasses all the steps of knowledge analytics, from knowledge access and filtering to data processing and sharing the produced data. Workflow-based data processing frameworks that run on cloud platforms and use a service-oriented approach provides versatile programming models, distributed task ability, and execution measurability that reduces data analytics completion time. Developers can implement huge knowledge analytics services through three models: knowledge analytics code as a service—which provides a well-defined data mining algorithmic rule or ready to use knowledge discovery tool as a web service to end users, for example organizations such as World Health Organization can access it directly online through a web browser; knowledge analytics platform as a service—provides a supporting platform that developers can use to make their own knowledge analytics applications or extend existing ones without worrying about the underlying infrastructure or distributed computing issues; and knowledge analytics infrastructure as a service—provides a collection of virtualized resources that developers can use as a computing infrastructure to run knowledge mining applications or to implement data analytics systems from scratch. End users whose goal is to perform complex knowledge analysis will make use of resources like Apache Hadoop and SciDB, whereas others can use proprietary solutions provided by firms like Google, IBM, EMC, BigML, Splunk Storm and Kognitio.

5 Cloud Computing in Bioinformatics and Big Data Analytics: Future Research

Cloud computing will play an important role in the bioinformatics research in coming future. Many places around the world lack infrastructure facilities required to support bioinformatics research. Bioinformatics research usually requires supercomputer for carrying out computations, but such facilities are not available for all researcher. Bioinformatics research can make use of cloud computing to meet its ever increasing computation demands by using the computational resources provide to it as a service via an Internet connection. The user has to pay only for the amount and time of services being used by it. Thus, cloud technology can be considered as a suitable candidate for meeting the future biomedical computing needs. Some of the reasons why cloud computing can act as important research tool in future are as follows:

5.1 Virtual Laboratory

Cloud computing can laid a ground for providing laboratory infrastructure required for carrying out bioinformatics computations. The advantage of using services provided by a cloud vendor is that they can cater to massive computational requirements through large datacenters with huge number of processors and other computational resources. It can provide users with a virtualized infrastructure. In this virtualized laboratory, resources can be accessed as services via an Internet connection. The users have to just connect to the respective cloud server offering their needs and perform computations in an on fly manner.

5.2 Scalability

Amongst the many advantages of cloud computing one very significant one is that of scalability. With varying workloads, cloud can also increase and decrease availability of resources in an elastic manner. Thus, with use of cloud researchers can demand more resources when they have high usage requirements and also shrink their resource usage when demand for resources diminishes. This scalable nature also leads to significant reduction in costs incurred on account of amount of usage of resources.

5.3 Computational Speedup and Time Effectiveness

Since, most of the technologies employed in cloud make use of parallelized technologies such as Hadoop MapReduce; therefore, use of cloud leads to the faster generation of results.

5.4 Data Management

Besides making available a huge range of softwares and tools as well as resources, cloud also offers data management capabilities. Several public cloud vendors such as Amazon offer services like S3 for storage. Many popular data sets such as GenBank, UniGene and HapMap are now available on Amazon. This removes the need for uploading data which is very time intensive.

Cloud computing also has significant potential in Big Data Analytics which is an upcoming field right now. Management of big data is a cumbersome task and an important issue. Individual research laboratories are generating several terabytes of data, and this data needs to be properly managed and analyzed. According to many renowned researchers, data is gold or similar to oil so providing security and management of data is an important issue. In the near future, cloud computing will play an important role in management as well as providing security to data with very low price. Cloud computing will be a very useful concept for big data analytics in the near future. Several scientific workflows are now available to researchers for meeting their big data analytic needs.

Thus, Cloud computing can be treated as a solution for meeting the big data needs in bioinformatics field. In this era of huge data sets and complex computations, we need to develop cloud platforms that can cater to needs of research communities consisting of data acquisition, storage and analysis. We also need services that can help in fast data transfers thereby reducing data uploading costs which can lead to a performance bottleneck. These services should also be available publicly to the entire research community.

6 Conclusion

Cloud computing is the latest technology prevailing in the information technology industry these days. It has gradually been recognized as an important tool for management of data. It has immense potential for handling complex computations and for meeting data storage requirements of an individual as well as an entire organization. This can be attributed due to the availability of a large number of resources at the Cloud service providers end. Due to the features such as elasticity, dynamic scalability, pay per usage and multitenancy, Cloud has several applications in different fields such as bioinformatics, signal processing and big data Analytics.

This manuscript discusses the role of cloud computing in the field of bioinformatics for management of huge data sets and for carrying out complex computations which eventually led to its application in big data analytics as well. We have also focused on how to manage big data using cloud computing. Thus, this paper is a survey of the current status of the usage of cloud computing as a technology in bioinformatics along with its applications on the basis of available bioinformatics platforms such as CloudBlast, Myrna and PeakRanger. It also discusses about the current state of the art of cloud computing in big data analytics along with the scope of future research based on cloud in both bioinformatics as well as big data analytics.

In future, we plan to work on analysis of electron microscopy images using publicly available cloud platforms such as Amazon EC2. We also plan to study its economy of scale in comparison with the existing research laboratories.

References

1. Alam, M., Shakil, K.A.: Recent developments in cloud based systems: state of art. arXiv preprint arXiv:1501.01323 (2015)
2. Taylor, R.C.: An overview of the Hadoop/MapReduce/HBase framework and its current applications in bioinformatics. BMC Bioinf. **11**(Suppl 12), S1 (2010)
3. Alam, M., Shakil, K.A.: Cloud database management system architecture. UACEE Int. J. Comput. Sci. Its Appl. **3**(1), 27–31 (2013)
4. Shakil, K.A., Alam, M.: Data management in cloud based environment using k-median clustering technique. In: IJCA Proceedings on 4th International IT Summit Confluence

2013-The Next Generation Information Technology Summit Confluence 2013, pp. 8–13 (2014)
5. Shakil, K.A., Alam, M., Sethi, S.: Exploring non-homogeneity and dynamicity of high scale cloud through hive and pig. arXiv preprint arXiv:1503.06600 (2015)
6. Alam, M., Shakil, K.A., Sethi, S.: Analysis and clustering of workload in Google cluster trace based on resource usage. arXiv preprint arXiv:1501.01426 (2015)
7. Alam, M., Shakil, K.A.: A decision matrix and monitoring based framework for infrastructure performance enhancement in a cloud based environment. arXiv preprint arXiv:1412.8029 (2014)
8. Alam, M., Shakil, K.A.. An NBDMMM algorithm based framework for allocation of resources in cloud. arXiv preprint arXiv:1412.8028 (2014)
9. Matsunaga, A., Tsugawa, M., Fortes, J.: Cloudblast: combining MapReduce and virtualization on distributed resources for bioinformatics applications. In: eScience, 2008. IEEE Fourth International Conference on eScience'08, pp. 222–229. IEEE (2008)
10. Leo, S., Santoni, F., Zanetti, G.: Biodoop: bioinformatics on Hadoop. In: Parallel Processing Workshops, 2009. International Conference on ICPPW'09, pp. 415–422. IEEE (2009)
11. Amin, N., Van Duijn, C.M., Aulchenko, Y.S.: A genomic background based method for association analysis in related individuals. PloS One **2**(12), e1274 (2007)
12. CloudStore File System. [Online] Available: http://kosmosfs.sourceforge.net (2015)
13. Dai, L., Gao, X., Guo, Y., Xiao, J., Zhang, Z.: Bioinformatics clouds for big data manipulation. Biol. Direct **7**(1), 43 (2012)
14. Calabrese, B., Cannataro, M.: Cloud computing in healthcare and biomedicine. Scalable Comput. Pract. Experience **16**(1) (2015)
15. Ahuja, S.P., Mani, S., Zambrano, J.: A survey of the state of cloud computing in healthcare. Netw Commun Technol **1**(2), 12–19 (2012)
16. Eugster, M.J.A., Schmid, M., Binder, H., Schmidberger, M.: Grid and cloud computing methods in biomedical research. Methods Inf. Med. **52**(1), 62–64 (2013)
17. Rosenthal, A., Mork, P., Li, M.H., Stanford, J., Koester, D., Reynolds, P.: Cloud computing: a new business paradigm for biomedical information sharing. J. Biomed. Inform. **43**(2), 342–353 (2010)
18. Hsieh, J.C., Hsu, M.W.: A cloud computing based 12-lead ECG telemedicine service. BMC Med. Inf. Decis. Making **12**(1), 77 (2012)
19. Dudley, J.T., Pouliot, Y., Chen, R., Morgan, A.A., Butte, A.J.: Translational bioinformatics in the cloud: an affordable alternative. Genome Med. **2**(8), 51 (2010)
20. Shanahan, H.P., Owen, A.M., Harrison, A.P.: Bioinformatics on the cloud computing platform Azure (2014)
21. Shanahan, H.P., Memon, F.N., Upton, G.J., Harrison, A.P.: Normalized Affymetrix expression data are biased by G-quadruplex formation. Nucleic Acids Res. **40**(8), 3307–3315 (2012)
22. Truong, H.L., Dustdar, S.: On analyzing and specifying concerns for data as a service. In: IEEE Asia-Pacific Services Computing Conference (Apscc 2009), pp. 83–90 (2009)
23. DaaS: The new information goldmine. http://online.wsj.com/article/SB125071202052143965.html. Accessed on Sept. 2015
24. NIST: http://www.nist.gov/itl/ssd/is/upload/NIST-stonebraker.pdf. Accessed on Sept. 2015
25. Wall, D.P., Kudtarkar, P., Fusaro, V.A., Pivovarov, R., Patil, P., Tonellato, P.J.: Cloud computing for comparative genomics. BMC Bioinf. **11**, 259 (2010)
26. Feng, X., Grossman, R., Stein, L.: PeakRanger: a cloud-enabled peak caller for ChIP-seq data. BMC Bioinf. **12**, 139 (2011)
27. Afgan, E., Baker, D., Coraor, N., Goto, H., Paul, I.M., Makova, K.D., Nekrutenko, A., Taylor, J.: Harnessing cloud computing with Galaxy cloud. Nat. Biotechnol. **29**(11), 972–974 (2011)
28. Afgan, E., Baker, D., Coraor, N., Chapman, B., Nekrutenko, A., Taylor, J.: Galaxy CloudMan: delivering cloud compute clusters. BMC Bioinf. **11**(Suppl 12), S4 (2010)

29. Yazar, S., Gooden, G.E., Mackey, D.A., Hewitt, A.W.: Benchmarking undedicated cloud computing providers for analysis of genomic datasets (2014)
30. Marx, V.: Biology: the big challenges of big data. Nature **498**(7453), 255–260 (2013)
31. Talia, D.: Toward Cloud-based Big-data Analytics, pp. 98–101. IEEE Computer, Science (2013)
32. Jung, G., Gnanasambandam, N., Mukherjee, T.: Synchronous parallel processing of big-data analytics services to optimize performance in federated clouds. In: IEEE 5th International Conference on Cloud Computing (CLOUD), 2012, pp. 811–818. IEEE (2012)
33. Truong, H.L., Dustdar, S.: Cloud computing for small research groups in computational science and engineering: current status and outlook. Computing **91**(1), 75–91 (2011)
34. Langmead, B., Hansen, K.D., Leek, J.T.: Cloud-scale RNA-sequencing differential expression analysis with Myrna. Genome Biol. **11**(8), R83 (2010)
35. Schatz, M.C.: Cloudburst: highly sensitive read mapping with mapreduce. Bioinformatics **25**(11), 1363–1369 (2009)
36. Feng, X., Grossman, R., Stein, L.: PeakRanger: a cloud-enabled peak caller for ChIP-seq data. BMC Bioinf. **12**(1), 139 (2011)
37. Zhao, S., Prenger, K., Smith, L., Messina, T., Fan, H., Jaeger, E., Stephens, S.: Rainbow: a tool for large-scale whole-genome sequencing data analysis using cloud computing. BMC Genom. **14**(1), 425 (2013)
38. Nordberg, H., Bhatia, K., Wang, K., Wang, Z.: Biopig: a hadoop-based analytic toolkit for large-scale sequence data. Bioinformatics **29**(23), 3014–3019 (2013)
39. Schumacher, A., Pireddu, L., Niemenmaa, M., Kallio, A., Korpelainen, E., Zanetti, G., Heljanko, K.: Seqpig: simple and scalable scripting for large sequencing data sets in hadoop. Bioinformatics **30**(1), 119–120 (2014)
40. Goecks, J., Nekrutenko, A., Taylor, J.: Galaxy: a comprehensive approach for supporting accessible, reproducible, and transparent computational research in the life sciences. Genome Biol. **11**(8), R86 (2010)
41. Khan, M.W., Alam, M.: A survey of application: genomics and genetic programming, a new frontier. Genomics **100**(2), 65–71 (2012)
42. Shakil, K.A., Sethi, S., Alam, M.: An effective framework for managing university data using a cloud based environment. In: 2nd International Conference on Computing for Sustainable Global Development (INDIACom), 2015, pp. 1262–1266 (2014)

Generalized Query Processing Mechanism in Cloud Database Management System

Shweta Malhotra, Mohammad Najmud Doja, Bashir Alam and Mansaf Alam

Abstract This is an epoch of Big data, Cloud computing, Cloud Database Management techniques. Traditional database approaches are not suitable for such colossal amount of data. To overcome the limitations of RDBMS, Map Reduce codes can be considered as a probable solution for such huge amount of data processing. Map Reduce codes provide both scalability and reliability. Users till date can work snugly with traditional Database approaches such as SQL, MYSQL, ORACLE, DB2, etc., and they are not aware of Map Reduce codes. In this paper, we are proposing a model which can convert any RDBMS queries to Map Reduce codes. We also gear optimization technique which can improve the performance of such amalgam approach.

Keywords Cloud database management system · CDBMS · MapReduce · Hadoop · Optimized algorithm · Cross rack communication · Data processing

1 Introduction

Cloud Database is based on distributed, parallel, grid computing. There are several companies like Yahoo, Microsoft, Amazon, and many more that are providing Cloud Database services. Cloud Database service provided by the Cloud provider is heterogeneous in nature. Heterogeneity is provided in the number of forms as follows and shown in Fig. 1.

S. Malhotra (✉) · M.N. Doja · B. Alam · M. Alam
Jamia Millia Islamia, New Delhi, India
e-mail: Shweta.mongia@yahoo.com

M.N. Doja
e-mail: mndoja@gmail.com

B. Alam
e-mail: babashiralam@gmail.com

M. Alam
e-mail: Mansaf_alam2002@yahoo.com

V.B. Aggarwal et al. (eds.), *Big Data Analytics*, Advances in Intelligent Systems and Computing 654, https://doi.org/10.1007/978-981-10-6620-7_61

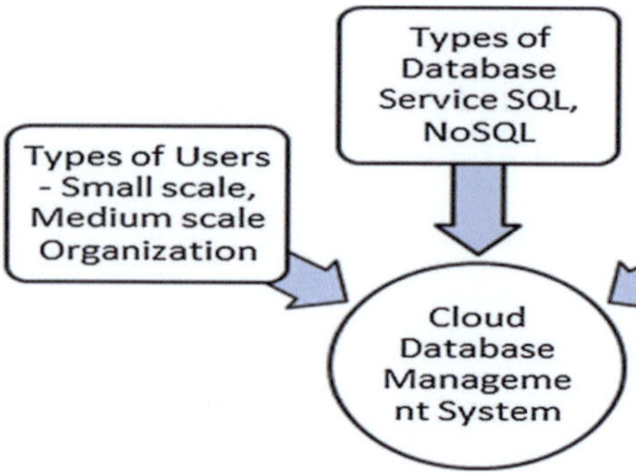

Fig. 1 Heterogeneous cloud database management system

- Types of users are different which includes simple, small-scale organization, medium-scale organization users.
- Types of data that are processed on Cloud differ which includes structured, unstructured, or semi-structured data.
- Types of Database service include RDBMS type SQL-based service or NOSQL.

An IDC report [1] predicts that by 2020 the global data volume will grow up to 40 zettabytes, and data is doubling every two years. Cloud Database Management System and Big data are integral terms. Cloud providers cannot handle such heterogeneous data with traditional Database Management Systems. RDBMS is not suitable because it has limited capacity and, moreover, it cannot explore original high fidelity data due to the different layers available for storage and processing. For such Cloud Databases as well as Big data problems, companies are now coming up with many solutions; one of the simple solution among many is MapReduce.

MapReduce codes are more suitable for such situations due to the following reasons:

- Map Reduce provides scalability.
- Map Reduce codes are in the form of simple Key-Value pairs.
- Large and complex data processing is being done with the help of simple two functions, i.e., Map and Reduce.
- Map reduce codes can be used to store data in an encrypted form.

In this paper, we have proposed one Generalized Model as a solution for such Cloud Databases as well as Big data processing problems. This system takes up queries in any Database languages, and the model converts the queries into simple Map Reduce codes. Actual processing is being done with the help of Map Reduce codes as shown in Fig. 2.

Below are the segments of the proposed model

- Firstly, the user interface which can take up the Database queries of the user.
- Secondly, compiler which converts the codes written in Database languages to the Map Reduce codes.

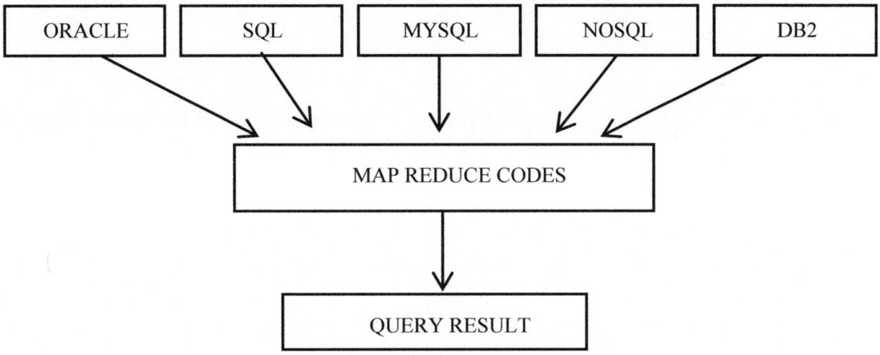

Fig. 2 System architecture

- Lastly, optimization technique is being proposed for MapReduce codes.

Rest of the paper is organized as follows. Current state of the work is described in Sect. 2. Layerwise System Model, architecture, and optimization technique are explained in Sects. 3 and 4. Lastly, Sect. 5 concludes the paper.

2 Related Work

2.1 MapReduce Functions

MapReduce programming paradigm based on parallel and distributed computing in which the Map and Reduce functions consists of Key-Value pairs [2, 3]. Parallelism or the concept of pipelining is used to enhance the MapReduce functionality. Authors in [4] described that MapReduce consists of several intermediate phases like shuffle, sort, and merge. These phases play an important role with respect to effective resource allocation. MapReduce codes are used for data analysis on the similar kind of data sets, hence authors in [5] proposed one cloud view framework which is used for processing, analyzing, and maintenance of the massive data sets. This framework uses the Map-Join-Reduce phases. Map Reduce task [6] deals with many problems; one of the problems is scheduling the Map Reduce task in an effective manner. Author in [6] emphasizes on two important factor, i.e., energy consumption and simulation time.

Author in [7] described one system SQLMR which coverts SQL queries into MapReduce codes and compared the performance of this system with HIVE, HadoopDB. This paper is also based upon the same notion and applicable for all the Databases.

There are several Databases available for Cloud Databases but with limited query capabilities, one of the issues came where data need to be integrated with local Databases as well as Cloud Databases hence author in [8] proposed

BigIntegrator [8]; one system which is used to process the data present at the local Databases and data located at the cloud repositories.

2.2 *Optimization Technique for MapReduce*

Author in [9] described one optimal algorithm to minimize the cross rack communication. In optimization, they discussed about reducer placement problem and explained one function for data coming in and coming out from the rack in terms of reducer. Authors in [10] described one improved algorithm for data load balancing in Hadoop. They implemented the algorithm which can balance the data at overloaded racks in preference.

3 System Design

Cloud Database Management System and Big data are related to each other as the data which are being present on the Cloud Databases are also recognized as Big data. Big data can be characterized by three ways, i.e., large amount of data in terms of Quintilian bytes, secondly, data in the form of structured or unstructured form and data that cannot be processed with the help of traditional RDBMS.

Traditional RDBMS are not suitable for Cloud Databases as they cannot process large amount of such complex data. Users till date are well-known to traditional Databases but, MapReduce, a simple programming model which works at Hadoop [11] framework is considered to be the suitable choice for such huge amount of data for the following reasons:

- MapReduce codes provide parallel processing on large and complex data.
- MapReduce provides scalability.

The Generalized Model proposed in this paper fulfills this gap.

3.1 *System Architecture*

There is a need of one system that can process the massive data presented at Cloud Database repositories without having much difficulty on user side. Figure 3 shows the complete structure and step by step working of such system called Generalized System.

Firstly, users send the queries through user interface; compiler converts the queries into MapReduce codes. Then optimized algorithm for the placement the Map and Reduce function is applied in such a way to minimize the cross rack communication for getting the best results in terms of running time.

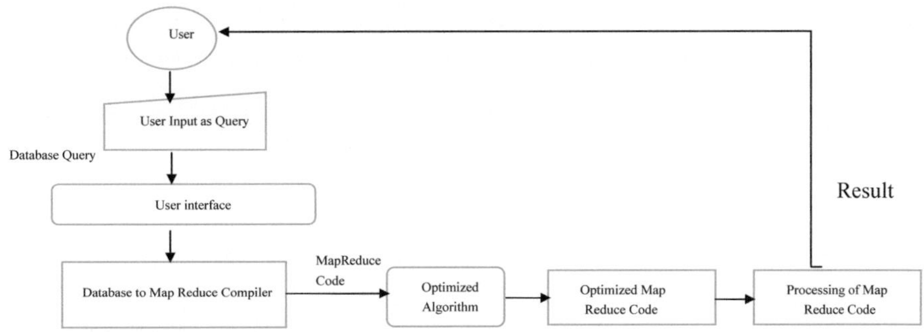

Fig. 3 System architecture

3.2 *Layerwise System Model*

System Architecture explained in the above section is described in terms of Cloud Database layers [12]. Figure 4 shows the Layerwise System Model. Cloud Database Management System consists of five layers [12], i.e., external layer which deals with the user interface, conceptual middleware layer and physical middleware layer provide virtualization, conceptual layer deals with processing of data, and lastly, physical layer deals with the effective storage of data present at Cloud repositories.

In this paper, the working of the proposed Generalized Model which is defined with the help of Cloud Database layers as follows:

External layer provides the user interface; here, the user writes queries in any Database languages like SQL, Oracle, DB2, etc. Then at conceptual middleware layer, queries written in different languages are converted into MapReduce codes.

Fig. 4 Layer wise working of model

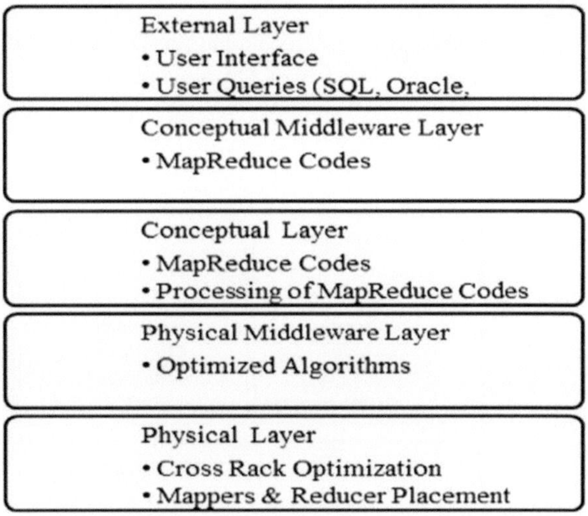

Actual processing is being done at conceptual layer. MapReduce codes can be further improvised at physical middleware and physical layer with the help of algorithms like cross rack communication for mappers and reducers.

4 Optimization Technique

Author in [9] described optimal algorithm for cross rack optimization in which they discussed about reducer placement problem and explained one function for data coming in and coming out from the rack in terms of reducer.

That is,

$$f_i(r_i) = m_i(R - r_i) + r_i(M - m_i). \quad (1)$$

They assumed that mapper function is placed at the same rack where data are placed to keep the data locality and then finding out the effective position of reducer function on the racks so that to minimize the cross rack communication.

In this paper, we have used the same optimal algorithm for cross rack optimization as shown in Fig. 5 but with the difference that it is considering the placement of both the mapper function and reducer function on the DataNodes of the racks. Earlier while placing reducer function on the racks, DataNodes were not considered. Here, following is the assumptions that have been considered in this paper:

- *N* is the number of racks,
- *D* is the DataNodes present at racks,
- *M* is the mapper function,
- *R* is the reducer function,

For example, if data is located at the DataNode1 of Rack1, then 90% probability is that mapper is placed over the same DataNode of same rack where the data are present. About 7% probability is that mapper is placed at the other DataNode of

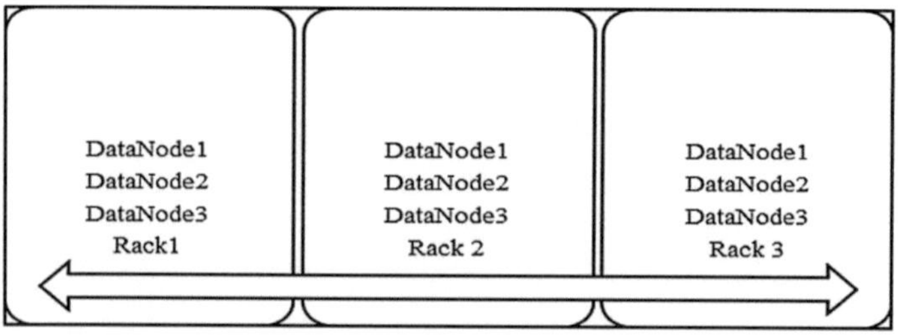

Fig. 5 Cross rack communication

same rack where data are presented, and only 3% probability is that mapper is placed at the DataNode of other rack. Same applies for reducer.

Now, for each rack S_i, the amount of data sent from or coming into one rack to another is defined based on Eq. 1, but these functions are defined in terms of mapper and reducer.

$f_i(m_i, r_i) = 0.9m_id_{ij}(R - r_i) + 0.9r_id_{ij}(M - m_i)$, if mapper and reducer are placed at the same DataNode of same rack where data are present,

$f_i(m_i, r_i) = 0.9m_id_{ij}(R - r_i) + 0.07r_id_{ij}(M - m_i)$, if mapper is placed at the same DataNode where data are present, but reducer is placed at the other DataNode of same rack.

$f_i(m_i, r_i) = 0.9m_id_{ij}(R - r_i) + 0.03r_id_{ij}(M - m_i)$, if mapper is placed at the same DataNode of the same rack where data are present but reducer is placed at the different DataNode of the different rack.

Where $i = 1, 2, 3, \ldots, p$ are the number of racks.

In this way, a simple MapReduce functions can be placed based on these functions can improve the performance of the proposed model as these functions are considering both the placement of mappers and reducer function into account.

5 Conclusion

We have proposed a model that can effectively process data at Cloud repositories to overcome the limitations of an existing traditional RDBMS system. Proposed model consists of three modules. Firstly, user interface where the users can put their queries in any Database language. Secondly, the complier that converts the queries into MapReduce codes, and lastly, the enhanced optimal cross rack algorithm to minimize the cross rack communication which considers the placement of both mapper as well as reducer. In future, the proposed model can be implemented with the help of existing programming language.

References

1. Gantz, J., Reinsel, D.: The digital universe in 2020: big data, bigger digital shadows, and biggest growth in the far east. Proc. IDC iView IDC Anal. Future (2012)
2. Dean, J., Ghemawat, S.: MapReduce: simplified data processing on large clusters. Commun. ACM **51**(1), 107–113 (2008)
3. Dahiphale, D., Karve, R., Vasilakos, A.V., Liu, H., Yu, Z.: An advanced Mapreduce: Cloud Mapreduce, enhancements and applications. IEEE Trans. Netw. Serv. Manag. **11**(1), 101–115 (2014)

4. Zhang, Q., Zhani, M.F., Yang, Y., Wong, B.: PRISM: fine grained resource-aware scheduling for MapReduce. IEEE Trans. Cloud Comput. **3**(2), 182–194 (2015)
5. Bhardwaj, R., Mishra, N., Kumar, R.: Data analyzing using map-join-reduce in cloud storage. In: IEEE 2014 International Conference on Parallel, Distributed and Grid Computing, 2014, pp. 370–373 (2014)
6. Althebyan, Q., Qudah, Q., Jaraweh, Y., Yaseen, Q.: Multi-threading based map reduce tasks scheduling. In: 2014 IEEE International Conference on Information and Communication Systems (ICICS), pp. 1–6 (2014)
7. Hsieh, M., Chang, C., Ho, L., Wu, J., Lui, P.: SQLMR: A scalable database management system for cloud computing. In: International Conference on Parallel Processing (ICPP) 2011, pp. 315–324 (2011)
8. Zhu, M., Risch, T.: Querying combined cloud-based and relational databases. In: International Conference on cloud and service computing (CSC) 2011, pp. 330–335 (2011)
9. Li-Yung, H., Jan-jan, W., Pangfeng, L.: Optimal algorithm for cross-rack communication optimization in map reduce framework. In: IEEE International Conference on Cloud Computing 2011, pp. 420–427 (2011)
10. Liu, K., Xu, G., Yuan, J.: An improved Hadoop data load balancing algorithm. J. Netw. **8**(12), 2816–2822 (2013)
11. Apache Hadoop: http://hadoop.apache.org
12. Mongia, S., Doja, M.N., Alam, B., Alam, M.: 5 Layered architecture of cloud database management system. AASRI Conf. Parallel Distrib Comput. Syst. **5**, 194–199 (2013)

Deliberative Study of Security Issues in Cloud Computing

Chandani Kathad and Tosal Bhalodia

Abstract Cloud computing is an intact new archetype that offers a non-conventional computing exemplar for association to take up information technology and respected utility. Cloud computing provides platform for entrance to numerous, boundless site from flexible work out to on require provision to active storage and computing prerequisite execution. It is observed that potential gain attained in the course of cloud computing is at rest uncertain for generously reachable resources and open-ended resources which blow cloud implementation. Design, level dependency, flexibility, and multi-tenancy are such factors which penetrate new dimension of cloud form. Study of cloud problems is discussed in this article. Varying, active, and secure cloud model implementation face so many challenges which are covered in this paper. Any proposed security for cloud is enclosed, and derivative aspect of cloud security are denoted by this survey.

Keywords Cloud security · Cloud computing

1 Introduction

Currently, cloud security has turned into a very vivacious problem in the computing world. One major part on which the present era business depends on outsourcing of computational services and resources, which are speeding up due to progressive cloud computing. Distributed system divided subsequently into a cloud computing which presents for extremely elastic resource group, storage, and computing resources. By the time, the major approach to get accessibility of software and stored information in the value addition to exited process on the cloud explains how they can influence the distributed cloud computing model. Is it your cloud secure?

C. Kathad (✉) · T. Bhalodia
Atmiya Institute of Technology and Science, Rajkot, India
e-mail: kathadchandani@gmail.com

T. Bhalodia
e-mail: tosalbhalodia@gmail.com

V.B. Aggarwal et al. (eds.), *Big Data Analytics*, Advances in Intelligent Systems and Computing 654, https://doi.org/10.1007/978-981-10-6620-7_62

Elsewhere is there any deliberative examination for its security? Whenever the matter of connectivity of cloud with external world it would be suspect or might be damaged through exploiting by threats and attacks of vulnerabilities. Cloud provides low-load services and applications which are aggravated business, engineering, and academic to use cloud as host. At the different side with various types of technical resources, there are various attack surface with their oddity can negotiate security in presented model of cloud computing. Some of the numerous problems are:

- Cloud security
- Multi-tenancy
- Dealer lock-in
- SLA administration
- Service portability
- Protected information management.

These are prime problems which become obstacles for cloud computing model. Now, the cloud contributor and further so from clients point of view. Following reasons denote that approval of cloud model is obstruct because cardinal factor security.

- SLA: Required data becomes non-accessible threat where it is lacking prospective at service layer concurrence.
- Multi-tenancy: Same physical and rational medium accessed by the unusual occupants.
- Loss of control: Unawareness of storing and accessing of data from third party which is referred as subcontract security administration.

Inside this manuscript, it is analyzed that security concerns implicated in the cloud computing models. The purpose is to recognize the variety of attack vectors and security issues significant to cloud models. This article depicts complete study designed for every weakness to underline its source reasons. This research should assist cloud consumers and providers to include an insight to understand the cloud security issues and how they can oppose these issues. This paper is well thought-out as follows. Respective security problems are covered in Sect. 2. Cloud security implications and linked research challenges significant issues that bother cloud computing model is included in Sect. 3. Section 4 denotes the exploration conclusions and summary. Finally, Sect. 5 winds up the paper with future work and subsequent steps.

2 Cloud Computing Security Issues

Cloud computing exemplar provides 3 service delivery and deployment model. The delivery models are as given below:

1. Private cloud: Particular body included in the private cloud platform.
2. Public cloud: It is accessible toward freely by civic consumers to enroll and utilize the obtainable infrastructure.
3. Hybrid cloud: Confidential cloud which expands for utilization of equipments, services, and application in unrestricted clouds.

The deployment models are as follows:

1. Infrastructure-as-a-service (IaaS): Computer component like network equipments, servers, and memory space which delivered as service is known as IaaS.
2. Platform-as-a-service (PaaS): To build up, install, and control the application users need platform, equipments, and business which are provided by cloud.
3. Software-as-a-services (SaaS): The necessity of application execution in cloud infrastructure which becomes platform for hosting application and is contributed by cloud.

This additional factor enhances the requirement to have security issues, addresses and probably mitigation for threats to cloud design, as enclosed in this study paper. Survey done on these cloud computing issues:

- Multi-tenancy
- Elasticity
- Availability of Information(SLA)
- Cloud secure federation (Fig. 1).

As it is relevant, the review performed by IDC venture board, Fig. 2 reveals the pinnacle cloud security concerns and problems that associations face at what time they look frontward to embrace cloud's advantages. Cloud computing has a set of propose related to its supple and flexible [1] structural design. When it comes to transportation of protected information, the cloud purchaser and contributor should have equally shared dependability in the form of faithful affiliation and harmonize.

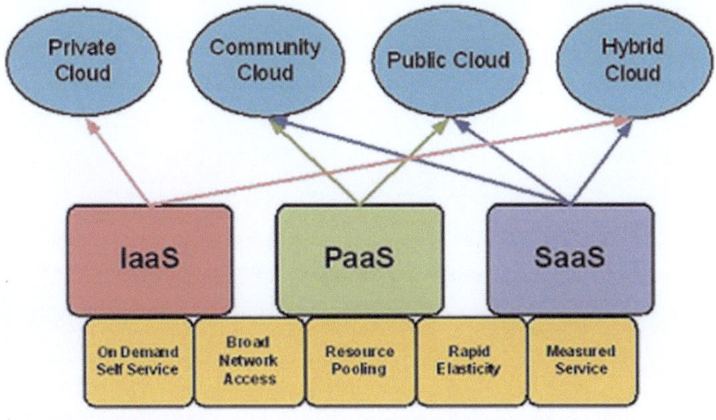

Fig. 1 Cloud deployment model

The next part denotes the cloud security implications based on fundamental issues discovered in this part.

3 Cloud Security Implications and Remediations

Cloud is eternally changing and vibrant as well as composite, principally for the reason that of a variety of aspects such as: storage on demand, computing on demand, virtualization requirement, elastic computing, multi threading/processing, multi-tenant atmosphere and so on. Due to limitations and requirements, it moves from right place to affect correct security in time.

1. **Cloud Multi-tenancy**

Cloud was constructed and used for a number of reasons of which some of the most cardinal reasons were shared computing, shared memory, storage, and access resources. Cloud suppliers install multi-tenancy as de facto norms to accomplish proficient usage of resources, though reducing price. Resources, storage, services, and applications of all residents who live at similar platform of supplier's site can be included in multi-tenancy. Multi-tenancy can be best denoted in Fig. 3.

2. **Elasticity**

Elasticity is an additional significant factor of cloud computing which expands capabilities of customers from top-to-bottom level different resources accessed for services which are highly on demand. For suppliers, increasing and decreasing the level of resident's equipments propose view of neighbors for using the space before

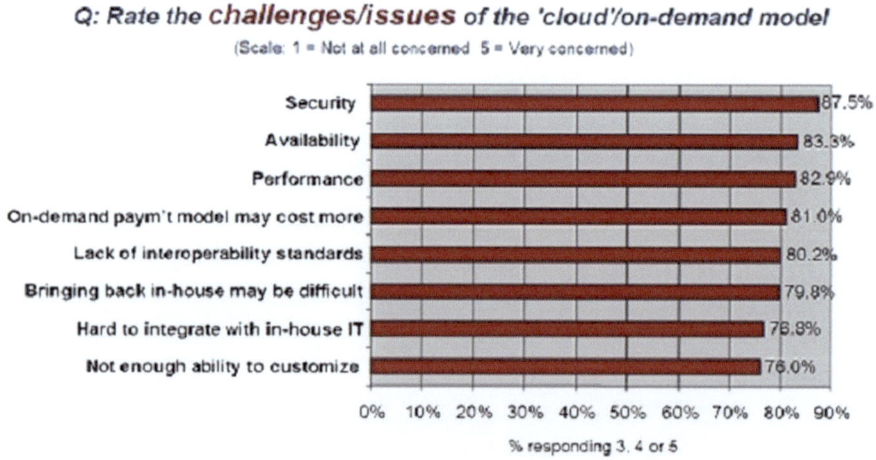

Fig. 2 Cloud computing security issues. *Source* IDC Enterprise panel, 3Q09, n = 263

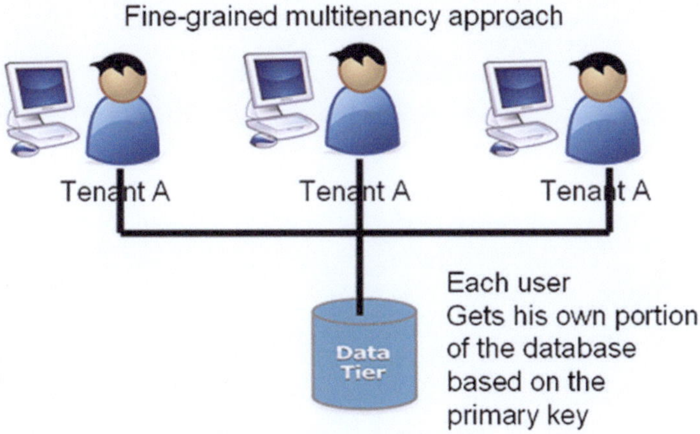

Fig. 3 Cloud multi-tenancy model

occupied. Data or information is unwrap and misplace then it becomes extremely damaging situation for association and industry (Fig. 4).

3. **Availability of Information**

Because of numerous problems, highly required data or information cannot be accessed as soon as needed that become threatening for association while porting services, procedures, and applications of cloud. Because of necessity of any country with respect to physical data storage from specific organizer's computing and storage resources getting off and destroy. In this era, information is everything overlooking still the minimum feature can escort competition winning the client. Figure 5 explores cloud service level agreement.

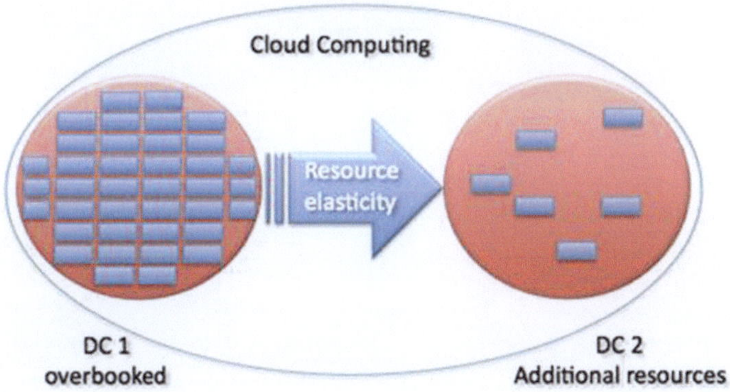

Fig. 4 Cloud resource elasticity

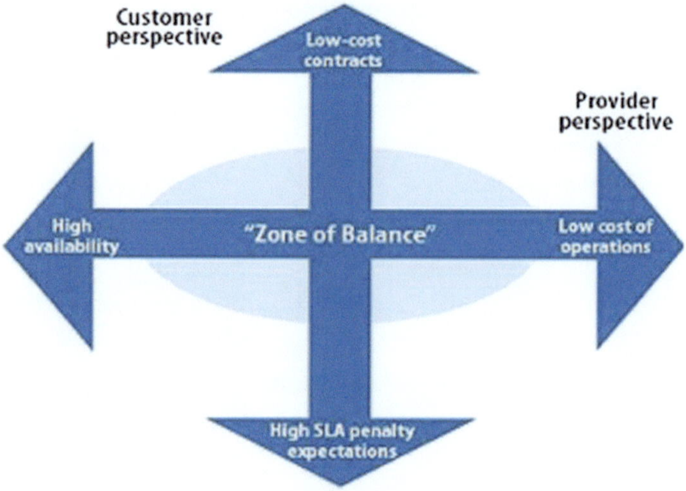

Fig. 5 Cloud service level agreement

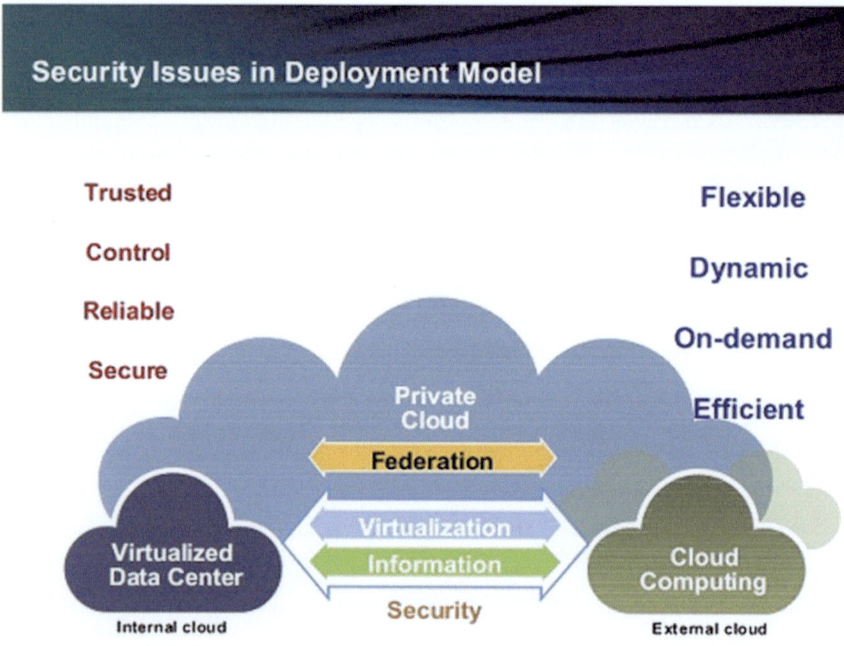

Fig. 6 Secure federation

4. **Cloud Secure Federation**

As soon as a cloud user leverages application and information that depend on services from vivid clouds, it will require to sustain its security necessities imposed on both clouds and in between. This represents a range of problems as when numerous clouds collaborate together to transport a larger pool of resources or incorporated services, their security requirements need to be federated and forced on physically and rationally various cloud platforms whether it would be IaaS, PaaS, or SaaS (Fig. 6)

4 Conclusion

Cloud is vivacious which has countless facets together good as well as bad. Although qualities provide like you go through model, flexibility of resource adoption or reduction, lower total cost of ownership (TCO), and approximately no upfront investment, there are a lot of issues, despite of its merits which can prohibit adoption of cloud by business, data security which ported to cloud. There are many safety implications appropriate to cloud model of which this manuscript has attempted to focus on top of the majority serious ones.

All these issues stem for the incoherence of consumers skirting cloud models which bar them to leverage power of cloud.

To excellently use the model, we need to chunk the offered security issues and speak to the security anxieties/implications. Based on the facts and particulars searched above, we can go over the main point the cloud security concerns as below:

A. A few of the security suggestions are derived as of the expertise which structures the especially essential of cloud like virtualization.
B. Multi-tenancy is one more area which needs greatest awareness to control some attacks on victim resources from malicious users cloud security include prime issue is tenant segregation that provides solution of SaaS level bottom to physical communication.
C. Cloud security management is extremely vital to organize and handle the client facing data and the way supplier's infrastructure (material/rational) roles.
D. The cloud model be supposed to enclose a security binding as denoted in Fig. 7, so that every access to any item of the cloud proposal ought to get ahead through multilayer security solution.

By this conversation, it is suggested that cloud computing security is at least integrate the subsequent solution(s) to make certain that supplier is at equality with in-house hosting despite the fact that, end user/tenant is secured of its data confidentiality and reliability.

Fig. 7

A. Flexible engine, cloud APIs, and CML like systems which provide elastic platform for security. These should be based on industry encryption and certification rules.
B. Support for multi-tenancy with separation in place somewhere each one occupant can simply perceive its data, information and security configurations. Separation at logical VM and hypervisor level as well as physical level, for example, different blades on the existing circumstance be supposed to offer in a delicate approach such that only an occupant has right of access to its resources, through license to clean the data before release resources to supplier pool. This will make sure that any resources being reassigned are appropriately scrubbed for data.
C. Suppliers should support combination and synchronization by way of tenant's managerial security policy [16] next to variety of levels to deliver incorporated security. This into twist involves that the security pertained is layered.
D. Suppliers should be adjustable to meet regular environmental alterations and stakeholders requested to guarantee that the cloud security build is upheld irrespective of where some modification acquire place.

5 Future Work

Article concludes the assorted cloud security challenges and purpose can be signified clarification about vivid cloud security problems wherever alleviation are often ported as of Infrastructure, platform- and software-as-a-service, and generously accessible to fusion to confidential cloud designs. Association such while Cloud Security Alliance (CSA) [2] and NIST are trying to set collectively standards for cloud computing security and resolution the concerns discussed in this research paper. It is recommended to accept an adaptive approach in undertaking the cloud security issues which will assist in the difficult conception and combing of security requirement of different stakeholders at various levels of details. As next steps, we would collect data inseminated from a variety of stakeholders (providers, consumers, vendors) such that different cloud models with their limitations and qualities can be modified to security issue mitigation techniques, which are neither inactive nor single time (security is always long-lasting phenomena).

References

1. ENISA: Cloud computing: benefits, risks and recommendations for information security. www.enisa.europa.eu/act/rm/files/deliverables/cloud-computing-risk-assessment/at_download/fullReport/
2. Cloud Security Alliance (CSA): http://www.cloudsecurityalliance.org/
3. Velte: Cloud Computing—A Practical Approach. Tata McGraw-Hill Edition (ISBN-13:978-0-07-068351-8)
4. Sosinsky, B.: Cloud Computing Bible. Wiley Publishing Inc. (ISBN 13:978-0470903568)
5. IDC: IDC ranking of issues of cloud computing model. http://blogs.idc.com/ie/?p=730/
6. Kretzschmar, M., Golling, M.: Security management spectrum in future multi-provider inter-cloud environments—method to highlight necessary further development. In: 5th International DMTF Academic Alliance Workshop on Systems and Virtualization Management (SVM), pp. 1–8 (2011)
7. Guitart, J., Torres, J.: Characterizing cloud federation for enhancing providers' profit. In: IEEE 3rd International Conference on Cloud Computing (CLOUD), pp. 123–130 (2010)
8. Uttam Kumar, T., Wache, H.: Cloud broker: bringing intelligence into the cloud. In: IEEE 3rd International Conference on Cloud Computing (CLOUD), pp. 544–545 (2010)
9. Lampe, U., Wenge, O., Müller, A., Schaarschmidt, R.: Cloud computing in the financial industry—A road paved with security pitfalls? In: 18th Americas Conference on Information Systems (AMCIS). Association for Information Systems (AIS) (2012)

An Overview of Optimized Computing Approach: Green Cloud Computing

Archana Gondalia, Rahul N. Vaza and Amit B. Parmar

Abstract Distributed computing is an exceptionally versatile and techno-financial structural planning for running high-performance computing (HPC), venture, and Web applications. As the utilization of tremendous server farms (DC) and immense group jumps up step by step, vitality utilization by these DC is raising speedier. This high vitality utilization influences the high operational expense as well as results in high carbon discharges. Ideal vitality arrangements are obliged to check the effect of Cloud processing on the earth. Expanded processor chips usage frees more warmth. This pointless warming requires furthermore cooling, and cooling again makes warm; then, we move to a stage where we have to change the structure by getting the same registering speed at lessened impressiveness use. Cloud computing with green calculation can empower more vitality upgraded utilization of figuring force.

Keywords Green computing · High-performance computing (HPC)

1 Introduction

Distributed computing is an exceedingly versatile and financially savvy construction modeling for running HPC, undertaking, and Web applications. It utilizes colossal server farms (DC) and enormous bunch is expanding step by step so vitality utilization by these DC. This high vitality utilization influences the high operational expense as well as results in high carbon outflows. Ideal vitality

A. Gondalia (✉)
Department of Computer Engineering, AITS, Rajkot, India
e-mail: 13mcen30@nirmauni.ac.in

R.N. Vaza · A.B. Parmar
AITS, Rajkot, Gujarat, India
e-mail: rnvaza@gmail.com

A.B. Parmar
e-mail: abparmar@gmail.com

V.B. Aggarwal et al. (eds.), *Big Data Analytics*, Advances in Intelligent Systems and Computing 654, https://doi.org/10.1007/978-981-10-6620-7_63

arrangements are obliged to check the effect of Cloud processing on nature. So this huge measure of CO_2 dissemination in environment has created the need for Green computing [5]. Cloud computing with green calculation can empower more vitality effective utilization of registering force.

Distributed computing or Cloud computing, being a developing innovation likewise, brings up huge issues about its natural maintainability. Through the utilization of huge shared virtualized data centers, Cloud figuring can over huge vitality reserve funds. Then again, Cloud administrations can likewise further expand the Web movement and its developing database which could lessen such vitality funds. A Green Cloud system for lessening its carbon-foot-shaped impression in wholesome way without yielding the nature of administration (execution, responsiveness, and accessibility) is offered by the different Cloud suppliers (Fig. 1).

2 Requirement of Green Computing

Present-day server farms, working under the Cloud registering model, are facilitating a mixed bag of uses running by keep running for a few moments (e.g., provide solicitations for the applications of Web, like e-business and interpersonal organizations gateways with short-term loads of work) which keep running for more spans of time (e.g., recreations or huge information set handling) on allocation equipment stages. The requirement to deal with different applications in a server farm makes the test of on-interest asset provisioning and allotment in light of time-shifting workloads. Typically, server farm assets are statically apportioned to applications, in light of crest burden qualities, keeping in mind the end goal to keep up seclusion and give execution ensures. Up to this point, elite has been the sole concern in server farm arrangements, and this interest has been satisfied without

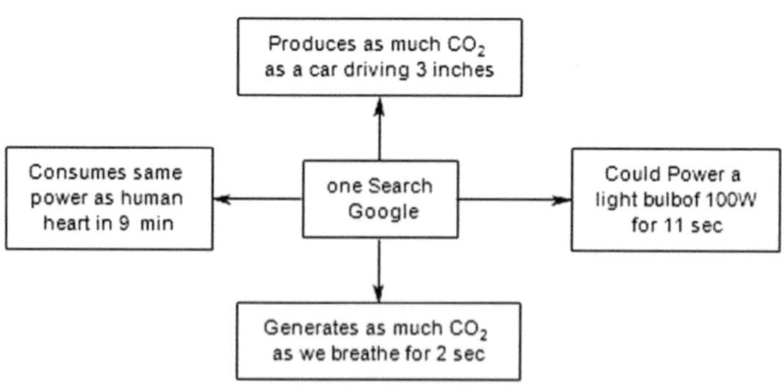

Fig. 1 Energy utilized in one Google search

giving careful consideration to vitality utilization. Data focuses are costly to keep up and antagonistic to the earth. High vitality costs and immense carbon-foot-shaped impressions are acquired because of enormous measures of power expected to power and cool various servers facilitated in these server farms. Cloud administration suppliers need to receive measures to guarantee that their net revenue is not drastically decreased because of high vitality costs. It is a high time a specialized workforce ought to comprehend the need of "GREEN COMPUTING" while utilizing ICT. Numerous innovation organizations have taken the activity to advance the thought and institutionalize the utilization and make a stride ahead toward green figuring.

3 Architecture of Green Cloud Computing

The point of this paper is to address the issue of empowering vitality productive asset designation, thus prompting Green Cloud processing server farms, to fulfill contending applications' interest for registering administrations, and to spare vitality. Figure demonstrates the abnormal state building design for supporting vitality proficient administration allotment in Green Cloud processing framework. There are fundamentally four primary elements included:

Presently, building design of green registering is demonstrated in Fig. 2. In green Cloud structural planning, administrations are given to clients. It has taken after primary elements including:

1. Brokers: Cloud customers or their intermediaries submit administration demands from anyplace on the planet to the Cloud. Notice that there can be a distinction between Cloud buyers and clients of conveyed administrations. For example, a shopper can be an organization conveying a Web application, which introduces changing workload as indicated by the quantity of "clients" getting to it.

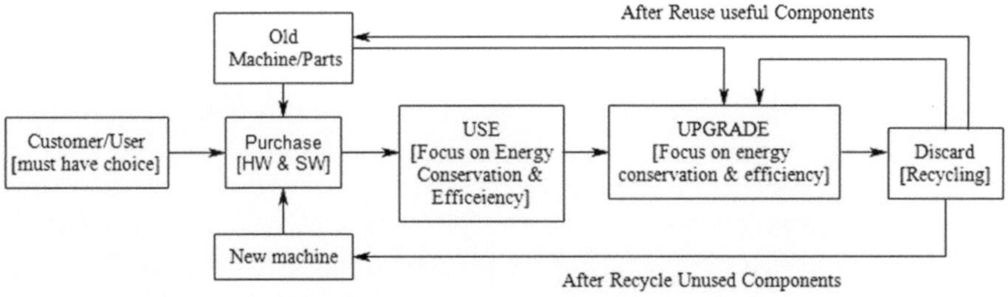

Fig. 2 Green computing cycle

2. Green resource allocator: The Cloud base and shoppers are the interfaces. It needs the connection of the accompanying parts to bolster vitality proficient asset administration:

   - Scheduler: The task will be scheduled by the user.

     – Task selector: Task selection will be performed by task selector.
     – Application master filer: Select particular qualities of buyers so that imperative shoppers could be conceded uncommon benefits and organized to different buyers.
     – Resource information: It is an interface between consumers and Cloud infrastructure.
     – Cost calculator: Calculation of cost is performed by cost calculator.
     – Carbon emission calculator: How much carbon dioxide absorbed will be calculated with this calculator.

3. Allocation of various resources will be provided to Private Cloud.
4. At last required services are provided to the user (Fig. 3).

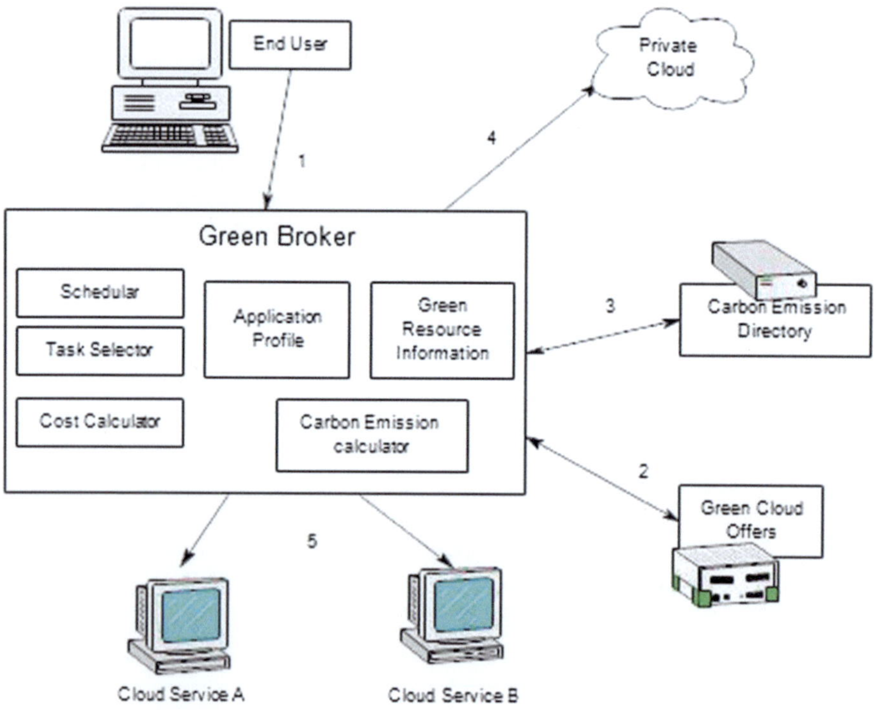

Fig. 3 Green broker

4 Energy Efficiency of Cloud Computing

4.1 Usage

Software as a Service model has altered the applications, and programming is circulated and utilized. Further, organizations are changing to Software as a Service Clouds to minimize their cost of IT. Hence, it turned out to be essential to address the vitality productivity at application level itself. Be that as it may, this layer has gotten next to no fascination since numerous applications are as of now on utilization, and the greater part of the new applications is generally overhauled form of or created utilizing already executed instruments. To accomplish vitality productivity at application level, SaaS suppliers ought to focus on sending programming on right sort of framework which can execute the product most effectively. This requires the exploration and examination of exchange o_ in the middle of execution and vitality utilization because of execution of programming on numerous stages and equipment.

4.2 Virtualization

In the stack of Cloud, all works in the writing address the difficulties at the Infrastructure as a Service (IaaS) supplier level where examination center is on booking and asset administration to lessen the measure of dynamic assets executing the workload of client applications. The combination of VMs, VM movement, booking, interest projection, heat administration and temperature mindful designation, and burden adjusting is utilized as essential systems for minimizing force utilization. As examined in past area, vitalization assumes a vital part in these strategies because of its few components, for example, combining, lives movement, and execution disengagement. Combining aides in dealing with the exchange off between execution, asset use, and vitality utilization. Additionally, VM movement permits adaptable and dynamic asset administration while encouraging shortcoming administration and lower support cost. Because of different levels of deliberations, it is truly difficult to keep up arrangement information of each virtual machine inside of a Cloud data center. In this manner, different backhanded burden estimation systems are utilized for combining of VMs. Albeit above combination routines can lessen the general number of assets used to serve client applications, the movement and migration of VMs for coordinating application interest can affect the quality of service administration prerequisites of the client. Since Cloud suppliers need to fulfill a certain level of administration, some work concentrated on minimizing the vitality utilization while diminishing the quantity of SLA infringement. One proposal of a streamlining for capacity vitalization is known as Sample-Replicate-Consolidate Mapping (SRCMap) that empowers the vitality rate for element input/output loads of work by uniting the combined load of work on a part of physical volumes relative to the input/output workload power. Since force is scattered in Cloud data center because of warmth created by the servers, a few works additionally have been proposed for element booking of VMs and applications which consider the warm states or the warmth dissemination in a server farm. The thought of warm figure booking likewise enhances the unwavering quality of underline foundation.

4.3 Network Infrastructure

At system level, the vitality effectiveness is accomplished either at the hub level or at the foundation level. The vitality productivity issues in systems administration are normally alluded to as "green systems administration," which identifies with implanting vitality mindfulness in the outline, in the gadgets, and in the conventions of systems. There are four classes of arrangements offered in writing, to be specific asset combining, vitalization, particular connectedness, and relative registering. Asset union aides in regrouping the underused gadgets to lessen the worldwide utilization. Like merging, specific connectedness of gadgets comprises of dispersed components which permit the single bits of hardware to go unmoving for quite a while, as straightforwardly as could be allowed from whatever is left of the arranged gadgets. The distinction of asset solidification is that the combining applies to assets that are allocated inside of the system foundation, while particular connectedness permits killing unused assets at the edge of the system. Vitalization as talked about before permits more than one administration to work on the same bit of equipment, in this way enhancing the equipment use. Relative processing can be connected to a framework all in all, to network conventions, and to individual gadgets and parts. Adaptive link and dynamic voltage scaling rate are average samples of relative figuring. Dynamic voltage scaling lessens the vitality condition of the CPU as an element of a framework burden, while adaptive link rate applies a comparative idea to network interfaces, diminishing their ability, and in this way their utilization, as a component of the connection load.

5 Various Approaches to Make Cloud More Green

For the most part, three methodologies have been gone for to make distributed computing situations more natural neighborly. These methodologies have been gone for in the server farms under trial conditions. The down-to-earth utilization of these techniques is for further study. The systems are shown below:

1. Dynamic voltage recurrence scaling technique: Electronic circuitry has a working clock connected with it. Subsequently, system intensely relies upon equipment. The force investment funds are likewise low contrasted with

different methodologies. The force investment funds to cost brought about proportion are likewise low.
2. Resource allotment relocation systems: Every machine which is physical has various virtual machines whereupon the applications will run in Cloud computing. The virtual machine relocation system emphasis on moving virtual machines in a manner that the force increment is minimum. This strategy is managed in point of interest later.
3. Algorithmic methodologies: It has been experimentally established that a perfect server devours around 70% of the force used by a completely used server. Utilizing a neural system predictor, the green booking calculations first gauges obliged element workload on the servers. At that point, superior's servers are killed keeping in mind the end goal to minimize the quantity of running servers, consequently minimizing the vitality use at the purposes of utilization to give advantages to every other level. Various servers are further appending to help guarantee administration-level assertion. While guaranteeing nature of administration, the main issue is to secure the earth and to decrease the aggregate expense of possession.

6 Conclusion

This paper introduces new thoughts for enhancing force execution of Cloud application, server farms, and so on. To start with, we investigated different measurements for breaking down force execution of distributed computing and server farm; we have suggested conceivable procedures to decrease the force prerequisite. Green Cloud computing is for the further innovation that backings environment, again use expended vitality and power, then enhance assets productively. Green figuring spotlights on decrease of carbon dioxide discharge in environment and in this way makes IT industry environment well disposed. What's more, make your whole association Green inside and out conceivable. Comprehend the life cycle of IT items. Lessen, however, much paper as could reasonably be expected and reuse it when you can. How about we begin taking a shot at it and grasp what's to come.

References

1. Yamini, R.: Power management in cloud computing using green algorithm. In: 2012 International Conference on Advances in Engineering, Science and Management [1] (ICAESM), pp. 128–133, 30–31 Mar 2012
2. Jain, A., Mishra, M., Peddoju, S.K., Jain, N.: Energy efficient computing—green cloud computing. In: 2013 International Conference on Energy Efficient Technologies for Sustainability (ICEETS), pp. 978–982, 10–12 Apr 2013

3. Garg, S.K., Buyya, R.: Green Cloud computing and Environmental Sustainability. Harnessing Green IT: Principles Pract. 315–340 (2012)
4. Sheikh, R.A., Lanjewar, U.A.: Green computing—embrace a secure future. Int. J. Comput. Appl. **10**(4), 0975–8887 (2010)
5. Murugesan, S.: Harnessing green IT: Principles and practices. IT Prof. **10**(1), 24–33, Jan–Feb 2008

A Literature Review of QoS with Load Balancing in Cloud Computing Environment

Geeta and Shiva Prakash

Abstract Cloud computing is a type of computing technology which can be considered as a new model of computing. It also can be considered as a speedily emerging new technique for providing computing as a service. In cloud computing, many cloud users demand various services as per their daily new needs. So the function of cloud computing is to provide all the desired services to the cloud users. But due to limited resources, it is very difficult for cloud providers to provide all the users desired services. From the cloud providers, perception cloud resources must be allotted in a rational manner. So, it is a major issue to meet cloud users satisfaction and QoS requirements. The aim of this paper is to present a study of previous works in load balancing and QoS methods used in the cloud computing environment. This paper mainly addresses key performance challenges and different modeling with their applications for QoS management and simulation toolkits in cloud computing.

Keywords Cloud computing · QoS management · Load balancing · Virtual machine

1 Introduction

Cloud computing field has spread in finding in recent years owing to its rapid user demand. It is an emerging computing technology in the field of information technology (IT). Many cloud operators have activated in the market to provide a rich offering, including Platform as a Service (PaaS), Infrastructure as a Service (IaaS),

Geeta (✉)
UPTU, Lucknow, India
e-mail: geetasingh02@gmail.com

S. Prakash
Department of Computer Science & Engineering, Madan Mohan Malviya University of Technology, Gorakhpur, India
e-mail: shiva.plko@gmail.com

V.B. Aggarwal et al. (eds.), *Big Data Analytics*, Advances in Intelligent Systems and Computing 654, https://doi.org/10.1007/978-981-10-6620-7_64

and Software as a Service (SaaS) solutions. The QoS within the case of flash and also the like, storage of our digital pictures is, from the buyer purpose of read, wherever inside the cloud. We do not have to be bound to pick up wherever, specifically, we have an affinity to just would like our flash login identification and an Internet affiliation. We will see this model as evident in Web-based e-mail too.

There are some important characteristics of the cloud computing [1].

Self Service on demand—the cloud users can use on-demand services such as server time and network storage without human interaction with, respectively, service provider.

Location independence—customer generally has no knowledge or control over the specific location of the provided resources but may be able to specify location at a higher level of abstraction e.g., data center, country, or state. Examples of resources include storage, network bandwidth, processing, memory, and virtual machines.

Broad network access—the cloud computing capabilities are available over the Internet and accessed through standard techniques that promote use by various thick or thin client platforms (e.g., laptops, mobile phones, and PDAs).

Rapid elasticity—the cloud computing capabilities can be elastically and rapidly helped in some cases automatically, to quickly scale in and rapidly released to quickly scale in. The capabilities available often seem to be infinite and can be bought at anytime in any quantity, to the user.

Measuring service—the usage of cloud computing resource can be controlled, reported, and monitored by the cloud providers.

The cloud technology stack is a flexible and easy way to retrieve and store huge data without worrying about the software and hardware needed. As the number of consumers on cloud increases, automatically, the existing resources decreases which creates the problem of delay between the consumers and the service providers. The traffic over the Internet must be dealt.

To rise above this problem, a lot of load balancing techniques are intended by researchers. However, cloud computing has significantly straightforwarded the ability provisioning method although there are many challenges in the field of QoS management. QoS shows the strength of concert, availability, and consistency presented by the platform as well as an application. This paper presents the thoughts of previous load balancing algorithms, the monitoring of workload in the system, and their modeling to the management of QoS in cloud computing environment [2].

The rest of the paper is carefully intended as follows: In Sect. 2, we describe the research challenges of cloud computing environment. In Sect. 3, we review previous cloud computing work focused on load balancing, QoS management. Section 4 presents overall discussion about the QoS work in cloud computing. Finally, Sect. 5 concludes the paper.

2 Research Challenges in Cloud Computing

There are several research challenges which indicate the need of further improvement. The main challenges are as follows:

I. **Security and Privacy**: Security and privacy is the biggest issue in cloud. It occurs because of movement of networks data and application, loss of control on data, various natures of resources, and several security policies.

II. **Performance**: The performance is also a big issue in cloud computing. It deliberates the capability of the cloud organization. The outcome may be poor due to not have appropriate assets viz. limited bandwidth, memory, diminutive CPU speed, etc.

III. **Efficient Load balancing**: By this method, workload has been distributed equally across all the nodes in cloud environment. Load balancing is used to reach good consumer contentment and examine the ratio of resources, and ensure that no any particular node is overloaded, therefore refinement of the whole performance of the cloud.

IV. **Resource Management and Scheduling**: it can be considered at several levels viz. software, hardware, virtualization level with performance, privacy, security, and other attributes being dependent on the resources and management. It includes the management of disk space, memory, CPU's, cores, VM images, threads, I/O devices etc.

V. **Require a constant and Fast Internet speed**: With the help of cloud system, business gets the capability to save money on software and hardware but still requires spending additional on the bandwidth. This is not possible to fully exploit the services of cloud without high-speed communication channels.

VI. **Data center Energy Consumption**: With the help of a survey done by Amazon, the cost consumption of its data centers is 53%, and the total cost is used by the servers for a 3-year amortization period while cooling and energy requirements use 42% of the total budget including both the cooling requirements (23%) and direct power consumption ($\sim$19%) for amortization period of fifteen years.

VII. **Scale and Quality of Service Management**: Although loud computing has significantly eased the competency based method, a lot of challenges of quality of service management. Quality of service means the levels of concert, availability, and reliability on hand by the platform and a use or infrastructure that hosts it. Quality of service is elementary for cloud consumers and to be expecting from the providers to provide the declared features.

3 Literature Review

In this survey, we cover the works related to quality of service and load balancing in cloud computing. Quality of service can be increased by balancing the load on different machine, so delay will be decreased, such research work based on modeling of workload, quality of service management, and load-balancing algorithms in cloud computing environment. The meaning of system modeling is analyzing the concert of a cloud computing whichever at runtime or at design time. The values of quality of service such as reliability, availability, and response time are calculated using these system models. The most common aspects of load balancing of cloud computing are as first, resource pooling in which cloud service provider used the on-demand services using virtualization concepts and multi-tenancy to make readily available resources to the numerous consumers. Second, quick elasticity and flexibility permit the cloud system to balance up and down quickly as per desires of the cloud users and provide the capability to free the resources as soon as no longer desired. Third, scalability facilitates on-demand services and resources in the cloud computing environment. Fourth aspect is efficiency to accomplish extremely scalable system, able to balance the loads as soon as the load increases by a huge amount and a user of cloud computing, user demands more resources online rapidly is very important. An appropriate allocation of responsibilities among the processors can attain these features for the cloud systems environment. At last, Dynamic and Static Resource Allocation in this ways, the load is assigning across cloud computing system, moreover, statically or dynamically. Literature shows that the resource distribution in dynamic ways is better than the static one to retain the dynamic requirements of a cloud user.

Di et al. [3] presented workload guess and pattern analysis that is validated for long-term basis based on a Bayesian algorithm. Here, there are several workloads-based key features to find the possibility of the next features, a Bayesian classifier is used. The researchers defined several workload-based key features and used a Bayesian classifier to evaluate the next possibility of each feature. The tests, however, require resources such as thousand of machines and a large number of related contents or data which is collected from Google data center. In Caprarescu et al. [4], gave a self-organizing approach and also considered Decentralized methods. This approach is able to give proper robust solutions for resource provisioning, load balancing, and service deployment in the cloud infrastructure.

In order to forecast and get temporal correlations between loads of various computer clusters in the cloud, a Hidden Markov Models is used by Khan et al. [5]. Various proposals have been made by the authors such as a technique to forecast and classify workloads in cloud systems in order to supply proper cloud resources. A co-clustering algorithm has also been developed by the authors to find servers that have scheme of equal workload which is developed by analyzing and researching the correlations performance for applications on various servers.

In a similar manner, a data center simulation tool DCSIM [6] focused on the dynamic resource management of infrastructure as a service. Each host can run a large number of virtual machines and has a model or power model to give the power consumption of the entire data center.

Pattern recognition techniques are presented by Gmach et al. [7] to cloud workload and data center. Based on pattern recognition and trend analysis, the researchers proposed a workload prediction algorithm whose goal is to find a procedure to allocate servers to various workloads by using the resource pool properly. The synthetic workloads are created to reflect the later or following activities of the workload but the design and trend are analyzed first.

A best practice guide proposed in [8] by Trivedi is to build empirical models. In this paper, major matters involved are the gathering of the very useful content or data, variable-selection procedure, and the modeling technique. The benefits of various prediction approaches have also been properly described by the researchers.

A Demand Estimation with Confidence (DEC) method has been proposed by Kalbasi et al. [9] to solve the issues of multi-collinearity in regression approaches. Proper enhancement of the estimation accuracy can be achieved through DEC. A service demand estimation from exploitation and end to end response times have proposed by Liu et al. [10]. The issue is evaluated as quadratic optimization programs which are based on queuing formula, and results achieved can be backed out with experimental data. A simulator based on the event GROUDSIM [11] is used for certain applications arranged on large-scale grids and cloud. In cloud computing environment [12], different methods of resource allocation and their applications are discussed. Also, differentially adapted dynamic proportion-based network resource allocation in cloud computing was discussed. The resources are allocated in cloud computing environment via different parameters like maximum efficiency, maximum energy, SLA aware, elevated throughput, highest efficiency, QoS aware, highest energy, and consumption of power. Calbasi [13], presents a method to evaluate online resource demand based on evaluation of least absolute deviations, regression techniques—least squares, and support vector regression. Casale et al. [14] presented an optimization-based inference approach and expressed as a robust linear regression problem which uses open- and close-based queuing network performance models. This approach sums up measurements (i.e., utilization of the servers and system throughput), generally retrieved from log files, to estimate service times.

A proposed resource allocation model [15] deals the consumer's job to an appropriate data center. Their implementation is based on an agent-based test bed using Java Agent. This is adaptively find a proper data centre based on (a) the geographical distance is man-made from network delay stuck between a user and data centers, and (b) every data centres' workload. The coordinator, monitoring agents, and users are agents in this system. The game theory-based method was proposed by author Guiyi et al. [16] to provide solution for recourse allocation in cloud computing environment. The QoS constrained based recourse allocation problem. The binary integer programming method has proposed for preliminary optimization for cloud services. This method has designed an evolutionary mechanism on the basis of initial results by which it is able to achieve reasonable solution and final best possible. In totality, authors focused on the complicated parallel computing problem on distinct machines associated across the Internet.

A resource allocation and management algorithm of cloud were presented by Bacigalupo et al. [17]. This algorithm is based on forecasting. LQNs methods are used to evaluate the completion of an application install on the systems with strict SLA desires based on data from the past. The researchers also gave the advantage and disadvantage of key the practical use of LQNs in the cloud systems.

The relations between resource consumption and workload for cloud Web applications are studied by Desnoyers et al. [18]. Queuing scheme are useful for representation of various elements of the system, data mining, and machine learning approaches in order to assure flexibility of the model to work under various system conditions. Through the proposed method, great accuracy for forecasting usage of resources and workload is achieved.

To enhance the throughput by means of minimum response time is possible by using new load balancing techniques [19] in the network. The servers can sent and received data in minimum delays by dividing the traffic in between the servers. Lot of algorithms is presents that balance the traffic load between the servers [20]. The well known example of traffic load balancing in our day today life can be related to internet websites. Long response time and more delays experience by the users in earlier server systems without load balancing. Load balancing techniques are plays major role in enhancing quality of services in multimedia applications typically concern redundant servers which help a better allocation of the communication traffic consequently that the website ease of use is categorically advanced [19].

An economic model have presented by Ye et al. [21] based on discrete Bayesian Networks to classify end-users long-term performance considering cloud service supply of an end user. Then, by using effective diagrams, simulation, and analytical experiments, the composition QoS aware service is resolved. Susana proposed [22] a queuing theory-based technique of dynamic load balancing strategy to offer differentiated services. To achieve the differentiated services-based solution, use the key attribute of intensity of concurrency in servers. For maintaining the required distance in normal service times among the service classes by using dynamic load balancing technique based on self-adaptive nature. Markov and Fault Trees models are also used by Jhawar and Piuri et al. in [23] to evaluate the availability and the reliability of the fault tolerance patterns of a cloud environment under the different deployment contexts. The authors have also proposed an approach based on the above evaluation to identify the best approach which is according to the user's requirements. The QoS in cloud computing is enhanced on proper implementing load balancing techniques on the basic of dynamically monitoring the load of the system.

4 Discussion

The research work proposed by authors on the QoS in cloud computing has greatly increased the various services provided by cloud computing service providers. QoS field aims to improve the QoS by keeping the delay to small quantity by balancing the load in cloud computing. Multimedia, audio, video conferencing, etc. are considered the main applications of this area where enhancement in the delay may be useless.

Cloud has greatly simplified the capacity provisioning method; however, it creates several issues in the management of QoS. Quality of service includes the levels of performance, availability, and reliability offered by the platform or the application or the infrastructure that hosts it. Research in workload modeling and its application in QoS management in cloud computing. Few well-known load balancing techniques via which QoS can be improved in cloud computing

- Dynamic Load Balancing that results fault tolerance, low overhead, high scalability can be used in enhancing performance in cloud computing.
- Approaches related to load balancing based on Weighted Active Monitoring to enhance processing time and response time.
- Load balancing based on round-robin technique assigns the virtual machines in circular order; by these methods, some nodes may be under loaded/overloaded and can result in decreasing resource utilization.
- The multiple workflows in cloud computing for dynamic works deal by load balancing technique to improve quality of service.
- A lot of load balancing techniques get evaluated on the basis of different metrics of QoS like throughput, cost, resource utilization, and results show the improvement over existing others works.

This survey shows a lot of improvement over authors works with own works but there are several assumptions. So without considering assumptions taken at the time of evaluation, their improvement may not be considerable. Even though there are many existing works that show improvement, they have disadvantages also. Therefore, we say that there is no any single approach to give better solution in all conditions.

5 Conclusion

This paper surveyed the various research efforts that are being carried out in the workload modeling, system modeling, their different applications to QoS management, and its load balancing algorithms in the cloud computing environment. We have also discussed the major challenges that are faced by cloud computing environment and designing of many load balancing algorithm and various modeling techniques for the QoS management in cloud systems. We have discussed the proposed algorithms, but the research work opens many research opportunities to us in the area of load balancing in cloud computing.

References

1. Mell, P., Grance, T.: The NIST definition of cloud computing, Technical report published in NIST Special Publication 800-145 at 25 Oct 2011
2. Petcu, D., Macariu, G., Panica, S., Craciun, C.: Portable cloud applications: from theory to practice. Future Gener. Comput. Syst. **29**(6) 1417–1430 (2013)
3. Di, S., Kondo, D., Walfredo, C.: Host load prediction in a Google compute cloud with a Bayesian model. Proceedings in the international conference for high performance computing, networking, storage and analysis, SC, pp. 1–11 (2012)
4. Caprarescu, B.A., Calcavecchia, N.M., Di Nitto, E., Dubois, D.J.: Sos cloud: Self-organizing services in the cloud. In: Bio-inspired models of network, information, and computing systems, vol. 87, pp 48–55. Springer, Berlin, Heidelberg (2012)
5. Khan, A., Yan, X., Shu, T., Anerousis, N.: Workload characterization and prediction in the cloud: A multiple time series approach. In: Proceedings of the IEEE Network Operations and Management Symposium, Maui, HI, USA NOMS NOMS 2012, pp. 1287–1294 (2012)
6. Keller, G., Tighe, M., Lutfiyya, H., Bauer, M.: DCSim: A data Centre simulation tool. In: Proceedings of the 2012 8th international conference on network and service management, and 2012 workshop on systems virtualization management, CNSM-SVM 2012, Las Vegas, NV, USA, pp. 385–392 (2012)
7. Gmach, D., Rolia, J., Cherkasova, L., Kemper, A.: Workload analysis and demand prediction of enterprise data center applications. In: Proceedings of the IEEE 10th international symposium on workload characterization, IISWC, pp. 171–180, Boston, MA, USA (2007)
8. Hoffmann, G.A., Trivedi, K.S., Malek, M.: A best practice guide to resource forecasting for computing systems. IEEE Trans. Reliab. **56**(4), 615–628 (2007)
9. Kalbasi, A., Krishnamurthy, D., Rolia, J., Dawson, S.: DEC: Service demand estimation with confidence. IEEE Trans. Softw. Eng. **38**(3), 561–578 (2012)
10. Liu, Z., Wynter, L, Xia C, Zhang F, "Parameter inference of queueing models for it systems using end-to-end measurements". Perform Eval. **63**(1), 36–60 (2006)
11. Ostermann, S., Plankensteiner, K., Prodan, R., Fahringer, T.: Groudsim: An event-based simulation framework for computational grids and clouds. In: Proceedings of the conference on parallel processing, Euro-Par 2010, Ischia, Italy, pp. 305–313 (2010)
12. RamMohan, N.R., Baburaj, E.: Resource allocation techniques in cloud computing-research challenges for applications. In: Fourth international conference on computational intelligence and communication networks (2012)
13. Kalbasi, A., Krishnamurthy, D., Rolia, J., Richter, M.: MODE: Mix driven on-line resource demand estimation. In: Proceedings of the 7th international conference on network and services management, international federation for information processing, pp. 1–9 (2011)
14. Casale, G., Cremonesi, P., Turrin, R.: Robust workload estimation in queueing network performance models. In: Proceedings of Euromicro PDP, pp. 183–187 (2008)
15. Vignesh, V., Sendhil Kumar, K.S., Jaisankar, N.: Resource management and scheduling in cloud environment. Int. J. Sci. Res. Publ. ISSN **3**(6), 2250–3153 (2013)
16. Wei, G., Vasilakos, A.V., Zheng, Y., Xiong, N.: A game-theoretic method of resource allocation for cloud computing services. In Springer, J. Supercomput. pp. 252–269 (2010)
17. Bacigalupo, D., van Hemert, J., Chen, X., Usmani, A., Chester, A., He, L., Dillenberger, D., Wills, G., Gilbert, L., Jarvis, S.: Managing dynamic enterprise and urgent workloads on clouds using layered queuing and historical performance models. Simul. Model. Prac. Theory **19**, 1479–1495 (2011)

18. Desnoyers, P., Wood, T., Shenoy, P.J., Singh, R., Patil, S., Vin, H.M.: Modellus: Automated modeling of complex internet data center applications. TWEB **6**(2): 8 (2012)
19. Shimonski, R.: Windows 2000 & windows Server 2003 clustering and load balancing, p. 2. McGraw-Hill Professional Publishing, Emeryville, CA, USA (2003)
20. Brian, A.: Load balancing in the cloud: tools, tips, and techniques. A Technical white paper in Solutions Architect, Right Scale
21. Ye, Z., Bouguettaya, A., Zhou, X.: QoS-aware cloud service composition based on economic models. In: Proceedings of the 10th international conference on service-oriented computing, ICSOC'12, Shanghai, China, pp. 111–126 (2012)
22. De Saram, S.L., Perera, S., Jayewardene, M.: QoS aware load balancing in multi-tenant cloud environments, published in Int. J. Next Gener. Comput. **4**(1) (2013)
23. Jhawar, R., Piuri, V.: Fault tolerance management in IaaS clouds. In: Proceedings of 2012 IEEE first AESS European Conference on Satellite Telecommunications, ESTEL 2012, Rome, Italy, pp. 1–6 (2012)

WAMLB: Weighted Active Monitoring Load Balancing in Cloud Computing

Aditya Narayan Singh and Shiva Prakash

Abstract Nowadays, cloud computing is an amazing and fast-growing area in research industry. It provides IT-related service through Internet. Load balancing is an essential feature in cloud computing environments, and without proper load balancing, we cannot expect better response time. In traditional active monitoring load balancing techniques in which they generally check least loaded virtual machine and those who are least loaded selected for execution of task, some authors are also select the virtual machine randomly. In our proposed strategy for assigning the virtual machine, we calculate weight factor on the basis of physical memory, bandwidth, number of processor, and processor speed. After calculating the weight of each virtual machine, we select those virtual machine that is highest weight and available for execution of the task. We also verified our results with existing work through CloudAnalyst that is CloudSim-based simulator; our result shows the improvement over existing one.

Keywords Cloud computing · Virtual machine · Load balancing · CloudSim · CloudAnalyst

1 Introduction

Cloud computing is newly introduced model that recently came popular in computer industry and academia. It provides computing as an utility to meet end-user requirement. Broadly, it can be defined as an on-demand computing system where various hardware, software, and applications share their resources with anyone having Internet facilities [1] . Many people use Google drive, Mi cloud, etc., and

A.N. Singh (✉) · S. Prakash
Department of Computer Science and Engineering,
Madan Mohan Malviya University of Technology, Gorakhpur, India
e-mail: aditya905014@gmail.com

S. Prakash
e-mail: shiva_pkec@yahoo.com

V.B. Aggarwal et al. (eds.), *Big Data Analytics*, Advances in Intelligent Systems and Computing 654, https://doi.org/10.1007/978-981-10-6620-7_65

these are cloud services. Various documents such as photographs, contact, SMS, call log, notes that are stored in our devices like mobile phone, desktop are also stored in servers that are occupied by the third parties. These are the different cases of cloud services.

Cloud provider's offers computing, storage, and software as services. Cloud computing is on-demand service provision technique where various organizations are avoiding the setup cost of hardware and software installation. In spite of fact that there are magnificent coming times of cloud computing, still there are many critical problems arising. Whenever the size of cloud scales up, cloud service provider requires handling massive request. These requests handled in this way keep the performance same or provide better when this type of situations arises. Various critical issues still should be unraveled. Load balancing is one of the issues.

Load balancing in cloud environment is very challenging task. Load balancing is a technique where workload of various systems is distributed to another system in such a way performance of the system is never decreased and user gets better response time.

Load balancing is also categorized as two types, static load balancing and dynamic load balancing. In static load balancing, we are checking the current state of the node and distribute the load to various nodes through given predefined rules for the input request. The various load balancer algorithms such as round robin, weighted round robin, and shortest job first algorithm are some static algorithms. Dynamic load balancer is based on the current state of the system, and no prior knowledge is required. Throttled algorithm, modified throttled, genetic algorithm, particle swarm optimization, etc., are some of dynamic load balancer. Dynamic load balancing gives better results than static load balancing because its takes run time statics in load balancing and another features, and it is also provide to user that easily modify the changing requirements at run time that occur.

This paper mainly focuses on the implementation of weighted active monitoring load balancing strategy which can use the combined weight of various parameters like physical memory, number of processor, processor speed, and bandwidth. We choose that available virtual machine which has highest weight. These strategies show that it gives better response time to the user request.

The remaining section of paper is arranged as follows: Sect. 2 provides the literature review, Sect. 3 provides proposed algorithm and previous algorithm and what is the problem associated with previous algorithm, Sect. 4 shows experimental setup through CloudAnalyst simulator, Sect. 5 shows simulation result and analysis, and Sect. 6 concludes the paper.

2 Literature Review

In this section, we discuss some known contribution in earlier effort for load balancing in cloud computing.

Brototi et al. in [2] proposed load balancing approach based on soft computing approach. Stochastic Hill Climbing is a local optimization search that is used for allocating the arriving user request to virtual machines. It does not provide the global solution. In this, author searches for the virtual machine randomly. If finds the virtual machine. It allocates the request to virtual machine, and if virtual machine is found allocated, then search another virtual machine randomly for execution of request and each iteration; if virtual machine does not perform as expected, then decreases the cost value of virtual machine in the next iteration.

Zhen et al. in [3] proposed an automated resource management system that uses the virtualization technology to allocate the resources of data center dynamically. In this way, they achieve two goals: load balancing and less energy consumption. They developed future prediction algorithm that can keep record of the future resource requirement of any applications. They also developed the skewness algorithm that can measure the unevenness utilization of a server in multidimensional environment. They also defined a server as cold spot if the utilization of any of its resources is below a specified value and as hot spot if the utilization of all its resources is above a specified value.

Vikas et al. in [4] proposed modified active monitoring load balancing algorithm in cloud computing. In this algorithm, the author checks for the least loaded virtual machine with CPU utilization of each virtual machine and selects that virtual machine which has the least CPU utilization for performing any task in cloud computing environment. In this way, it gives better response and data processing time in cloud computing environment.

Shridhar et al. in [5] proposed modified throttled load balancing algorithm. In this approach, they first maintained index table of virtual machines and configure the position of virtual machine busy or available similar to throttled algorithm. In this approach, virtual machine is initially selected depending on the availability. If it is available it selects the virtual machine otherwise send to message not available. When other request is arrived then virtual machine at index next already assigned virtual machine is choose. This process is repeated until the size of index table is reached. If the size of index table is reached, then this process is repeated from top of the index table.

Kousik et al. in [6] proposed a genetic-based novel load balancing strategy for cloud computing. This algorithm performed three operations: selection, genetic, and replacement. Advantage of this algorithm is that it cannot stuck in local optimal solution, fits for very large task, and is valid for the complex objective function. In this algorithm, every processing unit consists of a processing unit vector and job submitted by cloud user is represented by job unit vector. Various analysis results show that it gives higher response time and data center processing time in comparison with the traditional algorithm and also guarantees quality of service.

3 Proposed Work

3.1 Problem Statement

In the paper [7], Shridhar et al. proposed an optimal load balancing algorithm by modifying the active load balancing strategy. In this strategy author added a condition in active monitor load balancer that picked least loaded virtual machine is utilized instantly as a part of the last cycle if yes then that virtual machine is not selected for next execution of the task otherwise it is selected.

The proposed strategy of the author does not work with the heterogeneous environment because every virtual machine does not have same capacity in heterogeneous environment. Then, why we cannot choose same virtual machine in next iteration if capacity of virtual machine is able to handle that task easily. We proposed a weighted active monitor load balancing policy through which we can calculate weight of each virtual machine through parameters such as RAM, bandwidth, number of processor, and processor speed using the following equation.

3.2 Proposed Strategy

Calculate the weight W of each virtual machine using the following formula:

$$W = W_1[R_1 + R_2 + \cdots] + W_2[B_1 + B_2 + \cdots] + W_3[Np_1 + Np_2 + \cdots] + W_4[Ps_1 + Ps_2 + \cdots];$$

where W_1, W_2, W_3, and W_4 are the predefined weights of corresponding system parameter, R_1, R_2 are RAM, B_1,B_2 are bandwidth, Np_1, Np_2 are the number of processors, and Ps_1, Ps_2 are the processor speed of the corresponding system. It is very difficult to decide the weights. One approach is more general the factor larger is the weight. Another approach was that it gives the user preference over the other. In this later approach is used and weights are consider in the following manner: $W_1 = 0.2$, $W_2 = 0.1$, $W_3 = 0.4$, and $W_4 = 0.3$ in such a way that their summation became one.

3.3 Flowchart for Proposed Weighted Active Monitoring Load Balancing (WAMLB) Algorithm

Figure 1 shows that the various steps are involved in the proposed algorithm.

Whenever a cloudlet request coming to data center controller, data center controller (DCC) passes that request to virtual machine (VM) load balancer. Load balancer checks for the availability of VM and selects that virtual machine which has highest weight value. Send that VM id to data center controller. DCC assigns

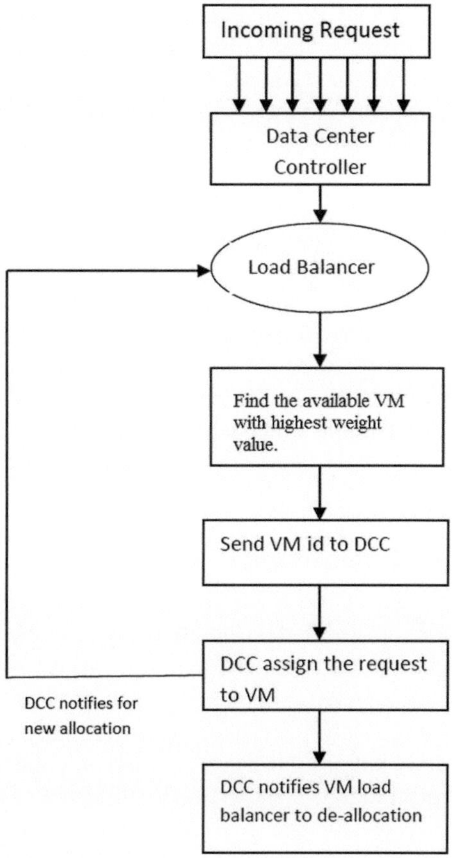

Fig. 1 Flowchart of the proposed weighted VM assign algorithm

that request to the VM. It also notifies the load balancer to update the allocation table. After finding the appropriate response incoming request (cloudlet), it notifies the virtual machine load balancer for deallocating the appropriate virtual machine.

3.4 Proposed Weighted Active Monitoring Load Balancing Algorithm

Input: Number of incoming requests (cloudlets) x1, x2, x3, x4, … xn.
Available virtual machines y1, y2, y3, y4, … ym.
Output: All incoming requests x1, x2, x3, x4, … xn are allocated to available VM with highest weight value among the available VM y1, y2, y3, y4, … ym.

1. WAMLB maintains index table of each VM, and check the status of each virtual machine that is busy or available and weight value of each VM. Initially, all VMs has available.
2. Whenever DCC receives requests, it parses the index table and selects available VM with highest weight value. First identified is selected if more than one virtual machines are found.
3. WAMLB returns the virtual machine id to DCC.
4. DCC sends the requests to that VM.
5. DCC notifies WAMLB for new allocation.
6. WAMLB updates the allocation table of requests hold by each VM.
7. DCC receives the response when VM finishes the request, and it notifies VM deallocation.
8. WAMLB updates the allocation Table
9. Continue from step 2 for next request.

4 Experimental Setup

The proposed algorithm in this paper is implemented in CloudAnalyst [8] simulator that is based on the CloudSim [9]. As cloud infrastructure is distributed in nature and requests are coming from various regions, it should be handled smartly. The CloudAnalyst is extending functionality of CloudSim and built on top of CloudSim tool kit. It is GUI-based simulation tool that also gives simulation result in graphical form. Figure 2 shows the architecture of CloudAnalyst simulator.

CloudAnalyst gives the real-time scenario with six user bases representing six different continents of the world. The number of specific user is identified through particular application like Facebook users from Africa, Asia, and North America, etc. This simulator is also very flexible, and it gives data center, bandwidth, virtual machine, processor, and many more for experiment purpose. Figure 3 shows the graphical user interface (GUI) of CloudAnalyst simulator.

A typical application that can benefit from cloud is social networking sites like Facebook, Twitter, Google plus, etc. Facebook is most popular social networking site that has 1.49 billion monthly users as of the second quarter of 2015. Hypothetical application, like Facebook user, Twitter user, Internet user, is considered for experimentation. Six user bases represent six different geographical

Fig. 2 Architecture of CloudAnalyst simulator

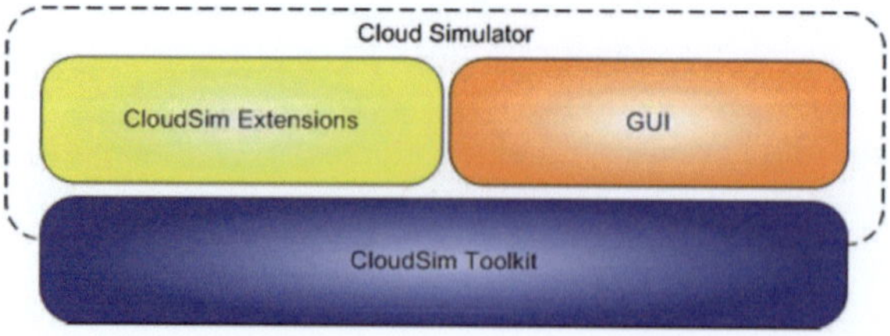

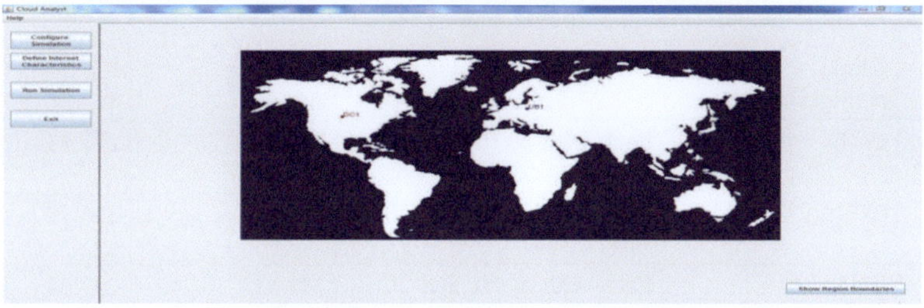

Fig. 3 GUI of CloudAnalyst simulator

Table 1 Simulation configuration

User base	Region	Simultaneous online user during peak hours	Simultaneous online user during off-peak hours
UB1	0—N. America	6000	600
UB2	1—S. America	2000	200
UB3	2—Europe	5000	500
UB4	3—Asia	7000	700
UB5	4—Africa	1000	100
UB6	5—Oceania	1500	150

locations of world. For simplicity of simulation, we can consider each user is single time zone, and out of total register users, only 5% users are online during pick hour and only one-tenth users online in off-peak hours. For experimental purpose, six different user bases containing six different regions, number of peaks, and off-peak users are given in Table 1. The same data is used in different load balancing algorithm for experimental purpose and also considered for result analysis.

Each data center has capability to host number of virtual machines which are used for application execution. Each machine has different capacity like storage space, CPU, processor speed, and RAM.

5 Simulation Result and Analysis

For simulation purpose, we consider three data centers (DCs) in same region having 5, 10, and 20 virtual machines (VMs) which have different sizes like 512 MB, 1 and 2 GB RAM capacity. Machines have different bandwidth and have different number of processors like dual-core, quad-core, and octa-core processor with different processing speed. We first set all machine in region 0 in North America then after region 2 and 3 of the same configuration and find the following result that given in Table 2 with overall average response time (RT) in millisecond (ms). Performance analysis graph is shown in Fig. 4.

Table 2 Average overall average response time in (ms)

S. no.	Cloud configuration	DC specification	RT using AMLB	RT using WAMLB
1	CC1	Each with 5, 10, and 20 VMs	221.82	217.81
2	CC2	Each with 5, 10, and 20 VMs	230.83	226.77
3	CC3	Each with 5, 10, and 20 VMs	243.71	237.68

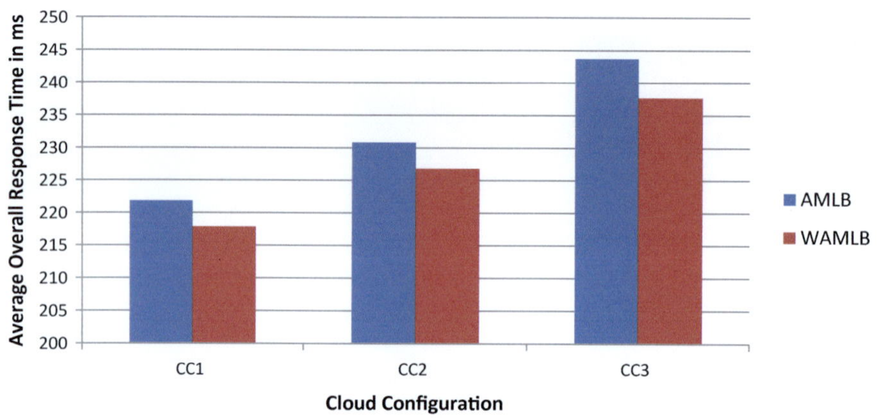

Fig. 4 Performance analysis graph

6 Conclusion

Our weighted active monitor load balancing technique focuses on effective utilization of VM by assigning the virtual machine on the basis of weight factor. Our proposed algorithm manages the load at server by intelligently assigning the incoming request by seeing the current status of VMs with weight value. We also compared our results with existing work through CloudAnalyst, and it shows that our result shows improvement over existing one.

As a future work we also improved our proposed algorithm taking more parameter in index table like CPU utilization of each VM calculate then assign the request in that way so further it gives improved response time.

References

1. Darak, M.S., Dr. Pawar, V.P., Lohiya, S., Darak, S.: Cloud computing and its applications in various sector. Asian J. Manage. Sci. **02**, 07–11, ISSN: 2348-0351 (2014)

2. Mondal, Brototi, Dasgupta, Kousik, Dutta, Paramartha: Load balancing in cloud computing using stochastic hill climbing—A soft computing approach. Procedia Technol. **4**, 783–789 (2012)
3. Xiao, Z., Song, W., Chen, Q.: Dynamic resource allocation using virtual machines for cloud computing environments. In: IEEE transaction on parallel and distributed systems, (2012)
4. Kumar, Vikas, Prakash, Shiva: Modified active monitoring load balancing with cloud computing. Int. J. Sci. Res. Dev. **2**(9), 184–189 (2014)
5. Domanal, S.G., Ram Mohana Reddy, G.: Load balancing in cloud computing using modified throttled algorithm. In: Cloud Computing in Emerging Markets, IEEE International Conference on Bangalore, (2013)
6. Dasgupta, K., Mandal, B., Dutta, P., Mondal, J.K., Dam, S.: A genetic algorithm based load balancing strategy for cloud computing. Procedia Technol. **10**, 340–347, (2013)
7. Domanal, S.G., Reddy, G.R.M.: Optimal load balancing in cloud computing by efficient utilization of virtual machines. In: COMSNETS, IEEE Sixth International Conference on Bangalore, 978-1-4799-3635-9, (2014)
8. Wickremasinghe, B., Calheiros, R.N., Buyya, R.: Cloudanalyst: A cloudsim-based visual modeller for analysing cloud computing environments and applications. In: Proceedings of the 24th International Conference on Advanced Information Networking and. Applications, Perth, Australia, (2010)
9. Calheiros, R.N., Ranjan, R., Beloglazov, A., Rose, C., Buyya, R.: Cloudsim: A toolkit for modeling and simulation of cloud computing environments and evaluation of resource provisioning algorithms. In: Software: Practice and experience (SPE), vol. 41, no 1, ISSN: 0038-0644. Wiley Press, New York, USA, pp. 23–50, (2011)

Applications of Attribute-Based Encryption in Cloud Computing Environment

Vishnu Shankar and Karan Singh

Abstract Cloud computing is becoming very popular and has very good future, but it has various security issues and that need to be addressed. Storing data at some other place have serious problems of privacy and data misuse. Attribute-based encryption has addressed there issues. In this paper, we are discussing about cloud computing and its stacks and growth of cloud computing. We have seen what is the present work going on and then concluded.

Keywords Attribute-based encryption · Cloud security · Encryption

1 Introduction

In electricity plug point, we just plug the electrical appliances and use it; we are not concerned about how the electricity is generating and how it is coming to that plug point. It has given a virtualization of electricity and hides the unwanted details from the user. In early days, factories use to have their own power generation systems but now they are outsourcing it. Similar virtualization is required for information technology in place of having their own huge resources they should try to have fully virtualized resources and pay as they use them. It makes free from infrastructure investment and maintenance of their resources (Fig. 1).

Vaquero et al. [1] have stated "Clouds are a large pool of easily usable and accessible virtualized resources (such as hardware, development platforms, and/or services). These resources can be dynamically reconfigured to adjust to a variable load (scale), allowing also for an optimum resource utilization. This pool of resources is typically exploited by a pay-per-use model in which guarantees are

V. Shankar (✉) · K. Singh
School of Computer and Systems Sciences, Jawaharlal Nehru University,
New Delhi 110067, India
e-mail: vishnuok@gmail.com

K. Singh
e-mail: karancs12@gmail.com

V.B. Aggarwal et al. (eds.), *Big Data Analytics*, Advances in Intelligent
Systems and Computing 654, https://doi.org/10.1007/978-981-10-6620-7_66

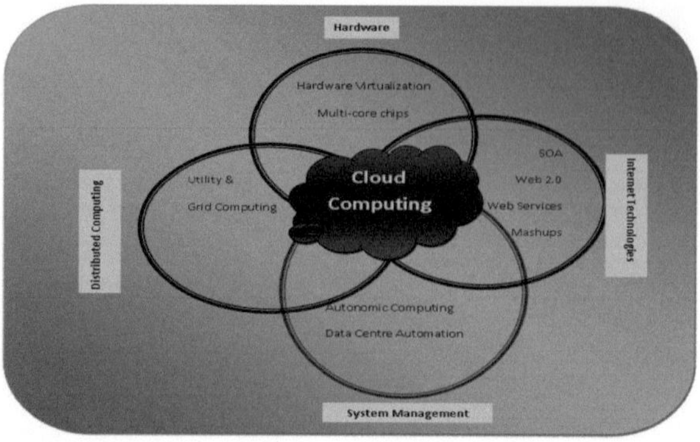

Fig. 1 Cloud computing technologies

offered by the infrastructure provider by means of customized service-level agreements." Service-level agreement is a contract for measuring service between service provider and consumer.

2 Classes of Cloud Computing

Cloud computing can be classified based on the services they provide as IaaS, PaaS, SaaS. IaaS stands for infrastructure as a service, PaaS is platform as a service, SaaS is software as a service. Infrastructure as a service offers virtualized computation, virtualized storage, and virtualized communication as per demand. Raw computing and storage services are provided by infrastructure as a service. Higher level of abstraction is provided by platform as a service that makes cloud simply programmable. In PaaS, developers can develop applications without warning about a number of processors, and amount of memory will be required by application. In the cloud stack, the applications are at the top, users are more inclined toward online software services then program installed on local machines. Word processing and spreadsheet applications can be used in the form of web service. This is software as a service it releases users from maintenance, and the work of developing and testing will be easier.

3 Motivation

Motivation of cloud computing is its growth. The growth of cloud computing is very fast. In Asia, the growth of cloud computing is even faster. Presently, various techniques have been proposed so far for making data on cloud to be secure, but there is still an improvement and scope for making more efficient way need to be explored.

4 Literature Survey

Tysowski et al. [2] are focusing on security of data stored on cloud computing, and specifically, when it is used by mobile devices. Owner of sensitive data wants the security of their data when they store it in cloud. Attribute-based encryption is used for doing this, and it is done in a way that mobile user must have minimum computation on its part. It controls the access based on certain attributes that are possessed by requesting user. Group key mechanism is used for providing additional security by the data owner. Data re-encryption was provided for efficient revocation of user, data stored at CSP will not be converted into plaintext in place of it encrypted data will be again encrypted such that only authorized person should have access.

Liang et al. [3] are focusing on improvement of CP-ABE as it has a problem in revocation. In CP-ABE, if any user has been given access to some resources and he is misusing it there is no mechanism to stop him, when these are detected then system manager need to reconstruct the whole system. CP-ABE is similar with role-based access control system. Designing a revocation scheme is a difficult task for CP-ABE, as it is works on different sets of attributes than individual characteristics. In place of CP-ABE, author has proposed CP-ABE-R in this user has a unique id. There will be a revocation list has information about revoked user where revocation will be with the help of time stamp. Author has used binary tree technique to update information for reducing computational and communicational cost. In this user has unique key with personalized factor t and t', attribute related and revocation related personalized factor relatively.

Bethencourt et al. [4] have proposed a technique by which data stored in distributed systems can be kept confidential, if the storage server is not trusted. In this technique, there is provision of describing who will be able to decrypt the data. This thing who will be able to decrypt is specified with the help of attributes. This is quite similar to the role-based access control. This approach is CP-ABE called ciphertext policy attribute-based encryption. In this ciphertext is accessible by the user only if his attributes passes through access tree. It is collusion resistance.

It was having following algorithms setup, encrypt, key generation, decrypt, and delegate. Author has implemented it in CP-ABE package.

Liu et al. [5] have given a new concept of clock-based proxy re-encryption scheme for not reliable could. As we know, storing data in could have a problem of security and that is why various organizations still hesitate to put their sensitive data on the cloud. In this paper, author has achieved fine-grained access and scalable user revocation. CP-ABE and PRE are used in this with time tree concept. In HABE, data owner was sending re-encrypt command and PRE keys to the cloud, but it was having problem of delays. In C-PRE, the re-encryption key will be sent in advance and it will not have communication delay and by PRE the workload also will be reduced from data owner.

Do et al. [6] have focused on confidential and fine-grained access in cloud computing with five important things that cloud have milt tenancy, massive scalability, elasticity, pay-per-use, and self provisioning of resources. Earlier KP-ABE and PRE were good for confidentiality and user revocation, respectively, but suffer from collusion attack. In this paper, author has proposed to divide file into two parts namely header and body. Header was having key encrypted with KP-ABE, and body was having message in this symmetric encryption was used. Body was stored in cloud server and privilege manager to manage header. The user who is not authorized by privilege manager will not have key to encryption and will not be able to access data in the body.

Jahid et al. [7] are focusing on online social networks that provide people a way to have communication and express them. Here, the privacy of a user is a great concern on social media and there are various privacy violations coming in picture that is a serious issue. Even though social networking sites providing access control policies for each articles and provision for having data for a set of friends or groups, this can be done by ABE, and user having desired set of attributes can decrypt it. As persons social life changes with that friend and their groups also changes so it needs changes in the group too. If we are deleting someone from a group, then we must change key and then re-distribute it to all other members, and data will be again re-encrypted. It will have an issue a problem if the size of group is large and users frequently leave the group. Author has given EASIER that will have fine-grained access control and will manage dynamic groups. Old OSN were having only one relation friend but in EASIER user have a provision to define a relationship by attribute. It has been implemented on CP-ABE toolkit.

Zhao et al. [8] have focused on trusted data sharing on cloud. Stack of cloud having three layers and basic of cloud has briefed, confidentiality and integrity have been raised as an issue. Author said data must be encrypted before storing it on cloud. Here, if A has issued a key to B and data is intended to be used by B at any cost even if C gets the key or any other way it must not be accessible to C. Progressive elliptic curve encryption scheme has been proposed in this data can be encrypted multiple times, but it will be decrypted just in one round by one key.

Wang et al. [9] have proposed HABE by the combination of HIBE and CP-ABE. Here is focus on confidential data must be accessed efficiently with efficient encryption and fine-grained access control. In CP-ABE, author said following issues as in cloud the client may have limited bandwidth and resources so performance will be an issue, then big organization needs attribute authorities and revocation also must be addressed efficiently. In HABE, we have RM as TTP and similar to PKG in HIBE, DM is as PKG in HIBE and AA in CP-ABE. DM will have arbitrary no of attributes and have full access over them. DM will have ID and user will have ID and attribute both. For doing revocation in HABE, proxy re-encryption and lazy re-encryption are used. Attributes have ID and when a user is revoked ID no is increased. It can have in future full under standard model and its performance can be done better.

Ming et al. [10] have explored problem in CP-ABE one is revocation and another one is data owner is bound to trust on attribute authorities. In this paper, attributes will be managed by jointly with data owner and attribute authority by an access tree that will have one side attribute sub-tree and another side permission sub-tree they will be, respectively, controlled by attribute authority and owner of data. This approach is good for practical implementation. Improvement in this is required as it disclosed attribute information if we use proxy re-encryption.

Yu et al. [11] have suggested improvement in CP-ABE using proxy re-encryption. Authors have taken attribute as index values and it will have positive, negative and do not care occurrences. Authors have used in access structure AND. This work is secure for ciphertext attack and most of the load at the time of revocation is shifted to proxy servers. In the paper, authors have discussed KP-ABE that is similar to CP-ABE. KP-ABE will use the reverse of CP-ABE here key will be for access structure and ciphertext for attributes.

5 Conclusions

We have seen various attribute-based encryption techniques that are presently there. We have pros and cons with the existing techniques. In revocation, we have seen various issues. Still, we need some better technique that can address current issues.

References

1. Vaquero, L.M., Rodero-Merino, L., Caceres, J., Lindner, M.: A break in the clouds: towards a cloud definition. ACM SIGCOMM Comput. Commun. Rev. 39(1):50–55 (2009)
2. Tysowski, P.K., Hasan, M.A.: Hybrid Attribute-Based Encryption and Re-Encryption for Scalable Mobile Applications in Clouds. Technical Report 13, Centre for Applied Cryptographic Research (CACR), University of Waterloo (2013)
3. Liang, X., Lu, R., Lin, X.: Ciphertext Policy Attribute Based Encryption With Efficient Revocation. Technical Report BBCR, University of Waterloo (2011)
4. Bethencourt, J., Sahai, A., Waters, B.: Ciphertext-policy attribute-based encryption. In: Proceedings of IEEE Symposium on Security and Privacy (SP '07), pp. 321–334 (2007)
5. Liu, Q., Wang, G., Wu, J.: Clock-based proxy re-encryption scheme in unreliable clouds. In: Proceedings of 41st International Conference on Parallel Processing Workshops (ICPPW), pp. 304–305, Sept 2012
6. Do, J.-M., Song, Y.-J., Park, N.: Attribute based proxy re-encryption for data confidentiality in cloud computing environments. In: Proceedings of First ACIS/JNU International Conference on Computers, Networks, Systems and Industrial Engineering (CNSI), pp. 248–251, May 2011
7. Jahid, S., Mittal, P., Borisov, N.: EASiER: encryption-based access control in social networks with efficient revocation. In: Proceedings of Sixth ACM Symposium on Information, Computer and Communications Security (ASIACCS '11), pp. 411–415 (2011)
8. Zhao, G., Rong, C., Li, J., Zhang, F., Tang, Y.: Trusted data sharing over untrusted cloud storage providers. In: Proceedings of IEEE Second International Conference on Cloud Computing Technology and Science (CLOUDCOM '10), pp. 97–103 (2010)
9. Wang, G., Liu, Q., Wu, J.: Hierarchical attribute-based encryption for fine-grained access control in cloud storage services. In: Proceedings of 17th ACM Conference on Computer and Communications Security (CCS '10), pp. 735–737 (2010)

10. Ming, Y., Fan, L., Jing-Li, H., Zhao-Li, W.: An efficient attribute based encryption scheme with revocation for outsourced data sharing control. In: Proceedings of First International Conference on Instrumentation, Measurement, Computer, Communications and Control, pp. 516–520 (2011)
11. Yu, S., Wang, C., Ren, K., Lou, W.: Attribute based data sharing with attribute revocation. In: Proceedings of Fifth ACM Symposium on Information, Computer and Communications Security (ASIACCS '10), pp. 261–270 (2010)

Query Optimization: Issues and Challenges in Mining of Distributed Data

Pramod Kumar Yadav and Sam Rizvi

Abstract The technique of finding the optimal processing method to answer a query is called Query optimization, whereas a collection of various sites, distributed over a computer network is called Distributed Database. In Distributed Database, the site communicates with each other through networks. There are various issues arise during evaluation of query cost, among which the processing cost and a transmission cost are important. There are several algorithms developed to find the best possible solution for a particular query, but they all have their certain limitations. The optimizer is mainly concern on search space, search strategy, and the cost model. It primarily focuses on these three factors. The mining cost of a query depends on the order of evaluation of the operators, for the same query we can have different cost if the order is changed. Hence, to find the optimal cost for a particular query is emerging as an open challenge for many researchers. Therefore, the cost-based query optimization technique has emerged as an important concept for dealing with the query optimization. This paper explores the issues and challenges of query optimization in mining of distributed data.

Keywords Query optimization · Distributed database · Cost-based optimization

1 Introduction

The optimizer is mainly concerned on search space, search strategy, and the cost model. It primarily focuses on these three factors. These factors play a vital role in evaluating the cost of a query. The search space includes the number of options for a single user query. These options when executed produce the same results [1]. The

P.K. Yadav (✉)
Krishna Institute of Engineering and Technology, Ghaziabad, India
e-mail: pramodyadavster@gmail.com

S. Rizvi
Jamia Millia Islamia, New Delhi, India
e-mail: samsam_rizvi@yahoo.com

V.B. Aggarwal et al. (eds.), *Big Data Analytics*, Advances in Intelligent Systems and Computing 654, https://doi.org/10.1007/978-981-10-6620-7_67

variation in the results totally depends on the order of the execution of the operation and the way they are implemented. The primary task of a search strategy is to find the best execution plan. The cost of each plan is predicted by the cost model. One of the important problems in a centralized database is the central point failure. Since the data in a centralized database is stored and maintained at a particular node, therefore the failure of the central point will result to poor reliability of the system. This along with other problems lead to the development of the distributed database. There are several advantages of the distributed database over centralized database [2]. The first and the foremost benefit is that the distributed database will not stop working though the entire network goes down, as in case of centralized Database. The communication overhead may be reduced in Distributed Database by replicating data on different sites [3, 4]. High reliability and availability are the second important advantage of the distributed database over centralized database [5].

A. Search Space: The search space consists of the collection of all possible query execution plans. It primarily focuses on finding the optimal query execution plan. The query execution plans developed by the search space produces the similar results after execution [6]. The query tree is used to represents the solution of the plan for executing the join expression and cost is associated with the every point of search. The major role of the cost function is to maps the query tree to their respective costs [7]. Due to the large number of relations required for processing a distributed query, searching an optimal query plan is difficult, which ultimately increases the search cost. This problem can be solved by generating plans that minimize the cost of the search [3].
B. Search Strategy: The main task of the search strategies is to find the execution plans in an efficient and cost effective manner. For most of the search strategies, the Dynamic programming forms the base [3]. There are basically two approaches which can be used to solve the problems related to search strategy [5]. The first and foremost approach is a deterministic approach which builds a plan on base relations and then joins it with one or more relation at each step until the complete plan is obtained. The partial plan that may not produce the optimal plans is pruned [3, 5], due to which the reduction in the optimization cost is achieved. The second approach which is referred to as randomized strategy is implemented. In this, it is mainly concern on finding the optimal solution around some particular point, though it does not guarantee the optimal solution. Randomized strategy does not cost much for optimizing the optimal plans in terms of memory and time consumption. The working tradition of randomized strategy is that it starts with some randomly selected plans and then tries to find the neighbor plan and then compare the cost of the plan with a neighbor plan. If the cost of the neighbor plans is less than the starting plan, then the neighbor plan is considered as a solution plan [4]. This phenomenon continues till it finds a plan which has no neighbor having lesser cost, for a predefined number of neighbors. Constant space overhead is one of the most important advantages of random strategy [3].

2 Query Optimization Techniques

Query Optimization is emerging as one of the important areas of research, as the size of the databases increases from terabyte to zeta byte. The need of various optimization techniques is in high demand. Optimization plays a vital role in finding the solution from large databases [1, 3]. With the help of query optimization, it would be possible to find optimal execution plans, with minimum cost. A group of all possible execution plans for a query which is considered by the optimizer is the execution space of the query whereas the cost function is used to evaluate the cost of an execution plan in the execution space. The Optimizer plays an important role in selecting a minimal cost plan from the execution space [5, 8]. Some of the important approaches for finding the optimal cost query plan are Dynamic programming, Iterative dynamic programming, Randomized Optimization and Greedy algorithms.

2.1 Dynamic Programming

The Optimizer in the Dynamic programming plays a vital role in finding the optimal query cost plans as they can be easily extended. One of the key components of a query optimizer is its search strategy. The primary task of the optimizer is to determine which plans to enumerate, and the classic enumeration algorithm is based on the concepts of dynamic programming [3, 4]. The concept of Dynamic programming produces efficient results when all queries are standard and simple. However, it is not efficient for complex queries. In order to optimize queries in a distributed database, the complex queries techniques need to be integrated into the system. In such conditions, the search space may become very large which may not be suitable for Dynamic programming, because of its very high complexity [3].

2.2 Iterative Dynamic Programming

The Iterative Dynamic Programming concept is very much similar to dynamic programming. In this, we apply dynamic programming iteratively to optimize the query plans. IDP results to a polynomial complexity and it produces best plans in most of the situations [3, 8]. In comparison to Dynamic programming, IDP produces good plans than any other algorithm during high complexity situations [3, 5]. There are several advantages of Iterative Dynamic Programming over Dynamic programming. One of the important benefits of IDP is the adaptation to the optimization problem. The result of the adaptation totally depends on the query, if the query is simple; these IDP variants produce an optimal plan similar to the Dynamic programming utilizing the same amount of time as dynamic programming [4]. The second benefit of IDP is that all IDP variants can be easily integrated into an existing query optimizer which is based on the concepts of Dynamic programming [3].

2.3 Randomized Optimization

Constant space overhead is one of the key benefits of randomized algorithms. Due to the in the deterministic behavior of many randomized algorithms, it is difficult to estimate the running time. In case of simple queries randomized algorithms are slower than heuristics and dynamic programming, but in case of a very large database, it works better than both algorithms [2, 5]. The Two-Phase Optimization is one of the best-known randomized algorithms and is obtained by the combination of applying iterative improvement and simulated annealing [3]. These both algorithms are based on the concept of randomized algorithms. In order to find the solution of a distributed optimization problem, these techniques are used. For a given user query, the iterative improvement and simulated annealing, both use the same heuristic function for generating the optimal query plans. Since data in the distributed database are scattered across the multiple sites in the distributed form [4, 5]. The efficiency of the algorithms depends upon the location of data storage. If the data is located nearby on the distributed site than the efficiency would be high, otherwise, it would be low. As it is known that query, processing will be more efficient when the required data is very close to each other, i.e., it resides at the same site. On the other hand, if the data required to answer user query resides in disparate sites, then the query processing efficiency would be low, as it would require joining data from each site to generate the result. The closeness is defined in terms of number of sites participating to answer the query. The efficiency of the algorithm will totally depend upon the number of sites participating. If the number of sites is less than query processing will be more efficient and if the number of sites participating is more than the query processing will be less efficient [3].

2.4 Greedy Algorithm

Greedy algorithm is one of the important emerging algorithms and it has emerged as an alternative to dynamic programming. These algorithms execute much faster as compared to the dynamic programming, but they produce worse plans. The working of greedy algorithms comprises of three phases and constructs plans in a bottom-up way. In the first phase, the greedy algorithm also makes use of the same access Plans, join Plans, and finalize Plans functions in order to generate plans. In the second phase, it carries out a very simple and rigorous selection of the join order. In order to find the next best join, the greedy algorithm applies a plan evaluation function [3].

3 Issues and Challenges

In order to estimate the cost of a plan, we have to evaluate the cost of every individual operator of the plan, followed by additions of these costs. The cost of an operator in a centralized system is composed of CPU costs and disk Input/output costs. The disk I/O costs are further composed of seek, latency, and transfer costs [1]. Where as in a distributed system, the cost of processing a query is expressed in terms of the total cost measure or the response time measures. The total cost measure is the sum of all cost components. In the distributed system, the total cost measure includes the local processing cost, only if no relation is fragmented and the given query contains selection and projection operations. However, the communication costs between different sites may be incurred in addition to the local processing cost, when join and semi join operations are executed [8]. It assigns an estimated "cost" to each possible query plan and selects the plan with the lowest cost [1, 9].

4 Conclusion

Since errors play a vital role on the actual execution cost estimation, therefore the accurate cost estimation in distributed databases is very important. Generally, we select an execution plan that is good for large queries with multiple joins or multiple indexes in the cost-based approach. It also improves the productivity by eliminating the need to tune database statements on our own. Since Dynamic programming does not provide a feasible solution due to its large space complexity and complicated objective functions, a new set of techniques like Genetic Algorithm, Ant Colony Optimization Algorithm, and Hybrids of various Evolutionary Algorithms are now being explored for solutions to Distributed Queries. The Two-Phase Optimization is a combination of applying iterative improvement and simulated annealing, and is one of the best-known randomized algorithms. It can be used to find out the best optimal query cost.

References

1. Kossmann, D.: The state of the art in distributed query processing. ACM Comput. Surv. **32** (4):422–469 (2000)
2. Lew, M.S., Sebe, N., Djeraba, C., Jain, R.: Content-based multimedia information retrieval: state of the art and challenges. ACM Trans. Multimedia Comput. Commun. Appl. **2**(1):1–19 (2006)
3. Kossmann, D., Stocker, K.: Iterative dynamic programming: a new class of query optimization algorithms. ACM Trans. Database Syst. **25**(1):43–82 (2000)
4. Kumar, T.V.V., Singh, V., Verma, A.K.: Distributed query processing plans generation using genetic algorithm. Int. J. Comput. Theor. Eng. **3**(1):1793–8201 (2011)

5. Chaudhuri, S., Shim, K.: Optimization of queries with user defined predicates. ACM Trans. Database Syst. **24**(2):177–228 (1999)
6. Drenick, P.E., Smith, E.J.: Stochastic query optimization in distributed database. ACM Trans. Database Syst. **18**(2):262–288 (1993)
7. Chen, B.C., Ramakrishnan, R.: Bellwether analysis: searching for cost-effective query-defined predictors in large databases. ACM Trans. Knowl. Discov. Data. **3**(1), Article 5 (2009)
8. Patil1, R., Chen, Z., Shi, Y.: Database keyword search: a perspective from optimization. In: 2012 IEEE/WIC/ACM International Conferences on Web Intelligence and Intelligent Agent Technology, pp 30–33
9. Kosala, R., Blockeel, H.: Web mining research: a survey. ACM SIGKDD **2**(1):1–15 (2000)
10. Pentaris, F., Ioannidis, Y.: Query optimization in distributed networks of autonomous database systems. ACM Trans. Database Syst. **31**(2):537–583 (2006)
11. Liao, S.H., Chu, P.H., Hsiao, P.Y.: Data mining techniques and applications—a decade review from 2000 to 2011. Expert Syst. Appl. **39**:11303–11311 (2012)
12. Smeulders, A.W.M., Worring, M., Santini, S., Gupta, A., Jain, R.: Content-based image retrieval at the end of the early years. IEEE Trans. Pattern Anal. Mach. Intell. **22**(12) (2000)
13. Barrena, M., Jurado, E., Márquez-Neila, P., Pachón, C.: A flexible framework to ease nearest neighbor search in multidimensional data spaces. J. Data Knowl. Eng. **69**:116–136 (2010)
14. Ozsoyoglu, G., Altingovde, I.S., Al-hamdani, A., Ozel, S.A., Ulusoy, O., Ozsoyoglu, Z.M.: Querying web metadata: native score management and text support in databases. ACM Trans. Database Syst. **29**(4):581–634 (2004)

Comprehensive Study of Cloud Computing and Related Security Issues

Manju Khari, Manoj kumar and Vaishali

Abstract Cloud Computing is a global technology changes in order to accomplish the phenomenon that shifts traditional IT services to modern IT services as it provides computing services through a simple internet connection. Also the characteristics of "Pay per use" and on-demand services of cloud model attract the consumers more toward cloud computing. These characteristics can help us to access a shared pool of resources such as storage, networks, servers, etc., without actually, in reality, acquiring them. A lot of big IT Leaders organization such as Microsoft, Google, sales-force, Amazon, and others generate cloud computing structures and provide related services to customers. Even though advantages of cloud computing are clear in front of global computing system but there is a need for security model in cloud computing. This paper discusses and presents a comprehensive study of cloud computing and related security issues.

Keywords Cloud computing · Computing services · Cloud computing security · Security issues · Security requirements

1 Introduction

Considering the earlier computing model vs. the cloud computing model, cloud computing has several possible benefits. Nowadays the main barrier for compelling cloud computing services is the security and security measures provided with these services. The main security challenge with cloud services is that the proprietor of the data may not have a tool to regulate where the data is physically located. So, if

M. Khari · M. kumar (✉) · Vaishali
Department of Computer Science, AIACTR, Geeta Colony, Delhi, India
e-mail: mnj_gpt@rediffmail.com

M. Khari
e-mail: manjukhari@yahoo.co.in

Vaishali
e-mail: vaishalig1012@gmail.com

V.B. Aggarwal et al. (eds.), *Big Data Analytics*, Advances in Intelligent Systems and Computing 654, https://doi.org/10.1007/978-981-10-6620-7_68

someone desires to exploit the benefit of using cloud computing services, another one might also desire and utilize the advantages of cloud computing services. Mahmood and Zaigham [1] say "global public used cloud computing in the form of internet". (e.g., Hotmail since 1996; YouTube since 2006; and Gmail since 2007, etc.), Hotmail is possibly the earliest cloud computing mail server that permitted the common public to keep their data in the form of files at physically distance servers. This gives power to data and facility to users that data is delivered and managed by others. In the last decade, many organizations spread their IT establishment by using cloud services. As in the last few years, many of other matching services have been developed for cloud computing [1]. The remaining structure of this paper is as follows: Sects. 2 and 3 describe a study on the cloud computing architecture and highlight the NIST model of cloud computing. In Sect. 4, we list out cloud computing security issues based on service models and deployment model and relation between them focusing on general security issues. Conclusion and related future work are represented in Sect. 5.

2 Cloud Computing Component

The cloud brings the basic setup characteristics that are useful to organize the cloud services in a fast and cost-effective way. Mell and Grance [2] state five essential characteristics of cloud computing which are listed in Table 1.

In general, there are four different cloud deployment models specifically public cloud, private cloud, community cloud and hybrid cloud. Alexa and James [3] stated these as given in Table 2.

Table 1 Essential characteristics of cloud computing

Essential characteristics	Concept applied
On-demand self-services	A cloud customer (CC) can individually take computing capabilities such as network storage, virtual machines, and server time, etc., as needed spontaneously without requiring human interaction with each service's provider
Measured services	Billing is counted and delivery as a utility service such as storage, bandwidth, processing, and active user accounts, etc., service usage can be monitored, controlled, and reported providing transparency for both CC and cloud provider (CP) of the utilized service
Broad-network access	Facility to access the service via standard platforms such as desktop, mobile, laptop, or by using other distributed system
Resource pooling	CP pool their resources are then imparted by numerous clients. Thus cloud services can support millions of concurrent CC such as memory, network, bandwidth, etc.
Rapid elasticity	A CC can rapidly gain more resources from the cloud by scaling out and can scale back in by quitting those resources once they are no more needed

Table 2 Deployment model of cloud computing

Deployment model	Concept applied
Public cloud	Public cloud services can be retrieved by the associated consumer with the help of simple but high speed of internet connection
Private cloud	A private cloud is well known for a precise group and bounds access to just that group
Community cloud	A community cloud is mutual among two or more groups that have need of similar cloud services desires
Hybrid cloud	A hybrid cloud is fundamentally combinations of at least two different cloud deployment models

Table 3 Cloud computing service models

Service model	Concept applied	Examples of commercial cloud systems
Software as a services (SaaS)	A SaaS CP gives CC access to both services and applications. While using these services then there is no need to install a physical copy of the software on your devices. The disadvantage of this service is CC has the least control over the cloud	Sales-force customer relation management (CRM) system, Microsoft Live Mesh and Google apps, etc.
Platform as a service (PaaS)	A PaaS system Consider as next level of the SaaS setup. A PaaS CP gives CC access to the component that they need to create and run applications over the web	Sales-force Apex system and Google App Engine, etc.
Infrastructure as a service (IaaS)	IaaS CP gives physical and virtual equipment to develop software application environments with a supply using based rating model to CC	Amazon (elastic cloud computing) EC2, amazon (simple storage service) S3 and microsoft (connected service framework) CSF, etc.

In order to select the probable satisfactory service model or combination of service models, CC fully recognize what each service model is and what responsibilities the CP assume versus the responsibilities the CC assumes. Alexa and James [3] state service model and there use, and we also provide examples from where these services can be commercially consumed by CC in Table 3 listed below.

3 Cloud Computing Model

In the last section we studied about definition approved by NIST of cloud computing under which we stated all components of that definition but before we move on to its model diagram, it is more important to understand few points of the NIST cloud model [4]:

- While taking services first SaaS and then PaaS or moving from SaaS to PaaS and vice versa, CC can have better security mechanism on more resources.
- While taking deployment model services first as a public cloud and then community cloud or moving toward the left to right and again from right to left in NIST model, CC can have better security mechanism over more resources.

Figure 1 denotes NIST cloud computing model and all components of this model are explained in Sect. 2.

4 Security Issues Based on Cloud Computing Model and Its Component

4.1 Security Issues Based on Service Models

It is very clear about cloud computing technology that CC will never be able to control everything with cloud computing because there are always two problems (your problem) CC and (their problem) CP. The duties related to security challenges and issues in cloud computing can be understood by separating between the CP and the CC. Such as, the CP must promise to CC that their borrowed services and data

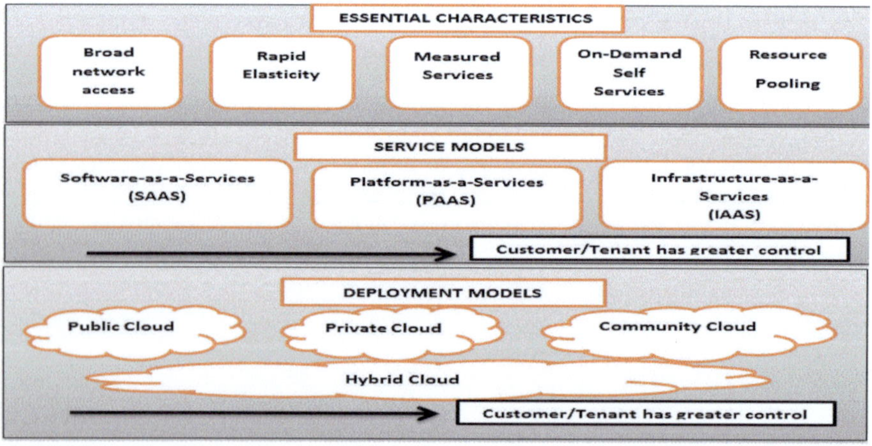

Fig. 1 Cloud computing NIST model

associated with those services will be fully safe and protection mechanism will be applied to it. Also, the physical location or infrastructure where this data is located needs to be secure.

- Challenges in SaaS: Choudhary [5] states that the main issues in SaaS are that CC needs to rely on the CP for fitting efforts to establish safety. The CP must do the work to keep numerous CC from seeing one another's information. Thus, it gets tough for the CP to make this promise to the CC that right efforts to establish safety will be set up. Furthermore, it is hard to get confirmation that the application will be accessible when required.
- Challenges in PaaS: According to Subhashini and Kavitha [6]. In PaaS, the administration supplier may provide limited access to the CC to manufacture Softwares on top of the stage. PaaS is offered to permit designers to collect their specific particular applications/software's on top of the platform. As a result, it tends to be more extensible than SaaS, at the expense of customer-ready features [6].
- Challenges in IaaS: As stated by Subhashini et al. [6] and Gajek [7], in IaaS, "the developers have good control over the security as long as there is no security hole in the virtualization manager". One more factor for the same concern is that physical location of CC data is placed in CP hardware.

To conclude the security accountabilities according to services, Huglory [8] stated that selecting cloud services and cloud deployment models state are responsibilities that are owned by the CP and which are owned by the CC. Once a CC determines what the CP is answerable for, it should then evaluate the provider's security controls and authorizations to determine whether the CP can meet the desired security needs. In Table 4 (R stands for Responsible), (SR stands for Shared Responsibility), (CP stands for Cloud Provider), (SP stands for Service Provider), (CC stands for Cloud Customer), (SOA stands for Service Oriented Architecture).

Table 4 Responsibilities on cloud security

Service model	Responsibility of	CP	SP	CC
IaaS	VM's security	–	–	R
IaaS	Secured VM image repository	R	–	–
IaaS	Securing VM boundaries	R	–	–
IaaS	Hypervisor security	SR	SR	–
PaaS	SOA related security	SR	–	SR
PaaS	API security	–	R	–
SaaS	SaaS security	SR	SR	–
SaaS	Web application security	R	–	–

Table 4 analysis as follows with SaaS, the liability of security lies with the CP. Focus on PaaS model proposes better CC control but fewer higher level features. IaaS offers greater tenant or CC control over security as compared with other service models.

4.2 Security Issues Based on Deployment Models

Anjum et al. [9] recognize that there are three major groups involved in cloud security:

- The First group is the CP's of deployment models namely public and hybrid model.
- The Second group is the group or persons which use cloud services either by transferring and hosting their applications that are data binaries or by having an interface or a joint connected to an external cloud to do few activities such as a module or to route messages through the cloud or downloading cloud public data.
- The third group is the administration and other Third-Party regulatory entities that may have important roles such as audit, forensic, etc.

Mutum and Anita [10] state consistent nature of resource pooled of cloud computing makes CP focus on all their security resources on securing the cloud pattern. The execution of cloud often contains modern security methods, generally, occurs due to the reason of location or centralization of data with global pattern. Thus acceptance of this pattern may introduce a number of new and variety of security services. Discussed security services are based on the cloud deployment model through which it is being provided. The public cloud shows major risk where as the private cloud has kind of lesser impact. While talking about the hybrid model, the data location is outside of the infrastructure premise at some time. So, the hybrid cloud security is not just about the data but also its location. Hence, it is required to ensure that location of the data has the right logical and physical security, and consider all its relevant standards [10]. The cloud deployment model and the probable security level are illustrated in Table 5.

In Table 5 (ORG stands for the organization), (TP stands for the third party), and (B stands for both), also Mahmood and Zaigham [1] describe and characterize ownership, management, location, and security level. It also describes the security

Table 5 Cloud deployment model

Deployment model	Ownership	Management	Location	Security
Public cloud	TP	TP	Off-site premises	Low
Private cloud	ORG or TP	ORG or TP	On-site premises	High
Community cloud	B	B	B	Medium
Hybrid cloud	ORG or TP	ORG or TP	On-site premises	High

range low, medium, and high by the help of deployment model location and summarizes all the characteristics of deployment models in one place. Each Deployment model presents its own challenges and issues which are described briefly one by one as below:

- Challenges in Public Cloud: In public clouds, networks are generally distributed and cloud services are allocated by other TP's and managed or hosted by the CP. The CP takes all the accountabilities and provides installation, management, provisioning, and maintenance.
- Challenges in Private Cloud: In private clouds all copyrighted networks normally within the premises and use mostly for the regular purpose of the organization. Also in private clouds, the organizations are in charge of maintaining the cloud and also answerable for security. As compared with the public cloud, data is more secure in the private cloud.
- Challenges in Community Cloud: Community clouds are kind of replica of public cloud except for the condition that it focuses on particular community and operations. Community cloud is also called semi-private cloud in that they are delivered services to particular CC with common backgrounds and to fulfill a similar purpose.
- Challenges in Hybrid Cloud: Hybrid Cloud is created by the combination of some part of public and private clouds. Thus, accountability responsibilities are generally separated between the organizations and the public cloud CP, thus it may lead toward it to one of the issues of a security breach.

4.3 General Security Issues and the Relation Between Their Service and Deployment Models

An ideal protected cloud computing model should state and fulfilled some general level of security as well thus international standards organization (ISO 7498-2) state some agenda of information security which cloud computing security also do follow. So, service models and deployment models require some different security levels. Figure 2 denotes the traditional security requirements with service and deployments models of cloud computing [11]. In Fig. 2 Asterisk mark means an essential requirement of security whereas a dash indicates optional requirements of security. Thus while taking a combination of the particular type of services (e.g., if CC take public cloud as a deployment services and PaaS as service model then it is necessary to give priority to the authorization security).

As can be seen from Fig. 2, it summarizes that the hybrid cloud requires less security properties as compared to other deployment models. Thus, it indicates that other deployment models need to address more security aspects. One more analysis of Fig. 2 indicates that the integrity is a common loop hole of security in all the deployment models.

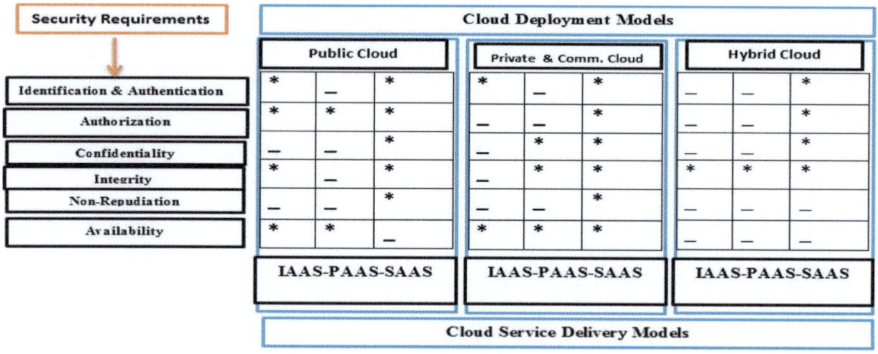

Fig. 2 Security requirements for cloud deployment-delivery model

5 Conclusion

In this paper, the main focus is on overall security requirements in cloud computing and its respective components. We concisely describe in this paper about cloud computing along with all its components with the help of NIST cloud computing model. The role of CC and CP in cloud computing is also briefly explained in this paper as most of the security agenda depends upon it. Every existing technology has some advantages and disadvantages. With the increase in popularity of cloud computing more security challenges and issues occur and are presented in front of us which may lead to limiting the popularity of cloud computing. We also classify and distinguish in between different service providers on different cloud services. As the development of new services in cloud computing takes place, some areas of cloud computing do require latest possible solutions such as data protection measures, new cloud storage technologies and physical security of cloud requirements. If we want to maintain demand and assets of cloud computing then it is necessary to deal with these challenges and issues in regular interval of time and we should try and find out possible ways to deal with it.

References

1. Zaigham, M.: Data location and security issues in cloud computing. In: International Conference on Emerging Intelligent Data and Web Technologies, IEEE (2011)
2. Mell, P., Grance, T.: The NIST definition of cloud computing. In: National Institute of Standards and Technology, Information Technology Laboratory, Version 15 (2009)
3. Alexa, H., James, C.: The basics of cloud computing. In: Camegie Mellon University produced for US-CERT (2011)
4. Vic Winkler, J.R.: Cloud computing architecture book. In: Securing the cloud (2011)
5. Choudhary, V.: Software as a service: implications for investment in software development. In: 40th Annual Hawaii International Conference on System Sciences, IEEE (2007)

6. Subashini, S., Kavitha, V.: A survey on security issues in service delivery models of cloud computing. In: Journal of Network and Computer Applications (2011)
7. Gajek, S.: Breaking and fixing the inline approach. In: ACM Workshop on Secure Web Services, ACM (2007)
8. Huaglory, T.: Security issues in cloud computing. In: IEEE International Conference on Systems, Man and Cybernetics, COEX, Korea (2012)
9. Anjum, A., Mousmi, C., Hala, M.: Cloud computing security issues. In: International Journal of Application or Innovation in Engineering & Management (IJAIEM) (2012)
10. Mutum, M., Anita, G.: Security issues in cloud computing. In: 5th International Conference on Bio-Medical Engineering and Information (BMEI) (2012)
11. Ramgovind, S., Eloff, M., Smith, E.: The management of security in cloud computing. In: Conference on Information Security for South Africa, Proceedings of IEEE (2010)

Healthcare Data Analysis Using R and MongoDB

Sonia Saini and Shruti Kohli

Abstract Big Data Analysis in the healthcare domain is an upcoming and nascent topic. The data that can be analyzed from the healthcare domain is typical of huge volume and is quite varying in nature. The Electronic Health Records (EHRs) of just one year for a major hospital can typically run into terabytes and since these records are both structured as well as unstructured, they are a good fit for being analyzed using Big Data tools like Hadoop, R, and Python, etc. Twitter, with its brevity of messages, is one the sources of fast moving information. Real-time information sharing has made healthcare organizations, hospitals, medical institutes, research companies to come out with their respective Twitter "handle", from which the respective organization can share it's official information, can be reached for information, clarifications, and even grievance redress. Such all information is unstructured with links, video, text all being shared and proper data analysis tools are required to gather meaningful data from the tweets. In this paper, we focus on Twitter (Social) data analysis using R and MongoDB. We discuss the data analysis packages available in R, which can be used to analyze tweet and EHR data. We discuss how MongoDB helps map tweets to documents, provides basic operations like aggregation and what all analysis features/packages R provides for analyzing the medical domain data.

Keywords Data analytics · Electronic health record (EHR) · R · MongoDB · Healthcare · Streaming data

S. Saini (✉)
Birla Institute of Technology, Ranchi, India

S. Kohli
Faculty of Computer Science & Engineering,
Birla Institute of Technology, Ranchi, India

V.B. Aggarwal et al. (eds.), *Big Data Analytics*, Advances in Intelligent Systems and Computing 654, https://doi.org/10.1007/978-981-10-6620-7_69

1 Introduction

The healthcare industry has multiple sources from which it generates large volumes of data. Most of this data is generated as a part of compliance with record keeping, regulatory requirements, and data generated by way of patient care [1]. Until now, a large part of this data was being stored either in tapes or in disks and also offline as log books and record books, but the rapidly generated data and large volumes of data have spurred the need for digitization of data. Though it is a difficult task to digitize all the hard copy data but driven by the surge in the generated data, healthcare norms compliance, the possibility of improving the overall quality of healthcare delivery and reducing the overall costs at the same time, these "big data" silos of information are fundamental supporting multitude medical healthcare functions, like clinical decision support systems, surveillance of diseases, and health management of population [2–5]. According to the reports released by the IDC, it is estimated that the U.S. healthcare system, by year 2011, has generated 150 Exabyte of data. It will be no surprise if the U.S. healthcare data volume will soon be to tune of zettabyte. Lab data may soon be in the volumes of yottabyte too. As per a statistic, a premier health network, based out of California, and estimated to have 9 million members, is believed to hold 25–50 petabytes of information data from Electronic Health Records (EHRs), medical images and annotated data [6].

1.1 Introduction to Data Analytics and Its Applications

Data analytics is a statistical analysis of the data from which meaningful conclusions can be inferred thus enabling efficient use of manpower and resources. Some of the prominent data analytics applications in Health Care Organizations are mentioned below:

Clinical decision support—Data analytics help provide support in decision making by clinicians.

Dispensation of real-time information—An example to cite may be providing decision support on in-patient data, which may help move medical equipment on an urgent need basis if a stipulated threshold is reached or breached.

Suggestion of probable diagnoses—If the input data gives ambiguous symptoms, or patient history is incomplete, or other missing data, then data analytics may help provide suggestions for probable diagnoses based on similar cases from historical data.

Population health management—Data Analytics may help in determining effective interventions and preventive medical and healthcare practices for patients who are high-risk and also helps to anticipate future adverse health events.

Administration and planning—It helps to assess the administrative functions of a healthcare facility in order to understand likely resource requirements, staffing levels, infrastructure necessities, and service availability (like diagnostic imaging, specialized check-up, etc.)

Fraud prevention—To detect pattern using previous data and to apply that learning in real time to recognize, warn or even avert suspicious actions before any cash is administered or any such fraudulent transactions take place.

2 Related Works

Many studies have been done previously for social media analysis and text mining used for medical purposes. Some of the areas in which healthcare data analytics has been researched on include the following:

- Predicting increase of pandemics
- Modeling hospital structure network
- Biomedical text mining
- Reduction of healthcare costs by analysis and remedial actions for preventing re-admission.

Existing studies and implementations are done in the field of healthcare data analytics prove the efficiency brought about by the analytics in terms of cost or efforts saved to an organization. The Michigan University Health department standardized blood transfusions administration by infusing analytics into their processes, combining big data analytics research and existing domain expertise, which resulted in a thirty-one percent reduction in transfusions and a consequential reduction of $200,000 per month in expenses [6].

Data is already being produced at a humongous scale within the healthcare domain, with electromagnetic data, sensor records, radiograph films data, MRI, and CT scan data. Some of the data is very critical in nature such as real-time streaming data which is monitoring the neonatal births referred to the ICU and possibly alerts about life-threatening infections quickly [6].

The data in healthcare can come from various sources and in various forms such as structured Electronic Health Record (EHR) data. Structured data has characteristics of easy storage, query, recall, analysis, and manipulation by machine. Data is also in an unstructured manner in the form of clinical notes, hand-written prescriptions, transcriptions, logs, etc. A typical HC Analytics platform can do feature extraction from structured and unstructured EHR in the context of patient representation which can then be fit to a predictive model for classification, regression, and similarity. According to a research by IBM [7], focused on the areas in where data analytics yields clearly advantageous results, is the identification of the patients who are prominent in consumption of health resources or subject to increased risk for adverse outcomes. Data Analytics helps the average individual by providing information required to make informed decisions for the management of their own health and to adopt and track healthy lifestyle habits; selecting treatments, programs, and processes that are cost-optimized; reducing re-admissions of earlier patients by identifying the lifestyle factors contributing to the increased risk of adverse events and adjusting the treatment plans accordingly [8]; improving outcomes by examining vital data from individual health monitors; managing population health by detecting vulnerabilities within patient populations during disease outbreaks or disasters; and orchestration of clinical, operational and finance data together to analyze resource utilization productively and in real time [7].

3 Proposed Model for Healthcare Analytics with R and MongoDB

In our approach of data analysis for social network data which may have vital information pertaining to medical domain or healthcare in general, we hypothesize a model for providing R with preprocessed aggregated analytics data with the MongoDB NoSQL data store doing simple analytics on which R will build further either by loading the preprocessed CSV to a data-frame or data-table in R or by using the RMongo package to directly query MongoDB. The model approach is according to the input nature of the data to be analyzed. We analyzed an offline (Static Nature) Data Model. In this model, we have an (offline) dump of data files that we want to analyze. These (data files) could be anything from archived records, OPD logs, equipment reading logs, or EHR data. This model does I/O to read and write files read into and written from the NoSQL data store. The NoSQL data store, on its part, can provide some analytics which can readily be used further on.

While R provides a range of packages and functions to do the data analytics pertaining to healthcare data, R has certain limitations as the entire dataset has to fit the primary memory or RAM only. For large datasets to be analyzed using R, packages such as "**bit**" and "**ff**" can be used, which can help manage large objects in R. Reading and writing of large CSV files can be done using the chunked sequential access with the package "**ff**" [9].

MongoDB provides an apt fit for storing unstructured healthcare data. The machine generated data (of hospital equipment) is variably structured (for example some sensors may provide reading 24-by-7 and other (non-critical or not required any further) are shut-off). Similarly, social media data from social sharing sites is also very voluminous and variably structured. For such data, a low latency access, high read throughput, and distributed data store such as MongoDB seems fit.

In our analysis, we extracted 15,000 tweets from Twitter via the R twitteR package. A Tweet can easily be stored as a BSON document in MongoDB. For the tweet data, simple aggregation analytics can be done in MongoDB, like top-n Hashtags, queries on geospatial data (like longitude and latitude attributes in the Tweet structure here), stemming, stopword removal, and basic Full Text Search capability. R can further deduce meaningful results like co-occurrence of text (for

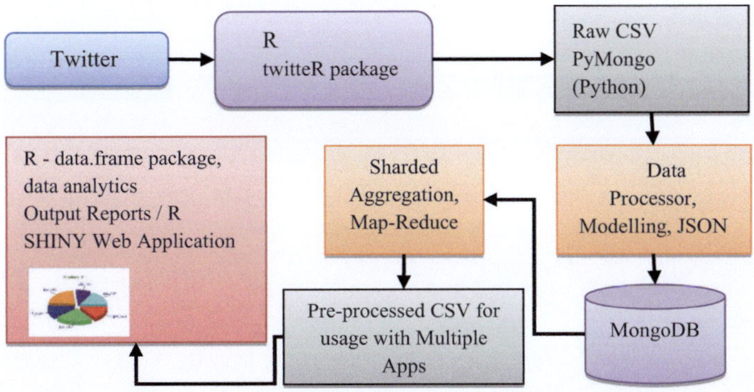

Fig. 1 An "offline" (static-nature) off-loading preprocessed analytics model

example, finding co-occurrence of words "Doctor" and "Vaccination", "Hospital" and "Flu", etc.), word count and building a word-cloud to study the prominent text tweeted (Fig. 1).

3.1 Experimental Result

From the analysis of a Twitter corpus of 15,000 tweets, which were stored in a MongoDB data store, we analyzed the source of tweets and got results like 1112 Tweets were from Twitter Client for IPhone. Further queries to get tweets containing the text "**Vaccination**" we got 4579 records in the corpus. result.db. getCollection("segment").find({"text": { $regex: /Vaccination/, $options: "i"}}).-count() (Fig. 2).

Here, in the above-mined data, we see a tweet indicating that vaccination program implementation improved in the recent times. Word-cloud is an important indicator which informs us about top words in the data. R libraries "**plyr**", "**stringr**", "**tm**", and "**wordcloud**" were used (Fig. 3).

4 Conclusion and Future Research

This study used social media data with focus on healthcare topics and how it can be stored in MongoDB and analyzed in R. Up-front analytics by a NoSQL data store like MongoDB can help by acting as an accelerated analytics platform to further analysis in R, thus potentially "off-loading" resource-intensive analytics in R. Temporal extract of social media data can run into several thousand tweets or posts. Analyzing such massive datasets directly off a data-stream in R can either be

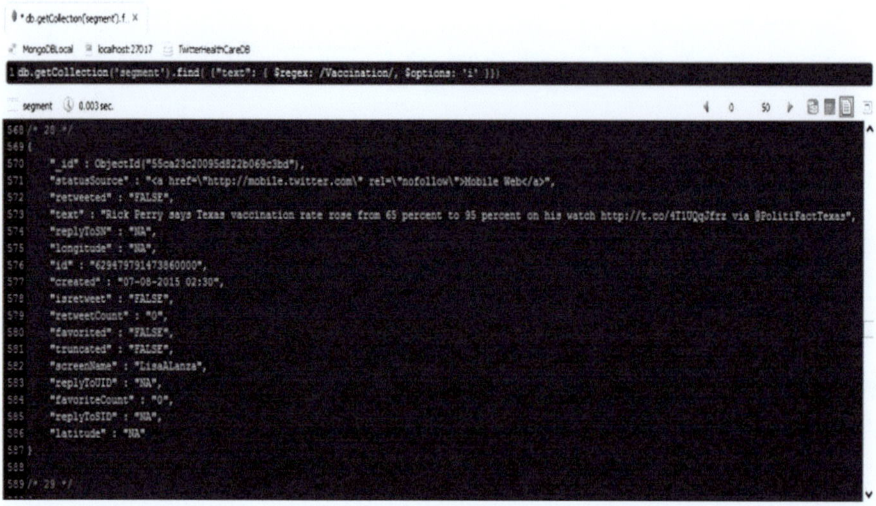

Fig. 2 Regular expression or even full text-based search can filter out data as a part of preprocessed analytics

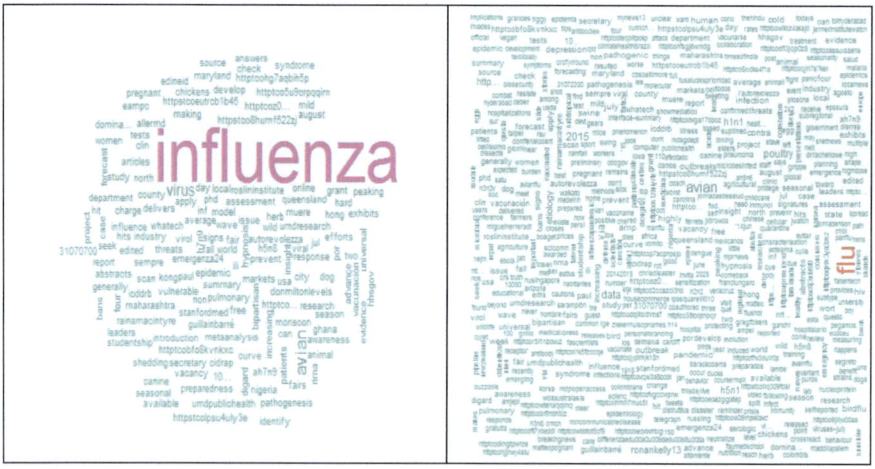

Fig. 3 Word-cloud generated in R from tweet data with healthcare specific filtered text data in the corpus

achieved with the "ff" and "bit" packages or we can use this model approach (discussed here) to provide R with an off-loading analytics platform. The result is that more analytics can be done within shorter rendering and processing times.

References

1. Raghupathi, W.: Data mining in health care. In: Healthcare Informatics: Improving Efficiency and Productivity, pp. 211–223 (2010)
2. Burghard, C.: Big data and analytics key to accountable care success. In: IDC Health Insights (2012)
3. Dembosky, A.: Data Prescription for Better Healthcare, Financial Times, p. 19. http://www.ft.com/intl/cms/s/2/55cbca5a-4333-11e2-aa8f-00144feabdc0.html-website (2012)
4. Feldman, B., Martin, E.M., Skotnes, T.: Big Data in Healthcare Hype and Hope. http://www.west-info.eu/files/big-data-in-healthcare.pdf-website (2012)
5. Fernandes, L., O'Connor, M., Weaver, V.: Big data, bigger outcomes. J. AHIMA, 38–42 (2012)
6. IHTT: Transforming Health Care through Big Data Strategies for Leveraging Big Data in the Health Care Industry. http://ihealthtran.com/wordpress/2013/03/iHT2-releases-big-data-research-report-download-today/-website (2013)
7. IBM: Data Driven Healthcare Organizations Use Big Data Analytics for Big Gains. http://www03.ibm.com/industries/ca/en/healthcare/documents/Data_driven_healthcare_organizations_use_big_data_analytics_for_big_gains.pdf (2013)
8. IBM: Harvard Medical School. http://public.dhe.ibm.com/common/ssi/ecm/en/imc14685usen/IMC14685USEN.PDF (2011)
9. Oehlschlägel: Managing Large Datasets in R–ff Examples and Concepts. Vienna (2010)

Data Mining Tools and Techniques for Mining Software Repositories: A Systematic Review

Tamanna Siddiqui and Ausaf Ahmad

Abstract A software repository contains a historical and valuable wealth of information about overall development of software system (project's status, progress, and evolution). Mining software repositories (MSR) are one of the interesting and fastest growing fields within software engineering. It focuses on extracting and analyzing the heterogeneous data available in software repositories to uncover interesting, useful, and actionable information about software system and projects. Using well-established data mining tools and techniques, professionals, practitioners, and researchers can explore the potential of this valuable data in order to better understand and manage their complicated projects and also to produce high reliable software system delivered on time and within estimated budget. This paper is an effort to discover problems encountered during development of software projects and the role of mining software repositories to resolve these problems. A comparative study of data mining tools and techniques for mining software repositories has been presented.

Keywords Mining software repositories (MSR) · Heterogeneous data · Software mining

1 Introduction

Nowadays, software plays a very important role in the life of human and according to day-to-day needs and requirements it is going to enhance and evolve. Software evolution has been introduced as one of the most vital theme in software engineering and maintenance. It generally deals with spacious amounts of data that engenders from different sources such as source code repositories, bug tracking

T. Siddiqui (✉) · A. Ahmad
Department of Computer Science, Aligarh Muslim University, Aligarh, India
e-mail: ja_zu_siddiqui@hotmail.com

A. Ahmad
e-mail: ausafahmad.cs@gmail.com

V.B. Aggarwal et al. (eds.), *Big Data Analytics*, Advances in Intelligent Systems and Computing 654, https://doi.org/10.1007/978-981-10-6620-7_70

systems, version control system, issue tracking system, mailing and project discussion lists. One of the key points of software development and evolution is to design theories and models that make it possible for understanding the past and present, as well as help in predicting future characteristics related to software maintenance, and therefore support software maintenance tasks [1]. In this concern mining software repositories (MSR) contribute important role. Mining software repositories is a new emerging research field that attempts to gain a deeper understanding of the development process in order to build better prediction and recommendation systems [2]. Historical and valuable information stored in software repositories provide a great opportunity to acquire knowledge and help in monitoring complex projects and products without interfering with development activities and deadlines. Source code control system store source code and changes in it as development progress, bug tracking system keeps records of reported software defects in software development projects, issues tracking system manages and maintains lists of issues, and archive communication between project personnel record rationale for decision throughout the entire life of a project. Such wealth of information helps researchers and software project personnel to understand and manage the development of complex projects within estimated budget and time deadline. For example, historical information can assist developers in understanding the rationale for the current structure of the software system [3].

2 Software Repositories

The software repositories are a storage location maintained online or offline by several software development organizations where software packages, source code, bugs, and many other information related to software and their development process are maintained. Due to open source, the number of these repositories and its uses is increasing at a rapid rate. Anyone can extract many types of data from here, study them, and can make changes according to their need. The examples of software repositories are the following

2.1 Historical Repositories

Such repositories contain a heterogeneous and huge amount of software engineering data generated between long periods of time; some of them are following:

Source control repositories (SCR). SCR record the development history of a project. These repositories keep all the changes made to the source code together with metadata about each change during maintenance, e.g., developer name who made the change, the time at which change was made and a short message describing the intention of change, and the changes performed. The most commonly available, accessible, and used repositories for software projects are source control repositories. Some widely used source control repositories are Perforce, ClearCase, CVS (Concurrent Versions System), subversion, etc.

Bug repositories (BR). BR keep the track of bugs/faults encountered in different phase of software development life cycle maintained by the developers of different organizations. E.g., Jira and Bugzilla are bug repositories maintained by Atlassian and Mozilla community respectively. The benefits of maintaining these repositories are to improve communication, increase product quality, ensure accountability, and increase productivity.

Archived communications (AC). These repositories record the discussion carried out between developers and project managers about various features of a project throughout its entire life cycle. Some examples of archive communication are instance messages, emails, mailing lists, and IRC chats.

2.2 Run-Time Repositories

These repositories contain information related to the execution and the usage of an application at a single or multiple different deployment site such as deployment logs.

Deployment Logs (DL). Software deployment is a complete set of activities that make a software product available for use [4]. These activities can occur at the producer or consumer or both sides. The information related to execution of a particular deployment of a software project or heterogeneous deployments of the same projects are recorded in this type of repositories. For example, the error message expressed by an application at different single or multiple deployment sites may be recorded in deployment logs. The availability of deployment logs continues to increase at a rapid rate due to their use for remote issue resolution and due to recent legal acts [5].

2.3 Code Repositories

CR repositories are maintained by the collection of source code of a large number of heterogeneous projects. Sourceforge.net, GitHub, and Google code are example of CR.

3 Related Work

Mining software repositories is a new emerging field and focus on extracting of both elementary and valuable information regarding software attributes from heterogeneous extant software repositories [6]. These types of repositories are mined to extract the hidden facts by different contributors with regards to accomplishing the different targets. The use of data mining is gaining continuous popularity in software engineering environments due to satisfactory results since last decade [7, 8] and its application include area as bugs prediction [9], Co-evolution of production and test code [10], impact analysis [11], effort prediction [12, 13], similarity analysis [14], prediction of software architectural change [15], software intelligence [5], also used to reduce complexities in Global Software Development [16] and many more.

According to Hassan and Xie [5], "Software Intelligence (SI) is a software developed to analyze source code to clearly understand the Information Technology scenarios. It offers a set of software tools and methods for extracting the valuable information. It keeps software experts up to date and relevant extracted information used to enhance the decision making." Before decade, mining software repositories (MSR) investigations were essentially subjected to industrial level. Consequently, research efforts were reasonably limited to a select few software systems and application domains, or restricted due to lack of historical software data that were not openly available like open source. Recently, there has been a rapid trained shift with respect to the above-noted situation; all these are because of vogue and development of open source software. Consequently, availability of the open source paradigm has been successful in producing excellent and high-quality products that continue to use and evolve.

As we reviewed many research papers, we observed that comparison of techniques used by different researchers is very hard because different researchers used different frameworks, techniques, and data sets. Some use their own private datasets that not accessible to all. Some papers are discussed in Table 1.

4 Challenges in Software Development

Some challenges faced by project managers and programmers are following.

4.1 Faults Encountered

At present time, all software companies essentially focus on handover high-quality products to their customers because of quality leads to customer satisfaction. To achieve the end user satisfaction, these companies targeting to produce high reliable and quality products which must be free from bugs. Therefore, for every software manager, delivering bags free software products to the customers has become the first priority. For example, United States Department of Defense (DOD) losses nearly four billion dollars per year basis because of software failures [17].

A study carried on 104 software projects developed by many developers in different parts and location indicate that end user reports 0.15 faults per 1 KLOC

Table 1 Techniques used in software mining by the various authors

S. No.	Task	Technique used	Data sets	Authors	Refs.
			Private/public		
1	Fault prediction	Statistical prediction rule	Private	Xuemei Zhanga, Hoang Phamb	[24]
2	Fault prediction	K-means clustering method	Private	Shi Zhong, Khoshgoftaar T.M., Seliya N.	[25]
3	Fault prediction	J48 & linear regression	Public	Menzine T., Di Stefano J., Chapman R.M	[26]
4	Fault prediction	CRB & data clustering	Private	Taghi M. Khoshgoftaa, Naeem Seliya	[27]
5	Fault prediction	AntMiner + classification	N.A.	Olivier V., David M., Bart B., Mues C., Manu B.	[9]
6	Detecting half-done change	Apriori association rule	Public	Qinbao S., Martin S., Michelle C., Carolyn M.	[28]
7	Detecting half-done change	FP-growth association rule	Public	Ying A.T., Murphy G.C., Chu-Carroll M.C.	[29]
8	Effort prediction	Linear regression rule	Public	Rahul P., Martin S., Barbara K., Pekka F.	[30]
9	Effort prediction	Decision tree (M.M.)	Public	Martin S., Michelle C.	[31]

(thousand lines of code) during the initial year after delivering of projects to customers; which means for a 100 KLOC project, 15 faults may occur that cannot be ignored [18, 19]. High reliable software to meet user requirements can be achieved by introducing the well-organized development process and structured testing process. In many cases, the results of testing process at development site may differ from user site where the project actually run which also leads to faults.

4.2 Half-Done Changes

A requirement also leads to changes in already developed projects, mostly in source code. Typically, a software project is developed and maintained by a group of developers. Especially in the case of open source software (OSS) these developers are not from the same geographical location. For example, a case study conducted on open source Apache Server, state that the core of this project, including new functionalities is developed by approximately 15 developers [19].

However, for changes in large project is done by a group of programmers. More programmers cooperate in carrying out changes to the source code also create a problem. As programmer that make changes in one module probably do not predict its effect on other modules that changed together, points to half-done change or incomplete change. Due to source code written in different programming languages, it is probably difficult to discover coherence between parts [20] which is also a cause of the half-done change.

5 Software Mining: A Solution

Software mining involves the concept of data mining to build a model or extract information that support and improve the continuous development process of software projects. In this, software artifacts are used as input data and output gives a systematic pattern that helps in prediction of further changes and help practitioners in addressing the challenges discussed above section.

5.1 A Solution of Fault Prediction

The end user always expects that the software system always fulfil the requirement and being free of bugs. While we know that software testing in an exhaustive way is infeasible. Testing phase of development process takes a lot of time and effort. In this concern software mining (SM) provides a solution by modelling software quality predictions and classification. For software quality prediction, software metrics and regression techniques are used to predict the various types of bugs in modules and in quality classification, modules are classified as a fault-prone and non-fault-prone by using classification mining techniques [19].

Therefore, based on the results of SM algorithm, managers allocate budget to the module that contains more bugs and programmers gives more concentration on it rather that module that contain no or some errors. Definitely, this is a better and efficient approach for budget allocation than traditional approach to allocate the budget to whole projects.

5.2 A Solution of Half-Done Change

Half-done change is also a major cause of bugs/faults. Pattern extracted from change histories repositories helps in fault prevention caused by half-done change in source code. Association mining techniques are applied on these repositories that gives warning like "Developers who change the function A, along with the suggested change in related function B, C [21] etc." This task is done by using mining techniques as a plugin in the programing framework by programmers that suggest the related change in source code at once. Source code of some software projects are nearly written in different languages, especially in open source software, to make the changes in such types of source code could be very challenging for a normal programmer, such types of changes can made easily and successfully by software mining.

A notable point is that classification techniques are used for fault prediction and concern of management while association techniques used for half-done change and a concern of programmers.

6 Comparative Study of MSR Tools

A number of mining tools have been developed for the extraction of information or pattern from the different heterogeneous datasets stored in various type software repositories discuss in Sect. 2. Some tools specially used for software mining are Softchange, Hipikat, Dynamine, Kenyon, Chianti, and Apfel. The dimensions of comparison of these tools are intent, information, infrastructure, effectiveness, interaction, input data, and language dependency (Table 2).

Parameter	Description
Intent	It describes expected user like managers, programmers, testers, maintainers, researchers, etc. [22]
Information	The specific data that tool extract for analysis as change management, source code, defect tracing, informal communication, etc. [22]
Infrastructure	A requirement needed to run the tool such as operating system, IDE, store backend, etc. [22]
Effectiveness	Describe the feasibility of proposed such as status, cost, evaluation [23]
Interaction	Describes interactivity and the life tools [23]
Input data	Refers to the input data require by a particular tool
Language independency	Describes the nature, whether the tool is depend on programing language or not

Table 2 A comparative study of MSR tool based on their characteristics and support

List of tools ⟶		DME	SCG	CHI	HKT	AFT	KYN
↓ List of parameters							
User	Manager	…	YES	…	…	…	…
	Programmer	YES	YES	YES	YES	YES	…
	Tester	YES	…	YES	…	…	…
	Maintainer	YES	YES	YES	YES	YES	…
Time	Past	YES	YES	YES	YES	YES	YES
	Present	YES	…	YES	…	…	…
	Future	…	…	…	…	…	YES
Information source	CVS	YES	YES	YES	YES	YES	YES
	Issue tracking	…	YES	…	YES	…	YES
	S/W release	…	YES	…	…	…	…
Change management		YES	…	YES	…	YES	YES
Defect tracking		…	YES	YES	YES	…	YES
Archive mailing lists		…	…	…	YES	…	…
Infrastructure requirement		YES	YES	YES	YES	YES	…
Online/offline		Both	Offline	Offline	Offline	Offline	Both
Storage required		…	YES	YES	…	YES	YES
Input data		SMC	MCB	EP	CVSV	EP	PMVC
Language dependency		…	YES	YES	YES	YES	…

Notations

SCG Softchange; *HKT* Hipikat; *DME* Dynamine; *KYN* Kenyon; *CNI* Chianti; *AFL* Apfel; *EP* Eclipse; *MCB* Metadata from CVS & Bugzilla; *SMC* Set of methods & calls, programs; *CVSV* CVS Data version; *PMVC* Program metadata from various kind of system

7 Conclusion

The present era is the era of software, everything is going computerizing. This is not possible without software. Development of high-quality software on time, within the estimated cost and effort is very challenging task for the software organizations. In this concern, mining software repositories play an important role. In this paper, we have discussed some problem faced by the project personnel and researcher and their expect solution in terms of software mining. The technique used to resolve the challenges is mentioned in this paper and a comparative study of software mining tools has done. This paper helps the project personnel and researchers to understand the basic working of mining software repositories (MSR).

References

1. Novais, R.L., Torres, A., Mendes, T.S., Mendonca, M., Zazworka, N.: Software evolution visualization: a systematic mapping study. Inf. Softw. Technol. **55**, 1860–1883 (2013)
2. Connor, A.M.: Mining Software Metrics from the Jazz Repository. ARPN J. Syst. Soft. **1**(5), ISSN 2222-9833 (2011)
3. Hassan, A.E., Holt, R.C.: Using development history sticky notes to understand software architecture. In: Proceeding of the 21st International Workshop on Program Comprehensive, Italy, June (2004)
4. Software deployment, https://en.wikipedia.org/wiki/Software_deployment
5. Hassan, A.E., Xie, T.: Software intelligence: the future of mining software engineering data. In: Proceedings of the FSE/SDP Workshop on Future of Software Engineering Research, ACM, pp. 161–166 (2010)
6. Keivanloo, I.: A linked data platform for mining software repositories. In: 9th IEEE Working Conference on Mining Software Repositories (2012)
7. Halkidi, M.: Data mining in software engineering. Intell. Data Anal. **15**(3), 413–441 (2011)
8. Xie, T., Pei, J., Hassan, A.E.: Mining software engineering data. In: 29th International Conference on Software Engineering Companion, ICSE (2007)
9. Vandecruys, O.: Mining software repositories for comprehensible software fault prediction models. J. Syst. Softw. **81**(5), 823–839 (2008)
10. Zaidman, A., Van Rompaey, B., Demeyer, S., van Deursen, A.: Mining software repositories to study co-evolution of production & test code. In: 1st International Conference on Software Testing, Verification, and Validation, pp. 220–229 (2008)
11. Canfora, G., Cerulo, L.: Impact analysis by mining software and change request repositories. In: 11th IEEE International, Symposium on Software Metrics (2005)
12. Moser, R.: A model to identify refactoring effort during maintenance by mining source code repositories. In: Product Focused Software Process Improvement, pp. 360–370. Springer, Berlin (2008)
13. Weiss, C.: How long will it take to fix this bug? In: Fourth International Workshop on Mining Software Repositories, ICSE Workshops MSR '07 (2007)
14. Sager, T.: Detecting similar Java classes using tree algorithms. In: Proceedings of the 2006 International Workshop on Mining Software Repositories, ACM, pp. 65–71 (2006)
15. Ratzinger, J.: Mining software evolution to predict refactoring. In: First International Symposium on Empirical Software Engineering and Measurement (2007)

16. Kandjani, H., Tavana, M., Bernus, P., Wen, L., Mohtarami, A.: Using extended axiomatic design theory to reduce complexities in global software development projects. Comput. Ind. **67**, 86–96 (2015)
17. Dick, S., Meeks, A., Last, M., Bunke, H., Kandel, A.: Data mining in software metrics databases. Fuzzy Sets and Systems, pp. 81–110. (2003)
18. Cusumano, M., MacCormack, A., Kemerer, C., Crandall, W.: Software development worldwide: the state of practice. IEEE Comput. Soc. **20**(6), 28–34 (2004)
19. Vandecruys, O., Martens, D., Baesens, B., Mues, C., De Backer, M., Haesen, R.: Mining software repositories for comprehensible software fault prediction models. J. Syst. Softw. **81**, 823–839 (2008)
20. Ying, A., Murphy, G., Ng, R., Chu-Carroll, M.: Predicting source code changes by mining change history. IEEE Trans. Softw. Eng. **30**(9), 574–586 (2004)
21. Zimmerman, T., Weissgerber, P., Diehl, S., Zeller, A.: Mining version histories to guide software changes. In: Proceedings of International Conference on Software Engineering (ICSE), pp. 429–445 (2005)
22. German, M.D., Cubranic, D., Storey D.: A Framework for describing and understanding mining tools in software development. ACM, MSR'05 (2005)
23. Sunday, O.O., Syed, U.I., Yasser S.A., Jarallah S.A.: A mining software repositories—a comparative analysis. Int. J. Comput. Sci. Netw. Secur. **10**(8), 161–174 (2010)
24. Zhanga, X., Phamb, H.: Software field failure rate prediction before software deployment. J. Syst. Softw. **79**, 291–300 (2006)
25. Zhong, S., Khoshgoftaar, T.M., Seliya, N.: Analyzing software measurement data with clustering techniques. Intell. Syst. IEEE (2004)
26. Menzine, T., Stefano, D.J., Chapman, R.M.: Mining repositories to assist in project planning and resource allocation. In: 26th International Conference on Software Engineering, Workshop. doi:10.1049/ic:20040480 (2004)
27. Khoshgoftaar, T.M., Seliya, N.: Analogy-based practical classification rules for software quality estimation. Empirical Softw. Eng. **8**, 325–350 (2003)
28. Song, Q., Shepperd, M., Cartwright, M., Mair, C.: Software defect association mining and defect correction effort prediction. IEEE Trans. Softw. Eng. **32**(2) (2006)
29. Ying, A.T., Murphy, G.C., Ng, R., Chu-Carroll, M.C.: Predicting source code changes by mining change history. IEEE Trans. Softw. Eng. (2004)
30. Rahul, P., Martin, S., Barbara, K., Pekka, F.: An empirical analysis of software productivity over time. In: 11th IEEE Int. Softw. Metr. Symp. (2005)
31. Shepperd, M., Cartwright, M.: Predicting with sparse data. IEEE Trans. Softw. Eng. **27** (2001)
32. What is data preparation, http://www.datapreparator.com/what_is_data_preparation.html
33. Mockus, A., Fielding, R., Herbsleb, J.: A case study of open source software development: The apache server. In: Proceedings of the ICSE Conference, pp. 263–272 (2000)

SWOT Analysis of Cloud Computing Environment

Sonal Dubey, Kritika Verma, M.A. Rizvi and Khaleel Ahmad

Abstract Cloud computing is a technology which deals with the collection of a large number of computers connected together on communication networks, for example the Internet. Cloud computing, dynamically increases computing capacity or add capabilities with minimum intervention of humans and without much investment in new infrastructure. At this moment cloud computing is at infancy stage, with many groups of providers, delivering cloud-based services, from full-scale applications to storage services. In the present era, IT sector turned into cloud-based services independently, but cloud computing integrators and aggregators as of now up and coming. The virtual servers in cloud computing virtually exist and so they can be scaled on the fly without affecting the client, to some extent in spite of being physically objectified, cloud gets expanded or compressed. In this paper, an attempt is made to do a SWOT analysis of a cloud computing environment as many users are in dilemma whether to use it or not. What are the benefits and disadvantages in using the cloud? A critical and detail analysis is done by mapping its Strengths (S), Weakness (W), Opportunity (O), and Threat (T) in different ways.

Keywords Cloud computing · SWOT · CSP · SLA · SWOT analysis

S. Dubey · K. Verma
WET, Regional Institute of Education, Bhopal, India
e-mail: ersonaldubey@gmail.com

K. Verma
e-mail: vermakritika011@gmail.com

M.A. Rizvi
NITTTR, Bhopal, India
e-mail: marizvi@nitttrbpl.ac.in

K. Ahmad (✉)
Department of CS & IT, MANU University, Hyderabad, India
e-mail: khaleelamna@gmail.com

V.B. Aggarwal et al. (eds.), *Big Data Analytics*, Advances in Intelligent Systems and Computing 654, https://doi.org/10.1007/978-981-10-6620-7_71

1 Introduction

Cloud computing is an important improvement in the delivery of information and services. According to National Institute of Standards and Technology (NIST) definition, "*Cloud computing is a model for enabling ubiquitous, convenient, on-demand network access to a shared pool of configurable computing resources (e.g., networks, servers, storage, applications, and services) that can be rapidly provisioned and released with minimal management effort or service provider interaction*" [1].

There are three service models, five key characteristics, and four deployment models [2].

1.1 Key Characteristics of Cloud Computing

Self-Service On-Demand: It provides need-based services to end users who request resources at real time. The user can scale up and scale down the required infrastructure up to a desired level without disturbing the host job.
Broad Network Access: The capabilities available at the network can be accessed by the clients with the help of Internet.
Pooling of Resource: With the help of multitenant model, grouping of provider's computing resources is grouped with the help of different physical and virtual resources.
Rapid Elasticity: On-demand elastically scaling of delivering and releasing of capabilities (inward and outward) is done.
Service Measurement: With the help of abstraction suitable to the type of service the control and optimization of resource is done automatically with the use of metering ability [2].

1.2 Service Models of Cloud Computing

Software as a Service (SaaS): The provider's application that runs on the cloud infrastructure is used by the client. Various client devices such as thin client interface (e.g., web browser) or a program interface. Have accessibility to applications through the Internet.
Platform as a Service (PaaS): The end user deploys the applications that are made or procured on the cloud infrastructure, which are built up using programming languages, libraries, tool, and services supported by the provider.
Infrastructure as a Service (IaaS): The end user that provisions the processing, networks, storage, and other essential computing resources for the deployment and running of arbitrary software, which may include operating systems and applications [2].

1.3 Deployment Models of Cloud Computing

Private cloud: The cloud infrastructure is owned by a single organization that comprises of multiple clients for private use.
Community cloud: Different organizations with common concerns (e.g., mission, policy, security requirements and compliance considerations) own this cloud infrastructure and are managed by a specific community of consumers of such organization.
Public cloud: General public can openly use the cloud infrastructure.
Hybrid cloud: The cloud infrastructure can be classified in at least two distinctive cloud infrastructures (private, community, public) that represent idiosyncratic units, however, are bound together by standardized or proprietary technology that allows data and application portability [2].

2 SWOT Analysis

As defined by Albert Humphrey, "*A SWOT analysis is a strategic planning tool used to evaluate the Strengths, Weakness, Opportunities, and Threats involved in a project or in a business venture or in any other situation of an organization or individual requiring a decision in pursuit of an objective*".

2.1 SWOT Definition

SWOT is an abbreviation for Strengths, Weaknesses, Opportunities, and Threats. SWOT is a simple model that evaluates what an organization can and cannot do as well as its possible opportunities and threats. As per the definition, Strengths (S) and Weaknesses (W) are the internal factors over which organization has some measure of control. Furthermore, by definition, Opportunities (O) and Threats (T) are measured to be external factors over which organization has basically no control [3]. The SWOT framework is represented in Fig. 1.

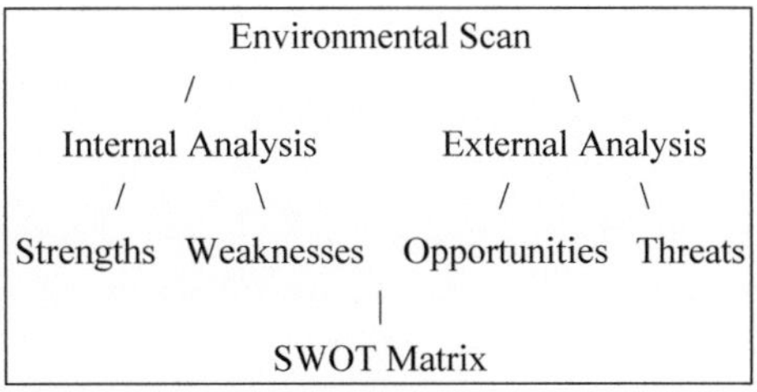

Fig. 1 SWOT analysis framework

The SWOT analysis includes the following segments as explained by Albert Humphrey.

- **Strengths** are usually internal features of an organization or business that gives it a benefit over its opponents. These are usually things like the quality, reputation, assets, people, value proposition, competitive advantages, geographical location, etc.
- **Weaknesses** are typically internal characteristics of an organization that place it as a weakness to the opponents. These are usually things like reputation or credibility, IT systems, financial aspects, people or business processes, loss of key staff, etc.
- **Opportunities** are external factors that present the opportunity to expand profits, sales, and/or get market share. This might include ingoing a marketplace wherein there may be excessive growth, developing new products, weak competition, improving marketing plans, or creating new partnerships.
- **Threats** are external factors which could present a hazard to the existing or future business. These threats may be outside the control of an organization. Examples of these threats may comprise price inflation or deflation, legal, financial conditions, competitive pricing or new competitors, or lack of key partners or contracts [4].

2.2 Need of SWOT Analysis of Cloud Computing

SWOT is a degree of analyzing a system to presentation its high-quality factors and awful factors for evaluation. Mostly, SWOT analysis is utilized to assess the state of affairs of marketplace when a person wants to enter in the market. Before moving into the cloud environment one needs to have some fare knowledge about the cloud and its services. Therefore, SWOT analysis gives few proofs; we are trying to assess the cloud computing on SWOT norm.

During our study of cloud computing we came across several opinions. Some of them were in favor of cloud computing while some were not, i.e., against cloud computing. Hence, due to the diversity in opinions about it, we tried to analyze it and thus we are doing a SWOT Analysis on cloud computing.

2.3 The SWOT Matrix

To flourish procedures taking into account the SWOT outline, a matrix of these aspects can be created. The TOWS matrix, also known as a SWOT Matrix is shown in Table 1.

Table 1 TOWS/SWOT matrix

	Strengths	Weaknesses
Opportunities	S-O strategies	W-O strategies
Threats	S-T strategies	W-T strategies

- **S-O approaches** practice opportunities that are appropriate to the organization's strengths.
- **W-O approaches** overcome weaknesses to follow opportunities.
- **S-T approaches** discover ways that an organization can use as its strengths to diminish its susceptibility to threats.
- **W-T approaches** set up a self-protective plot to thwart the organization's weaknesses from making it extremely vulnerable to threats.

2.4 *Strengths of Cloud Computing*

S1 Data sharing.
S2 Scalable storage space.
S3 Enhance availability of data and services.
S4 Development of OS-independent applications.
S5 Improved performances of services.
S6 Reliability of data and services.
S7 Reduced cost (pay-per usage).
S8 Work load diversity.
S9 Power-management flexibility.
S10 The cloud offerings are heterogeneous and without agreed interfaces.
S11 Increased security level for devices achieved by a centralized monitoring and maintenance of software.
S12 Number of new functionalities might be offered.
S13 Portability of application is possible.
S14 Enhance business agility while maintaining IT security and control.
S15 Attain cloud economics while leveraging existing IT investments.
S16 Pricing transparency.
S17 Controlled interface, ubiquitous access, location independence, sourcing autonomy, virtual professional environments, and hurried elasticity.
S18 Delivering variable costs, reduced capital expenditure, lower staff costs, cost efficient consolidation of physical resources.
S19 Simplifying access and management of applications and IT resources in a virtualized on-demand model.
S20 Flexible and resilient in disaster recovery.
S21 Service Level Agreement (SLA) guarantees the services from the cloud service providers to client.

2.5 *Weakness of Cloud Computing*

W1 Interoperability (communications between the cloud).
W2 Global compliance problem/different compliance in different regions.
W3 Open Standards.
W4 A bulk loads are limited by bandwidth.
W5 Cloud services are multi-vendors solutions by definition.
W6 Very few true hybrid cloud offerings exists today.
W7 Modification on maintenance model.
W8 Paradigm swing at present occupational and IT departments.
W9 No easy migration to another CSP (Cloud Service Provider).
W10 More and in depth knowledge is required for managing and implementing SLA contracts with CSP's.
W11 Third-party/CSP dependability for computing services.
W12 High-speed Internet connection essential to connect to cloud database.
W13 No precise method to select/find CSP.

2.6 *Opportunities of Cloud Computing*

O1 Overcoming latency limitations.
O2 Improving bandwidth utilization.
O3 Dynamic network monitoring.
O4 Technical issues resolution.
O5 CRM (Customer Relationship Management) has become one of the most accessible opportunity.
O6 Market entry or application deployment is cheaper, quicker repayment of improvement charges, and superior return on investment.
O7 Better comprehension of process and governance risk will transfer the preferences of IT owners toward the auditable and very professional security practices of CSPs.
O8 Customers will become more aggressive in dropping their cost of both business and personal computing, and will become far more accepting of lightweight client machines running free and open-source operating systems and applications.
O9 Overall growth in development demand will expand the significance of high-leverage application frameworks that allow quicker development of higher quality products.
O10 Adaptive to future needs.
O11 Cloud provides an excellent back-end for mobile applications.
O12 Optimizing the usefulness and proficiency of cloud computing environments.

O13 Mitigating identity, privacy, security, reliability, and manageability risks in cloud-based environments, as they vary from traditional data centers.
O14 Expansion and growth.
O15 The more effective use of computer resources to help the environment and encourage energy saving.
O16 Most of the cloud providers replicate user's data in multiple places. This multiplies redundancy of data and data independence from system failure offers a level of disaster recovery.
O17 CSP has the ability to relocate security resources for filtering, traffic shaping or encryption, dynamically, in order to increase the defensive measures.
O18 The organization can concentrate on serious tasks without having to experience additional costs with respect to IT staffing and training.
O19 The cloud computing approach speeds the deployment while preserving dynamic flexibility.

2.7 Threats of Cloud Computing

T1 Security issues (Privacy, Authentication, Malware, Confidentiality, Third party, Data integrity, Loss of data: Is foreseeable, thus backup for every usage has to be maintained on the PC).
T2 Management of data.
T3 Data ownership.
T4 Connectivity, Speed, Safety and Efficiency.
T5 Virtual security is critical and security concern must be addressed on the path to hybrid cloud deployments.
T6 Physical location of software and hardware is unidentified. Site investigations and inspections are hard.
T7 Quality problems with CSP.
T8 Measurement of useful resource utilization and end user activities lies in the hands of the CSP.
T9 Opaque cost structure because of greater flexible usage of cloud services.
T10 No or little insight in CSP uncertain procedures.
T11 Natural calamities.
T12 Migration from one cloud platform to another is difficult.
T13 Portability: porting of services/application at another location may be cumbersome.
T14 Vendor shutdown: the vendor may suddenly go out of business and close the shop. This would create a very unstable situation for consumer [5].

After going through a lot of data and analysis done in the above-mentioned Table 2, it is analyzed that to follow opportunities which are appropriate to the firm's strengths are:

Table 2 Mapping of strength with opportunities (S-O)

Strengths	Opportunities
S1	O1 + O2 + O11 + O19
S2	O9 + O12 + O14 + O19
S3	O1 + O2 + O11 + O16
S4	O9 + O10
S5	O1 + O2 + O3 + O11 + O13 + O17
S6	O13 + O16 + O17
S7	O6 + O8 + O18
S8	O3 + O16 + O19
S9	O12 + O15
S10	O9 + O10
S11	
S12	O9 + O17 + O19
S13	O3 + O11 + O13
S14	O5 + O6 + O7 + O8
S15	O6 + O8 + O18
S16	O5 + O7 + O8
S17	O1 + O2 + O3 + O10 + O11 + O12 + O13 + O16 + O17
S18	O6 + O18
S19	O3 + O19
S20	O16 + O17 + O19
S21	

- Security of the data will improve
- Data sharing with ease
- Scalability and availability is easier
- Business agility is increased
- Cost will be reduced
- Service Level Agreement guarantees the services
- Heterogeneous environment is enhanced.

It can be summarized that many opportunities will be open for the betterment for business and organizations with the arrival of a cloud computing environment.

After analyzing the above-mentioned data in Table 3, it is analyzed that when the cloud will establish itself in the marked and advancement done in the cloud technology, weakness will be overcome automatically there will be opportunities only with cloud. The future of the Internet is cloud only. The opportunities of the cloud are

- Communication between the clouds is established
- Global fixed standard is introduced
- Bandwidth is improved
- Maintenance model is enhanced.

Table 3 Mapping of weakness and opportunities (W-O)

Weakness	Opportunities
W1 + W6 + W9	O3 + O5 + O9 + O11 + O12 + O14 + O19
W2 + W3 + W5	O5 + O7 + O8 + O9 + O13 + O14 + O19
W4	O1 + O2 + O3 + O9 + O10 + O12 + O14 + O19
W7	O7 + O10 + O12 + O13 + O17
W8	O6 + O8 + O9 + O12 + O14 + O15 + O19
W10 + W11	O5

It can be summarized that many opportunities will be open for the betterment of a cloud computing environment.

By analyzing the mentioned Strengths and Threats in Table 4, it is analyzed that to reduce the vulnerabilities to external threats we have to concentrate on some strengths of cloud like

- Security of the cloud should be improved
- Data sharing, scalability, and availability should be simplified
- Business agility should be increased
- Cost should be reduced
- SLA guarantees the services
- Heterogeneous environment should be enhanced.

It can be summarized that improving all the above mentioned threats in turn cloud computing environment will more popular.

By analyzing the above-mentioned Weakness with Threats in Table 5, it can be said that to establish a self-protective plan to thwart the organization's weaknesses from making it highly susceptible to external threats are listed below

Table 4 Mapping of strength with threats (S-T)

Strengths	Threats
S5 + S6 + S8 + S11 + S14 + S21	T1
S1 + S2 + S3 + S19 + S20	T2
S14 + S17 + S21	T3
S2 + S4 + S8 + S17	T4
S6 + S14 + S15 + S17	T5
S5 + S17 + S18 + S20	T7
S21	T8
S7 + S15 + S16 + S18	T9
S21	T10
S6 + S13 + S20	T11
S10 + S13	T12 + T13
S21	T14

Table 5 Mapping of weakness with threats (W-T)

Weaknesses	Threats
W1 + W6 + W9	T1 + T4 + T12
W2 + W3 + W5	T2 + T3 + T9 + T12 + T13
W4	T2 + T4 + T7 + T13
W7	T1 + T2 + T4 + T5 + T7 + T12 + T13
W10 + W11 + W13	T1 + T2 + T3 + T5 + T7
W12	T2 + T4 + T7 + T12

- Communication between the clouds should be established
- Global fixed standard should be introduced
- Bandwidth should be improved
- Maintenance model should be enhanced.

It can be summarized that then most of the threats will be vanished for the betterment of a cloud computing environment.

3 Conclusion

After above-mentioned marathon analysis and discussion on Strength (S), Weakness (W), Opportunity (O), and Threat (T) of cloud computing. It can be concluded that cloud computing has yet not reached a maturity that leads it into a fruitful stage. However the majority of the key problems with cloud computing have been solved to a certain point that Cloud computing has become very popular for commercial and organizational utilization. This does not mean that all the problems listed above have been completely resolved, only that the accordingly risks can be accepted to a certain point. Cloud computing is thus still a very popular area for research. It can be summarized that although there are few threats and weaknesses in cloud computing, but on the contrary, there are various strengths and opportunities thus this technology is getting popular and the future is cloud. This technology will get better day by day as researches will take place.

References

1. Demarest, G., Wang, R.: Oracle cloud computing. An Oracle white paper. http://www.oracle.com/us/technologies/cloud/oracle-cloud-computing-wp-076373.pdf (2010)
2. Mell, P., Grance, T.: The NIST definition of cloud computing. NIST (National Institute of Standards and Technlogy) Special Publication 800-145
3. Sourabh, J., et al.: SWOT Analysis—Definition, Advantages and Limitations. http://www.managementstudyguide.com/swot-analysis.htm

4. Eversoll, L.: SWOT (Strengths, weaknesses, opportunities, threats). http://www.lizeversoll.com/2011/02/13/swot-strengths-weaknesses-opportunities-threats/ (2011)
5. http://www.quickmba.com/strategy/swot (2010)
6. Dimitrios, Z., Dimitrios, L.: Addressing cloud computing security issues. Future Gener. Comput. Syst. **28**, 583–592 (2012) (Elsevier)
7. Tanzim Khorshed, Md., et al.: A survey on gaps, threat remediation challenges and some thoughts for proactive attack detection in cloud computing. Future Gener. Comput. Syst. **28**, 833–851 (2012) (Elsevier)
8. Khan, A.N., et al.: Towards secure mobile cloud computing: a survey. Future Gener. Comput. Syst. **29**, 1278–1299 (2013) (Elsevier)
9. Changa, V., et al.: The development that leads to the cloud computing business framework. Int. J. Inf. Manag. (2013)
10. Marston, S., et al.: Cloud computing—the business perspective. Decis. Support Syst. **51**, 176–189 (2011)

A Review on Quality of Service in Cloud Computing

Geeta and Shiva Prakash

Abstract Cloud Computing is a computing technology that uses remote control servers and Internet to maintain applications and data. It is an emerging technology. Today's Cloud computing is a wide area in research and industry. It is a term, which involves networking, virtualization, software, web services and distributed computing. In cloud computing environment there are various challenges like efficient load balancing, real benefits/business outcome, resource scheduling, datacenter energy consumption, etc. Quality of Service (QoS) plays an important role in distributed computing for multimedia and other essential applications. Aim of this paper to provide a survey of the QoS modeling approaches and other frame works suitable for cloud systems and describe their implementation details, merits and demerits. This paper supports new researchers to be able to understand main techniques used and their limitations in environment of cloud computing for providing QoS.

Keywords Cloud computing · Quality of service · Load balancing · QoS parameters

1 Introduction

Cloud Computing [1] is a computing technology that uses remote control servers and Internet to maintain applications and data. It is an emerging technology. Cloud provides resources over Internet using multi-tenancy, virtualization technology, web services [2], etc. Multi-tenancy is important for developing software as a service (SaaS) application. Multi-tenancy allows the same software platform to be

Geeta (✉)
UPTU, Lucknow, India
e-mail: geetasingh02@gmail.com

S. Prakash
Department of Computer Science & Engineering, MMMUT, Gorakhpur, India
e-mail: shiva.plko@gmail.com

V.B. Aggarwal et al. (eds.), *Big Data Analytics*, Advances in Intelligent Systems and Computing 654, https://doi.org/10.1007/978-981-10-6620-7_72

shared by multiple applications. Virtualization provides abstraction of independent hardware access to each virtual machine applications communicate over the Internet using web services. There are three models of cloud computing [3, 4]. Software as a Service (SaaS): it is also known as on demand service. It is an application that can be accessed from anywhere, any time on the world as long as you can have a computer with an internet connection. Platform as a service (PaaS): PaaS providers offer a predefined combination of Operating System and application servers. It is a platform for developers to write and create their own SaaS. Infrastructure as a Service (IaaS): The Cloud service providers provide computers, as physical or more often as virtual machines. Some common examples are Amazon, GoGrid, etc. There are four deployment of cloud service-Public Cloud: Public cloud makes services such as computing, storage, application, etc. available to general public. These services may be free or offered as payment as per public usage. Major public cloud providers are Amazon, Google, Microsoft, etc. Private Cloud: Private cloud is a cloud infrastructure operated only for a single organization. It is not available to general public. Community Cloud: Community cloud shared infrastructure between several organization with common concerns such as jurisdiction, compliance, etc. Hybrid Cloud: It is a combination of two or more clouds (public, private, or community).

In Cloud Computing the term QoS denotes the levels of availability, reliability and performance offered by the infrastructure and by the platform and or an application that hosts it. It is fundamental for cloud consumers, who expect cloud providers to deliver the quality features, and for cloud providers, who requisite to find the correct tradeoffs between operational costs and QoS levels. However, it is a difficult decision problem to find optimal tradeoff, often enraged by the presence of service level agreements specifying Quality of Service targets and economical penalties associated to violations of Service level agreement (SLA) [5].

Rest of paper organized as Sect. 2 presents detailed literature review of related work of QoS in environment of cloud computing. Section 3 presents comparative study of main works of QoS in environment of cloud computing. Finally, presents conclusion in Sect. 4.

2 Related Works of Quality of Service in Cloud Computing

Quality of Services plays an important role in making the cloud services acceptable to customers in cloud computing. Cloud computing systems may crowd thousands of internationally dispersed users at any given time. These users may access dissimilar types of services that have different requirements depending on the type of users, resources and services involved [6]. Several Authors have put forward their ideas for innovative and new solutions for handling this imperative area is management of resources.

In [7] Alhamazani et al. have described the importance of dynamically monitoring the Quality of Service of virtualized services. The Researchers explain the monitoring of the services which would help both the application developer and cloud provider to maximize there turn of their investments in terms of keeping hosted applications and the cloud services operating at peak efficiency, detecting changes in service and application performance, SLA violations, failures of cloud services and other dynamic configuration changes. Researchers mainly concentrate on SNMP based QoS monitoring which is a paper describing work in progress.

The effect of different factors on the QoE of multimedia users have presented by Mushtaq, and Mellouk et al. [8] in a cloud computing network (CCN). The Researchers have grouped the factors that affect the Quality of Experience (QoE) into four groups. These four groups are characteristics of videos, network parameters, types of user's profiles and terminal characteristics. The data collected through different methods have been classified using machine learning techniques such as Naive Bayes, Support Vector Machines, K-Nearest Neighbors, Decision Tree, Random Forest and Neural Networks and they have determined the best method for Quality of Service (QoS)/Quality of Experience (QoE) correlation after evaluating them. The QoE/QoS correlation is used to evaluate the machine learning techniques. Hence it can be concluded that this paper describes the capabilities of machine learning techniques.

In [9], Stoicuta have described a client application for monitoring cloud Quality of Service on iOS5. This application can be used to control the performance of their cloud provider by the client. But the designed application has been focusing on available transfer rate and one way delay very narrowly. Hence the application has limited applications.

In [10], Li have proposed a novel for cloud workflow scheduling model. The authors have incorporated trust in this model in addition to the QoS targets. In order to analyze the user's requirements and design a customized schedule, the authors proposed two stage workflow model where the macro multiworkflowstage is based on trust and micro single workflow stage classifies workflows into time sensitive and cost sensitive based on QoS demands. The fuzzy clustering technique is used to classify the workflows. The model restricts the Quality of Service parameters considered to bandwidth, storage, response time, reliability and cost. In this model the delivery of QoS is limited only to average values and no guarantee of service delivery is provided at least in terms of a predetermined confidence level. This is a strong limitation of the proposed model as the consumers do not have the ability to select their own Quality of Service parameters and no guarantee of the Quality of Service delivery at least a statistical validation.

In [11], Goyal have proposed a trust management model based on QoS. In this proposed model Author explains how to use multiple QoS attribute to calculate the trust value, but there is no prioritization between attributes and also there is no clear explanation how these attributes are combined.

Emeakaroha et al. [12] have presented a schedule that takes many SLA attributes for application deployments in the Cloud environment. The attributes considered in this application includes network bandwidth, storage capacity, and CPU time for deploying applications. These attributes have limited application in real world as they require to be considered during deployment. When the applications have been ready for user access once, the users would be more interested in performance attributes such as processing time, response time etc. Hence, in real world business this model may not have much practical significance.

An optimization framework proposed by Kouki, Ledoux, and Sharrock et al. [13] for cross layer cloud services. The proposed framework is acceptable for salespersons advertising gathering of facilities and also takes the changeable nature of cloud environment. An optimization across various layers has been carried out enforcing the Service Level Agreement dependencies between them. The proposal currently faces the problem of run time management of QoS performance.

Iyer and Veeravalli have proposed and formulated a resource allocation strategy for cloud infrastructure based on bargaining [14]. They have combined the Raiffa Bargaining Solution and Nash Bargaining Solution to appear at an optimal allocation strategy. This proposal monitors the dynamic environment of cloud very well during run time but it does not permit to manage resources from multiple sources. Hence if a single service supplier cannot meet all the desires of the user, he will be demanded to settle a sub optimal allocation of resources.

Chen and Zhang [15] have proposed a workflow scheduling algorithm which is based on Particle Swarm Optimization (PSO). The proposed method can optimize up to seven attributes specified the users and compared to traditional optimization methods that allow only for the workflow execution time. The weakness of the proposed method is lacking of monitoring scheme for catching Quality of Service violations.

den Bossche et al. [16], presented set of heuristics for scheduling deadline constrained applications. It is in a cost effective manner in a hybrid cloud system. This mechanism attempts to maximize local resources along with minimize the external resources without compromising the QoS requirements of the applications. This set of heuristics takes the cost of both data transfer and computation along with the estimated data transfer times. The main criteria in optimization is the maximization of cost saving. The effect of different cost factors and workload characteristics on the cost savings have been analyzed along with the sensitivity of the results to the different runtime estimates. The advantages of the proposed methodology are that an optimized set of resources can be selected from both in private and public cloud systems for meeting the QoS requirements. But it suffers from certain weaknesses. Though it is considered only the deadline concerned applications, it does not consider the failures that may occur after the scheduling has done. The failure will affect the application in terms of quality and increase the cost of execution.

A generic QoS framework have proposed by Liu et al. [17] for Cloud workflow systems which is consists of four components such as QoS aware service selection, QoS requirement specification, QoS violation handling and QoS consistency monitoring. However the knowledge sharing and data communication between the components for different Quality of Service dimensions is not suitable for solving difficult problems such as monitoring, multi based service selection and violation handling.

Some algorithms to equivalence the cost of hardware and SLA violations for resource allocation in cloud for SaaS providers have proposed by Buyya et al. [18]. These proposed algorithms takes certain Quality of Service attributes such as service initiation time and response time for satisfying the customer's while minimizing the use of hardware resources. All these algorithms are established to reuse the already created Virtual Machines in order to reduce cost and it may create security problems for users as the residual information in the VMs can be used against them.

QoS ranking prediction frameworks have been proposed for Cloud services by Zheng et al. [19], by taking past service usage experiences of users. This framework is used to avoid the time consuming, expensive real world service invocations and requires no extra invocations of Cloud facilities when making Quality of Service ranking prediction. In this framework Collaborative filtering technique is used to predict Quality of Service for web services, it can is also be used for cloud services. This framework is used Pearson Correlation Coefficient to calculate the similarity between users.

Garg have described a framework in [20], to measure the quality and prioritize Cloud service. This framework makes significant impact and creates fresh competition among Cloud providers to satisfy their SLA and enhance their QoS. They proposed an Analytical Hierarchical Process based ranking method that can be used to evaluate the Cloud services which is based on various applications depending on Quality of Services requirements. The presented method is used for quantifiable QoS attributes such as Assurance of Service, Cost, Accountability, Agility, Performance, Usability, Security, and Privacy. It is not suitable for non-quantifiable Quality of Service attributes such as Service Response Time, Transparency, Interoperability, Sustainability, Suitability, Accuracy, Availability, Reliability and Stability.

A service selection algorithms based on QoS aware have proposed by Ruozhou et al. [21] for composing diverse services offered by a Cloud. Using virtualization technology various types of resources require to be virtualized as a set of Cloud services. Customized Cloud services that occupy not only diverse types of computing services but also computing services of interconnecting networks in the Cloud End-users. So, the networking services and Cloud computing services has been modeled as combined customized Cloud service.

Ani [22–24] considered some QoS constraints, such as deadline, file size, budget, requested length, penalty and rate ratio. Penalty Rate Ratio is a ratio for consumer's compensation if the Software as Service provider misses the deadline. The maximum time a consumer would like to wait for the result is called Deadline. The size of input file provided by consumers called the Input File Size. Budget is the amount customer wishes to pay for the resources. Request Length is the Millions of Instructions required to be executed to server request.

A new system called Cloud Monitoring System (CMS) have described by Chitra et al. [25]. This is used to improve Quality of Service during Service Level Agreement negotiation. The negotiation between users and cloud Service provider's periodic polling is administered and reports are accomplished in an absolute manner. After detecting the local corrections, each element of network has to eject alarms in order to assure that global parameters are not violated. In this monitoring system the failed node can be noticed with the help of monitoring and it gradually improves the efficiency of the cloud and attracts the users. More QoS parameters can be considered.

An algorithm is proposed by Chen et al. [26], to help choose data centers and cloud providers in a various cloud environment for example a video service manager. Performances are evaluated with various video service workloads. Compared with using only one cloud provider, dynamically deploying services in multi cloud is better in aspects of both QoS and cost.

3 Comparative Study of Research Work

This section summaries main works of QoS in environment of cloud computing as the work discussed above in literature review on the basis of techniques used and their merits and demerits.

Table 1 Comparison study of research work

Sl. No.	Author and reference	Proposed model/framework	Merits	Demerits
1	Buyya [7]	SLA oriented resource provisioning for cloud and service computing	It integrates the market based resource provisioning with virtualization technologies for flexible resource allocation	It does not integrates in combined manner of IaaS, PaaS and SaaS
2	Liu [8]	A Generic QoS framework for cloud workflow systems	Author covers all four stages of cloud workflow in this framework	In this framework QoS metrics are not identified
3	den Bossche [9]	A set of Heuristics scheduling deadline constrained workloads on hybrid cloud system	It takes the cost of both data transfer and computation along with estimated data transfer times, different cost factors and workload characteristics	In this method, failures may occur after the scheduling does not consider
4	Chen [10]	Trust-based and QoS demand clustering analysis customizable cloud workflow scheduling strategies	In these strategies multiple parameter optimizations are possible	No monitoring mechanism is implemented for catching violations

(continued)

Table 1 (continued)

Sl. No.	Author and reference	Proposed model/framework	Merits	Demerits
5	Iyer [11]	Resource allocation in a compute cloud through bargaining approach	It handles the dynamic nature of cloud during run time	It may lead to sub optimum solutions from a customer's perspective, if a single provider cannot meet all the requirements
6	Kouki [12]	An optimization framework for cross layer cloud services	Suitable for vendors selling products across multiple layers dynamic nature of cloud has been considered	There is a problem in the run time management of QoS performance
7	Emeakaroha [13]	A heuristic scheduling that takes multiple SLA parameters when deploying applications in cloud	Considers deployment attributes as storage capacity network bandwidth and CPU time, before installation of applications in the cloud system	It does not consider performance parameter as response time, performance time
8	Goyal [14]	A QoS based trust management model for cloud infrastructure as a service	It can be used multiple QoS parameters	There is no possibility to prioritize the parameters
9	Li and Zhang [15]	A set based discrete PSO for cloud workflow scheduling with user defined QoS constraints	The workflow scheduling mechanism breaking up into multiple stages and grouping the requests of the user requirements	There is absence of QoS delivery guarantees
10	Stoicuta [16]	An OpenNet Inf-based cloud solution for cross layer quality of service monitoring part using iOS terminal	It can be used by clients to monitor	It focuses only on available transfer rate and one way delay as QoS parameters
11	Mustaq [17]	Empirical study based on machine learning method to access the QoS/QoE correlation	It has been studied using a selected set of machine learning method	The Qos/QoE correlation is a scheme for evaluating the machine learning methods
12	Alhamazani [18]	Cloud monitoring for optimizing the quality of service of hosted applications	This work is based on concept and idea only	There is no evaluation

(continued)

Table 1 (continued)

Sl. No.	Author and reference	Proposed model/framework	Merits	Demerits
13	Zheng [19]	QoS ranking prediction for cloud services	Outperformed rating based schemes and greedy method	It has to be considered accuracy of ranking method
14	Garg [20]	A framework for ranking and comparing cloud services	In this attributes are explained for consumers and providers	In this framework Non quantifiable QoS attributes are not used
15	Yu [21]	QoS aware service selection in virtualization based cloud computing	Virtualization increases QoS by monitoring system	It is considered single QoS parameter

As per Table 1 we see that each of the proposed model/framework have its merit and demerit. Explanation of each work is described in Sect. 2.

4 Conclusion

In this paper we have reviewed current proposed framework in workload and system modeling and applications to cloud QoS management. Managing QoS is a difficult job in making such an innovative method to larger customers. The findings of the Researchers in terms of the merits and demerits of the reviewed work have been presented in the table given above to find the references easily. It can be seen from Table that there is still a lot future work in this exciting and challenging area.

References

1. Buyya, R.K., Yeo, C.S., Venugopal, S., Broberg, J., Brandic, I.: Cloud computing and emerging IT platforms: reality, vision, and hype for delivering computing as the 5th utility. J. Future Gener. Comput. Syst. **25**(6), 599–616 (2009)
2. Armbrust, M., Fox, A., Griffith, R., Joseph, A.D., Katz, R., Konwinski, A., Lee, G., Patterson, D., Rabkin, A., Stoica, I., Zaharia, M.: A view of cloud computing. Mag. Commun. ACM **53** (4), 50–58 (2010)
3. Buyya, R., Vecchiola, C., Selvi, S.T.: Cloud Computing Architecture, pp. 111–140 (2013)
4. Ding, S., Yang, S., Zhang, Y., Liang, C., Xia, C.: Combining Quality of Service prediction and customer satisfaction estimation to solve cloud service trustworthiness evaluation problems. Knowl. Based Syst. **56**, 216–225 (2014)
5. Genez, TAL., Bittencourt, L.F., Madeira, E.R.M.: Workflow scheduling for SaaS/PaaS cloud providers considering two SLA levels. In: The IEEE/IFIP NOMS (2012)
6. Firdhous, M., Hassan, S., Ghazali, O.: A comprehensive survey on Quality of Service implementations in cloud computing. Int. J. Sci. Eng. Res. (IJSER). **4**(5) (2013)

7. Alhamazani, K., Ranjan, R., Rabhi, F., Wang, L., Mitra, K.: Cloud monitoring for optimizing the QoS of hosted applications. In: Proceedings of 4th International Conference on Cloud Computing Technology and Science, pp. 765–770 (2012)
8. Mushtaq, M.S., Augustin, B., Mellouk, A.: Empirical study based on machine learning approach to access the QoS/QoE correlation. In: Proceedings of 17th European Conference on Networks and Optical Communications (NOC), pp. 1–7 (2012)
9. Stoicuta, F., Ivanciu, I., Minzat, E., Rus, A.B.,: An OpenNetInf-based cloud computing solution for cross layer QoS: monitoring part using iOS terminal. In: Proceedings of 10th International Symposium of Electronics and Telecommunication, pp. 167–170 (2012)
10. Li, W., Hangzhou, Zhang, Q., Wu, J., Li, J.: Trust-based and QoS demand clustering analysis customizable cloud workflow scheduling strategies. In: Proceedings of International Conference on Cluster Computing Workshops, pp. 111–119 (2012)
11. Goyal, M.K., Gupta, P., Aggarwal, A., Kumar, P.: A QoS based trust management model for cloud Iaas. In: Proceedings of 2nd IEEE International Conference Parallel Distributed and Grid Computing, pp. 843–847 (2012)
12. Emeakaroha, V.C., Brandic, I., Maurer, M., Breskovic, I.: A Scheduling heuristic that takes multiple SLA parameters when deploying applications in cloud. In: Proceedings of 35th IEEE Annual Computer Software and Applications Conference Workshops, pp. 298–303 (2011)
13. Kouki, Y., Nantes, Ledoux, T., Sharrock, R.: Cross-layer SLA selection for cloud services. In: Proceedings of 1st International Symposium on Network Cloud Computing and Applications, pp. 143–147 (2011)
14. Iyer, G.N., Veeravalli, B.: On the resource allocation and pricing strategies in compute clouds using bargaining approaches. In: Proceedings of the 17th IEEE International Conference on Networks, pp. 147–152 (2011)
15. Chen, W-N., Zhang, J.: A set based discrete PSO for cloud workflow scheduling with user-defined QoS constraints. In: IEEE International Conference on Systems, Men and Cybermetics, pp. 773–778 (2012)
16. Van den Bossche, R., Vanmechelen, K., Broeckhove, J.: A set of Heuristics scheduling deadline constrained workloads on hybrid cloud System. In: Proceedings of the 3rd IEEE International Conference on Cloud Computing Technical and Science, pp. 320–327 (2011)
17. Liu, X., Yang, Y., Yuan, D., Zhang, G.: A Generic QoS framework for cloud workflow systems. In: Proceedings of the 9th IEEE International Conference Dependable, Automatic and Secure Computing, pp. 713–720 (2011)
18. Buyya, R., Garg, S.K., Calheiros, R.N.: SLA oriented resource provisioning for cloud and service computing: challenges, architecture and solutions. In: Proceedings of the 11th International Conference Cloud and Service Computing, pp. 1–10 (2011)
19. Zheng, Z., Wu, X., Zhang, Y., Lyu, M.R., Wang, J.: QoS ranking prediction for cloud services. In: IEEE Transactions on Parallel and Distributed Systems, vol. 24(6) (2013)
20. Garg, S.K., Versteeg, S., Buyya, R.: SMI Cloud: A framework for comparing and ranking cloud Services. In: Proceedings of the 4th IEEE International Conference on Utility and Cloud Computing (UCC) (2011)
21. Yu, R., Yang, X., Huangy, J., Duanz, Q., Ma, Y., Tanaka, Y.: QoS-aware service selection in virtualization-based cloud computing. In: Network Operations and Management Symposium (APNOMS), 2012 14th Asia-Pacific, pp. 1–8 (2012)
22. Mary, N.A.B.: Profit maximization for software as service using SLA based spot pricing in cloud computing. Int. J. Emerg. Technol. Adv. Eng. ISSN 2250-2459. An ISO 9001:2008 Certified Journal. **3**(1) (2013)
23. Mary, N.A.B.: Profit maximization for service providers using hybrid pricing in cloud computing. Int. J. Comput. Appl. Technol. Res. **2**(3), 218–223 (2013)
24. Mary, A.N.B., Jayapriya, K.: An extensive survey on Quality of Service in cloud computing. Int. J. Comput. Sci. Inform. Technol. **5**(1), 1–5 (2014)
25. Chitra, B., Sreekrishna, M., Naveen kumar,V.: A Survey on optimizing quality of service during service level agreement in Cloud. Int. J. Emerg. Technol. Adv. Eng. (IJETAE). **3**(3) (2013)

26. Chen, W., Cao, J.: Quality of service aware virtual machine scheduling for video streaming services in multi cloud. Tsinghua Sci. Technol. **18**(1), 308–317 (2013)
27. Chhabra, A., Singh, G., Waraich, E., Sidhu, B., Kumar, G.: Qualitative parametric comparison of load balancing algorithms in parallel and distributed computing environment. In: Proceedings of World Academy of Science, Engineering and Technology (PWASET), vol. 16 (2006)

Association Rule Mining for Finding Admission Tendency of Engineering Student with Pattern Growth Approach

Rashmi V. Mane and V.R. Ghorpade

Abstract Association Rule Mining is one of the important techniques in data mining. Generation of the rule involves two phases where the first phase finds the frequent itemsets and second phase generates the rule. Many algorithms are specified to find frequent item set from the sequential patterns. There are mainly two approaches for finding frequent item sets. First approach is with candidate sequence generation, i.e., Apriori approach and second is the pattern growth method. If the sequence length is less, pattern growth method performs better than that of Apriori approach. In this paper, we have analyzed the pattern growth approach for the database of an engineering student. With finding associations among the attributes we can find the tendency of taking admission and prioritizing an engineering branch. To find strong and valid association rules, different measures like minInterest, lift, leverage, and conviction are considered during finding rules.

Keywords Association rule mining · Pattern growth · Constraint · Measure

1 Introduction

Data mining is an important process where intelligent methods are applied to extract necessary and needed data patterns. Data mining is also called as KDD. Knowledge discovery in DB is mainly aimed to develop methodologies and tools which can retrieve useful information and knowledge from data required for analysis purpose and for decision making. It can provide tools for automation of data analysis.

R.V. Mane (✉)
Department of Technology, Shivaji University, Kolhapur, Maharashtra, India
e-mail: rvm_tech@unishivaji.ac.in

V.R. Ghorpade
D.Y.Patil College of Engineering, Kolhapur, Maharashtra, India
e-mail: vijayghorpade@hotmail.com

V.B. Aggarwal et al. (eds.), *Big Data Analytics*, Advances in Intelligent Systems and Computing 654, https://doi.org/10.1007/978-981-10-6620-7_73

Association rule mining plays a vital role in discovering useful information in most of the applications containing too large data for manual analysis. Finding really useful patterns from the data is hard for decision makers. Association rule mining is mainly developed to identify the relationships strongly associated among frequent itemsets. Association analysis is widely used in transaction data analysis for direct marketing, catalog design, and other decision making. Mining association rule can be done in two steps. The first step is to generate a set of all frequent itemsets and generate all rules from frequent itemsets. This uses a support-confidence framework.

Frequent pattern mining is one of the widely used techniques for finding frequent subsequence as patterns from a sequence database. It has got a wide variety and range of application in various areas as market basket analysis, stock market analysis, biomedical, DNA sequence, telephonic network, etc. This problem was first introduced by Agrawal and Srikant [1, 2]. Many recent studies have given a number of different ways for mining sequence patterns. Frequent pattern mining techniques aim to find all frequent subsequence with input as source sequence and minSupport value as the threshold. From these, frequent subsequences relationship among a set of items can be found.

In this paper, we have analyzed pattern growth approach for finding frequent subsequence. The input data is of first year engineering students. From the given set of sequence, rules are generated to state the tendency of the student for admitting in a particular branch of engineering.

2 Problem Definition

For a database D containing a set of transactions with sequences where each element of the sequence represents an attribute of a relation. The length of all sequence is same as each attribute represents one item of a sequence. Each tuple of a database is with <Sid, S> where Sid as Student_id and S represents a sequence with attributes as <Name, Gender, Caste, Address, 10th marks, 12th marks, CET Score, Name of Jr.college, Name of Admitted College, Branch>. From the given sequence database, with a minimum support ($minSup$) as threshold, frequent subsequence patterns are to be mined with pattern growth approach. Constraints are pushed in the algorithm to minimize the time. Any sequence is said to be frequent if it satisfies $Support\,(X) \geq minSup$ where X is a subsequence and $Support\,(X)$ represents with which percentile the sequence is present in a given number of transactions or the frequencies of occurring patterns. Rules are generated from the set of frequent itemsets. For a rule, $X \rightarrow Y$ if it satisfies $Supp\,(X \cup Y) \geq minSup$ and $\frac{Supp\,(X \cup Y)}{Supp\,(X)} \geq minConf$ then it can be extracted as a valid rule.

3 Pattern Growth Approach

Frequent item sets can be found with Apriori based or a pattern growth approach. Apriori-based algorithm uses candidate generation and test method, while pattern growth approach uses a divide and conquer strategy. This method focuses only on frequent prefixes instead of generating all the candidate sequence as priori-based, [3]. The main idea of pattern growth approach is to divide the search space and to project sequence databases. Frequent itemsets are found with itemsets satisfying $Support\,(X) \geq minSup$. Pattern growth approach uses a pattern growth property [4] where let α be the frequent item set in the database, B be α's pattern base. β be an item set in B. Then α ∩ β is a frequent item set in the database, if and only if β is frequent in B.

Algorithm executes in following steps

1. Find length-1 sequence patterns—In this step algorithm scans the database D and finds all frequent items with length-1.
2. The search space is divided into different subsets according to the prefixes found in the first step with length-1 sequence.
3. For the corresponding projected database, subsets of sequential patterns are found with recursive mining.

If the algorithm is applied to sequential patterns with attribute constraints, then it will find the frequent subset of sequences for specific postfix database (Fig. 1).

Let a sequence database is given as—(Tables 1 and 2).

The algorithm will work in such a way that it tries to first find the length-1 sequence and considers it as prefixes. Here in given sequence length-1 sequence are

Input: frequent prefixes α, i, projected Database D | α

Output: set of frequent itemsets

For each prefix α with length i

1. Scan each projected database .Find a set of frequent items b such that

    i. b can be assembled to last element of prefix α

    ii. < b >can be append to α

2. For each element b, append it to α to form sequence pattern α' and output α'.

3. For each α' repeat the process for (α', i+1, D | α') and goto step 1.

Fig. 1 Algorithm for finding frequent itemsets with Pattern Growth Approach

Table 1 Sequence database

Tid	Sequence
1.	PQQR
2.	QQR
3.	PQQQRS

Table 2 Projected database and sequence patterns

Prefix	Projected database	Sequential patterns
{P}	{_QQR} {_QQQRS }	{PQ}.{PQQ}, {PQQQ}, {PQQR}, {PQQR}, {PQQQRS}
{Q}	{_QR} {_QQRS}	{QQ}, {QQR}, {QQQ}, {QQQR}, {QQQRS}
{R}	{_S}	{RS}
{S}	{}	{S}

P, Q, R, and S. All four different prefixes are considered and for the respective projected database, subsets of sequential patterns are found.

The algorithm will perform better if we have restricted the prefixes for finding only user interesting patterns. Length-1 frequent items with attribute constraint will have nodes in the tree. The nodes are arranged in such a way that more frequently occurring nodes have a better chance than less frequently occurring ones. New patterns are generated in the second step with the concatenation of suffix pattern with projected postfix database.

4 Analysis of Pattern Growth Approach to Find the Admission Tendency of Student

The Frequent pattern mining techniques can be used for student database [5]. The pattern growth approach can be used to find the admission tendency of an engineering student for a particular branch. We have a student database from different engineering college where we have stored the database in the form of sequences containing the different attributes as Student_id, Name, Gender, Caste, Address, 10th marks, 12th marks, CET Score, Name of Jr.college, Name of Admitted College, and Branch. Let we have to find the association among student marks and branch in which he has taken the admission. We can restrict the length-1 prefix to user interesting attributes (Table 3).

After preprocessing this, CSV or text file is used as source sequence data set for algorithm. Once all frequent itemsets are found then the rules are generated with these frequent subsequences. The association among the attributes is found with support-confidence framework. This is a generally used framework for finding certain type of dependency or relation among the attributes or items. There are two measures of association rule, one is support and another is confidence.

Table 3 Attributes replaced with characters

S. No.	10th mark	Replaced by	12th marks	Caste	Replaced by	CET score	Replaced by	Branch	Replaced by
1.	40–50	f	F	Open	P	0–30	w	Computer	X
2.	51–60	e	E	SC	Q	31–60	v	Electronics	Y
3.	61–70	d	D	ST	R	61–90	u	Chemical	Z
4.	71–80	c	C	NT-1	S	91–120	z	Environment	W
5.	81–90	b	B	OBC	T	121–150	y	Food	U
6.	91–100	a	A	NT-2	U	161–200	x	Civil	V

Let I be the set of items in a database D where X, Y are item sets and $X \cap Y = \not\subset$ as x and Y are disjoint sets. Minimal Support and minimal confidence are given by users. If $\boldsymbol{X} \rightarrow \boldsymbol{Y}$ is a valid rule then it should satisfy.

1. $\boldsymbol{supp}\ (X \cup Y) \geq \boldsymbol{minsupp}$
2. $\boldsymbol{conf}(X \rightarrow Y) = \frac{\boldsymbol{supp}\ (X \cup Y)}{\boldsymbol{supp}\ (X)} > \ = \boldsymbol{minconf}$

where $\boldsymbol{supp}(X) = \frac{|X(t)|}{|D|}$ denotes an itemset X in a transaction database D has a support and X (t) = {t in D |t contains X} $\boldsymbol{conf}(X \rightarrow Y)$ Represents confidence of the rule $X \rightarrow Y$ [6, 7]. For a rule $\boldsymbol{X} \rightarrow \boldsymbol{Y}$, X specifies antecedent and Y specifies consequent of the rule. The support-confidence framework captures a certain dependence among the items but not sufficient to find all uncertainties of association rules. In order to generate valid rules, other measures are considered as lift, conviction, laplace, leverage, etc. [8].

The rule $\boldsymbol{X} \rightarrow \boldsymbol{Y}$ is of interest if $\left|\frac{\boldsymbol{supp}\ (X \cup Y)}{\boldsymbol{supp}\ (X)\boldsymbol{supp}(Y)} - 1\right| \geq \boldsymbol{minInterest}$ where minInterest is $1 > minInterest > 0$ [8–10] (Table 4).

Table 4 Different measures to find valid association rule

Measure	Definition	Measured by
Lift	Lift measures how far from independence are antecedent and consequence. It ranges within [0, +∞]	$\boldsymbol{lift}(X \rightarrow Y) = \frac{\boldsymbol{conf}(X \rightarrow Y)}{\boldsymbol{supp}(Y)}$
Conviction	Conviction is to tackle some of the weakness of confidence and lift. Unlike lift it changes as per the rule direction	$\boldsymbol{conv}(X \rightarrow Y) = \frac{1 - \boldsymbol{supp}(Y)}{1 - \boldsymbol{conf}(X \rightarrow Y)}$
Laplace	Laplace is a confidence estimator that takes support into account. It ranges between [0, 1]	$\boldsymbol{lapl}(X \rightarrow Y) = \frac{\boldsymbol{supp}(X \cup Y) + 1}{\boldsymbol{supp}(X) + 2}$
Leverage	Leverage is another measure called novelty. It ranges from [−0.25, 0.25]	$\boldsymbol{leve}(X \rightarrow Y) = \boldsymbol{supp}(X \cup Y) - (\boldsymbol{supp}(X) \times \boldsymbol{supp}(Y))$
Interest	It states that antecedent is approximately independent on consequent	$\boldsymbol{Interest}(X, Y) = \frac{\boldsymbol{supp}(X \cup Y)}{\boldsymbol{supp}(X)\boldsymbol{supp}(Y)}$

5 Experimental Results

The experiment is carried out on various transactions. Frequent itemsets are found with the use of the support-confidence framework. This implementation is carried out on JAVA Standalone application. All experiments were performed on 1.7 GHz Intel Core i5 CPU machine with 4 GB of main memory Microsoft XP and J2SE Runtime Environment 1.5.

The first experiment performed to find the memory needed for pattern growth approach with Minimum Support of 50 percentile. A number of transaction sequences is varied. The second experiment is carried out to find the time required for finding the frequent items. The experiment shows that more time needed as per more number of transactions (Figs. 2 and 3).

Following chart shows the number of rules obtained with different measures (Fig. 4).

The chart shows that unnecessary many rules are generated from a combination of the frequent patterns. Many of the rules are of uninteresting. These rules are pruned with different measures as confidence, lift, Laplace and conviction. Rules satisfying the measures as lift, conviction, and confidence are valid rules. Experimental study shows that time required finding frequent itemsets with the constraint for an algorithm is better.

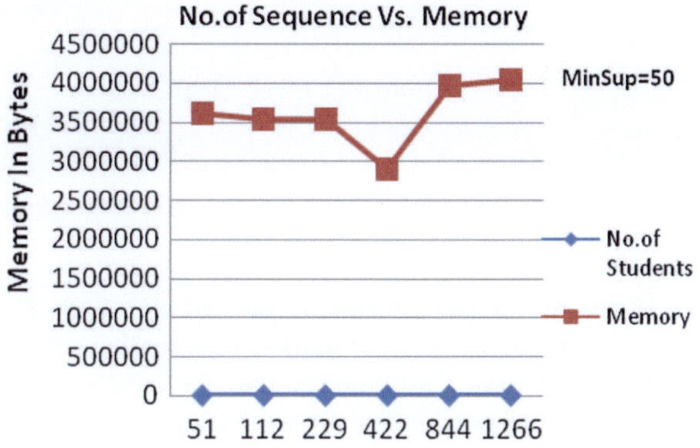

Fig. 2 Memory with varying number of sequences

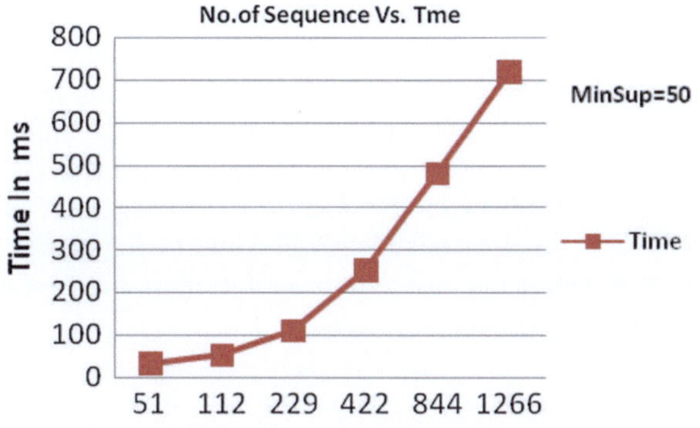

Fig. 3 Runtime performance with varying number of sequences and minsup = 50%

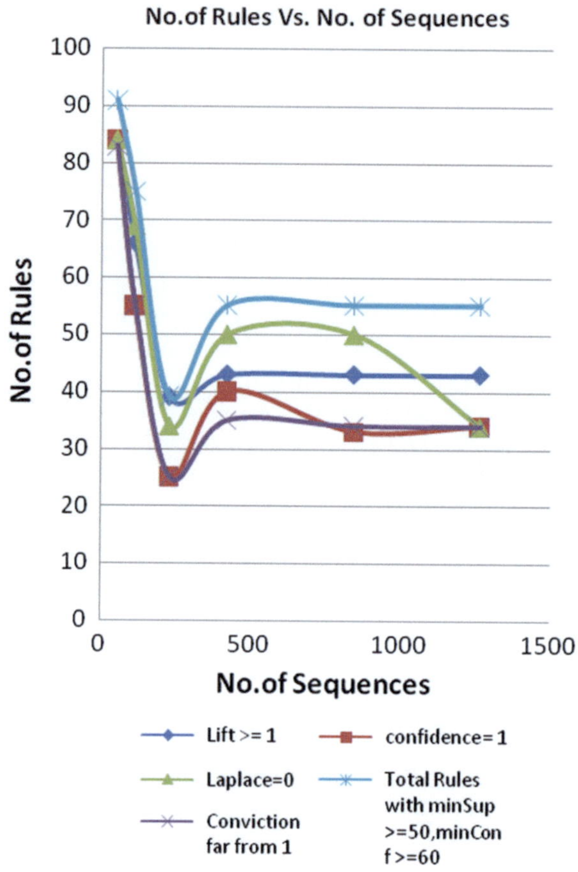

Fig. 4 Number of rules with varying number of sequences and different measures

Frequent itemset mining is carried out with Pattern Growth approach with attribute constraint as 10th marks, 12th marks, CET score, and branch. It finds the projected database for given prefixes. Let bBxX combination is a frequent sequence pattern, as $\boldsymbol{Support}\,(\boldsymbol{bBxX}) \geq \boldsymbol{minSup}$ where ***minSup*** is user specified threshold. For restricting the generation of unnecessary rules, antecedent and consequent are used with user specification [11]. For example, if we have to find the association among students marks and the admitted branch then antecedents are chosen as student's 10th marks, 12th marks, CET score and consequent as Branch name. From the above frequent sequence bBxX, the strong rule may be generated as—bBx $\rightarrow$ *X*, where the rule states that for a given sequence database, if 10th marks in range of 81–90, i.e., in b range, 12th marks in range 81–90, i.e., B and CET Score is 161–200, i.e., *x* then student will admit to branch *X*, i.e., Computer. In this way, by adding data item constraint to an algorithm, frequent itemsets are found in less time and valid rules are generated.

6 Conclusion

The problem of finding the tendency of taking admission for a particular branch of engineering is an association rule mining problem. Mining association rules are combination of two subproblems as generating all frequent item sets and generating all rules or finding associations among these frequent subsequences. The drawback of apriori-based algorithms for finding frequent item sets is generation of huge number of candidate sequences and a repetitive scan of database and is overcome by Pattern-growth approach [3, 12]. The major cost of this approach is the construction of prefix projected database. Experimental work shows that by adding data item constraints at the source sequence database only user interesting patterns can be found with less time than that of an algorithm without item constraint. Further, these itemsets are used for forming strong or valid rules.

References

1. Agrawal, R., Srikant, R.: Mining sequential pattern. In: Yu, P.S., Chen. (eds.) Eleventh International Conference on Data Engineering (ICDE 1995), pp. 3–14, IEEE Computer Society Press, Taipei, Taiwan (1995)
2. Srikant, R., Agrawal, R.: Mining sequential patterns: generalization and performance improvements, EDBT 1996, pp. 3–17, Avignon, France (1996)
3. Pei, J., Han, J., Mortazavi, B.: PrefixSpan: mining sequential patterns efficiently by prefix projected pattern growth, ICDE, pp. 215–224, Heidelberg, Germany (2001)
4. Han, H., Pei, J., Mortazavi-Asl, B., Chen, Q., Dayal, U., Hsu, M-C.: FreeSpan: frequent pattern projected sequential pattern mining. In: Proceedings of 2000 international conference on knowledge discovery and data mining, pp. 355–359 (2000)
5. Romero, C., Romero, J.R., Luna, J.M., Ventura, S.: Mining rare association rules from e-learning data. In: 3rd International conference on educational data mining, pp. 171–180 (2010)
6. Dunham, M.H.: Data mining introductory and advanced topics. Pearson Education (Book) (2006)
7. Zhang, C., Zhang, S.: Association rule mining models and algorithms. Springer(Book) (2002)
8. Azevedo, Paulo J., Jorge, Alipio M.: ECML 2007, LNAI 4701, pp. 510–517. Published in Springer-Verlag, Berlin Heidenberg (2007)
9. Brin, S., Motwani, R., Ullman, J., Silverstein, C.: Beyond market baskets: generalizing association rules to corelations. In:Proceedings of ACM SIGMOD International Conference on Management of Data, pp. 265–276 (1997)
10. Piatetsky-Shapiro, G., Matheus, C.: Knowledge discovery workbench for exploring business databases. Int. J. Intell. Syst **7**, 675–686 (1992)
11. Ng, R., Lakshamanan, L.V.S., Han, J., Pang, A.: Exploratory mining and pruning optimization of constrained association rules. In: Proceeding 1998 ACM, SIGMOD, pp. 13–24 (1998)
12. Pei, J., Han, J., Wang, W.: Mining sequential pat terns with constraints in large databases. In: CIKM '02, Proceedings of the eleventh international conference on Information and knowledge management, ACM Press, pp. 18–25, New York, USA (2002)
13. Zaki, M.J.: Spade: an efficient algorithm for mining frequent sequences. Mach. Learn. **42**, 31–60 (2001)

14. Zaki, M.: Sequential mining in categorical domains-Incorporating constraints. In: proceeding of CIKM'00, pp. 422–29 (2000)
15. Bonalis, E., Gagliero, L., Cerquitelli, T., Garza, P.: Generalized association rule mining with constraints. Inf. Sci. **194**, 68–84 (2012)
16. Bonchi, F., Giannotti, F., Lucchese, C.: A constraint based querying system for exploratory pattern discovery
17. Goethals, B., Zaki, M.: Proceedings of IEEE ICDM workshop on frequent itemset mining implementations FIMI 2003, Melbourne, USA (2003)
18. Pei, J., Han, J., Wang, W.: Constraint based sequential pattern mining: the pattern growth method. J. Intell. Inf. Syst. 133–160 (2007)
19. Campagni, R., Merlini, D., Sprugnoli, R.: Sequential pattern analysis in a student database (2013)
20. Olmezogullari, E., Ari, I.: Online association rule mining over fast data. In: Proceeding of IEEE international congress on big data. IEEE pp. 110–117 (2013)
21. Wang, K., Tang, L., Han, J., Liu, J.: Top down FP-growth for association rule mining. PAKDD 2002, LNAI 2336 pp. 334–340, Springer (2002)

Integrated Effect of Nearest Neighbors and Distance Measures in *k*-NN Algorithm

Rashmi Agrawal

Abstract Supervised learning or classification is the cornerstone of Data Mining. A well-known, simple, and effective algorithm for supervised classification is *k*-Nearest Neighbor (*k*-NN). A distance measure provides significant support in the process of classification and the correct choice of distance measure is the most influential process in the classification technique. Also, the choice of *k* in *k*-Nearest Neighbor algorithm plays an effective role in the accuracy of the classifier. The aim of this paper is to analyze the integrated effect of various distance measures on different values of *k* in *k*-Nearest Neighbor algorithm on different data sets taken from UCI machine learning repository.

Keywords *k*-Nearest neighbor · Classification · Distance measure · Euclidean · Cosine · Cityblock · Mahalanobis · Data sets

1 Introduction

Predictive Data Mining is used to predict the value of an unknown attribute which helps in classifying the data. Classification or supervised learning is an important technique of Data Mining. In supervised learning [1], a set of classes involved in analyzing the data is known apriori and this information is supplied with each record attached to a specific class in the training set itself. Various algorithms are used in object classification but *K*-Nearest Neighbor is considered as one of the most simple and accurate algorithms [2]. Despite its simplicity, it also suffers from the limitation of knowledge of a number of neighbors to be compared in advance and at each step, it repeats the same process. That is why, it is called as lazy learner [3, 4].

A distance measure provides significant support in the process of classification. For an individual problem, a particular distance measure may provide a better result

R. Agrawal (✉)
Faculty of Computer Applications,
Manav Rachna International University, Faridabad, India
e-mail: rashmi.sandeep.goel@gmail.com

V.B. Aggarwal et al. (eds.), *Big Data Analytics*, Advances in Intelligent Systems and Computing 654, https://doi.org/10.1007/978-981-10-6620-7_74

as compared to others. Therefore the correct choice of distance measure is the most essential step in the classification technique. Also, the choice of k in k-Nearest Neighbor greatly affects the accuracy of the classifier.

The purpose of this paper is to analyze the integrated effect of various distance measures and different values of k in k-Nearest Neighbor algorithm on different data sets taken from UCI machine learning repository.

2 Related Work

Ararthi and Govardhan [5] studied time series data classification algorithm for finding the shapelets within a data set and shown that if Mahalanobis distance measure is used in place of standard Euclidean measure, the accuracy of the algorithm is increased and algorithm runs faster than the existing measures.

Han and Park [6] studied two distance measures, Euclidean and Divergence, and applied them in image classification problem. They showed that the FCM algorithm with divergence distance measure gives more accurate results as compared to the FCM with the standard Euclidean measure. During his study, same training and test procedures were performed on the same data set.

Oleg and Stephen [7] studied the handwritten symbols on spaces of curves using different distance measures. They considered the Euclidean and Manhattan distances and prove experimentally that Manhattan distance gives better results as compared to Euclidean and provides an efficient implementation.

Madzaron and Gjorgjvikz [8] solved the classification problem using SVM based Binary Decision Tree Architecture (SVM-BDT). They considered Euclidean distance, Standardized Euclidean distance and Mahalanobis distance for clustering influence. After rigorous experiments, they proved that the performance of SVM-BDT is highly affected by the choice of distance measure used in the clustering process.

3 Methodology

Wilson and Martinez in [9] have discussed a variety of distance functions. In this paper, we shall use some of the popular distance measures and apply them on different real data sets taken from UCI machine learning repository.

If s and t are two input values and n is the total number of attributes, then various distance measures are defined as follows:

1. **Euclidean Distance**

$$d_{st}^2 = (x_s - x_t)(x_s - x_t)'$$

2. **Mahalanobis**

$$d_{st}^2 = (x_s - x_t)C^{-1}(x_s - x_t)'$$

3. **Cosine**

$$d_{st} = 1 - \frac{x_s x_t'}{\sqrt{(x_s x_s')(x_t x_t')}}$$

4. **Cityblock**

$$d_{st} = \sum_{j=1}^{n} |x_{sj} - x_{tj}|$$

5. Weighted Inverse Euclidean
6. Weighted Squared Inverse Euclidean
7. Weighted Inverse Mahalanobis
8. Weighted Squared Inverse Mahalanobis
9. Weighted Inverse Cosine
10. Weighted Squared Inverse Cosine
11. Weighted Inverse Cityblock
12. Weighted Squared Inverse Cityblock.

Data sets

We used the following data sets for our study from the UCI machine learning repository [10].

IRIS This is a common data set which is popular in pattern recognition. It contains 3 classes each of 50 instances where each class refers to a type of Iris plant.

GLASS This data set was motivated by the criminological investigation. It has 214 instances and 10 attributes. The output class may be any one out of the seven types of glasses.

WINE This data set is the result of a chemical analysis of wines. It is considered as a good data set for testing a classifier. It has 178 instances distributed over three classes.

HEART-STATLOG Heart disease data set from Statlog has 270 instances with 13 attributes.

A short description of the all the data sets used is given in the following Table 1.

Table 1 Data set description

Data set	#Instances	#Attributes
IRIS	150	4
GLASS	214	10
WINE	178	12
HEART-STATLOG	270	13

4 Results and Discussions

We performed fivefold cross-validation method in Matlab 2015a to classify the objects in these data sets using the *k*-NN algorithm.

We applied 12 distance measures discussed above on four data sets with varying value of *k* as 1, 2, 3, 4, 5 and 10. The following table describes integrated the effect of *k* and various distance measures on the accuracy of IRIS data set (Fig. 1).

We observe that the accuracy of classifier is neither k-dependent nor distance measure dependent, but it is an integrated effect of both the value of k as well as a distance measure.

The analysis of Table 2 also shows that the maximum accuracy (96%) for IRIS data set is obtained using Euclidean distance measure at $k = 2$ & 5, using Cityblock distance measure at $k = 10$, using inverse Euclidean measure at $k = 10$ and squared inverse Euclidean at $k = 10$ (Fig. 2).

Table 3 describes the accuracy of *k*-NN classifier on Glass data set at various values of *k* by computing distance of neighbor records using various distance measures.

Fig. 1 Accuracy (in %) of IRIS Data set

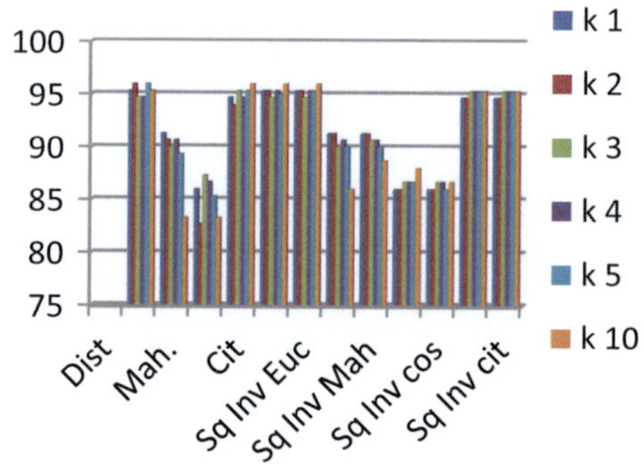

Table 2 Accuracy (in %) of IRIS Data set

k→Dist	1	2	3	4	5	10
Euc.	95.3	96	94.7	94.7	96	95.3
Mah.	91.3	90.7	90	90.7	89.3	83.3
Cos.	86	82.7	87.3	86.7	85.3	83.3
Cit	94.7	94	95.3	94.7	95.3	96
Inv Euc.	95.3	95.3	94.7	95.3	95	96
Sq Inv Euc	95.3	95.3	94.7	95.3	95.3	96
Inv Mah.	91.3	91.3	90	90.7	90	86
Sq Inv Mah	91.3	91.3	90.7	90.7	90	88.7
Inv cos	86	86	86.7	86.7	86.7	88
Sq Inv cos	86	86	86.7	86.7	86	86.7
Inv cit	94.7	94.7	95.3	95.3	95.3	95.3
Sq Inv cit	94.7	94.7	95.3	95.3	95.3	95.3

Fig. 2 Accuracy (in %) of GLASS Data set

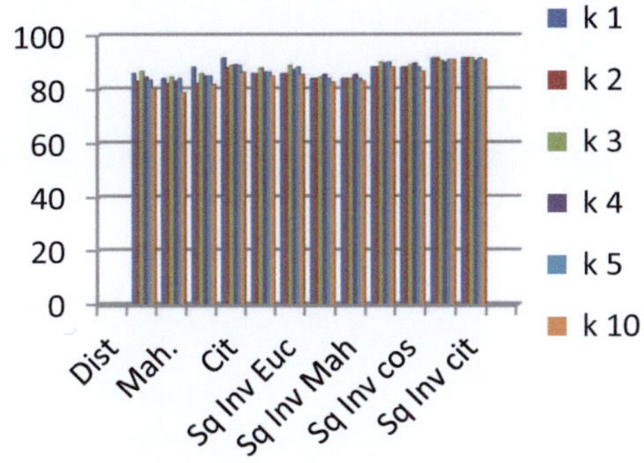

Table 3 Accuracy (in %) of GLASS Data set

k→Dist	1	2	3	4	5	10
Euc.	86	83.2	86.9	84.6	83.6	80.4
Mah.	84.1	82.2	84.6	83.2	84.1	79
Cos.	88.3	82.2	86	85	85	81.8
Cit	91.6	87.9	88.8	89.3	88.8	86.4
Inv Euc.	86	86	87.9	86.4	86.4	85
Sq Inv Euc	86	86	88.8	87.4	88.3	85.5
Inv Mah.	84.1	84.1	84.6	85.5	84.1	82.7
Sq Inv Mah	84.1	84.1	84.1	85.5	84.1	83.2
Inv cos	88.3	88.3	90.2	89.7	90.2	88.3
Sq Inv cos	88.3	88.3	89.3	89.7	88.3	86.9
Inv cit	91.6	91.6	90.7	90.2	91.1	91.1
Sq Inv cit	91.6	91.6	91.6	90.7	91.6	91.1

It is clear that for Glass data set, the best distance measure tuns out to be Cityblock and its variants which give the most promising results at $k = 1$. The next promising distance measure is Inverse Cosine which gives its best results at $k = 3$.

The analysis of Table 4 shows that the maximum accuracy for Wine data set is obtained using Inverse Euclidean distance measure at $k = 5$, using Square Inverse Euclidean measure at $k = 5$ and using City block distance measure at $k = 4$ (Fig. 3).

Table 5 shows that for Heart–Statlog data set the best distance measure for finding the accuracy of the classifier is Euclidean at $k = 10$ (Fig. 4).

It follows from the above analysis that the accuracy of the classifier cannot be determined at a fixed value of k and using a certain distance measure. Table 2 shows that at $k = 2$, some distance measure like Inverse Cosine and Squared Inverse Cosine predict only 86% accuracy whereas at the same value of k the other distance measure such as Euclidean gives 96% accuracy. Similar observations can be seen in Tables 2, 3, 4, and 5 at various values of k.

Table 4 Accuracy (in %) of WINE Data set

k→Dist	1	2	3	4	5	10
Euc.	94.4	94.9	95.5	96.6	96.6	96.6
Mah.	89.9	87.2	92.1	89.3	92.1	93.8
Cos.	93.3	94.9	94.6	94.9	95.5	96.6
Cit	96.6	96.6	96.6	97.2	96.6	98.3
Inv Euc.	94.4	94.4	95.5	94.9	97.2	95.5
Sq Inv Euc	94.4	94.4	95.5	94.9	97.2	96.1
Inv Mah.	89.9	89.9	92.1	92.1	91.6	93.8
Sq Inv Mah	89.9	89.9	92.1	92.1	92.1	93.8
Inv cos	93.3	93.3	94.4	94.4	95.5	96.1
Sq Inv cos	93.9	93.3	93.8	93.8	94.9	96.1
Inv cit	96.6	96.6	96.6	96.6	96.6	96.6
Sq Inv cit	96.6	96.6	96.6	96.6	96.6	96.6

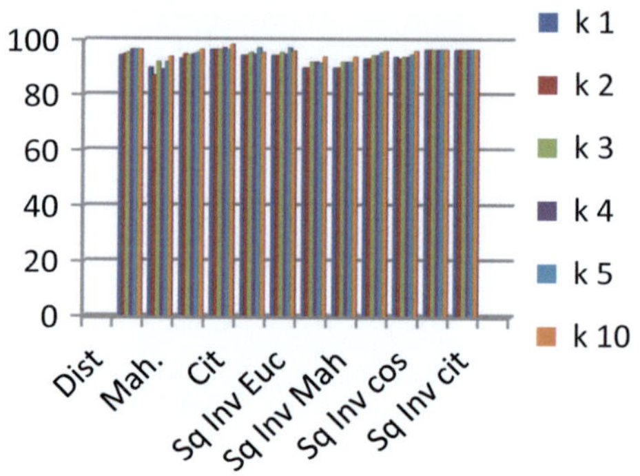

Fig. 3 Accuracy (in %) of WINE Data set

Table 5 Accuracy (in %) of HEART-STATLOG Data set

k→Dist	1	2	3	4	5	10
Euc.	75.2	75.2	81.1	81.5	84.1	85.2
Mah.	73.7	72.6	80.4	79.3	82.2	80
Cos.	77	77	83.3	83.3	83.7	84.4
Cit	75.9	75.9	82.2	81.1	83	84.4
Inv Euc.	75.2	75.2	81.1	81.5	83.7	84.8
Sq Inv Euc	75.2	75.2	81.1	81.9	83	84.1
Inv Mah.	73.7	73.7	80	79.3	82.2	79.6
Sq Inv Mah	73.7	73.7	80	78.5	81.1	79.6
Inv cos	77	77	82.2	81.9	82.6	83.7
Sq Inv cos	77	77	79.6	80.4	82.2	82.6
Inv cit	75.9	75.9	82.2	81.9	82.6	83.7
Sq Inv cit	75.9	75.9	80.7	81.1	83	83

Fig. 4 Accuracy (in %) of HEART-STATLOG Data set

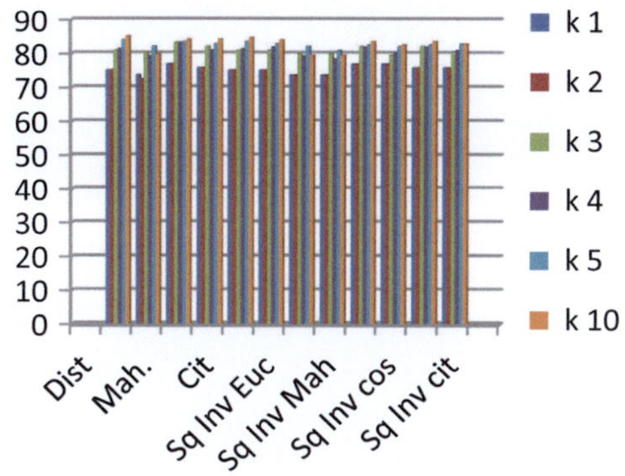

5 Conclusion

Through the above analysis, we conclude that accuracy of *k*-NN classifier is neither dependent on the value of *k* nor on a certain distance measure, rather there is an integrated effect of the number of nearest neighbors (k) and selected distance measure to get the maximum accuracy of a data set.

Experimental results were carried out in MATLAB 2015a using 12 distance measures and 4 real data sets taken from UCI machine learning repository. Further study is required to find new techniques to improve the classification accuracy of the *k*-NN classifier.

Acknowledgements My thanks are due to my supervisor, Dr. Babu Ram, for his kind guidance during the preparation of this paper.

References

1. Hastie, T., et al.: The elements of statistical learning: data mining, inference and prediction. Math. Intell. **27**(2), 83–85 (2005)
2. Wu, X., et al.: Top 10 algorithms in data mining. Knowl. Inf. Syst. **14**(1), 1–37 (2008)
3. Agrawal, R.: K-Nearest neighbor for uncertain data. Int. J. Comput. Appl. **105**(11) (2014)
4. Liu, Zhun-ga, Pan, Q., Dezert, J.: A new belief-based K-nearest neighbor classification method. Pattern Recogn. **46**(3), 834–844 (2013)
5. Arathi, M., Govardhan, A.: Performance of mahalanobis distance in time series classification using shapelets. Int. J. Mach. Learn. Comput. **4**(4), 339–345 (2014)
6. Han, J., Park, D., Woo, D., Min, S.: Comparison of distance measures on Fuzzyc-means algorithm for image classification problem. AASRI Procedia **4**, 50–56 (2013)
7. Golubitsky, O., Watt, S.: Distance-based classification of handwritten symbols. IJDAR **13**(2), 133–146 (2010)

8. Madzarov, G., Gjorgjevikj, D.: Evaluation of distance measures for multi-class classification in binary svm decision tree. Artificial Intelligence and Soft Computing. Springer, Berlin Heidelberg (2010)
9. Wilson, D.R., Tony, R.M.: Improved heterogeneous distance functions. J. Artif. Intell. Res. 1–34 (1997)
10. UCI machine learning repository. [online] Archive.ics.uci.edu. Available at: http://archive.ics.uci.edu/ml, Accessed 20 Aug 2015

FSC
www.fsc.org
MIX
Papier aus verantwortungsvollen Quellen
Paper from responsible sources
FSC® C105338

If you have any concerns about our products,
you can contact us on
ProductSafety@springernature.com

In case Publisher is established outside the EU,
the EU authorized representative is:
Springer Nature Customer Service Center GmbH
Europaplatz 3, 69115 Heidelberg, Germany

Printed by Libri Plureos GmbH
in Hamburg, Germany